1001909199

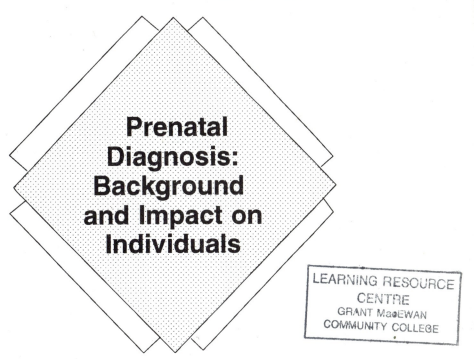

# Prenatal Diagnosis: Background and Impact on Individuals

LEARNING RESOURCE
CENTRE
GRANT MacEWAN
COMMUNITY COLLEGE

Volume 12 of the
Research Studies

Royal Commission on
New Reproductive Technologies

© Minister of Supply and Services Canada, 1993
Printed and bound in Canada

This volume is available in both official languages. Each volume is individually priced, but is also available as part of a complete set containing all 15 volumes.

Available in Canada through your local bookseller
or by mail from
Canada Communications Group — Publishing
Ottawa, Canada K1A 0S9

---

**CANADIAN CATALOGUING IN PUBLICATION DATA**

Main entry under title:

Prenatal diagnosis : background and impact on individuals

(Research studies ; no. 12)
Issued also in French under title: Le diagnostic prénatal, aperçu de la question et des personnes en cause.
Includes bibliographical references.
ISBN 0-662-21386-6
Cat. no. Z1-1989/3-41-25E

1. Prenatal diagnosis — Canada. 2. Fetus — Diseases — Diagnosis — Canada. 3. Obstetrics — Diagnosis — Canada. I. Canada. Royal Commission on New Reproductive Technologies. II. Series: Research studies (Canada. Royal Commission on New Reproductive Technologies) ; 12.

RG628.P73 1993              618.2'2'0971              C94-980079-1

---

The Royal Commission on New Reproductive Technologies and the publishers wish to acknowledge with gratitude the following:

- Canada Communications Group, Printing Services
- Canada Communications Group, Graphics

> Consistent with the Commission's commitment to full equality between men and women, care has been taken throughout this volume to use gender-neutral language wherever possible.

# Contents

| | |
|---|---:|
| Preface from the Chairperson | xi |
| Introduction | xv |

## ⟨1⟩ The History and Evolution of Prenatal Diagnosis
### Ian Ferguson MacKay and F. Clarke Fraser

| | |
|---|---:|
| Executive Summary | 1 |
| Introduction | 2 |
| Historical Milestones | 4 |
| The Evolution of Prenatal Diagnostic Techniques | 5 |
| Prenatal Diagnosis in Canada | 28 |
| Epilogue | 44 |
| Conclusions | 46 |
| Notes | 49 |
| Bibliography | 60 |

## ⟨2⟩ Risk Assessment of Prenatal Diagnostic Techniques
### RCNRT Staff

| | |
|---|---:|
| Executive Summary | 71 |
| Introduction | 72 |
| Risk Assessment | 73 |
| Conclusions | 84 |
| Bibliography | 86 |

## ⟨3⟩ A Survey of Research on Post-Natal Medical and Psychological Effects of Prenatal Diagnosis on Offspring
### Julie Beck

| | |
|---|---:|
| Executive Summary | 93 |
| Introduction | 94 |
| Amniocentesis | 94 |

| | |
|---|---:|
| Chorionic Villus Sampling | 97 |
| Diagnostic Ultrasound | 98 |
| Conclusions | 100 |
| Bibliography | 101 |

## 4. A Demographic and Geographic Analysis of the Users of Prenatal Diagnostic Services in Canada

**Patrick M. MacLeod, Mark W. Rosenberg, Michael H. Butler, and Susan J. Koval**

| | |
|---|---:|
| Executive Summary | 105 |
| Introduction | 106 |
| Literature Review | 106 |
| Methodology | 112 |
| Results of the Analysis | 119 |
| Conclusions | 146 |
| Appendix 1. Medical Genetics Centres in Canada Providing Prenatal Diagnosis | 148 |
| Appendix 2. Genetic Indications for Prenatal Diagnosis and the Expected Demand for Services | 149 |
| Notes | 180 |
| Bibliography | 180 |

**Tables**

| | |
|---|---:|
| 1. Summary of Referrals and Physicians Making Referrals to Prenatal Diagnostic Centres, by Region, Canada, 1990 | 114 |
| 2. Number of Referrals to Prenatal Diagnostic Centres, by Province and Census Division, Atlantic Provinces, 1990 | 122 |
| 3. Referrals to Prenatal Diagnostic Centres, by Health Region, Quebec, 1990 | 127 |
| 4. Referrals to Prenatal Diagnostic Centres, by Census Division, Ontario, 1990 | 131 |
| 5. Referrals to Prenatal Diagnostic Centres, by Province and Census Division, Prairie Provinces, 1990 | 136 |
| 6. Referrals to Prenatal Diagnostic Centres, by Census Division, British Columbia, 1990 | 143 |
| 2A. Genetic Indications for Prenatal Diagnosis and the Expected Demand for Services | 149 |

**Figures**

| | |
|---|---:|
| 1. Observed Utilization of Prenatal Diagnostic Services by All Women, Atlantic Provinces, 1990 | 150 |

2. Expected Utilization of Prenatal Diagnostic Services by All Women, Atlantic Provinces, 1990     151
3. Observed Compared with Expected Utilization of Prenatal Diagnostic Services by All Women, Atlantic Provinces, 1990     152
4. Obstetricians/Gynaecologists and Family/General Practitioners, Atlantic Provinces, 1990     153
5. All Physicians Making Referrals to Prenatal Diagnostic Centres Compared with Total Physicians, Atlantic Provinces, 1990     154
6. Total Referrals to Prenatal Diagnostic Centres per 100 Physicians, Atlantic Provinces, 1990     155
7. Observed Utilization of Prenatal Diagnostic Services by All Women, Quebec and Labrador, 1990     156
8. Expected Utilization of Prenatal Diagnostic Services by All Women, Quebec and Labrador, 1990     157
9. Observed Compared with Expected Utilization of Prenatal Diagnostic Services by All Women, Quebec and Labrador, 1990     158
10. Obstetricians/Gynaecologists and Family/General Practitioners, Quebec and Labrador, 1990     159
11. All Physicians Making Referrals to Prenatal Diagnostic Centres Compared with Total Physicians, Quebec and Labrador, 1990     160
12. Total Referrals to Prenatal Diagnostic Centres per 100 Physicians, Quebec and Labrador, 1990     161
13. Observed Utilization of Prenatal Diagnostic Services by All Women, Ontario, 1990     162
14. Expected Utilization of Prenatal Diagnostic Services by All Women, Ontario, 1990     163
15. Observed Compared with Expected Utilization of Prenatal Diagnostic Services by All Women, Ontario, 1990     164
16. Obstetricians/Gynaecologists and Family/General Practitioners, Ontario, 1990     165
17. All Physicians Making Referrals to Prenatal Diagnostic Centres Compared with Total Physicians, Ontario, 1990     166
18. Total Referrals to Prenatal Diagnostic Centres per 100 Physicians, Ontario, 1990     167
19. Observed Utilization of Prenatal Diagnostic Services by All Women, Prairie Provinces, 1990     168
20. Expected Utilization of Prenatal Diagnostic Services by All Women, Prairie Provinces, 1990     169
21. Observed Compared with Expected Utilization of Prenatal Diagnostic Services by All Women, Prairie Provinces, 1990     170

22. Obstetricians/Gynaecologists and Family/General
    Practitioners, Prairie Provinces, 1990 — 171
23. All Physicians Making Referrals to Prenatal Diagnostic
    Centres Compared with Total Physicians, Prairie
    Provinces, 1990 — 172
24. Total Referrals to Prenatal Diagnostic Centres per 100
    Physicians, Prairie Provinces, 1990 — 173
25. Observed Utilization of Prenatal Diagnostic Services by All
    Women, British Columbia, 1990 — 174
26. Expected Utilization of Prenatal Diagnostic Services by All
    Women, British Columbia, 1990 — 175
27. Observed Compared with Expected Utilization of Prenatal
    Diagnostic Services by All Women, British Columbia, 1990 — 176
28. Obstetricians/Gynaecologists and Family/General
    Practitioners, British Columbia, 1990 — 177
29. All Physicians Making Referrals to Prenatal Diagnostic
    Centres Compared with Total Physicians, British
    Columbia, 1990 — 178
30. Total Referrals to Prenatal Diagnostic Centres per 100
    Physicians, British Columbia, 1990 — 179

## 5  Perceptions, Attitudes, and Experiences of Prenatal Diagnosis: A Winnipeg Study of Women Over 35
### Karen R. Grant

| | |
|---|---|
| Executive Summary | 185 |
| Chapter 1. Introduction | 186 |
| Chapter 2. Prenatal Diagnosis in Ante-Natal Care | 189 |
| Chapter 3. Methodology | 202 |
| Chapter 4. Presentation of Findings: Part 1. A Qualitative Study of Women's Perceptions of Prenatal Diagnosis | 216 |
| Chapter 5. Presentation of Findings: Part 2. A Survey of Women's Attitudes Toward, and Perceptions of, Prenatal Diagnosis | 242 |
| Chapter 6. Discussion | 283 |
| Appendix 1. Information Sheets and Consent Forms | 293 |
| Appendix 2. Interview Guide | 297 |
| Appendix 3. Questionnaire | 302 |
| Notes | 328 |
| Bibliography | 331 |

**Tables**

| | | |
|---|---|---|
| 1. | Referrals to the Study and Number of Participants | 207 |
| 2. | Sample Distribution by Clinic Day of the Week | 208 |
| 3. | Distribution of Study Participants by Selected Sample Characteristics | 244 |
| 4. | Comparison of Interview/Questionnaire vs. Questionnaire-Only Subsamples on Selected Demographic Characteristics | 248 |
| 5. | Length of Genetic Counselling Sessions | 249 |
| 6. | Estimates of Risk of Bearing a Child with a Genetic Disorder and Self-Assessed Risk of a Genetic Abnormality | 250 |
| 7. | Women's Intended Use of, and Intended Use of Types of, Prenatal Testing | 251 |
| 8. | Cross-Tabulation of Chance of Risk by Intention to Use PND Tests | 251 |
| 9. | Reasons for Using or Not Using PND | 252 |
| 10. | Women's Perceptions Regarding the Information Received in Counselling | 255 |
| 11. | Women's Assessments of the Genetic Counselling Session | 257 |
| 12. | Satisfaction with Counselling by Selected Demographic Characteristics | 258 |
| 13. | Distribution of Respondents on Selected Indicators of General Well-Being | 262 |
| 14. | Correlations Between Measures of General Well-Being and Selected Demographic Characteristics | 265 |
| 15. | Mean Scores on Measures of Health Locus of Control | 267 |
| 16. | Women's Access to, and Satisfaction with, Social Support | 269 |
| 17. | Correlations Between Social Support Available and Satisfaction with Social Support | 270 |
| 18. | Correlations Between Social Support Measures (Quantity of Support and Satisfaction) and Selected Demographic Characteristics | 272 |
| 19. | Women's Support in Reproductive Decision Making | 274 |
| 20. | Independent Variables Entered into Regression Equations | 279 |
| 21. | Women's Perceptions That Genetic Counselling Satisfied Their Concerns | 280 |
| 22. | Women's Perceptions of Genetic Counselling as Informative | 280 |
| 23. | Women's Perceptions of Genetic Counselling as Helpful | 281 |
| 24. | Women's Perceptions of Genetic Counselling as Stressful | 281 |
| 25. | Women's Perceptions of Genetic Counselling as Reassuring | 282 |

### Figures
1. Research Model — 209
2. List of Questionnaire Items Used to Define Health-Specific Locus of Control Scales — 213
3. General Well-Being Schedule and Its Dimensions — 214
4. Measures of Social Support — 215

## 6. Manitoba Voices: A Qualitative Study of Women's Experiences with Technology in Pregnancy
### Sari Tudiver

| | |
|---|---|
| Executive Summary | 347 |
| Background, Goals, and Rationale | 350 |
| Methodology and Ethics | 355 |
| The Sample of Women | 358 |
| The Interview Process | 371 |
| Assessing the Reliability of the Interviews | 372 |
| The Women's Narratives | 376 |
| Major Themes | 389 |
| Recommendations of the Women Interviewed | 424 |
| Conclusions | 435 |
| Supplemental Recommendations of the Research Report | 440 |
| Appendix 1. Consent Form for Participants | 443 |
| Appendix 2. Topic Areas and Questions | 445 |
| Acknowledgments | 451 |
| Notes | 452 |
| Bibliography | 457 |

### Tables
1. Ages of Participants — 360
2. Pregnancy Outcomes — 361
3. Social Information — 363
4. Medical Conditions Identified by the Women — 364
5. Prenatal Tests and Birth Situations — 365
6. Women Having Amniocentesis or Related Procedures — 366
7. Women Refusing Prenatal Screening or Diagnostic Tests — 367
8. Women with Positive Maternal Serum AFP Results — 368

##  A Review of Views Critical of Prenatal Diagnosis and Its Impact on Attitudes Toward Persons with Disabilities
### Joanne Milner

| | |
|---|---|
| Executive Summary | 461 |
| Introduction | 462 |
| Social Context of Congenital Disability and Prenatal Diagnostic Technologies | 466 |
| Medical Attitudes and Influences | 469 |
| Counselling and Informed Choice | 474 |
| Proliferation of PND Technologies | 477 |
| Conclusion | 479 |
| Notes | 480 |
| Bibliography | 489 |

##  Parental Reaction and Adaptability to the Prenatal Diagnosis of Genetic Disease Leading to Pregnancy Termination
### Louis Dallaire and Gilles Lortie

| | |
|---|---|
| Executive Summary | 495 |
| Introduction | 496 |
| Materials and Methods | 496 |
| Results | 500 |
| Discussion | 510 |
| Recommendations | 513 |
| Appendix 1. Questionnaire | 515 |
| Appendix 2. Consent Form | 525 |
| Appendix 3. Letter of Endorsement | 526 |
| Appendix 4. Project Personnel | 527 |
| Bibliography | 527 |

**Tables**

| | |
|---|---|
| 1. Distribution of Patients by Maternal Age | 500 |
| 2. Parity, Marital Status, and Sterilization in the Study and Comparison Groups | 501 |
| 3. Distribution of Patients According to the Number of Pregnancies | 501 |
| 4. Diagnoses in the Study and Comparison Groups (Leading to Pregnancy Termination) | 502 |
| 5. Fetal Anomalies | 503 |

6. Number of Months Elapsed at the Time of Interview Since Pregnancy Termination 504
7. Origin of Information Received Prior to the Prenatal Diagnostic Procedure 504
8. Perception of an "Elevated Risk of Recurrence" 507

# Preface from the Chairperson

As Canadians living in the last decade of the twentieth century, we face unprecedented choices about procreation. Our responses to those choices — as individuals and as a society — say much about what we value and what our priorities are. Some technologies, such as those for assisted reproduction, are unlikely to become a common means of having a family — although the number of children born as a result of these techniques is greater than the number of infants placed for adoption in Canada. Others, such as ultrasound during pregnancy, are already generally accepted, and half of all pregnant women aged 35 and over undergo prenatal diagnostic procedures. Still other technologies, such as fetal tissue research, have little to do with reproduction as such, but may be of benefit to people suffering from diseases such as Parkinson's; they raise important ethical issues in the use and handling of reproductive tissues.

It is clear that opportunities for technological intervention raise issues that affect all of society; in addition, access to the technologies depends on the existence of public structures and policies to provide them. The values and priorities of society, as expressed through its institutions, laws, and funding arrangements, will affect individual options and choices.

As Canadians became more aware of these technologies throughout the 1980s, there was a growing awareness that there was an unacceptably large gap between the rapid pace of technological change and the policy development needed to guide decisions about whether and how to use such powerful technologies. There was also a realization of how little reliable information was available to make the needed policy decisions. In addition, many of the attitudes and assumptions underlying the way in which technologies were being developed and made available did not reflect the profound changes that have been transforming Canada in recent decades. Individual cases were being dealt with in isolation, and often in the absence of informed social consensus. At the same time, Canadians were looking more critically at the role of science and technology in their lives in general, becoming more aware of their limited capacity to solve society's problems.

These concerns came together in the creation of the Royal Commission on New Reproductive Technologies. The Commission was established by the federal government in October 1989, with a wide-ranging and complex mandate. It is important to understand that the Commission was asked to consider the technologies' impact not only on society, but also on specific groups in society, particularly women and children. It was asked to consider not only the technologies' scientific and medical aspects, but also their ethical, legal, social, economic, and health implications. Its mandate was extensive, as it was directed to examine not only current developments in the area of new reproductive technologies, but also potential ones; not only techniques related to assisted conception, but also those of prenatal diagnosis; not only the condition of infertility, but also its causes and prevention; not only applications of technology, but also research, particularly embryo and fetal tissue research.

The appointment of a Royal Commission provided an opportunity to collect much-needed information, to foster public awareness and public debate, and to provide a principled framework for Canadian public policy on the use or restriction of these technologies.

The Commission set three broad goals for its work: to provide direction for public policy by making sound, practical, and principled recommendations; to leave a legacy of increased knowledge to benefit Canadian and international experience with new reproductive technologies; and to enhance public awareness and understanding of the issues surrounding new reproductive technologies to facilitate public participation in determining the future of the technologies and their place in Canadian society.

To fulfil these goals, the Commission held extensive public consultations, including private sessions for people with personal experiences of the technologies that they did not want to discuss in a public forum, and it developed an interdisciplinary research program to ensure that its recommendations would be informed by rigorous and wide-ranging research. In fact, the Commission published some of that research in advance of the Final Report to assist those working in the field of reproductive health and new reproductive technologies and to help inform the public.

The results of the research program are presented in these volumes. In all, the Commission developed and gathered an enormous body of information and analysis on which to base its recommendations, much of it available in Canada for the first time. This solid base of research findings helped to clarify the issues and produce practical and useful recommendations based on reliable data about the reality of the situation, not on speculation.

The Commission sought the involvement of the most qualified researchers to help develop its research projects. In total, more than 300 scholars and academics representing more than 70 disciplines — including the social sciences, humanities, medicine, genetics, life sciences, law, ethics, philosophy, and theology — at some 21 Canadian universities and 13 hospitals, clinics, and other institutions were involved in the research program.

The Commission was committed to a research process with high standards and a protocol that included internal and external peer review for content and methodology, first at the design stage and later at the report stage. Authors were asked to respond to these reviews, and the process resulted in the achievement of a high standard of work. The protocol was completed before the publication of the studies in this series of research volumes. Researchers using human subjects were required to comply with appropriate ethical review standards.

These volumes of research studies reflect the Commission's wide mandate. We believe the findings and analysis contained in these volumes will be useful for many people, both in this country and elsewhere.

Along with the other Commissioners, I would like to take this opportunity to extend my appreciation and thanks to the researchers and external reviewers who have given tremendous amounts of time and thought to the Commission. I would also like to acknowledge the entire Commission staff for their hard work, dedication, and commitment over the life of the Commission. Finally, I would like to thank the more than 40 000 Canadians who were involved in the many facets of the Commission's work. Their contribution has been invaluable.

*Patricia A. Baird*

Patricia Baird, M.D., C.M., FRCPC, F.C.C.M.G.

# Introduction

The practice of prenatal diagnosis involves a complex relationship between technology and individuals, partly because of the seriousness of the choices that may have to be made because of the technology's use. This relationship provides the context for the studies in the next three volumes examining prenatal diagnostic technologies. This volume outlines the development of prenatal diagnosis in Canada and what is known about its risks and long-term effects. It goes on to provide some data relevant to the demographics of women in Canada using prenatal diagnosis and then explores in depth the views of some of these women.

An understanding is needed of what the technologies are, and the volume begins with a description of them. Prenatal diagnosis is predicated upon the existence of diagnostic procedures that are capable of providing accurate and timely information about the status of the fetus; in light of such information, subsequent choices may be made. The nature of these choices — whether to terminate or to continue a pregnancy in the event that a congenital anomaly or genetic disease is detected — is difficult and, ultimately, personal. The second half of this volume consists of studies presenting the views and insights of some people who have faced such choices.

Knowing how the major diagnostic tests were developed, tested, and put into use, and how they are used by women and couples at higher risk of having an affected child helps in understanding how the current system of prenatal diagnosis operates — the subject of Volume 13 — and how it is likely to develop in the future, the subject of Volume 14.

## The Studies

The description of the history and evolution of prenatal diagnosis by Ian MacKay and Clarke Fraser is important not only for its introduction to the technologies themselves, but also for the way in which it relates the

Canadian experience and approach to technology development in this area. The collaborative process of multicentre trials, which was used to establish the safety and effectiveness of both amniocentesis and chorionic villus sampling (CVS), has made Canada a world leader in this area, and it provides a model for the practical application of the concept of evidence-based medicine in other areas. Their study is important for anyone interested in understanding where prenatal diagnosis has come from and how it has evolved from a peripheral activity by some doctors in response to concerned couples into a widely accepted activity involving highly sophisticated techniques in 22 genetics centres across Canada.

One of the topics that Mr. MacKay and Dr. Fraser discuss is the risks associated with prenatal diagnosis. The next two studies in this volume then go on to offer a more detailed elaboration of this discussion. They assess data on the risks associated with specific prenatal diagnostic techniques and examine data regarding possible post-natal medical and psychological effects of prenatal diagnosis on offspring.

In the first study, Commission staff assess the three categories of risk present in prenatal diagnosis: procedural complications that are a direct result of the technology and could cause harm to the mother or fetus; uncertainties relating to the fact that results in some cases must be stated in terms of probabilities rather than certainties; and human error in laboratory analysis and interpretation.

The results of this assessment are reassuring. In the case of second-trimester amniocentesis, which is still the most commonly used invasive prenatal diagnostic procedure, the authors found that risks to the woman are extremely low and that fetal injuries or loss are rare. The next most commonly used invasive procedure, CVS, which has the advantage of being carried out earlier in a pregnancy, was found to carry a somewhat greater risk of maternal complications, higher rates of fetal loss, and more diagnostic complications than amniocentesis. For this reason, physicians and researchers are currently exploring a first-trimester alternative to CVS in the form of early amniocentesis.

While there are abundant data relevant to evaluating the short-term risks associated with prenatal diagnosis, there are, as yet, fewer rigorous data on whether these tests may have long-term neurological effects on offspring. Julie Beck examines what is known about longer-term outcomes in children for the three most prevalent prenatal diagnostic techniques: amniocentesis, CVS, and diagnostic ultrasound. The most rigorous study on long-term effects of amniocentesis is still underway and is being carried out by Canadian researchers. Children exposed to amniocentesis were examined when they were six months old and again at age four years, and the researchers report that they have found no evidence of adverse effects from the procedure on either cognition or behaviour.

Ms. Beck notes that there have been no studies done on the long-term medical and neurobehavioural status of children exposed to CVS. With regard to exposure to diagnostic ultrasound, there have been no neurologic or cognitive problems found to be associated with it in children up to nine years old. Her findings regarding amniocentesis and diagnostic ultrasound are reassuring. She also points to the need both to conduct rigorous, well-designed, large-scale studies to evaluate any long-term effects of exposure to current prenatal diagnostic techniques, and to ensure that such studies are an intrinsic part of the introduction and dissemination of any new techniques in the future.

The intensive examination of the effectiveness and safety of prenatal diagnostic services in this country that has gone on prior to their widespread dissemination is a result of close collaborative work among those involved in this field in Canada. Another result of this collaboration has been the development of clear and explicit guidelines regarding eligibility for prenatal diagnosis. Yet, as Patrick MacLeod and colleagues demonstrate in their demographic and geographic analysis of prenatal diagnosis in Canada, women who live in rural and northern communities receive prenatal diagnostic services at lower rates than expected. This is because genetics centres tend to be located in larger urban areas, and also because physicians play a key role in access to prenatal diagnosis. Physicians in rural and northern locations refer their pregnant patients to genetics centres less frequently than do their colleagues in more urban settings. There is also evidence to suggest that utilization of prenatal diagnostic services increases with women's levels of education and income. Despite the existence of clear guidelines stating that all pregnant women who meet the specified conditions should be offered referral for prenatal diagnosis, prenatal diagnosis is much more likely for women in urban areas. This merits attention in terms of equitable access to services by women living outside major urban centres.

Karen Grant's analysis of the perceptions and attitudes of 122 Winnipeg women referred for prenatal diagnosis for advanced maternal age, that is, because they were over 35, confirms Patrick MacLeod's finding that education and affluence increase the likelihood that a woman will have access to prenatal diagnosis. Her study goes beyond the statistics generated by Dr. MacLeod, exploring the women's perceptions, attitudes, and experiences, primarily of the counselling that precedes the actual provision of prenatal diagnosis. Dr. Grant's study confirms and illustrates the difficult dilemmas and choices raised by the nature of prenatal diagnosis for the women undergoing it. Most patients found the genetic counselling provided to be useful. Some women would have liked to have had more than the presentation of medical facts. Many patients felt subtle pressures to proceed with testing, to do "what any responsible mother would do," though none reported overt persuasion or coercion.

Dr. Grant places these findings within the broader context of the prenatal diagnostic experience and finds a need for clear information and more sensitivity and support through every stage of the referral, counselling, and testing processes — this, despite the fact that the majority of respondents to the survey tended to be educated and affluent, with more resources and skills to inform themselves and to be effective consumers and patients.

This finding is of particular interest in the context of Sari Tudiver's in-depth qualitative study of the experiences with prenatal diagnosis of 37 women, also from Manitoba. The women she interviewed came from diverse backgrounds, but, in general, could be said to be unlikely to have the same skills and resources as the women interviewed by Dr. Grant. They included poor women, women with lower education levels, immigrant and refugee women, women with disabilities, deaf women, and teenaged mothers. Their views and experiences echo many of the themes developed in Dr. Grant's study, but with particular emphases stemming from these women's specific cultural and social backgrounds.

The study demonstrates vividly how complex and difficult a task of interpretation and communication prenatal diagnosis presents, and makes clear that these women do not want a fragmented health care system with practices and structures that isolate prenatal care from other aspects of their lives. For these women, pregnancy is a complex physical, cultural, social, and psychological life event. They describe how many medical encounters, including testing, assume a medicalized, disease-oriented view of pregnancy. They also detail the delicate balance in the physician-patient relationship and the need for a respectful exchange of information to facilitate informed choice and informed consent. Practitioners seeking an understanding of how prenatal care, including prenatal testing, is perceived by their patients will gain great insight from the stories told by these women in their own voices.

The experiences and views of the women with disabilities and the deaf women interviewed by Dr. Tudiver are particularly interesting in light of the next study in this volume, Joanne Milner's review of views critical of prenatal diagnosis. One of the concerns raised by some regarding prenatal diagnosis is that, by its very existence and with its expanding network of services, it will have increasingly negative implications for the way in which society views disabilities and will further marginalize persons with disabilities. This broader social concern regarding prenatal diagnosis must be addressed and carefully considered. Ms. Milner's assessment of medical attitudes and influence, and of counselling and informed choice, raises questions about whether women considering prenatal diagnosis are offered a wide range of views on disability. Her findings lend support to the calls made in the studies of Drs. Grant and Tudiver for sensitive counselling and support services for women undergoing prenatal diagnosis.

While these three studies focus on the counselling that precedes the provision of prenatal diagnosis, Louis Dallaire and Gilles Lortie have focussed on the other end of the process — what happens when prenatal diagnosis detects a severe genetic disease or congenital anomaly. Their study of two groups of patients demonstrates that, despite its shortcomings, the current system of counselling patients is helpful and of value. The first group, which consisted of patients who had received amniocentesis because they were known to be at risk of having a child with a genetic anomaly or disease, found the counselling that is part of the process helpful in dealing with the situation. The second group, which consisted of those who had had a pregnancy termination after a routine ultrasound detected a major anomaly, had not had counselling. Their reaction was, overall, one of shock, denial, and guilt. Drs. Dallaire and Lortie show that patients from both groups required a great deal of support at all stages of the process, beginning with the decision to continue or to terminate the pregnancy, through the termination if that was the decision, and for some time afterward.

## Conclusion

The studies in this volume provide useful insights and data regarding prenatal diagnosis and how it has developed and is practised in this country. Prenatal diagnostic techniques have been introduced in Canada with care and with due attention to safety and effectiveness. A low level of risk is found to be associated with it, in both the short and long term. Nevertheless, the choices facing women and couples concerning whether to undergo prenatal diagnosis and what to do if a genetic disease or birth anomaly is identified are difficult. The recommendations contained in the studies provide invaluable information about what potential parents expect from the counselling process. Staff at Canada's 22 medical genetics centres would be well advised to give these recommendations a close and careful reading. It is essential that complete, non-biased information about the options available be provided, as well as sensitive and caring support that respects the different choices that individual Canadians will make.

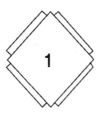

# The History and Evolution of Prenatal Diagnosis

### Ian Ferguson MacKay and
### F. Clarke Fraser

**Executive Summary**

Like many other areas of diagnostic medicine, prenatal diagnosis (PND) has seen remarkable growth over a short period of time. Beginning with the discovery of the sex chromatin during the early 1950s and continuing with recent advances in deoxyribonucleic acid (DNA) technology, PND has evolved into a sophisticated service within the practice of medical genetics. While the development of PND technologies is generally regarded as favourable, the technologies also present a variety of ethical, moral, social, and legal challenges that are not easily solved. The purpose of this report is to provide a historical perspective of PND to assist the Royal Commission on New Reproductive Technologies to evaluate the role of PND technology in modern medicine and modern society.

This report documents the history of PND from three perspectives. First, the development of PND services and guidelines is reviewed from a Canadian perspective. Attention is given to describing Canadian research initiatives, and the role of government in the delivery of genetic services. Second, the history of the reaction to, and debate over, developments in PND is discussed. Included in this discussion are

---

This paper was completed for the Royal Commission on New Reproductive Technologies in September 1991.

public, professional, governmental, and legal reactions to the evolution of PND technology. The evolution of the debate over the impact of PND and genetic screening is also discussed. Third, the evolution and present status of each of the techniques are described in some detail. Together, these perspectives give some insight into the events that underlay the evolution of PND technology.

# Introduction

## Prenatal Diagnosis

Before the application of modern diagnostic techniques to the field of obstetrics, the development of the fetus was very much a mystery. It was generally not until birth that the health or the sex of the child could be determined. Expectant couples were aware that maternal complications and the birth of a child with a disability were in the realm of possibility, but they and their physicians were limited in their ability to detect them. In contrast, diagnostic techniques now allow physicians to peer into the womb in order to monitor pregnancy, detect disorder, and predict complications.

The ability to detect fetal disorders is generally regarded as a significant advance in medicine. Using techniques of amniocentesis, chorionic villus sampling (CVS), and ultrasound scanning, many aspects of the genetic and developmental status of the fetus can be evaluated. At the present time, over 4 000 genetic disorders[1] and a large number of birth defects have been identified. Well over 300 such conditions can be diagnosed prenatally, and the list grows with increasing speed.

Before prenatal diagnosis (PND) was available, parents who were known to be at risk for having a child with a particular disorder would have to decide whether to refrain from pregnancy, take a chance, or (if already pregnant) have an abortion because their baby might have the condition. PND, for the most part, makes it possible to replace a probability of being affected with a definitive yes or no.

A stated purpose of PND and the accompanying counselling is to reduce suffering and anxiety caused by the occurrence of genetic disorders and other conditions present at birth. In the case of normal findings on testing, a couple can continue the pregnancy reassured that the fetus does not have the condition of concern. This encourages many at-risk couples, who otherwise would not have done so, to have a child.

When the fetus is found to be affected, the mother or couple has three choices: pregnancy continuation, therapeutic intervention, or pregnancy termination. There are a number of considerations that will assist the couple to make a decision that is informed and appropriate. Discussion and explanation of risks, benefits, and consequences are the main function of the genetic counselling that is recommended to accompany PND.

## Pregnancy Continuation

Couples may decide to continue the pregnancy and consider the diagnosis as advance notice of the birth of a child with a disability. PND in these cases can assist the family to prepare for the birth of a child with a disability and allow for delivery in a high-risk centre to reduce the risk of birth injury and institute early supportive management. For example, in the case of a fetus diagnosed with spina bifida, plans can be made for a special delivery to reduce the risk of injury to mother and child.

## Pregnancy Termination

The decision to terminate can be made for a variety of reasons, including the severity of the condition, the couple's attitude toward abortion, their family situation, and their ability to cope, emotionally and practically, with a disabled child.

## Therapeutic Intervention

In cases where a condition can be corrected or its effects mitigated, couples may choose therapeutic intervention rather than natural continuation or termination. Although there is little doubt that the future for the *in utero* treatment of genetic conditions holds some promise, very few disorders are amenable to *in utero* treatment at present. Many disorders may never be treatable. For instance, because of the nature of chromosomal disease, the choices after a diagnosis probably will be limited to either continuation or termination.

PND has seen remarkable growth over a short period of time. Although the advances in technology are generally regarded as beneficial, they present a variety of ethical, moral, social, and legal challenges. As understanding of genes and disease increases, the potential to use genetic diagnosis in general and PND in particular will increase. Because this will be accompanied by a parallel increase in the ethical challenges posed, the Royal Commission on New Reproductive Technologies, as part of its mandate, is charged with examining the various implications of PND and making recommendations concerning the appropriate use of these technologies. To appreciate what the future may hold for PND, it is important to understand the history and evolution of the diagnostic techniques, the professional guidelines adopted in Canada for PND services, and the public and professional debate that has accompanied their rapid development. This report, therefore, is to provide an historical perspective to aid the Commission's evaluation of the role of PND in modern medicine.

## Historical Milestones

An outline of important events provides a framework for the description of the technological developments on which the science of PND rests.

1880s
- Amniocentesis (puncture of the amniotic sac with a needle) was used to remove excess amniotic fluid during late pregnancy.

1930s
- Amniocentesis was used to inject a contrast medium into the amniotic sac to permit monitoring of the fetus using X-ray, and to identify the position of the placenta. It was also used to inject saline when a third-trimester termination was indicated.

1950s
- Amniocentesis was used to monitor amniotic fluid for indication of fetal distress in late pregnancy.
- Sex chromatin that enabled identification of sex of the fetus from microscopic study of stained cells was discovered.
- Amniocentesis was used to obtain fluid containing fetal cells from which fetal sex could be identified in cases in which the mother was a carrier of an X-linked disease (i.e., when male offspring were at high risk).
- Using cultured fibroblasts, the discovery that patients with Down syndrome have an extra chromosome was made.

1960s
- Techniques for culturing fetal cells from the amniotic fluid were developed, making prenatal diagnosis of chromosomal disorders possible.
- Techniques to detect certain enzyme deficiencies were developed.
- CVS of fetal membranes was attempted, using an endoscope and biopsy apparatus.

1970s
- The discovery that amniotic fluid alpha-fetoprotein (AFAFP) was elevated in cases of neural tube defect and certain other disorders was made.
- The discovery that maternal serum alpha-fetoprotein (MSAFP) was elevated in association with the presence of fetal neural tube defect was made. The development of screening programs to detect neural tube defects followed this discovery.
- Ultrasonography was employed to locate the placenta and the position of the fetus prior to amniocentesis.

- Real-time ultrasonography was used to follow the needle as it was introduced into the uterus and to identify a pocket of amniotic fluid from which to draw a sample during amniocentesis.
- Ultrasonography was used to diagnose major fetal malformations such as anencephaly and spina bifida.
- Fetoscopy was used to obtain fetal blood for diagnosing haemoglobinopathies such as sickle cell anaemia (SCA), thalassemia, and other blood disorders (e.g., haemophilia).
- Deoxyribonucleic acid (DNA) technology was used to demonstrate alteration in gene structure and hence diagnose certain single-gene disorders from amniotic fluid cells.

1980s
- CVS techniques were used to diagnose most disorders detectable with amniocentesis, but at an earlier stage of pregnancy.
- It was discovered that levels of MSAFP are depressed in trisomic pregnancies.
- Polymerase chain reaction (PCR) was developed, permitting diagnostic studies from very small amounts of DNA and greatly increasing the number of disorders eligible for PND as well as the speed of the test.

1990s
- Preimplantation diagnosis (PID) began on a trial basis.

## The Evolution of Prenatal Diagnostic Techniques

The prenatal diagnosis of a genetic condition is a two-step procedure. The first step involves gathering information or material from which a diagnosis can be made. This may require an invasive procedure, such as sampling amniotic fluid in the case of amniocentesis, or taking a biopsy of the chorionic plate in the case of CVS. Ultrasonography is also a first-step technique that can yield substantial information on the status of the fetus, and of the pregnancy in general. The second step involves the laboratory analysis and interpretation of the information to reach a diagnosis. From an historical perspective it is interesting to note that the two steps have evolved in different ways, though they are linked procedurally.

### Sampling Techniques

The sampling techniques (e.g., amniocentesis, CVS, and fetoscopy) have evolved gradually. That is, their present status is the result of stepwise modifications from previous techniques. Many of the techniques originated before PND was established as a specialty; they were borrowed from other disciplines and modified to suit the requirements of PND. Their gradual evolution improved the efficacy of the techniques and the safety of the procedures.

## Analytical Techniques

In contrast to the gradual evolution of the surgical and imaging techniques is the punctuated evolution of the analytical techniques. Their present efficacy and widespread application can be traced to five major advances, each of which was responsible for dramatic increases in PND capabilities during the past three decades. These are (1) the ability to extract and grow cells from amniotic fluid; (2) the ability to make high-quality chromosome (cytogenetic) preparations from these cells; (3) the ability to measure relevant enzymes in these cells to identify certain inborn errors of metabolism; (4) the discovery of the association between alpha-fetoprotein (AFP) and fetal disorder; and (5) the ability to use DNA from small numbers of cells to identify single-gene disorders.

The history of PND dates back to the early 1950s and the discovery of the sex chromatin by a group of Canadian anatomists, headed by Murray Barr. They were investigating the effects of prolonged fatigue in air crews by studying the brain cells of tired cats.[2] The brain cells of some cats had a relatively large mass of chromatin, not present in the cells of other cats. The differences did not relate to the degree of fatigue, and it eventually emerged that this mass was present in the brain cells of the female but not the male cats. Using cells from skin biopsies and the oral mucosa, it became possible to analyze the chromatin to establish the chromosomal sex of individuals who had errors of sex development.[3] It was further recognized that if one can distinguish male from female cells, one could determine the sex of a human fetus by studying fetal cells present in the amniotic fluid. This would be useful to do when a pregnant woman was known to carry a deleterious gene on the X-chromosome, which would put male but not female fetuses at risk for a severe disease such as Lesch-Nyhan syndrome (severe mental retardation with self-mutilation). By the mid-1950s, it was reported that the sex of a human fetus could indeed be determined by examining amniotic fluid cells for the presence or absence of the sex chromatin; the procedure was used in several European centres to test for a number of X-linked conditions.[4]

The next major advance was the development of techniques for culturing human cells (i.e., fibroblasts) and obtaining preparations that allowed accurate counts of chromosomes (karyotyping). Much of this work was done by groups interested in the treatment of radiation sickness following the first atomic explosions in the 1940s. In 1958 a young French paediatrician, Jérome Lejeune, found that the cells of children with Down syndrome had an extra chromosome, revealing a new category of genetic disease — chromosome disease.[5] Not long afterward, it was discovered that the fetal cells found in amniotic fluid could be cultured and their chromosomes examined.[6] This advance opened the way, during the late 1960s, for the prenatal detection of chromosomal abnormalities — Down syndrome in particular.[7]

It was then demonstrated that certain enzyme deficiencies and other metabolic disorders could be detected through biochemical assays of cells cultured from the amniotic fluid.[8] Within a few years, a variety of inborn errors of metabolism resulting in mental retardation and physical aberrations were detectable (e.g., galactosemia, and the mucopolysaccharidoses — inherited enzyme deficiencies leading to severe mental retardation).[9] The early 1970s also brought the discovery of the relationship between elevated amniotic fluid levels of AFP and the occurrence of neural tube defects (see section entitled "Alpha-Fetoprotein Testing and Screening"). Later a similar though less direct relationship was found between MSAFP and the occurrence of neural tube defects and, more recently, the occurrence of chromosomal aberrations.

The next important advance was the development of DNA technology, which began during the mid-1970s. Using DNA technology the sequence of base pairs that represents a particular gene could be defined; a number of genetic diseases could be diagnosed by demonstrating a specific alteration of a base pair or a small deletion in the DNA. Diseases that could hitherto be diagnosed only by study of fetal blood could now be diagnosed by analysis of amniocyte DNA (fetal cells extracted from the amniotic fluid). DNA hybridization was first applied in prenatal diagnosis of the hereditary anaemia, alpha-thalassemia.[10] Diagnosis of sickle cell disease, beta-thalassemia, and haemophilia was also greatly simplified,[11] and diseases that did not have any biochemical expression in amniocytes (e.g., Duchenne muscular dystrophy, phenylketonuria (PKU), and cystic fibrosis) could also be diagnosed. The advent of DNA amplification techniques (PCR) during the late 1980s allowed diagnosis to be done using a very small number of cells, thus removing the need for culture of amniocytes and greatly increasing the speed of the procedure.

Because of the potential of DNA technology, both diagnostically and therapeutically, it has been the focus of intense study. Many authorities consider it to be the great hope for the future, although applications are hotly debated.

## Amniocentesis

Amniocentesis is the invasive technique most commonly used for the prenatal diagnosis of genetic disease and other birth defects. Prior to its application to PND, it was used for a variety of indications. Among its earliest uses was the treatment of polyhydramnios over a century ago, by removal of excess amniotic fluid around the fetus.[12] Later, during the 1930s, amniocentesis was used to inject a contrast medium into the amniotic sac to monitor the developing fetus by X-ray and to identify the position of the placenta.[13] In the same decade, it was used to inject saline into the amniotic sac for pregnancy termination during the third trimester.[14] It was not until the 1950s that amniocentesis was used to obtain amniotic fluid for PND. Since that time the use of amniocentesis has grown remarkably, to a point where it is now the most widely employed PND technique.

### *The Technique*

The basic procedure of amniocentesis for PND has not changed much since the 1950s and 1960s; it involves withdrawal of a small amount of amniotic fluid from the amniotic sac. It is generally done as an outpatient procedure and, until recently, was almost exclusively performed between the fourteenth and seventeenth week of pregnancy (i.e., during the second trimester). During this time there is sufficient amniotic fluid to permit safe withdrawal of a small sample through a needle inserted through the abdominal wall, uterus, and amniotic sac.[15] This is also the period when amniotic fluid contains the greatest number of viable fetal cells usable for subsequent culture.[16] Some centres are investigating the possibility of doing amniocentesis earlier in pregnancy, between 10 and 12 weeks, although the circumstances under which early amniocentesis might be appropriate are limited. Reports suggest that it is probably a safe and reasonable alternative to mid-trimester amniocentesis.[17]

The first reports of amniotic fluid being used for PND date back to the early 1950s, when amniocentesis during the third trimester of pregnancy was used to obtain amniotic fluid to monitor the level of bilirubin, a biochemical indicator of Rh disease, which results from Rh incompatibility between the fetus and mother.[18] After the discovery of the sex chromatin, amniocentesis was used during the second trimester to diagnose the sex of fetuses in cases where males were at high risk for X-linked genetic disease.[19] Living cells were not required. After the techniques of cell culture and karyotyping were perfected, amniocentesis was used to obtain living fetal cells from the amniotic fluid to be used for culture and chromosome analysis.[20] Amniocentesis was rapidly recognized as a valuable technique for PND, and by the end of the 1960s it was being performed in many centres throughout the world.

During the early years of development, amniocenteses were performed blindly. That is, the aspiration needle was inserted by the feel as the needle went through the various barriers it transversed without visualization of the needle's path. The procedures were done on women who were about to have abortions for social reasons, and who volunteered to participate in exploratory trials.[21] As ultrasonography became available, scans were used to locate the placenta and the position of the fetus. The ultrasound was usually done days or hours before the amniocentesis, which was performed blindly.[22] With the development of real-time imaging (which allowed movement to be observed) and increased resolution, ultrasound scanning was used to follow the needle as it was introduced into the uterus. High-resolution imaging allowed the operator to select an optimal pocket of amniotic fluid from which to draw a sample.[23] It is generally agreed that real-time ultrasonography increases the efficiency and enhances the safety of amniocentesis by decreasing the risks and complications associated with the invasive procedure.

In addition to using ultrasound scanning to follow the needle during amniocentesis, the obstetrician often takes the opportunity to carry out a detailed ultrasonographic examination of the fetus. Gestational age is confirmed, the position of the developing fetus and placenta are noted, and major malformations may be detected. Ultrasound technology has consequently become an integral part of the amniocentesis procedure.

## *Indications*

The indications for amniocentesis have evolved during the past 25 years, adapted to the increase in the kinds and numbers of diseases and conditions that can be detected by amniocentesis and cytogenetic, biochemical, or DNA analysis. The fact that the number of detectable diseases has increased markedly over the past 20 years has increased the overall diagnostic value of the technique.

As noted previously, amniocentesis was first employed to monitor the fetus for Rh incompatibility and later to determine, by study of the sex chromatin, the sex of the fetus when male fetuses were at risk for X-linked disorders. After karyotyping techniques were developed, it became possible to diagnose Down syndrome and other chromosomal aberrations. The increase in frequency of Down syndrome with advancing maternal age had been recognized for many years, and it was also known that following the birth of a child with Down syndrome there was a significant, though small (around 1 percent), risk of recurrence (at any maternal age); thus both of these conditions became indications for amniocentesis. By the late 1960s indications included being at risk for a number of biochemical diseases and metabolic disorders that could be detected by enzyme measurement in the amniocytes. More recently the ability to diagnose genetic conditions by analysis of amniocyte DNA has greatly extended the list of detectable disorders.

The discovery that amniotic fluid AFP was associated with the occurrence of neural tube defects made presence of a neural tube defect in a close relative an indication for PND. When it was shown that the AFP was also elevated in the mother's serum when the fetus has a neural tube defect, elevated MSAFP was added to the list of indications. Very recently it has been shown that a decrease in MSAFP levels coupled with an increase in certain hormone levels are an indication that the fetus carries a chromosome disorder; it is likely that this indication will soon be added to the list.

Following the appearance of coordinated genetic services, centres began to develop standards for the appropriate use of PND. Because amniocentesis carried some procedural risk and was expensive, it was recognized that it should be offered only to women at increased risk of carrying a fetus with a diagnosable disorder.

At present the following criteria are recognized indications for the use of amniocentesis:

- advanced maternal age (i.e., 35 years of age or over);
- previous child or abortus with a chromosome abnormality;
- either parent a carrier of a chromosomal anomaly;
- previous child or other first-degree relative with a neural tube defect;
- maternal or paternal exposure to irradiation (referral for genetic evaluation recommended);
- abnormal ultrasound results;
- abnormal MSAFP levels;
- mother a known or presumed carrier of an X-linked recessive disorder; and
- both parents carriers of the gene for diagnosable inborn error of metabolism, or other serious disorders detectable using DNA analysis.[24]

By far the most common reason for doing amniocentesis is advanced maternal age; the second most common is the risk of having a child with a neural tube defect. Single-gene disorders are a small proportion. In most centres, a disorder of some kind is found in about 2 percent of fetuses tested.

The criteria listed above are considered unequivocal indications for amniocentesis; other indicators that have been implicated as risk factors for chromosomal aberrations are without general agreement,[25] either because the observed risk is not considered by some to be high enough to justify amniocentesis, or because the data are equivocal. Equivocal indications include maternal age approaching 35 years of age (where the risk may be somewhat above that for the general population), advanced paternal age, delayed fertilization, induced ovulation, donor insemination, or intrauterine growth retardation. Other factors identify risks of direct developmental damage to the embryo. Examples include maternal metabolic derangements (diabetes, PKU) and exposure to potentially teratogenic drugs or chemicals. These are indications for high-level ultrasound screening, rather than amniocentesis. Maternal anxiety is generally considered not to be an indication for amniocentesis, though it is occasionally done. Prenatal diagnosis of sex for non-medical reasons is explicitly stated not to be an indication.

## Safety

The justification for the use of genetic amniocentesis is always weighed against the risks of the procedure to the mother and fetus.[26] Maternal risks are now very low and, at most, can be considered minor complications. Transient vaginal bleeding and amniotic fluid leakage are among the most common complaints. Abdominal cramping and nausea have also been reported, although these are seldom severe.

Risks to the fetus include needle puncture, damage to the umbilical cord, placental separation, infection of the amnion and placenta, premature labour, and, the most serious, spontaneous abortion. Although the technique is considered relatively safe, the risk of spontaneous abortion as a result of the procedure is real and is among the most important information that counsellors impart to couples who are considering amniocentesis.

Many studies have been carried out on the safety of amniocentesis and, in particular, have addressed the rates of spontaneous abortions. Among the most widely cited are the Medical Research Council of Canada (MRC) study, the British collaborative study, and an American National Institutes of Health collaborative study.[27] Various studies have reported rates of spontaneous abortion ranging from 0.25 percent to 5 percent. Several reported a learning curve with better results as experience was gained. At present, professional opinion recognizes that, in experienced hands, the average added risk of spontaneous abortion as a result of the procedure is about 0.5 percent and that risks to the mother are minimal. This is part of the information that couples considering amniocentesis must weigh against the desire to know the genetic status of their fetus. The birth of a child with a disability may be regarded by the parents and others as a far more formidable outcome than a miscarriage.

## Chorionic Villus Sampling

CVS is the sampling of tissue from the membranes that surround the fetus. This tissue, which is fetal in origin, can be biopsied between the eighth and twelfth weeks of gestation. CVS detects the same disorders as amniocentesis, except for neural tube defects, but it can be done at an earlier stage than amniocentesis. It is considered an attractive alternative to amniocentesis and has been adopted worldwide.

Although amniocentesis during the second trimester of pregnancy was a successful method, it was not considered optimal. CVS, by comparison, had a number of advantages.[28] Chorionic villi contain cells that are actively dividing, and, therefore, they can be used immediately for cytogenetic analysis without the need for culture. This permits much earlier diagnosis, saving weeks of anxious waiting for results. Earlier diagnosis means the couple may not have to reveal the pregnancy to anyone but their doctor. If the fetus is affected and abortion is chosen, it is generally a much safer and less stressful procedure when done in the first rather than the second trimester. However, mosaicism (the presence of two cell lines in the culture) is more frequent, leading to difficulties of interpretation and the need for clarification by amniocentesis.

### *The Technique*

CVS is usually performed between the eighth and twelfth weeks of pregnancy. During this time the chorionic villi that project from the fetal sac begin to invade the uterine wall. This area of proliferation is destined to become the placenta later in gestation. Sampling involves a biopsy, by forceps or aspiration, of bits of this tissue to obtain viable cells for cytogenetic or DNA analysis.

Although there is the belief that CVS is a new, recently accepted procedure, it was first developed for PND purposes at about the same time as amniocentesis (during the late 1960s). CVS was first carried out in Scandinavia, by using an endoscope that was passed through the cervix, to provide direct visualization of the biopsy procedure.[29] Early attempts were not entirely successful, and there were technical problems resulting from the use of relatively large instruments.[30] Various modifications of instruments and procedures were tried without much success,[31] then interest in CVS began to wane while amniocentesis gained worldwide usage and was seen to be very safe and reliable.[32]

There was a resurgence of interest when a group of investigators from China, whose aim was to use PND to identify fetal sex for social reasons, reported success with a blind sampling technique (i.e., without optical guidance).[33] Using a cannula and syringe, they were able to aspirate placental tissues and then perform cytogenetic analysis on non-cultured cells. They reported minimal complications and were able to identify the sex of the fetus accurately for 94 of the first 100 patients who underwent the procedure.

With the advent of high-resolution and real-time ultrasonography, ultrasound technology could be used to monitor and guide the introduction of biopsy forceps or a suction catheter through the cervix and into the uterus. The use of ultrasound scanning to locate and sample chorionic villi was first reported in 1980.[34] Later, the same group reported 100 percent success in obtaining chorionic villi between the sixth and twelfth weeks of gestation.[35]

Researchers at the University of Milan reported similar results when four sampling techniques were compared. Ultrasound guidance improved the retrieval rate to 96 percent (from the 65 percent obtained with endoscopic guidance and blind aspiration).[36] Development of a process for direct and rapid karyotyping was another advance; in the same year, Tay-Sachs disease was diagnosed from uncultured villi using a biochemical assay.[37]

Concerns over potential bacterial and viral contamination with the transcervical method prompted development of a technique for sampling chorionic villi that involved passing the needle through the abdominal wall.[38] Although the advantages have yet to be fully explored, the latter may become the method of choice, and eventually supplant the transcervical approach.[39] The abdominal approach is less time consuming, can be employed later than the twelfth week of gestation, and is said to be easier to learn.

In an effort to provide diagnosis even earlier than the tenth to twelfth weeks, some centres perform CVS as early as 56 to 66 days; however, recent complications (i.e., a possible increase in craniofacial and limb anomalies) have caused investigators to reassess the safety of diagnosis at this earlier stage.[40]

### *Indications*

The first use of CVS centred around the desire to diagnose the sex of the fetus, as the technique was evaluated as a family planning tool in China, and many pregnancies were electively terminated because the fetus was of the unwanted sex (i.e., female). However, CVS can be used to diagnose any conditions detectable by examination of fetal cells, as is the case for amniocentesis; it is used in Canada for these indications. It cannot be used for conditions (e.g., neural tube defects) detected by study of the amniotic fluid or ultrasound.

CVS is contraindicated when there is an abnormal ultrasound appearance of the gestational sac, presence of an intrauterine device, pathological narrowing of the cervical canal, infection, or uterine contractions. There are also a number of factors that may be associated with adverse consequences such as miscarriage, maternal bleeding, or infection. Some of these include: first-trimester bleeding, Rh sensitization, and uterine fibroids (depending upon their position). Any of these situations may lead a physician to postpone or cancel the procedure.[41]

### *Safety*

As with amniocentesis, the risks and complications associated with CVS were not well documented during its early development, because early attempts at CVS were performed on volunteers who were planning to have abortions for non-medical reasons. In fact this was the case in some studies even as late as 1983.[42] As confidence with the procedure grew, investigators were able to delay termination in volunteer mothers for up to six weeks after the procedure to monitor both mother and fetus and assess the safety and complications of the procedure.

In the early days, procedural complications were a problem. For example, in one series during the early 1970s, CVS led to intrauterine infection and abortion in 2 of 26 patients.[43] In another 28 patients, almost half experienced complications including bleeding and leaking fluid that would probably have led to miscarriage if the pregnancy had been allowed to continue.[44] On the other hand, in 1975 the Chinese group reported no maternal morbidity and stated that only 4 percent of the pregnancies were lost to miscarriage. Others have also reported no major complications in relatively small series.[45]

In the early years, procedural discomfort was notable, especially when dilation of the cervix was necessary to permit the introduction of relatively large instruments.[46] More recently, the degree of discomfort is thought to be no greater than that of patients undergoing amniocentesis or a routine gynaecologic examination.

The advent of ultrasound guidance dramatically lessened the chance of unsuccessful sampling, and ultrasonography is considered to be an integral part of CVS. It is universally employed in centres around the world.[47]

As with amniocentesis, the early investigators/practitioners were exploring largely uncharted territory. If a technique seemed to work, it would be used until someone claimed to have a better one. Large comparative studies were not set up because it was not clear which procedures should be compared. By the mid-1980s, however, consensus was developing, and efforts to establish CVS as an alternative to amniocentesis were well under way. Calls for comparative studies were made, which prompted a flurry of reports comparing the rates of fetal loss and other complications in the two procedures. Some reports were individual small studies and assessments;[48] others were large-scale, expensive, prospective collaborative studies (e.g., the Canadian Collaborative CVS-Amniocentesis Clinical Trial Group and an American collaborative study).[49] The Canadian trial was one of the first in which the safety of the two techniques was compared, and it was the only one in which patients were assigned at random to one procedure or the other.

Current research suggests that fetal loss following CVS is slightly higher than that for amniocentesis. Patients considering PND are counselled that CVS entails a slightly higher risk of procedural failure and spontaneous abortion (i.e., there is a 0.6 percent higher loss rate that is considered to be procedure related), and this has to be weighed against the advantages of earlier diagnosis.

## Ultrasonography

The origins of ultrasound (unlike those of other techniques used in PND) lie far from the field of medicine. Ultrasound scanning was developed for use in anti-submarine warfare during the First World War. By sending ultrasonic waves into the water and recording their reflection off the hulls of submarines, surface ships were able to detect the underwater position of enemy vessels and act appropriately. The same principle was later employed in medicine during the 1950s, using the reflections of pulsed waves of sound directed at the body to elucidate internal structure and function.[50] Computer technology later made it possible to convert the patterns of the reflected waves to visual images. This application to diagnostic medicine, particularly to obstetrics, is regarded as a major medical milestone.[51] There has been such an exponential increase in its use that ultrasonography is now a routine part of obstetric care. It is widely used for diagnostic purposes by many medical specialists; it is not unique to obstetrics.

**The Technique**

Ultrasonography involves passing high-frequency, low-intensity sound waves through the body and recording the differential reflection from tissues of varying density. Reflected waves are converted into electronic signals that are displayed on a video screen. The resulting image represents a section through the anatomical structures under examination.

Early models of ultrasonographic equipment were capable of providing only "still" or static images for diagnostic interpretation. The resolution of these early models was poor. But resolution improved to permit detection of surprisingly subtle structural details. Computer technology made real-time scanning possible, allowing the operator and the patient to see moving images during the scanning procedure. Real-time scanning and higher resolution made it possible to show images of various physiological events such as heart and renal activity.

The use of ultrasonography for PND has three main purposes: (1) direct examination of the external and internal anatomy of the fetus, to estimate its size and look for malformations of skeletal and other major organ systems; (2) as an adjunct to other PND techniques to enhance their safety and accuracy — for example, to guide the needle during amniocentesis; and (3) to yield general information about the course of pregnancy, such as gestational age, location of the placenta, and presence of multiple fetuses. As a corollary, ultrasonography usually provides reassurance and relief to an expecting couple that the pregnancy is advancing normally. Visualization of the fetus can improve bonding of the mother to the fetus, which is considered important psychologically.

Ultrasonography was first used in PND to detect anencephaly (absence of skull and upper brain).[52] This was followed by the diagnosis of other neural tube defects, including spina bifida and hydrocephalus (water on the brain). Ultrasonographic examinations of the fetus were soon widely employed and used to detect increasingly subtle structural and functional abnormalities such as gastrointestinal tract anomalies,[53] urinary tract anomalies,[54] congenital heart defects,[55] and skeletal dysplasia.[56] By 1988, diagnostic ultrasonography had been used to detect over 200 specific disorders.[57] The number of detected disorders continues to grow each year as experience with the technique increases and the equipment improves.

The clinical value of ultrasonography prior to or accompanying amniocentesis, CVS, or fetal blood sampling is widely accepted.[58] Its value in enhancing safety and accuracy of these procedures has been well documented. Although there was some early controversy about whether ultrasonography improves the safety of sampling procedures,[59] all centres now employ it as an integral part of PND procedures.[60]

The use of ultrasonography with amniocentesis led to dramatic reductions in the frequency of bloody taps (blood in the amniotic fluid) and dry taps (failure to obtain fluid),[61] feto-maternal haemorrhage,[62] and multiple needle insertions.[63] At first, the ultrasound examination was done hours or days before the procedure. Because the position of the fetus can change, even in a short period of time, the pre-amniocentesis scanning was not entirely reliable. Using real-time imaging, ultrasound could be used during amniocentesis to locate a suitable pocket of amniotic fluid and guide the needle to that pocket.

Ultrasonography has also been important in the safe development of CVS, which requires accurate sampling of specific tissue from a specific site. Earlier attempts at CVS involved sampling through an endoscope, a flexible tube with a light source on the end, but these efforts were not particularly successful.[64] The use of ultrasound guidance greatly improved the accuracy and safety of the CVS technique. Moreover, ultrasonic guidance allows a single operator to perform the procedure; the operator can hold the ultrasound transducer in one hand and guide the cannula or forceps to the point of biopsy with the other.

Fetal blood sampling involves obtaining blood at a specific site, usually the umbilical cord (cordocentesis). The use of fetal blood sampling was more common before it was possible to analyze the DNA from amniocytes for diagnostic purposes, when pure blood sampling was the only way to obtain cells for the diagnosis of certain blood disorders. Today it is indicated only in certain rare circumstances, and these are diminishing as other techniques improve. During the early attempts when an endoscope was used to guide the needle to the cord, success was limited.[65] Real-time ultrasonographic imaging enhanced the safety and accuracy of the procedure, and it is now a necessary adjunct to fetal blood sampling.

Ultrasound has been employed to guide needles to the fetal heart[66] and placenta[67] to obtain blood samples for PND and for selective abortion. However, these methods of fetal blood sampling have not received much attention and are not considered standard techniques. In the rare event that skin or liver biopsies are required to diagnose specific congenital skin conditions[68] or liver-specific enzyme deficiencies, ultrasonography is used to guide biopsy forceps.[69]

In response to developments in the field of *in vitro* fertilization (IVF) and the recognition that rates of ectopic pregnancies are increasing, obstetricians have begun to evaluate early pregnancy more frequently and critically.[70] Ultrasonographic examinations for congenital anomalies have been largely confined to the second and third trimesters, but the use of transvaginal sonography (TVS) has significantly increased the ability to evaluate fetuses, and even embryos, in the first trimester of gestation. TVS is said to have specific advantages over traditional transabdominal sonography (TAS), including higher-resolution imaging of the fetus; it may be used a full week earlier in the pregnancy than TAS. This permits earlier confirmation of intrauterine pregnancy and exclusion of ectopic pregnancy.

TAS examinations are often technically limited, for example in cases of obesity, uterine retroversion, gas-filled bowel, or inability to achieve full bladder distension. TVS can be employed in these circumstances with relative success.[71]

### *Indications*

Ultrasonic screening is used routinely during pregnancy (Level I), to estimate fetal age by measuring body and femur length and head size, to look for placental abnormalities, to confirm the presence of multiple fetuses, and as an adjunct to PND sampling techniques. Level II ultrasonography is used to examine fetuses at risk for anatomical defects, involves a detailed examination of the fetus, section by section, and may last an hour or more.

The indications for the use of ultrasonography for PND include the following:

- a family history suggesting the fetus is at risk for neural tube defect or other demonstrable malformation;
- elevated MSAFP levels (ultrasonography may be as an alternate to or precede amniocentesis);
- suspicious findings from a routine ultrasound screening;
- exposure to potential teratogens in early pregnancy (e.g., maternal alcoholism or diabetes); and
- to guide instruments during amniocentesis, CVS, or fetal blood sampling.

Ultrasound scanning can detect both open and closed neural tube defects with remarkable accuracy. This has led to the recommendation that patients at risk for having a child with a neural tube or other craniospinal defect, and patients who have an elevated serum AFP during routine screening, should be referred for a complete ultrasonographic examination prior to, or perhaps instead of, amniocentesis.[72] This is currently an issue of debate.

### *Safety*

The safety of ultrasonography has been the subject of debate and worry. Some authors contend that the widespread, virtually indiscriminate use of routine ultrasound scanning has proliferated without extensive critical assessment. However, the literature suggests otherwise.[73] Reports of the safety of ultrasound are legion, including large collaborative studies.[74] These studies show no confirmed deleterious effects on mammalian tissue from low-intensity diagnostic ultrasound. Over 50 million women have been subjected to diagnostic ultrasound, but there is no epidemiological evidence of increased fetal death, abnormality, or intrauterine growth retardation. No adverse behavioural or neurological consequences have been demonstrated in the millions of children born after *in utero* exposure to ultrasound.

Although there is little to no evidence of adverse effects of ultrasonography to patients, their offspring, or equipment operators, many statements and commentaries emphasize the concerns people have.[75] One review concludes that the current scientific evidence is confusing in terms of both the goals of studies and their experimental design.[76] The lack of long-term follow-up and coordinated research led some investigators to conclude that ultrasonography has not been proven to be totally innocuous, since its effects, if they occur, may be subtle and delayed in expression. Others see the lack of evidence as reassuring.[77]

A recent exhaustive review concludes from human epidemiology, secular trends, and animal studies that ultrasonography as used in PND presents no measurable risk. Nevertheless, because exposure to ultrasound at higher levels can raise body temperatures to potentially hazardous levels, there should be guidelines relating to the number of sonograms per patient, and to the design of equipment to ensure dangerous levels are never reached.[78]

In summary, the advantages of ultrasound over other imaging techniques such as X-ray and magnetic resonance imaging are numerous. Ultrasonography is relatively cheap, is easily operated, and, unlike X-ray imaging, does not involve ionizing radiation. Real-time imaging has uses beyond diagnosis and is seen to promote bonding of mother to fetus. Furthermore, it can yield a wealth of information regarding the health of the fetus and the course of pregnancy.

## Fetoscopy

Fetoscopy is an invasive technique that uses a specialized endoscope to visualize the fetus *in utero*. The fetoscope can be used either to visualize the fetus for direct observation of malformations or to locate suitable biopsy sites for other PND techniques such as fetal blood sampling and, more rarely, skin and liver tissue sampling. Before real-time ultrasonography became available, fetoscopy was used for CVS. Because of the comparatively high rate of adverse reactions (bleeding and abortion) fetoscopy was never much used, and as ultrasound became progressively more effective, fetoscopy was used only under special circumstances and for certain rare indications.

### *The Technique*

The first reported use of an endoscope for the visualization of the fetus was a 10-mm endoscope, introduced into the uterus through the cervix.[79] The patients were women at mid-trimester, who were about to have a termination of pregnancy, and who volunteered for this experimental procedure. Later, in 1967, an amnioscope was used to look inside the amniotic sac, but the equipment was bulky, requiring separate introduction of a light source and the endoscope.[80] A Scottish obstetrician, Scrimgeour, coined the term fetoscopy in 1973. He used a fibre-optic endoscope with a smaller diameter than that previously used, and he was the first person to use the technique to diagnose neural tube defects.[81]

Scopes for peering into various body cavities had been available for some time. But scopes, needles, forceps, and optical systems better suited to PND were developed through the initiative of a few researchers who had to lobby equipment manufacturers to produce appropriately modified equipment according to their specifications. For example, the scope had to be so close to the fetus that a very wide angle lens was required, and even then the field visualized would encompass no more than a few fingers of one hand. Because usage was not expected to be high, companies did not have much incentive to advance technical development.

The next major development in fetoscopy was its use for aspiration of fetal blood to diagnose biochemical and metabolic genetic disorders that were not expressed in amniocytes — in particular hereditary anaemias in which the haemoglobin is abnormal.

Blood was first sampled from the umbilical cord in the early 1970s. It was done while the patient was under anaesthesia, introducing the fetoscope through an abdominal incision.[82] Fetoscopy was also used to take fetal skin biopsies and to photograph the fetus *in utero*. Further refinements were introduced in Canada, and in the United States, using a needlescope (smaller diameter) introduced through the abdominal wall to sample fetal blood.[83] Vessels were punctured and allowed to bleed into the amniotic fluid, then the blood-stained fluid was aspirated, or blood was drawn from the umbilical cord at its insertion into the placenta (cordocentesis). Cordocentesis was more successful than previous methods because it yielded pure fetal blood, uncontaminated with maternal blood or amniotic fluid.[84] Cordocentesis carried out under ultrasound guidance remains in use today. With increasing experience and improved equipment, fetoscopy success rates improved and adverse effects diminished, but the results were never as accurate as those of amniocentesis or CVS.

A variety of syndromes associated with fetal deformities have been diagnosed by fetoscopy, including cleft lip and palate, lobster claw hands and feet, and other deformities.[85] Prenatal diagnoses were done at 13 to 17 weeks of gestation and then confirmed at abortion immediately following the procedures. Fetoscopy has also been used to diagnose congenital skin disorders through direct observation and by skin biopsy.[86] Scalp biopsies also provide hair for biochemical analysis,[87] and fetoscopy has been used to biopsy fetal liver for diagnosis of metabolic disorders that are not diagnosable with other techniques.[88]

The fetoscope figured prominently in the development of first-trimester CVS, which has become an important PND technique. The original work on CVS was carried out in the late 1960s using an endoscope to visualize the transcervical biopsy of chorionic villi with little success.[89] Fetoscopes with smaller diameters had greater success, but after the widespread use of ultrasonography to guide the biopsy instruments, CVS became a major approach to PND, removing the need for fetoscopy.

### *Indications*

The main indications for fetoscopy are for fetal blood sampling, tissue biopsy, and direct fetal visualization.[90] The indications for the use of fetoscopy to examine the fetus are a risk of anatomical deformities of joints, limbs, head, face, back, or trunk. With the development of real-time ultrasonography, increased resolution, and a wider field of view, the need for fetoscopy for such examinations has decreased greatly. At present fetal blood sampling is indicated for the diagnosis of haemoglobinopathies that are not amenable to diagnosis by DNA analysis, diagnosis of blood type, fetal infection, and a few other conditions.

The need to sample blood at all has steadily decreased in recent years owing to the broad capabilities of DNA analysis and increased use of CVS. CVS allows earlier diagnosis than does fetal blood sampling, which is limited to the second trimester. Although ultrasound guidance is the method of choice, fetoscopy is still employed in CVS in a few centres.

The use of fetoscopy is contraindicated in a variety of circumstances, including operator inexperience, low genetic risk, gestational age less than 16 weeks, insufficient or discoloured amniotic fluid, and anterior placenta.

### *Safety*

The risks of fetoscopic methods are greater than those of amniocentesis and other PND techniques. As with the early development of the other techniques, the first attempts at fetoscopy were made on patients immediately prior to termination of pregnancy. Consequently, information on the associated risks was limited. As data accumulated, fetal loss was reported to be as high as 10 percent to 15 percent. This caused concern and prompted further efforts to improve instrumentation and technique.[91]

Fetal deaths subsequent to fetoscopy are generally the result of infection of the amnion, excessive fetal blood loss, or spontaneous abortion. In early years, individual centres reported loss rates as high as 16 percent, but in centres with experience of greater than 100 cases, loss rates were less than 5 percent. More recently this has improved to 3 percent or less.[92] A Greek study demonstrated similar decreases in fetal loss rates as experience with the technique increased.[93] There is a significant risk of pre-term labour and delivery; some reported rates are as high as 10 percent.[94]

The most important maternal complication following fetoscopy is infection of the placental membranes. Other complications include bleeding, (rarely) bowel or bladder injury, and recurrent leakage of amniotic fluid as the result of the amnion being punctured.

## Alpha-Fetoprotein Testing and Screening

Abnormal levels of AFP in the amniotic fluid (AFAFP) are associated with a variety of congenital disabilities and malformations. Most notable is the association between high levels of AFAFP and neural tube defects. These are among the most common and most serious congenital malformations with bleak clinical outlooks, and AFAFP testing has become an important aid toward their prenatal identification. Only those mothers known to be at increased risk by having a previous child with a neural tube defect can be tested; therefore, a minority, perhaps 10 percent, of all fetuses who are affected can be detected by this method.

The discovery that AFP may also be elevated in the maternal serum when the fetus has a neural tube defect has led to the measurement of MSAFP as a safe, relatively cheap, and easily performed method of screening pregnancies for neural tube defects. Although there are appreciable numbers of false positives and false negatives requiring further investigation, MSAFP screening can identify about 70 percent of fetuses with neural tube defects — a much higher proportion than that detected by AFAFP testing since, as noted above, most women at risk will not be identified for AFAFP testing.

### *AFAFP Screening*

AFP is a fetal-specific protein that is synthesized primarily by the fetal liver, but also produced by the yolk sac, gastrointestinal tract, kidney, and placenta. It is detectable in fetal plasma within the first month of gestation, and peak concentrations are found between the tenth and thirteenth weeks of pregnancy. Beyond this time, levels decline until term. From the fetal plasma, AFP is passed along to the kidneys and is excreted in small quantities with the urine into the amniotic fluid. The low concentration of AFAFP peaks between the twelfth and fourteenth weeks of pregnancy and, like that of the fetal plasma, declines until term. When there is an abnormal opening, such as an open neural tube defect, amniotic fluid AFP levels are greatly increased.

The association between increased AFAFP and neural tube defects was discovered by looking retrospectively at frozen amniotic fluid samples that had been stored and later found to have come from offspring with neural tube defects.[95] AFP was the only fetal-specific protein in the amniotic fluid, and it was postulated that in cases of open neural tube defects such as anencephaly, open spina bifida, and other defects involving an abnormal opening to the exterior, the opening allows cerebral spinal fluid to leak into the amniotic fluid. Following the development of appropriately sensitive assays, the test was used for PND in pregnancies known, by virtue of the family history, to be at increased risk for a neural tube defect.

The accuracy of AFAFP testing for neural tube defects was further enhanced by the discovery and subsequent development of acetylcholinesterase (AChE) assay. Like AFP, AChE is a protein constituent of amniotic fluid, levels of which are associated with open neural tube defects.

AChE assays are sometimes used to corroborate AFP measurements when results are ambiguous.[96]

*The Technique*

After obtaining a sample of amniotic fluid with amniocentesis, the concentration of AFAFP is measured and compared with normal values based on levels in large samples of unaffected pregnancies. The confidence of the result is based on how much the concentration exceeds a specified upper limit. Because means and standard deviations vary somewhat from centre to centre, this limit is usually expressed as a number of multiples of the median (MoM) above the average level, which shows less variation between labs. For instance, in many centres the odds are extremely high that a fetus has a neural tube defect or other abnormality if concentrations of AFAFP exceed 2.5 MoMs. With values that fall below this cutoff point, the odds are correspondingly diminished. The sensitivity of AFAFP permits the detection of about 98 percent of open neural tube defects.[97]

*Indications*

AFAFP testing is used primarily for the detection of neural tube defects, although conditions other than neural tube defects have elevated levels of AFAFP, including a variety of gastrointestinal and urinary tract malformations, and multiple pregnancies. The major indications for AFAFP testing are a previous child or other near relative with a neural tube defect, or an elevated MSAFP concentration. However, the AFAFP is also assayed in samples of amniotic fluid obtained for other reasons since it is a simple, cheap test and the amniotic fluid is already at hand.

*Safety*

Because AFAFP testing uses amniocentesis to obtain a sample of amniotic fluid, the risks are those associated with amniocentesis. The risk of spontaneous abortion as a result of an amniocentesis procedure is currently in the order of 0.5 percent.

Early AFAFP testing was associated with a number of technical problems. For example, amniocentesis without ultrasound guidance often led to bloody taps. Because both fetal and maternal blood contain AFP, contamination of the amniotic fluid with blood would elevate the concentration of AFAFP, leading to false-positive diagnoses and in some cases the abortion of unaffected fetuses. This problem has been all but eliminated with the widespread and effective use of ultrasound to guide needles during amniocentesis. Abnormally high levels of AFAFP also occur in multiple pregnancies, which would lead to a false-positive diagnosis of a defect, if not further investigated by ultrasound.

Similarly, normal AFAFP levels may not always mean that the pregnancy is unaffected, particularly in cases of closed neural tube defects. However, closed lesions constitute less than 10 percent of neural tube defects, and today the complementary use of AFAFP, AChE assay, and ultrasound yields a very high degree of accuracy, in the order of 98 percent,[98] in diagnosing all types of neural tube defects.

AFAFP testing has been offered as part of genetic services since the early 1970s, and it has become routine in virtually all countries that offer PND services. The laboratory and diagnostic experience with AFAFP testing involving many thousands of cases has been extensively reviewed and evaluated. These reviews (some based on individual experiences and others on the collective experience in a number of centres) are comprehensive and involve many thousands of cases. Retrospective studies have also provided valuable epidemiological information on the incidence of neural tube defects in various countries — information that is necessary in planning for diagnostic services and programs.

### MSAFP Screening

Soon after AFP was first observed in maternal serum, it was shown to be elevated during normal pregnancy,[99] beginning at the tenth to twelfth weeks, due, in part, to the ability of AFP to cross the placenta into the maternal circulation. Levels of MSAFP peak between 28 and 32 weeks of gestation. Abnormally elevated concentrations were found in cases of fetal death or spontaneous abortion, anencephaly, and other neural tube defects.[100] With the advent of more sensitive assays, it was felt that MSAFP could be a basis for non-invasive screening for neural tube defects and other malformations, and there were calls for its wide employment. Screening maternal blood for AFP could, even with less than perfect sensitivity, detect many more cases of neural tube defects than amniocentesis done for a positive family history. This is because between 85 percent and 90 percent of all infants who have neural tube defects are delivered by women who have not had a previous affected child, and who are not known to be at risk so they do not have the test.[101] Within a very few years screening programs were developed and implemented in a number of countries.

*The Technique*

MSAFP screening is a relatively simple technique that involves drawing maternal blood at about 16 weeks of pregnancy. Because the concentration of MSAFP is much less than that of AFAFP, more sensitive radioimmunoassay techniques are required to measure concentrations accurately.

The accuracy of MSAFP screening is less than that of AFAFP testing because of the overlap in the distributions of normal values and those where there is a neural tube defect or other relevant condition. Furthermore, the data must be adjusted for maternal age, weight, race, gestational age, and other variables, so each laboratory must establish normative values based on extensive testing. The upper cutoff value reflects an arbitrary compromise between missing open neural tube defects and performing unnecessary amniocentesis on pregnancies with normal fetuses. Calculating the odds that a woman is carrying a fetus with a neural tube defect from her MSAFP value is a complex process.

Probabilities are calculated as a function of the ratio of MSAFP in the normal and neural tube defect distributions for the measured value, adjusted for the patient's age, weight, race, and a priori risk based on family history and population frequency. This is the reason that MSAFP screening is undertaken in centres rather than in doctors' offices. The results have to be presented as probabilities, rather than positive or negative. For this reason, programs aim only to identify a subgroup of pregnant women who are at increased risk for carrying a fetus with a neural tube defect who can then be tested by the more definitive procedures of ultrasonography and AFAFP evaluation.

*Safety*

There are no reports of complications arising from sampling blood for the purposes of screening for MSAFP. Most of the concerns expressed over the technique have focussed on the validity of the test results (i.e., that it does not completely discriminate between pregnancies carrying normal and abnormal fetuses).

Early reports about the value of MSAFP screening were quickly followed by many studies of the effectiveness and accuracy of the technique. Some studies reported occasional abortions of normal fetuses, but more recent reviews report that with complementary AFAFP testing and ultrasound, the chances of aborting a normal fetus or missing an abnormal one are slim.

*MSAFP Levels and Trisomic Pregnancies*

Recently, retrospective studies have shown that MSAFP not only tends to be elevated in the presence of a fetal neural tube defect, but may be diminished when the fetus has trisomy 21 (Down syndrome) or another extra chromosome trisomy.[102] Sensitivity and specificity have been improved by concurrent measurements of certain hormones (human chorionic gonadotropin and estrogen) that tend to be higher in the presence of trisomy.[103] Test results for a woman of a particular age are stated in terms of the age that a woman in the general population would be to have the same odds. For example, test results from a 32-year-old woman may show that there is 1 chance in 70 that her fetus has a chromosomal abnormality. These results are equivalent to the odds that a 37-year-old woman has in the general population. Routine MSAFP screening may well replace the maternal age criterion for amniocentesis, but some think it premature to introduce such mass screening programs.[104] In Canada, the province of Manitoba uses MSAFP testing to screen for chromosomal trisomies in addition to neural tube defects.

## Magnetic Resonance Imaging

The use of magnetic resonance imaging (MRI) in PND is a relatively recent application of what is fast becoming an important tool in many areas of diagnostic medicine. MRI is similar to X-ray examination in its ability to peer into the body and depict internal structures. It does not, however, involve the use of ionizing radiation such as X-ray. Rather, it uses magnetism and radio frequency fields to examine the physical properties of the elements that make up the tissues of the body. In many respects, it is superior to other forms of imaging because of its ability to define soft tissues and organs.[105] It can also be used to provide information on the biochemical status of fetal tissues. It does not, however, reveal movement.

## *The Technique*

MRI is based on the phenomenon of nuclear magnetic resonance (NMR), which was discovered by a German physicist, Bloch, in 1946.[106] The property of nuclear magnetism is characteristic of some but not all atomic nuclei. Many of the elements that possess nuclear magnetism are biologically significant, including the ubiquitous hydrogen and carbon. The first applications of NMR were in physics and elemental chemistry, where it was used to study atomic structure and atomic interaction. Biochemists soon realized that NMR could be used to elucidate molecular structure and interactions in biochemical processes,[107] and it has since been used to explore a broad range of biological questions and to reveal internal anatomy.[108] The possibility of applying it to prenatal diagnosis of fetal anomalies and other birth defects was realized in the early 1980s.

MRI for PND involves exposing the subject to electromagnetic radiation and obtaining a series of images that, as with ultrasonography, appear as "slices" through a section of the pregnant woman's body. Visualization depends on the differences in the chemical composition of the various tissues rather than differences in density. Images show the relative position of organs and tissues within the body of the pregnant woman and reveal the position of the fetus and its developing organs and tissues as well as the position and structure of the placenta.[109]

MRI may have several advantages over ultrasonography during pregnancy. Its ability to define soft tissues of both the mother and the fetus can be useful in diagnosing specific congenital defects. Also, because MRI does not require distension of the bladder, as does ultrasound, anatomical relationships can be visualized without distorting tissues in the process.

MRI has been used to detect a number of fetal anomalies. It can be especially useful in defining the anatomy of the central nervous system, and has been used to diagnose a number of defects associated with the brain,[110] as well as other conditions including intrauterine growth retardation[111] and lung, renal, and heart defects.[112]

One of the major distinctions between MRI and ultrasonography is that MRI produces still images whereas ultrasonography is capable of both real-time and still imaging. Fetal movement during the MRI scanning procedure can result in artifacts that obscure resolution and complicate the assessment of the fetus.

## Indications

*Indications*

Recently, a number of areas have been suggested in which MRI could be a diagnostic adjunct.[113] It may be used in place of indicated maternal or fetal X-ray or ultrasound, or as an adjunct to ultrasonography, providing additional information on fetal structure, development, or growth, organ development, and location and structure of the placenta, or for confirmation of fetal anomalies and obstetric complications.

*Safety*

The safety of MRI has not yet been definitively established; its future applications will depend on prospective and retrospective studies on both the short- and long-term effects of exposure to magnetic and radio frequency fields. Prevailing opinion suggests that it has few hazards, which are minimal at most. Nevertheless, until the safety of MRI is established, it should be used only for clear indications, and fetal and placental exposure should be minimized.[114] The U.K. National Radiological Protection Board advises against imaging during the first trimester, during the period of organogenesis, unless the patient is undergoing termination of pregnancy.[115]

MRI is an expensive technique and is not widely available. While its potential uses are well documented, its widespread use depends heavily on economic, demographic, and safety considerations. It is unlikely that MRI will ever replace other imaging techniques such as ultrasound, which has established value and broad applications in the field of PND. However, the use of MRI in PND is barely a decade old, and it is likely that its use will grow as experience with the technique increases.

## Preimplantation Diagnosis

Preimplantation diagnosis is the newest technique for the prenatal diagnosis of genetic disorders and has its roots in three areas. Early embryos such as those of amphibia were discovered to have remarkable powers of reorganization after being manipulated. The early embryo could be split, for example, and each half would develop into a normal individual. Anne McLaren, a British embryologist and reproductive biologist, first speculated that this regulative power could allow successful biopsy of the early embryo for genetic diagnosis.[116] The second root was the ability to recover human eggs or early human embryos by the technique of IVF. The third and most recent was the development of DNA amplification techniques, which allowed diagnostic analysis of the DNA from very small amounts of tissue, even from single cells.[117]

*The Technique*

The development of preimplantation diagnosis stems from the concern that ordinary PND implies the option of abortion if a positive diagnosis is made. In particular, later abortions (e.g., second trimester) are associated with notable physical stress and psychological trauma for the mother.[118]

Screening the embryo prior to its implantation in the uterus would provide a method of PND that did not require abortion.[119] Because the technique is carried out on the embryo outside the uterus, it would mean only that the embryo would not be transferred into the uterus if it were found to be affected. If the test result were normal, the embryo could be transferred to the uterus for implantation and (it is hoped) continuation of the pregnancy.[120]

Preimplantation diagnosis is very much in an experimental state, but the technique appears to hold some promise in certain circumstances — if the pitfalls and complications are worked out. The success of the technique depends on a number of factors, the most important of which is the accessibility of early embryos. There are two methods under consideration. The first involves the techniques of IVF. Eggs are obtained from the donor, fertilized *in vitro* (i.e., outside the woman's body), and allowed to proceed through several cell divisions, after which a few cells are removed to provide DNA for genetic analysis. If the disorder in question is not present, the embryo is placed in the uterus. The early embryo appears to be able to reorganize itself and continue to develop normally. This method is costly and carries with it the low success rates associated with IVF.

The second method of obtaining embryos is their recovery, after conception, by the technique of uterine lavage.[121] In this case the early embryo is recovered by flushing the uterus and examining the washings. This method, however, has associated dangers and is not a recommended approach. It is considerably cheaper than IVF but much less efficient, as only one embryo, if any, can be recovered at any one cycle. Data on safety and efficacy are being collected but are still scant, and it is not recommended by the Society of Obstetricians and Gynaecologists of Canada (SOGC) at this time.

### *Indications*

At present preimplantation diagnosis can be done for any condition that can be diagnosed by analysis of the DNA, but the difficult, stressful, and expensive techniques of assisted reproduction are required to obtain the early embryo for testing. Furthermore, the reliability of the techniques of DNA diagnosis has not been fully established, and the method must still be considered experimental.

Women at risk for a genetic disorder who reject abortion on moral grounds but accept destruction of a preimplantation embryo constitute one group who might choose preimplantation diagnosis. A second group appears to be women who have had amniocentesis or CVS and endured the termination of a wanted pregnancy because of a genetic disorder, and who feel they cannot face the prospect again. However, given its limited capabilities, it seems unlikely that preimplantation diagnosis will ever seriously compete with other methods of PND.

In Canada, at least one centre, University Hospital in London, Ontario, has announced plans to establish a preimplantation diagnosis screening program to be known as Early Preimplantation Cell Screening. The intended program was developed in consultation with the Westminster Institute for Ethics and Human Values and plans to focus on couples with a family history of severe mental retardation. Other inherited diseases may be included at a later stage.

## Prenatal Diagnosis in Canada

### Beginnings

The history of PND in Canada dates back to the late 1960s and the introduction of amniocentesis in a few hospitals. Because use for genetic analysis was very much a new technique, its introduction was limited to teaching hospitals and university research facilities in a few Canadian cities. The early services were limited by the scarcity of trained personnel, laboratory facilities, and experience with the techniques; because of limited awareness on the part of the public, there was less demand for PND services at that time.

By 1970, medical genetics centres were established in major Canadian cities including London, Montreal, Winnipeg, Halifax, Vancouver, and Calgary. There were 13 centres doing PND by the end of 1971, each capable of diagnosing cytogenetic disease and some inborn errors of metabolism. As national and international experience with amniocentesis and laboratory techniques grew, so too did the capabilities of PND. Further research led to an expanding list of detectable diseases and, therefore, an increased demand for the services.

Despite the expansion of services, there were no guidelines for the use of amniocentesis; its practice relied heavily on methods and procedures gleaned from the international literature and by word of mouth. During the exploratory phase, procedures were done on volunteers who were going to have an abortion for social reasons, or who were at high risk for having a child with a serious disorder. There were failures in the form of dry taps (failure to obtain fluid) and bloody amniotic fluids, but no one knew how many. There were miscarriages following the procedure, but it was difficult to distinguish between those induced by the procedure and those that would have happened naturally. There were occasional reports of damage to the umbilical cord or placenta, infection, or needle puncture of the fetus, but no one knew how many. Of course, there was an increasing number of successful prenatal diagnoses. Early on, some obstetricians would do amniocentesis in their offices, on only a few patients a month; however, their failure rates were unacceptably high. As the demand for testing grew, obstetricians and geneticists agreed that the procedure should be done in centres by a few obstetricians who would do many cases, and who would thus become expert with the technique.

## Establishment of the Canadian Working Group

By 1971, there was serious concern that the use of amniocentesis was increasing on a haphazard basis, with no data on how effective or how risky it was. It was clear that its safety and effectiveness had to be evaluated. With the initiative and support of Dr. Malcolm Brown, the first president of the MRC, a working group was appointed in 1971 to look into the matter.

Although the working group was given a broad mandate, its most immediate task was to study the safety and efficiency of amniocentesis as well as its benefits and limitations. To accomplish this, the working group developed a protocol for a large collaborative study of the safety and effectiveness of amniocentesis. The study, which was funded by the MRC, invited all Canadian centres performing amniocentesis to take part. By 1976, all 13 centres participated in the collaborative effort by providing information and data collected in a consistent manner on their respective experiences with amniocentesis. The data were then pooled and analyzed in order to document the Canadian experience with amniocentesis.

The final report was published in 1977 and, in addition to presenting data, it made a number of recommendations regarding the delivery of PND services.[122] It outlined the indications for the use of amniocentesis for PND and concluded that it was an effective technique with a small, but not negligible, associated risk. Amniocentesis, in conjunction with adequate and appropriate counselling, was considered to be an effective tool for the detection of genetic disease. Facilities and funds within provincial health services were recommended to ensure efficient and equitable delivery of PND services.

The MRC report was, and still is, widely cited internationally. Thus Canadian investigators played an important role in the development of amniocentesis as a PND technique. Studies in other countries yielded similar results.[123] Together, these studies established amniocentesis as the foremost PND technique and changed its status from an experimental procedure to one of standard clinical practice.

In the years between the beginning and the publication of the MRC study, two events took place that were central to the development of PND services in Canada. The first Canadian guidelines for the practice of amniocentesis were published, and the Canadian College of Medical Geneticists (CCMG) was established.

## First Canadian Guidelines

Following the introduction of PND services in the early 1970s, there was concern that PND services were expanding without supervision, and without guidelines to ensure that amniocentesis was not used irresponsibly. Three professional organizations — the Canadian Paediatric

Society (CPS), the SOGC, and the Genetics Society of Canada (GSC) — decided to study the practice of amniocentesis and recommend guidelines for its use in Canada. After three years of study, these three organizations published a joint statement recommending that amniocentesis be performed for specific indications and stating how the techniques should be performed.[124] This was the first step in the development of Canadian guidelines for the safe and responsible delivery of PND services. These 1974 guidelines were not meant to pre-empt the MRC report, which would not appear until 1977, but they were drafted to provide some guidance to practitioners until the MRC report could recommend more substantial and comprehensive guidelines to standardize practice in Canada.

## Canadian College of Medical Geneticists

In the same year, at the annual meeting of the GSC, a small working group of those involved with genetic counselling services decided that a professional organization representing medical geneticists was needed to oversee the burgeoning medical genetics services, including PND. The concern was, in part, a response to the fact that a few ill-qualified geneticists were offering counselling that was inadequate, inappropriate, and sometimes erroneous. This meeting set in motion the chain of events that led to the formation of the CCMG and its incorporation in 1975. Since its incorporation, the CCMG has taken responsibility for the accreditation of medical geneticists, and of centres providing genetic services, and has been a central force in developing standards for the delivery of prenatal genetic services in Canada. Medical geneticists accredited by the CCMG can be physicians or persons with doctoral degrees who have proven themselves proficient in the provision of genetic services. The Royal College of Physicians and Surgeons of Canada, in response to long-standing and persistent requests from the CCMG, has recently recognized medical genetics as a specialty, and hence will share responsibility for the training of physicians in that field.

## Provincial Initiatives

Because health care in Canada is primarily a provincial responsibility, expansion of PND services depended largely on individual provinces to fund facilities, personnel, and programs. Provinces have played a pivotal role in developing programs to support these services. Among the first to initiate coordinated genetic services were Quebec, Ontario, and British Columbia. Other provinces have developed similar programs, and PND services are now offered at 21 centres and are available in every Canadian province except Prince Edward Island.

Ontario was an exemplary model of negotiation between geneticists and the provincial government for the allocation of funds for genetic services. The provincial government struck a task force in the early 1970s to study the need for genetic services. In 1976 the task force on genetic services reported to the Ontario Council of Health, recommending that Ontario develop and implement province-wide medical genetic services. The Council subsequently adopted the recommendations, which led to the development of a system for genetic services in the province. The system is based on a number of regional hospitals such that various regions of the province have more or less equal access to the services. Many of these centres are large and self-contained while others are smaller and rely on larger centres for professional and laboratory support. For instance, a service is offered in Sudbury, though amniotic fluid or CVS samples are sent to the clinic at the Children's Hospital of Eastern Ontario for laboratory analysis. To support these PND services, a global budget was allocated to be partitioned by an advisory committee on genetics made up of representatives from the various genetics centres. Genetic services in other provinces work on a number of more or less satisfactory variations of this model.

The necessary government involvement in the development of prenatal diagnostic services was, and continues to be, organizational and administrative, related to the provision and distribution of funds to ensure that services are available to the population. The quality of services, including counselling and laboratory diagnosis, is largely monitored by the CCMG through their published guidelines, standards, and accrediting procedures for member professionals and centres. Neither the federal nor provincial governments provide guidelines for the performance of PND. The only exception is the national guidelines that have been established by Health and Welfare Canada on the safe use of diagnostic ultrasound technology.[125]

MSAFP screening programs have been recognized as an effective method to detect neural tube defects (anencephaly, spina bifida) in the general population. In countries where MSAFP programs have been developed and implemented, the result has been a decrease in the number of babies born with neural tube defects. In Canada, only Manitoba offers MSAFP screening as a provincial program. Results from the five-year-old program show that the birth prevalence of neural tube defects in Manitoba has fallen by about 50 percent.[126] Similar programs are currently under consideration in other provinces, but no funding has yet been allocated.

## CCMG Guidelines

The early 1980s saw an increased demand for PND services in Canada. The CCMG, in cooperation with the SOGC and the CPS, responded by developing the first comprehensive set of guidelines for the use of PND techniques and for the delivery of PND services.[127] The 1983 guidelines were developed with wide consultation and relied on Canadian studies along with an evaluation of experience in other countries. The report of an international workshop on PND (Val David, Quebec, 1980) was also a

## Clinical Trials of Chorionic Villus Sampling

The early 1980s also saw renewed interest in first-trimester CVS as an alternative to amniocentesis, but obstetricians and gynaecologists felt that its safety and accuracy had to be measured before it was widely offered. To that end, a large-scale prospective study was launched in 1984 to compare the effectiveness, accuracy, and risks of CVS and amniocentesis. It was felt that a valid comparison could best be made by a trial where the women were assigned at random to one procedure or the other. This presented obvious difficulties, because the women might have strong feelings about their preferred procedures. The problem was largely overcome by including in the trial only women who were aware of the need for randomization and who consented to it. Those who did not wish to be assigned to receive the procedure at random could have amniocentesis, but not CVS. The study, under the direction of the Canadian Collaborative CVS-Amniocentesis Clinical Trial Group, was sponsored by the MRC. The report, which appeared in early 1989, concluded that CVS was an effective technique with specific advantages over amniocentesis, particularly that it could be used earlier in pregnancy, but that it carried slightly higher risks of spontaneous abortion.[129]

Similar (though not randomized) large-scale studies of the safety of CVS in countries such as the United States[130] reached more or less similar conclusions, though there may be some question of the safety of CVS before the tenth week of pregnancy (see the subsection on CVS in the section entitled "The Evolution of Prenatal Diagnostic Techniques").[131] CVS in Canada, as in other countries, is a technique that is firmly established in the clinical practice of PND.

## CCMG Update of 1983 Guidelines

The CCMG, along with the SOGC, has prepared an update of the 1983 guidelines, specifically to address the significant changes that have occurred during the past eight years.[132]

In addition to the guidelines for the operative procedures, the CCMG has published professional and ethical guidelines with respect to the practice of medical genetics.[133] These guidelines explicitly state the responsibilities of the geneticist to the patient, society, and the profession. These guidelines have teeth: a professional who transgresses could be censured and, if the CCMG Board considered it serious enough, could lose fellowship status in the CCMG as well as face disciplinary action from the provincial licensing body. The guidelines also establish reasonable standards of practice that could expose a transgressor to legal suit.

## Other National Guidelines

The operation of PND services in Canada does not differ appreciably from those in other countries of the developed world. The most noteworthy variation from country to country is the minimum age for women referred because of advanced maternal age. The cutoff age in Canada and other countries is 35 years, because the odds of having a fetus with a trisomy begin to increase sharply at that age, but some countries use 38 years of age as a minimum (e.g., Italy). Other centres allow lower age limits (e.g., a Texas clinic will consider any woman 33 years of age or more, and an Oregon clinic sets 34 years of age as the limit). It is reasonable to assume that economic factors play a large role in deciding these criteria. Where the cutoff is higher than 35 years of age, it is usually because funds are insufficient to provide the service for as many women; where it is lower than 35 years of age, the service may be paid for by the individual.[134]

The literature does not provide any evidence that countries legislate PND. There are, however, examples of jurisdictions that legislate that PND be available to women who choose to seek advice and testing. This is the case in Oregon in the United States, for example, where despite the lack of state-funded medical insurance the state will pay for PND services. However, even in jurisdictions where there is state funding, PND services tend to be concentrated in urban hospital centres, making it more difficult for members of rural populations to gain access.

In some countries, guidelines for the use of PND are developed and administered by groups similar to the CCMG — professional organizations that are responsible for regulating the practice of medical genetics. Such is the case in Sweden, Switzerland, and Great Britain.[135]

In the United States, the American Board of Medical Geneticists does provide some guidelines for the delivery of PND services, but individual states and institutions may further develop their own guidelines. For this reason, the delivery of PND may differ from state to state; however, the differences are minimal. For example, a centre in Houston, Texas, has developed its own guidelines and protocol for the delivery of services. These guidelines include indications for referral and criteria for termination procedures, among other things.[136]

The (American) Association of Cytogenetic Technologists has developed guidelines for chromosomal analysis. These were developed after a review of guidelines established by several states and regional genetics centres. Their intent is not necessarily to standardize laboratory procedures, but rather to provide institutions with a basis for developing laboratory standards of analysis.[137]

In Italy, there are no national guidelines for prenatal genetic services. Clinics and programs operate within the National Health Service System and follow, by and large, guidelines that are established in the international literature.[138]

In Hong Kong, genetic services are coordinated by the Department of Medical and Health Services of Hong Kong, and are under the direction of the Clinical Genetic Service and the Prenatal Diagnosis Service. These central bodies are responsible for the funding of programs. The Hong Kong Society of Medical Geneticists, which was established in 1986, is responsible for professional concerns including the promotion of its scientific programs. No mention is made of its role in establishing guidelines.[139]

It is important to note that professional organizations, with the support of governmental departments and agencies, have provided much direction with regard to the practice of medical genetics, particularly by advocating large-scale studies to establish the safety and accuracy of various techniques and to monitor their practice.

In countries where certain genetic disorders are unusually frequent, data on their prevalence have provided justification for special programs to identify carriers and to offer PND for high-risk couples. A number of programs that address such needs have been very successful in identifying carriers and affected fetuses. A case in point is the development of special programs in southern European countries where the prevalence of certain haemoglobinopathies (SCA, thalassemia) is high among certain ethnic populations. In these countries, successful screening programs have virtually eliminated these diseases in some regions and dramatically reduced their prevalence in others (e.g., Italy, Sardinia, and Cyprus).[140] In Canada, such programs exist for Tay-Sachs disease (a generative brain disease causing death in early childhood) in Ashkenazi Jewish and certain French-Canadian groups, for sickle-cell disease for persons of West African descent, and for thalassemias in Mediterranean and Oriental populations.

## Reaction to and Debate over Prenatal Diagnosis

The advent of PND has been regarded as breakthrough technology, and for many people has generated moral questions that are not answered easily. Consequently, personal, social, moral, and medical implications of PND continue to be the subject of public and professional debate.

During the formative years of PND toward the end of the 1960s, reaction to new developments was limited largely to discussions within the medical and research communities; public reaction, if any, was minimal. Even when amniocentesis began to be put into practice in the early 1970s, reaction was limited to professional concerns over specific techniques and the implementation of specific services. More recently, the impacts of PND on society, women in particular, and even the gene pool have been debated. Although there is concern over the safety and efficacy of specific techniques, much of the public discourse deals with major ethical dilemmas. The most notable example is the morality of using abortion as a means of avoiding the birth of a fetus with a congenital disorder.

One reason for the lack of widespread public debate and reaction to PND in its formative years may have been the absence of organized special interest groups that could respond to technological developments in the field. Even if individuals had concerns, for which there is little evidence, there was no means of publicizing them. Today, much of the public discourse is initiated by watchdog organizations and interest groups that have specific concerns about the development and impact of PND technology. Much of the debate over PND in Canada is led by groups representing women's interests, disabled people, the pro-choice movement, and the pro-life movement. These groups have significant political power and are regarded as major players in the debate.

Another possible factor contributing to the lack of public reaction during the early days of PND development was a lack of media attention. At that time, science and medicine did not seem to have the attention of the media that they enjoy today, and reports about breakthroughs in medicine, to say nothing of PND, were relatively few. Moreover, the technologies were considered experimental, and any published references to either the techniques or their impact were mostly buried in the scholarly literature.

Today the media follow events in the world of science and medicine closely, and are quick to report on any new developments. They also pay particular attention to controversial issues and new technologies. The increased profile of medicine and technology has led the media to provide a forum for the public and professionals to proclaim their views but, regrettably, few opportunities to exchange viewpoints and information.

## Public Debate

One of the first public debates over the use of preventive genetics concerned the development of screening and testing programs to identify carriers of the SCA gene in the United States. Because SCA is prevalent in the black population, these programs were aimed at black Americans so that they could be most effective in reducing the prevalence of the disease.

The aim of the SCA programs was to identify high-risk couples in which both parents could pass on the recessive gene. In such cases the chance was one in four that a child would manifest the eventually lethal anaemia. Unfortunately, in this first approach to genetic screening, the need for public education and for counselling services was not appreciated; their lack led to many misunderstandings about the nature of the disease. For example, there was the belief that anyone carrying the gene in a single dose was at risk for the disease, thus equating sickle cell trait and sickle cell carrier state disease. This misunderstanding led to unjustified anxiety, stigmatization of carriers, incidents of inflated insurance premiums, and even job losses. These unfortunate events greatly concerned black and civil rights organizations and geneticists. Even during the late 1970s, the U.S. government, through the Air Force Academy admission procedures, disqualified all candidates for aircrew who were found to be SCA gene carriers, despite the lack of proof that a carrier was any less fit to serve. After intense criticism from black action and civil rights groups and geneticists, state governments backed away from mandatory screening.[141]

Another major criticism of SCA screening programs was that there was nothing to offer high-risk couples except genetic counselling. After counselling, couples were still faced with the decision of whether to take the one-in-four risk, or not have children — PND was not practicable, as it required a fetal blood sample obtained by means of fetoscopy, which was not considered safe, effective, or widely available. Now the diagnosis can be done on cells from the amniotic fluid, or chorionic villi, so there is something definite to offer, and screening programs (with appropriate counselling and laboratory support) are functioning quite effectively in a number of countries.

More recently, concerns have been expressed over the use of genetic testing to identify genetic predisposition to disease and disability. Labour, civil, and public rights groups are concerned that diagnosing a genetic predisposition will lead to problems similar to those encountered with SCA testing (i.e., concerns about being labelled as a disease carrier).[142] People are also concerned about the confidentiality of personal genetic information and the potential of such information to be misused by insurance companies, leading to discrimination in the workplace. These concerns are not directly related to PND technology per se, but questions are also being asked about the potential use of PND for diseases of late onset (e.g., Huntington disease) or for genes that only increase susceptibility to a disease (e.g., diabetes or schizophrenia).

During the last decade, public and special interest groups have examined PND intensively, and have initiated public debate on a number of fronts and on a variety of issues. These include concerns over:

- the stigma of being labelled as a genetic disease carrier;[143]
- what it means to a woman to have her health and that of her fetus called into question;[144]
- whether older women are being stigmatized as being less fit to carry children;[145]
- whether programs to eliminate fetuses with certain disorders will adversely affect society's attitudes toward persons with disabilities;[146]
- whether the increasingly routine use of PND and prenatal screening alters women's perception and experience of pregnancy;[147]
- whether the proliferation of prenatal services diverts resources and attention from non-genetic causes of disability;

- whether the use of genetic technology, including PND, will result in biological differences between individuals being reduced to merely DNA codes, and loss of personal individuality;[148] and
- the medical, social, and biological impact of interfering with gene frequencies.

Many more arguments stem from special interests that advocate particular positions with regard to PND. Among the more widely publicized positions are concerns about abortion. Some argue that abortion should not be permitted under any circumstances. Others debate how serious the medical and social burden of a condition must be to justify abortion.

Some groups maintain that if an abnormality is diagnosed, women are either subtly or overtly pressured into terminating the pregnancy, and that such pressure impinges on the right of women to make personal choices with regard to pregnancy. They also point out that such pressure may discourage people who would consider having PND even if they would not have an abortion, but who wish to use a diagnosis to prepare themselves for the birth of a child with a disability.

It is a basic tenet of genetic counsellors in Canada that their counselling should be non-directive. Any pressure to influence a woman or couple to have (or not to have) an abortion would be contrary to the guidelines and leave the counsellor open to censure. There is little evidence that such coercion occurs in Canada; if it does occur, it is likely to come from over-authoritative physicians or friends and relatives rather than genetic counsellors.

Another concern is that some genetic conditions vary in severity, and that PND techniques cannot predict the degree to which a fetus will be affected by a particular disease. For instance, amniocentesis can be used to diagnose spina bifida but cannot test whether the child will have more or less severe manifestations of the disorder. This has raised some people's concerns that near-normal fetuses may be aborted. Uncertainty does exist in some diagnostic situations; it is the duty of the counsellor to try to ensure that the couple is aware of the risks and also of degrees of certainty, and that they understand the implications.

Similarly, there is the chance of error in diagnosis as the result of mistakes in laboratory work, or errors in record keeping. On the one hand, this has caused concern that a wrong diagnosis could lead to either a deformed child being carried to term (i.e., a false-negative result) or the abortion of a healthy child (i.e., a false-positive result).

False diagnoses of extra or missing chromosomes are exceedingly rare.[149] This is similar for enzymatic deficiencies. However, in some situations, such as mosaicism (i.e., the presence of two cell lines in the culture) or predictive testing where the DNA marker is close to the gene but not in it, the interpretation may involve some ambiguity. It is not that the diagnosis is wrong, but that if action is taken when the test has a recognized 5 percent probability of being inaccurate, the action may lead to the undesired result in 1 case in 20. Again, such uncertainties must be carefully explained to couples during genetic counselling.

There is also debate over the cost-benefit arguments that are used in some cases to justify PND. Some people react strongly to the notion that disability is costly to society, and they reject any material definition of ability or disability. Others define costs of disability broadly; they enter economic and social concerns as well as pain and suffering into cost-benefit equations. Such issues are complex, and there are no simple answers. However, there is some agreement that cost-benefit arguments should be considered in decision making concerning resource allocation.

Some groups have also expressed fears that new genetics research, including PND, is effectively old-style eugenics. Some groups believe that the promotion of PND, selective abortion, and encouraging or discouraging marriage and child bearing of individuals with certain traits are components of eugenic thought and thus to be discouraged. Some consider eugenics to be inherently evil and describe trends to use PND as "Hitler revisited."[150]

Apart from the political and moral overtones of eugenic concerns about PND, the basic eugenic question would be whether it increases the frequency of deleterious genes in the gene pool and what the long-term biological consequences would be. For example, would interfering with natural selection create a less adaptable genome? Those who support PND answer that it is not done for eugenic reasons. Whether it results in a decrease or increase in frequency of deleterious genes for different conditions, these changes will be slow and small. They hold that the purpose of PND is to alleviate the suffering, pain, and anguish both of the affected persons and of those who must support and care for persons with such disabilities.

Religious and other groups have had a significant impact on attitudes toward PND and the other new reproductive technologies; their opinions are important in shaping the debate about the impact of PND on individuals and society.

While abortion is prohibited under Jewish law and all Jews are taught not to treat abortion lightly, some Jewish legal authorities hold that in extenuating circumstances a pregnancy can be terminated. Severe genetic diseases that are amenable to PND are examples of extenuating circumstances.[151]

In contrast are the more stringent teachings and doctrines of the Roman Catholic Church. In a 1987 pronouncement, the Vatican urged governments to initiate legislative action to prohibit new reproductive technologies that are related to abortion. The statement specifically condemned the use of PND if the woman who requests it intends to have an abortion if an abnormality is found. The Vatican was concerned about the need to preserve the sanctity of human life and pointed out that a society, and indeed a civilization, can be measured by the respect shown to its weakest members.[152]

Measuring patients' reactions to and attitudes toward PND has been an important component of the research and development. In fact, many of the changes in techniques and programs are the result of problems and pitfalls identified through user surveys, and studies of patients' experiences. Patients' reactions, combined with the results from clinical trials, have provided the impetus for developing simpler and safer procedures and more effective services and programs.

An example of the importance of patients' reactions and attitudes was the development of CVS as a viable alternative to amniocentesis. CVS was primarily developed in response to concerns that mid-trimester amniocentesis, though safe and reliable, was not optimal because it could not be done before the second trimester. CVS had the advantage of providing earlier diagnosis and greater privacy with regard to the pregnancy and a possible decision to terminate. If abortion was chosen, the procedure was safer than the mid-trimester abortions associated with amniocentesis.

## Human Costs and Benefits of Screening Programs

In general, screening programs present greater problems and challenges than testing services such as amniocentesis, largely because of their wider public impact. Large-scale screening programs have costs and benefits in both economic and human terms. Although much attention has been paid to the economic impact of MSAFP screening, for example, fewer studies have attempted to assess its human impact. This is probably due to the difficulty of measuring intangibles such as parental distress or relief of anxiety. Human benefits and costs are not amenable to quantitative balancing, though psychological instruments are being developed to measure values such as quality of life.[153]

Different individuals will reach different conclusions regarding the relative costs and benefits of screening programs. Some view the reduction of suffering as a substantial benefit; others are influenced by the ability of screening to reduce the cost of supporting severely handicapped individuals who would otherwise be born. Some people regard the chance of accidental abortion of otherwise normal fetuses as indefensible. Yet others see the rare loss of a normal fetus as less of a cost than the long-term morbidity of a neural tube defect. In any event, wide discussions are required to enable society as a whole to decide the extent to which, if at all, a program should be implemented.[154]

## Professional Reaction

Professional reaction to developments in PND services, techniques, and programs has been fairly consistent from the early years to the present day. As noted previously, most of the early reactions to the advent of PND were from professionals whose attitudes and advice played a pivotal role in its early success. The support of professionals was contingent upon clinical studies to ensure the safety and effectiveness of the techniques before their acceptance into clinical practice. Professionals also recognized the need to ensure that the procedures were being performed by capable practitioners, who knew what conditions could be diagnosed. They recognized the need for organizations to oversee the expansion of medical genetics services in general and PND in particular. Organizations comparable to the CCMG began to appear around the world, along with governmental advisory bodies and research centres.

Professional organizations have responded to developments in the field of PND by advocating particular courses of action and responding to the need for clinical research trials and cost-benefit studies to justify programs and services. They continue to play a central role in this area by updating and revising the guidelines. In Canada, for example, the CCMG and other professional bodies keep pace with the ever-expanding field of PND by modifying guidelines to incorporate new technologies and new developments.

There is some professional debate over who should set guidelines for the delivery of PND services. Some people think that expansion of services has not always been in direct response to demand, and they suggest that other interests have fuelled development. A case in point is the expansion of ultrasound technology as part of standard obstetric care; it is said that at least some of the interests served are those of the medical supply companies.[155] Some authors suggest that the common cutoff ages for eligibility for PND are arbitrary and probably set for economic rather than sound medical reasons. They question the assumption that professionals should be the gatekeepers and suggest that consumers of the services and the public (particularly women) should have a seat at the table when such decisions are made.[156]

Professional organizations provide expert advice to governments, hospitals, and medical genetics clinics on the way programs should be implemented and funds allocated, and the kinds of research support required to sustain effective programs. Professionals have been involved in conducting and commenting on cost-benefit studies that may be helpful in justifying PND programs and services.[157]

Most of the formal professional reaction to PND in Canada is voiced by organizations such as the CCMG and the SOGC. However, individuals from the social and medical sciences have published viewpoints that differ from official stands on particular issues. They have, for example, commented extensively on attitudes toward disability and the impact of PND on these attitudes. Some persons advocate PND because disability is seen to be inherently destructive of productive life: people free from genetic disorders will be able to live full lives and contribute more productively to society. Others rebut this type of argument as one that presumes that disability per se is the source of non-productivity, rather than associated defeatism and the societal conditions that cause the lack of productivity.[158]

The recent attention given to a small number of physicians who wish to use PND to identify fetal sex for non-medical reasons has alarmed many professionals and members of the public. Most regard sex diagnosis for non-medical reasons as a thoughtless and dangerous application of PND. The medical community has, for the most part, reacted strongly against these developments and has stated (e.g., CCMG guidelines) that PND should not be used to identify sex for non-medical reasons. However, substantial arguments have been made in defence of sex diagnosis, in particular that couples have the right to make their own reproductive decisions.

Professional bodies have used their influence to prevent abuse in other ways, for example in the case of MSAFP testing kits. During the early 1980s regulatory agencies in the United States approved AFP testing kits for use in physicians' offices. It was claimed that these kits could be used to measure MSAFP levels and diagnose the presence of neural tube defects. Reaction from professional organizations was swift and vigorous. They strongly discouraged the use of such kits on the grounds that their unsupervised use would be dangerous and not consistent with the widely accepted fact that prenatal testing requires extensive normative data to allow proper interpretation of the results, and that counselling is needed to fully explain the purpose of the test. Uninformed use could lead to unnecessary anxiety, concern, and abortion.[159]

In Canada, and specifically Ontario, a similar controversy erupted in the mid-1970s over the question of office use of MSAFP testing kits. The Ontario Advisory Committee on Genetics was asked to recommend the conditions under which such screening should be permitted. In 1980, the Committee sought to oppose the unrestricted sale of the MSAFP kits. The decision was made because of a lack of data to document the need and appropriateness of such screening, and because educational, quality control, and ethical issues had not been considered. The Committee had the support of the Association of Genetic Counsellors of Ontario and the SOGC. As a result, the unrestricted sale of these kits was banned in Ontario and eventually in all of Canada.

As the public becomes more involved in the debate over new reproductive technologies, PND in particular, professionals are being called on to emerge from their hospitals and laboratories to explain their role in modern medicine and to justify the development of controversial technologies. Increasingly, scientists and health care professionals have to pay close attention not only to their professional interests but also to their societal responsibilities. By any measure, these challenges help to promulgate informed and expert opinion on complex and challenging issues.

One of the first comprehensive examinations of the impact of the new genetics is contained in a book by Israeli sociologist Amitai Etzioni published in 1973. The volume deals specifically with what he learned and felt after he participated in an international meeting of experts that reviewed the new scientific breakthroughs of the time.[160] Among other issues, Etzioni discussed the moral, social, and ethical impact of the new and potential genetic technologies. In surprising detail, he describes the consequences of being able to select the sex of a child, breed a healthier and superior race, detect genes that code for diseases that are manifested later in life, and detect genes that are "bad." He questions who should make decisions regarding the development and use of these technologies. Ultimately he called for a double antidote: a "stimulant" to energize the passive members of the community who allow science to shape society, and a "mild tranquillizer" for those who reject all technological advances. He also called for a greater ability to discriminate, judge, and review these new technologies, and to learn to use them for our own benefit rather than exploitation. Many of the issues Etzioni raised are exactly those that confront us today, the only difference being that at the time of Etzioni's writing the technologies were largely potential — today they are a reality.

## Government Reaction

Governments have responded to developments in the field of PND by developing and implementing PND services and programs, soliciting advice of experts and views from the public, and supporting research and development.

Governments, it may be assumed, are motivated to consider the best interests of the public and act in response to expert advice and prompting from special interest groups. Nevertheless, governments are constrained by competing interests, and complicating economic, social, and legal circumstances. They are required to balance prudently the best interests of the community with economic realities, and reflect common societal and community standards. This is a difficult task, one that requires wide consultation with the public and with experts in the field.

To assist them, governments commission task forces and set up bodies to advise them about scientific and economic realities, as well as the impact of particular public policy initiatives. In Canada, the federal government struck a commission (the Royal Commission on New Reproductive Technologies) to study, among other things, PND and genetic testing. Because technology tends to outpace the ability to deal with and comprehend the wider implications of its applications, the government is seeking a comprehensive study of these questions to gain the best advice on how to proceed with policy concerned with the new reproductive technologies. Commissions of inquiry in other countries have had a similar function.[161]

As is the case with any new health care technology and program, matters of economics and funding are important, especially in light of strains on the funding of health care. For this reason, governments may pay attention to cost-benefit and cost-effective arguments that predict the net gain, short- or long-term, to be realized if particular programs are implemented. These studies assist the government to translate attributes of programs and services into dollars; researchers can try to factor both tangible and non-tangible costs into the equation.

The predictions of cost-benefit analysis can vary between countries and even between regions within countries, and must take into account the local or regional epidemiology of genetic disease. For instance, in Canada, neural tube defects are more common in eastern than in western provinces. Cost-benefit analysis may reveal that PND programs may be economically justified in those areas where neural tube defects are common and not in areas where the incidence is low.

Government agencies (particularly the MRC) have been key supporters of basic and clinical research into the safety and efficiency of PND techniques. They have funded large-scale prospective and retrospective studies that have played a major role in incorporating new techniques into standard clinical practice.

Despite the best intentions to gather advice and counsel, governments have not always been successful in their attempts to implement prenatal genetic testing and screening programs and services. The U.S. experience with SCA testing is a classic example of how government attempts to implement programs may have untoward impact. The U.S. government endorsement of AFP kits by the Food and Drug Administration exemplifies the problems that can occur with product endorsement, and illustrates how governments can be at the mercy of limited data and information.

Notwithstanding these examples, the majority of government-supported programs have had the effect of reducing the incidence of a number of conditions. The screening programs that were set up to identify carriers of thalassemia (a hereditary anaemia) in Cyprus, Greece, and Italy resulted in dramatically reduced incidence of this severe disease. In some regions of these countries the disease has been almost totally eradicated through screening, testing, and selective abortion.

## Legal Concerns

As the ability to test and screen for genetic diseases continues to evolve, so too does the legal framework that defines the rights and responsibilities of parents, children, and fetuses. Governments, through their judicial and legal branches, have fiduciary responsibilities to interpret these rights to protect both the individual and society.[162]

The courts have been challenged to rule on a number of landmark cases that stem from the perceived implications of PND. These cases, known as "wrongful birth" and "wrongful life" suits, have focussed attention on legal definitions of the rights and responsibilities of patients, hospitals, and physicians.[163]

Wrongful birth suits are usually initiated by mothers whose doctors did not say that PND could be done to test the genetic status of a fetus when there was a risk of having a child with a genetic condition. As a result, the woman feels she was denied the opportunity to make an informed decision about whether or not to continue the pregnancy. Wrongful life cases[164] are brought on behalf of a child who would not have been born to experience the suffering caused by genetic disease if the doctor had properly informed the parents that this was likely to happen. In the few cases where these suits have been decided, courts have awarded costs to help attend to and care for a disabled child, and also punitive awards. No such suits have succeeded in Canada, as yet.

## Epilogue

PND has gradually become part of the system of genetic services. Many of the techniques were modified from other usages. The very early work on techniques for obtaining amniotic fluid for PND was done outside Canada, particularly in Israel, Great Britain, and the United States.

The procedures could not have been developed without the cooperation of pregnant women who were going to have abortions and who agreed to undergo experimental procedures before their pregnancies were terminated. Details are scant as to how these women became involved, their motives, and whether their consent was truly informed. Requirements for proof of informed consent, much less informed choice, were virtually non-existent in those days. It is likely that many, if not all, of the women who cooperated did so for altruistic reasons, but this cannot be documented some 30 years later. There is an opportunity to examine the question a little more closely in the case of women cooperating in the early development of fetoscopy in Montreal in the early 1970s. Personal recollections made it clear that these women did cooperate for altruistic reasons, and that they did sign consent forms.[165]

In Montreal, the first PND was done in 1968 by Dr. Louis Dallaire, whose doctoral research involved screening families with recurrent multiple malformations to look for chromosome rearrangements that might be the cause. Of the six discovered, one was found in a stillborn child whose mother carried a balanced chromosome translocation (a rearrangement that put her children at high risk). This diagnosis meant that her future offspring were at increased risk. The woman asked if there was any way to find out before birth if children were affected. When the woman became pregnant again, Dr. Dallaire found an obstetrician who was doing amniocentesis during late pregnancies for fetal monitoring, and who was willing to try it earlier — as soon as the uterus could be felt above the pelvic rim. The amniocentesis was successful, the culture grew, and the chromosomes were normal. In the following months doctors went on to do amniocentesis on women who were over 40 years of age or were carriers for X-linked diseases, and PND gradually began to be offered along with genetic counselling services.[166]

In Chicago, Dr. Henry Nadler, in his first job, was studying how inborn errors of metabolism might be expressed in cultured cells. He also worked in the genetics clinic, where he counselled a woman who had had two children with Down syndrome, and who was eight weeks pregnant. She carried a chromosome translocation, probably 21/21, which meant that any live-born child she had would have Down syndrome. In those days, however, it was impossible to be sure it was a 21/21 rather than 21/22, which carried a lower risk. Unfortunately her application for an abortion for genetic reasons was denied, and, following an illegal abortion, she died. As a result, Dr. Nadler committed himself to perfecting PND. He began learning how to grow cells from amniotic fluid, using fluid obtained during second-trimester abortions by an obstetrical colleague.[167]

In Winnipeg, PND was initiated after the Paediatrician-in-Chief, Dr. Harry Medovy, heard about it at the Bar Harbor course in Medical Genetics, a course that in those days was aimed primarily at physicians who had graduated from medical school without any exposure to genetics. The Winnipeg geneticists found some obstetricians willing to do the procedure and arranged that only a few would do it, to ensure that they had enough cases to become expert.

In Edinburgh, David Brock discovered the AFP connection with neural tube defects when his student, plagued with contaminations (from the manure the gardener was spreading outside the windows) that interfered with his attempts to grow cells from amniotic fluid, decided to study the proteins in amniotic fluid instead. The investigation revealed that all such protein came from the mother, with the exception of AFP. They guessed that for a fetus with an abnormal opening, the AFP might leak into the amniotic fluid. Subsequently, they measured the AFP in amniotic fluid that had been frozen and was later found to have come from anencephalic fetuses.[168]

In Vancouver, Dr. J.R. Miller recalls the frustrations of counsellors having to say no when asked whether there was any way of telling before birth whether babies would be abnormal. But when the first reports of PND appeared in the literature, he wrote a letter to the editor expressing concerns about the effects of amniocentesis on the human fetus. He was concerned that because the McGill group had demonstrated that amniocentesis in the mouse could cause cleft palate, it might also do so in human fetuses. However, it was shown that the palate closes before the stage at which the procedure is carried out in humans. PND seemed to become a logical extension of the existing services in Vancouver.[169]

In the early days, of necessity, a process of education and organization was required. In the beginning, for example, obstetricians would do amniocentesis, sometimes in their own offices, and then send the fluid to the cytogenetics laboratory without warning. One geneticist's first exposure to PND occurred when she was developing the techniques for growing cells in culture and examining their chromosomes — a woman arrived at her laboratory door with a test tube of amniotic fluid, still warm, for genetic analysis.[170]

Many physicians were not clear as to what conditions could be diagnosed by the study of the chromosomes. Samples were sent (inappropriately) for diagnosis of single-gene disorders such as achondroplasia (a type of dwarfism) and haemophilia (a bleeding disease) or simply for "genetic testing." The genetics centres had to decline to do tests without prior consultation. Fairly rapidly the present system evolved, in which amniocentesis is done by a limited number of physicians, at centres that must perform at least 50 procedures a year in order to be approved, and with the provision that women having the procedure are counselled beforehand.

Neither equipment manufacturers nor pharmaceutical houses seemed to have much opportunity to bring pressures to bear. The exception was the attempt to make AFP testing kits available for use in doctors' offices. U.S. professionals and the Canadian government, acting on professional advice, negated this effort.

The rapid evolution of PND and other genetic services has raised many questions that concern professionals, the public, and prospective users of these services. For example, concerns have been expressed over whether the use of PND at progressively earlier gestational stages will lead to referrals for progressively less severe conditions. Many concerns have been raised about the impact of PND on women and people with disabilities. Are women undergoing PND free of pressures to do so? Will the concept of screening for fetal abnormalities adversely affect society's attitudes toward people with disabilities? These concerns, among many others, are examples of what happens when technology evolves so rapidly that it outpaces the ability to grapple with its consequences. Most important, these concerns highlight the need for further study, debate, and a mechanism for public input into the regulation of PND services.

## Conclusions

- PND has seen remarkable growth over a short period of time. Rapid advances are due at least in part to the rapid conversion of scientific discoveries into applicable technologies, and the transfer of existing technology to specific uses in PND. Many of the scientific discoveries that made PND possible were made by scientists who were working on something else. The drive to develop services came from the synergism between the perceived need and the available techniques.
- Although prenatal sampling techniques (such as amniocentesis, CVS, and fetoscopy) and the analytical techniques (such as cell culture,

assays, DNA technology) are linked procedurally, they have evolved in different ways. The sampling and imaging techniques have evolved gradually as the result of stepwise modifications from previous techniques. In contrast, the analytical techniques have evolved in a punctuated progression. Their present success and widespread application can be traced to a number of important advances in laboratory technology and molecular biology.

- CVS was first developed in the late 1960s, at about the same time amniocentesis was gaining popularity in centres throughout the world as a PND procedure. CVS was developed to provide earlier diagnosis than was possible with other procedures (i.e., during the first trimester). Technical difficulties plagued early work, and no major efforts were made to further development until the early 1980s. Since that time CVS has been the subject of many studies, most of which conclude that the risks associated with CVS are slightly greater than those associated with amniocentesis, but there are advantages, particularly those related to its application earlier in pregnancy and the more rapid return of diagnostic results.

- Fetoscopy was first used to visualize the fetus *in utero*. Later it was used to sample fetal blood to diagnose genetic blood disorders (e.g., SCA, thalassemia). Because of the comparatively high frequency of complications and adverse reactions, fetoscopy never became widely used. To a great extent it has been replaced by ultrasound (for visualization of the fetus), and by amniocentesis and CVS (when PND of a particular haemoglobinopathy is required).

- The association of abnormal levels of AFP in the amniotic fluid with a variety of congenital anomalies was first made in the early 1970s. Soon afterward, it was recognized that AFP may also be elevated in maternal serum when the fetus has a neural tube defect. This discovery has led to the measurement of MSAFP as a safe, relatively cheap, and easily performed method of screening for neural tube defects, notwithstanding an appreciable number of false diagnoses that require further investigation for clarification. AFAFP testing combined with ultrasound screening offers very accurate diagnosis of the presence of neural tube defects (98 percent).

- Ultrasonography had its origins far from the field of medicine. It was developed for anti-submarine warfare during the First World War, and later applied to medicine and obstetrics. Since the 1950s there has been an exponential increase in the use of ultrasonography so that it is now a common part of obstetric care. It has played an important role in improving the success, accuracy, and safety of other PND techniques, including amniocentesis, CVS, and fetal blood sampling.

- The safety of ultrasound has been questioned. Although there is little evidence of adverse effects of ultrasound in patients, their offspring, or equipment operators, many statements and commentaries emphasize concerns for safety. Some people conclude that ultrasonography may not be totally innocuous, and that its effects, if they occur, may be subtle and delayed in expression. Most, however, conclude that the evidence available is reassuring and that dosages used for diagnosis are safe. A recent exhaustive review of human epidemiology, secular trends, and animal studies led to the conclusion that ultrasonography, as used in PND, presents no measurable risk.

- The possibility of applying MRI to prenatal diagnosis of fetal anomalies and other birth defects was realized in the early 1980s. MRI has a number of advantages over ultrasonography, in particular its ability to define soft tissues of both the mother and the fetus, which can be useful when diagnosing specific congenital defects. MRI is currently expensive and not widely available, and its safety has yet to be definitively established. It is unlikely that it will ever replace ultrasound, which has established value and broad applications in the field of PND.

- Preimplantation diagnosis is a new technique still in the experimental stage. It may hold some promise in the diagnosis of single-gene diseases in certain (rare) circumstances, but it must rely on the costly and stressful methods of IVF.

- The risks and complications associated with the major techniques (e.g., amniocentesis, CVS, and fetoscopy) were not well documented during their early development, because the women whose fetuses were diagnosed were having their pregnancies terminated for non-medical reasons. As confidence with the procedures grew, investigators were able to conduct clinical trials to assess the efficacy of the techniques, the safety of the procedures, and effects on both the mother and fetus. As the list of indications for PND grew, their use became more widespread; large-scale studies (retrospective and prospective) were carried out to assess the procedures and quantify risks and complications. Many observers report a learning curve as equipment improved and experience was gained.

- Canadian researchers have played important roles in the development of PND services. With the support of the MRC, investigators have conducted large-scale collaborative studies to determine the safety and efficacy of amniocentesis and CVS. These studies are widely cited, and are considered to be important contributions to the establishment of standards for clinical use of these techniques.

- Indications for the use of the various PND techniques grew as analytical techniques improved and as the cytogenetic, molecular, and biochemical bases of genetic diseases were identified.

- The first Canadian guidelines for PND were published in 1974 by the CPS, the SOGC, and the GSC. A more comprehensive set of guidelines was published by the CCMG, the SOGC, and the CPS in 1983. More recently, the CCMG and the SOGC have prepared an update of these guidelines in response to advances in the fields of PND and genetic research. The CCMG has published professional and ethical guidelines for the practice of medical genetics that explicitly state the responsibilities of the geneticist to patients, society, and the profession.

- During the latter 1960s, when PND was being developed, reaction was largely limited to discussions within the professional, medical, and research communities; public reaction, if any, was small. More recently there is wider debate over the impact of PND on society, women in particular, and even the gene pool. One reason for the lack of debate during the early years may have been the absence of organized special interest groups that could respond to technological developments in the field. Much of the debate over PND in Canada is led by women's interest groups, groups representing disabled people, and the pro-choice and pro-life movements. Today these groups have significant political power, and they are regarded as major players in the debate. In the early days, science and medicine did not always receive the same close attention from the media that they do now. Consequently, reports about breakthroughs in medicine, including PND, were relatively few, effectively limiting public debate. The technologies were considered experimental, and published references to either the methods or their impact were not widely accessible.

- Recent public debate and court challenges, known as wrongful birth and wrongful life suits, have focussed attention on the definition of rights and responsibilities of patients, hospitals, and physicians.

- As the public becomes more and more involved in the debate over new reproductive technologies, PND in particular, professionals are being called upon to explain their role in modern medicine and to justify the development of controversial technologies. Increasingly, scientists and health care professionals have to pay close attention not only to professional interests but also to their societal responsibilities. These challenges help to promulgate informed and expert information and opinion on complex and challenging issues.

## Notes

1. V.A. McKusick, "Mendelian Inheritance in Man," in *Catalogs of Autosomal Dominant, Autosomal Recessive, and X-Linked Phenotypes*, 8th ed. (Baltimore: Johns Hopkins University Press, 1988).

2. M.L. Barr and E.G. Bertram, "A Morphological Distinction Between Neurones of the Male and Female, and the Behaviour of the Nucleolar Satellite During

Accelerated Nucleoprotein Synthesis," *Nature* 163 (1949): 676-77; M.L. Barr, L.F. Bertram, and H.A. Lindsay, "The Morphology of the Nerve Cell Nucleus, According to Sex," *Anatomical Record* 107 (1950): 283-97.

3. K.L. Moore and M.L. Barr, "Smears from the Oral Mucosa in the Detection of Chromosomal Sex," *Lancet* (9 July 1955): 57-58.

4. D.M. Serr, L. Sachs, and M. Danon, "The Diagnosis of Sex Before Birth Using Cells from the Amniotic Fluid (A Preliminary Report)," *Bulletin of the Research Council of Israel* 5B (1955): 137-38; F. Fuchs and P. Riis, "Antenatal Sex Determination," *Nature* 177 (1956): 330.

5. J. Lejeune, M. Gautier, and R. Turpin, "Étude des chromosomes somatiques de neuf enfants mongoliens," *Comptes rendus hebdomadaires des séances de l'Académie des Sciences* (Paris) 248 (1959): 1721-22.

6. M.W. Steele and W.R. Breg, Jr., "Chromosome Analysis of Human Amniotic-Fluid Cells," *Lancet* (19 February 1966): 383-85; C.B. Jacobson and R.H. Barter, "Intrauterine Diagnosis and Management of Genetic Defects," *American Journal of Obstetrics and Gynecology* 99 (1967): 796-807.

7. W.Y.F. Hsu, "Prenatal Diagnosis of Chromosome Abnormalities," in *Genetic Disorders and the Fetus: Diagnosis, Prevention and Treatment*, 2d ed., ed. A. Milunsky (New York: Plenum Press, 1986); H.L. Nadler, "Antenatal Detection of Hereditary Disorders," *Pediatrics* 42 (1968): 912-18.

8. H.L. Nadler, "Patterns of Enzyme Development Utilizing Cultivated Human Fetal Cells Derived from Amniotic Fluid," *Biochemical Genetics* 2 (1968): 119-26.

9. A. Milunsky, *The Prenatal Diagnosis of Hereditary Disorders* (Illinois: Charles C. Thomas, 1973).

10. Y.W. Kan, M.S. Golbus, and A.M. Dozy, "Prenatal Diagnosis of $\alpha$-Thalassemia: Clinical Application of Molecular Hybridization," *New England Journal of Medicine* 295 (1976): 1165-67.

11. Y.W. Kan and A.M. Dozy, "Antenatal Diagnosis of Sickle-Cell Anaemia by D.N.A. Analysis of Amniotic-Fluid Cells," *Lancet* (28 October 1978): 910-11; Y.W. Kan and A.M. Dozy, "Polymorphism of DNA Sequence Adjacent to Human β-Globin Structural Gene: Relationship to Sickle Mutation," *Proceedings of the National Academy of Sciences* 75 (1978): 5631-35.

12. D. Lambl, "Ein seltener Fall von Hydramnios," *Centralblatt für Gynäkologie* 5 (1881): 329-34; F. Schatz, "Eine besondere Art von einseitiger Polyhydramnie mit anderseitiger Oligohydramnie bei eineiigen Zwillingen," *Archiv für Gynäkologie* 19 (1882): 329-69.

13. T.O. Menees, J.D. Miller, and L.E. Holly, "Amniography: Preliminary Report," *American Journal of Roentgenology and Radium Therapy* 24 (1930): 363-66.

14. M.E. Aburel, "Le déclanchement du travail par injections intra-amniotiques de sérum salé hypertonique," *Gynécologie et obstétrique* 36 (1937): 398-99.

15. M.S. Verp and J.L. Simpson, "Amniocentesis for Prenatal Genetic Diagnosis," in *Human Prenatal Diagnosis*, 2d ed., ed. K. Filkins and J.F. Russo (New York: Marcel Dekker, 1990).

16. A.E.H. Emery, "Antenatal Diagnosis of Genetic Disease," in *Modern Trends in Human Genetics I* (London: Butterworths, 1970).

17. M.I. Evans et al., "Early Genetic Amniocentesis and Chorionic Villus Sampling: Expanding the Opportunities for Early Prenatal Diagnosis," *Journal of Reproductive Medicine* 33 (1988): 450-52.

18. D.C.A. Bevis, "The Antenatal Prediction of Haemolytic Disease of the Newborn," *Lancet* (23 February 1952): 395-98; A.H.C. Walker, "Liquor Amnii Studies in the Prediction of Haemolytic Disease of the Newborn," *British Medical Journal* (17 August 1957): 376-78.

19. D.M. Serr and E. Margolis, "Diagnosis of Fetal Sex in a Sex-Linked Hereditary Disorder," *American Journal of Obstetrics and Gynecology* 88 (1964): 230-32.

20. Steele and Breg, "Chromosome Analysis of Human Amniotic-Fluid Cells."

21. H.L. Nadler, "Newer Procedures in the Preconceptional, Prenatal and Early Postnatal Diagnosis of Birth Defects," *Birth Defects: Original Article Series* 6 (1970): 26-31.

22. J.D. Curtis et al., "The Importance of Placental Localization Preceding Amniocentesis," *Obstetrics and Gynecology* 40 (1972): 194-98.

23. B.R. Benacerraf and F.D. Frigoletto, "Amniocentesis Under Continuous Ultrasound Guidance: A Series of 232 Cases," *Obstetrics and Gynecology* 62 (1983): 760-63.

24. Canadian College of Medical Geneticists and Society of Obstetricians and Gynaecologists of Canada, "Canadian Guidelines for Prenatal Diagnosis of Genetic Disorders: An Update," *Journal of the Society of Obstetricians and Gynaecologists of Canada* 13 (August 1991): 13-31; Verp and Simpson, "Amniocentesis for Prenatal Genetic Diagnosis"; S. Elias and J.L. Simpson, "Amniocentesis," in *Genetic Disorders and the Fetus: Diagnosis, Prevention, and Treatment*, 2d ed., ed. A. Milunsky (New York: Plenum Press, 1986); Hsu, "Prenatal Diagnosis of Chromosome Abnormalities."

25. Verp and Simpson, "Amniocentesis for Prenatal Genetic Diagnosis"; Hsu, "Prenatal Diagnosis of Chromosome Abnormalities."

26. Elias and Simpson, "Amniocentesis."

27. N.E. Simpson et al., "Prenatal Diagnosis of Genetic Disease in Canada: Report of a Collaborative Study," *Canadian Medical Association Journal* 115 (1976): 739-48; Medical Research Council of Canada, *Diagnosis of Genetic Disease by Amniocentesis During the Second Trimester of Pregnancy: A Canadian Study* (Ottawa: Minister of Supply and Services Canada, 1977); Medical Research Council (U.K.), Working Party on Amniocentesis, "An Assessment of the Hazards of Amniocentesis," *British Journal of Obstetrics and Gynaecology* 85 (Suppl. 2) (1978); NICHD National Registry for Amniocentesis Study Group, "Midtrimester Amniocentesis for Prenatal Diagnosis: Safety and Accuracy," *JAMA* 236 (1976): 1471-76.

28. N. Hahnemann and J. Mohr, "Genetic Diagnosis in the Embryo by Means of Biopsy from Extra Embryonic Membranes," *Bulletin of the European Society of Human Genetics* 2 (1968): 23-29; K.J. Blakemore and M.J. Mahoney, "Chorionic Villus Sampling," in *Genetic Disorders and the Fetus: Diagnosis, Prevention and Treatment*, 2d ed., ed. A. Milunsky (New York: Plenum Press, 1986).

29. J. Mohr, "Foetal Genetic Diagnosis: Development of Techniques for Early Sampling of Foetal Cells," *Acta Pathologica et Microbiologica Scandinavica* 73 (1968):

73-77; Hahnemann and Mohr, "Genetic Diagnosis in the Embryo by Means of Biopsy from Extra-Embryonic Membranes"; N. Hahnemann and J. Mohr, "Antenatal Foetal Diagnosis in Genetic Disease," *Bulletin of the European Society of Human Genetics* 3 (1969): 47.

30. R.J. Wapner and L. Jackson, "Chorionic Villus Sampling," *Clinical Obstetrics and Gynecology* 31 (1988): 328-44.

31. S. Kullander and B. Sandahl, "Fetal Chromosome Analysis After Transcervical Placental Biopsies During Early Pregnancy," *Acta Obstetricia et Gynecologica Scandinavica* 52 (1973): 355-59; S.A. Rhine et al., "Prenatal Sex Detection with Endocervical Smears: Successful Results Utilizing Y-Body Fluorescence," *American Journal of Obstetrics and Gynecology* 122 (1975): 155-60.

32. B. Brambati and A. Oldrini, "Methods of Chorionic Villus Sampling," in *Chorionic Villus Sampling: Fetal Diagnosis of Genetic Diseases in the First Trimester*, ed. B. Brambati, G. Simoni, and S. Fabro (New York: Marcel Dekker, 1986).

33. Tietung Hospital of Anshan Iron and Steel Co., Anshan, China, Department of Obstetrics and Gynecology, "Fetal Sex Prediction by Sex Chromatin of Chorionic Villi Cells During Early Pregnancy," *Chinese Medical Journal* 1 (1975): 117-26.

34. Z. Kazy, A.M. Stigár, and V.A. Bacharev, ["Chorionic Biopsy Under Immediate Real-Time (Ultrasound) Control,"] *Orvosi Hetilap* 121 (1980): 2765-66.

35. Z. Kazy, I.S. Rozovsky, and V.A. Bacharev, "Chorion Biopsy in Early Pregnancy: A Method of Early Prenatal Diagnosis for Inherited Disorders," *Prenatal Diagnosis* 2 (1982): 39-45.

36. G. Simoni et al., "Efficient Direct Chromosome Analyses and Enzyme Determinations from Chorionic Villi Samples in the First Trimester of Pregnancy," *Human Genetics* 63 (1983): 349-57.

37. E. Pergament et al., "Prenatal Tay-Sachs Diagnosis by Chorionic Villi Sampling," *Lancet* (30 July 1983): 286; E.E. Grebner et al., "Prenatal Tay-Sachs Diagnosis by Chorionic Villi Sampling," *Lancet* (30 July 1983): 286-87.

38. Simpson et al., "Prenatal Diagnosis of Genetic Disease in Canada."

39. G. Finikiotis and L. Gower, "Chorion Villus Sampling — Transcervical or Transabdominal?" *Australian and New Zealand Journal of Obstetrics and Gynaecology* 30 (1990): 63-65; B. Brambati, A. Lanzani, and L. Tului, "Transabdominal and Transcervical Chorionic Villus Sampling: Efficiency and Risk Evaluation of 2411 Cases," *American Journal of Medical Genetics* 35 (1990): 160-64.

40. H.V. Firth et al., "Severe Limb Abnormalities After Chorion Villus Sampling at 56-66 Days' Gestation," *Lancet* (30 March 1991): 762-63.

41. Blakemore and Mahoney, "Chorionic Villus Sampling."

42. D.H. Horwell, F.E. Loeffler, and D.V. Coleman, "Assessment of a Transcervical Aspiration Technique for Chorionic Villus Biopsy in the First Trimester of Pregnancy," *British Journal of Obstetrics and Gynaecology* 90 (1983): 196-98.

43. Kullander and Sandahl, "Fetal Chromosome Analysis After Transcervical Placental Biopsies During Early Pregnancy."

44. N. Hahnemann, "Early Prenatal Diagnosis: A Study of Biopsy Techniques and Cell Culturing from Extraembryonic Membranes," *Clinical Genetics* 6 (1974): 294-306.

45. S.A. Rhine, C.G. Palmer, and J.F. Thompson, "A Simple Alternative to Amniocentesis for First Trimester Prenatal Diagnosis," *Birth Defects: Original Article Series* 12 (3D)(1977): 231-47.

46. Hahnemann, "Early Prenatal Diagnosis."

47. Wapner and Jackson, "Chorionic Villus Sampling."

48. H. Brandenburg et al., "Fetal Loss Rate After Chorionic Villus Sampling and Subsequent Amniocentesis," *American Journal of Medical Genetics* 35 (1990): 178-80.

49. Canadian Collaborative CVS-Amniocentesis Clinical Trial Group, "Multicentre Randomised Clinical Trial of Chorion Villus Sampling and Amniocentesis," *Lancet* (7 January 1989): 1-6; G.G. Rhoads et al., "The Safety and Efficacy of Chorionic Villus Sampling for Early Prenatal Diagnosis of Cytogenetic Abnormalities," *New England Journal of Medicine* 320 (1989): 609-17.

50. I. Donald, J. MacVicar, and T.G. Brown, "Investigation of Abdominal Masses by Pulsed Ultrasound," *Lancet* (7 June 1958): 1188-95.

51. K.H. Nicolaides and S. Campbell, "Diagnosis of Fetal Abnormalities by Ultrasound," in *Genetic Disorders and the Fetus: Diagnosis, Prevention and Treatment*, 2d ed., ed. A. Milunsky (New York: Plenum Press, 1986).

52. S. Campbell et al., "Anencephaly: Early Ultrasonic Diagnosis and Active Management," *Lancet* (9 December 1972): 1226-27.

53. H.B. Zimmerman, "Prenatal Demonstration of Gastric and Duodenal Obstruction by Ultrasound," *Journal of the Canadian Association of Radiologists* 29 (1978): 138-41.

54. M. Matturri, B.E. Peters, and J.A. Kedziora, "Prenatal and Postnatal Sonographic Demonstration of Bilateral Ureteropelvic Junction Obstruction," *Medical Ultrasound* 4 (1980): 94-96; S. Campbell and J.M. Pearce, "Ultrasound Visualization of Congenital Malformations," *British Medical Bulletin* 39 (1983): 322-31.

55. L.D. Allan et al., "Echocardiographic and Anatomical Correlates in the Fetus," *British Heart Journal* 44 (1980): 444-51; J.W. Wladimiroff, P.A. Stewart, and H.M. Tonge, "The Role of Diagnostic Ultrasound in the Study of Fetal Cardiac Abnormalities," *Ultrasound in Medicine and Biology* 10 (1984): 457-63.

56. P. Jeanty et al., "Ultrasonic Evaluation of Fetal Limb Growth: Part I," *Radiology* 140 (1981): 165-68; P. Jeanty et al., "Ultrasonic Evaluation of Fetal Limb Growth: Part II," *Radiology* 143 (1982): 751-54; C.M. Rumack, M.L. Johnson, and D. Zunkel, "Antenatal Diagnosis," *Clinics in Diagnostic Ultrasound* 8 (1981): 210-30.

57. D.D. Weaver, "A Survey of Prenatally Diagnosed Disorders," *Clinics in Obstetrics and Gynecology* 31 (1988): 253-69.

58. Nicolaides and Campbell, "Diagnosis of Fetal Abnormalities by Ultrasound."

59. Medical Research Council (U.K.), "An Assessment of the Hazards of Amniocentesis."

60. Elias and Simpson, "Amniocentesis"; NICHD National Registry for Amniocentesis, "Midtrimester Amniocentesis for Prenatal Diagnosis."

61. A.J. Crandon and K.R. Peel, "Amniocentesis With and Without Ultrasound Guidance," *British Journal of Obstetrics and Gynaecology* 86 (1979): 1-3; T.D. Kerenyi and B. Walker, "The Preventability of 'Bloody Taps' in Second Trimester Amniocentesis by Ultrasound Scanning," *Obstetrics and Gynecology* 50 (1977): 61-64; M. Miskin et al., "Use of Ultrasound for Placental Localization in Genetic Amniocentesis," *Obstetrics and Gynecology* 43 (1974): 872-77.

62. R. Harrison, S. Campbell, and I. Craft, "Risks of Fetomaternal Hemorrhage Resulting from Amniocentesis With and Without Ultrasound Placental Localization," *Obstetrics and Gynecology* 46 (1975): 389-91.

63. D. McRobbie and M.A. Foster, "Pulsed Magnetic Field Exposure During Pregnancy and Implications for NMR Foetal Imaging: A Study with Mice," *Magnetic Resonance Imaging* 3 (1985): 231-34.

64. Hahnemann and Mohr, "Genetic Diagnosis in the Embryo."

65. C. Valenti, "Antenatal Detection of Hemoglobinopathies: A Preliminary Report," *American Journal of Obstetrics and Gynecology* 115 (1973): 851-53.

66. J. Bang, J.E. Bock, and D. Trolle, "Ultrasound-Guided Fetal Intravenous Transfusion for Severe Rhesus Haemolytic Disease," *British Medical Journal* (6 February 1982): 373-74; J. Bang, "Intrauterine Needle Diagnosis," in *Interventional Ultrasound*, ed. H.H. Holm and J.K. Kristensen (Copenhagen: Munksgaard, 1985).

67. Evans et al., "Early Genetic Amniocentesis and Chorionic Villus Sampling."

68. R.A.J. Eady and C.H. Rodeck, "Prenatal Diagnosis of Disorders of the Skin," in *Prenatal Diagnosis: Proceedings of the Eleventh Study Group of the Royal College of Obstetricians and Gynaecologists 1983*, ed. C.H. Rodeck and K.H. Nicolaides (Chichester: Royal College of Obstetricians and Gynaecologists and Wiley, 1984); Bang, "Intrauterine Needle Diagnosis."

69. W. Holzgreve and M.S. Golbus, "Prenatal Diagnosis of Ornithine Transcarbamylase Deficiency Utilizing Fetal Liver Biopsy," *American Journal of Human Genetics* 36 (1984): 320-28.

70. R.L. Bree and C.S. Marn, "Transvaginal Sonography in the First Trimester: Embryology, Anatomy, and hCG Correlation," *Seminars in Ultrasound, CT and MR* 11 (1990): 12-21.

71. E.B. Mendelson, M. Bohm-Velez, and M. Saker, "Transvaginal Sonography in the Abnormal First Trimester," *Seminars in Ultrasound, CT and MR* 11 (1990): 34-43.

72. Campbell and Pearce, "Ultrasound Visualization of Congenital Malformations"; NICHD National Registry for Amniocentesis, "Midtrimester Amniocentesis for Prenatal Diagnosis."

73. G. Neri, personal communication.

74. National Institutes of Health (NIH), *Diagnostic Ultrasound Imaging in Pregnancy. Consensus Statement*, Consensus Development Conference, Vol. 5 (1) (Bethesda, 1984); World Health Organization (WHO), "Ultrasound," in *Non-Ionizing Radiation Protection*, 2d ed., ed. M.J. Suess and D.A. Benwell-Morison (Copenhagen: WHO

Regional Office for Europe, 1989); Food and Drug Administration (FDA), *An Overview of Ultrasound: Theory, Measurement, Medical Applications, and Biological Effects* (Washington, DC: Food and Drug Administration, Bureau of Radiological Health, 1982).

75. H.B. Meire, "The Safety of Diagnostic Ultrasound," *British Journal of Obstetrics and Gynaecology* 94 (1987): 1121-22.

76. P.N.T. Wells, ed., "The Safety of Diagnostic Ultrasound: Report of a British Institute of Radiology Working Group," *British Journal of Radiology* (Suppl. 20) (1987).

77. NIH, *Diagnostic Ultrasound Imaging in Pregnancy*.

78. R.L. Brent, R.P. Jensh, and D.A. Beckman, "Medical Sonography: Reproductive Effects and Risks," *Teratology* 44 (1991): 123-46.

79. B. Westin, "Hysteroscopy in Early Pregnancy," *Lancet* (23 October 1954): 872.

80. B. Mandelbaum, D.A. Pontarelli, and A. Brushenko, "Amnioscopy for Prenatal Transfusion," *American Journal of Obstetrics and Gynecology* 98 (1967): 1140-43.

81. J.B. Scrimgeour, "Other Techniques for Antenatal Diagnosis," in *Antenatal Diagnosis of Genetic Disease*, ed. A.E.H. Emery (Edinburgh: Churchill Livingstone, 1973).

82. C. Valenti, "Endoamnioscopy and Fetal Biopsy: A New Technique," *American Journal of Obstetrics and Gynecology* 114 (1972): 561-64.

83. J.E. Patrick, T.B. Perry, and R.A.H. Kinch, "Fetoscopy and Fetal Blood Sampling: A Percutaneous Approach," *American Journal of Obstetrics and Gynecology* 119 (1974): 539-42; J.C. Hobbins and M.J. Mahoney, "In Utero Diagnosis of Hemoglobinopathies: Technics for Obtaining Fetal Blood," *New England Journal of Medicine* 290 (1974): 1065-67.

84. C.H. Rodeck and S. Campbell, "Umbilical-Cord Insertion as Source of Pure Fetal Blood for Prenatal Diagnosis," *Lancet* (9 June 1979): 1244-45; D.V.I. Fairweather, R.H.T. Ward, and B. Modell, "Obstetric Aspects of Midtrimester Fetal Blood Sampling by Needling or Fetoscopy," *British Journal of Obstetrics and Gynaecology* 87 (1980): 87-99.

85. A.J. Antsaklis, R.J. Benzie, and R.M. Hughes, "Fetoscopy: Fetal Visualization and Blood Sampling in Prenatal Diagnosis," in *Human Prenatal Diagnosis*, ed. K. Filkins and J.F. Russo (New York: Marcel Dekker, 1985); R.J. Benzie, "Fetoscopy in Toronto," in *Fetoscopy*, ed. I. Rocker and K.M. Laurence (Amsterdam: Elsevier/North Holland Biomedical Press, 1981); Rodeck and Campbell, "Umbilical-Cord Insertion as Source of Pure Fetal Blood"; M. Tolarová and A. Zwinger, "The Use of Fetoscopy by Inborn Morphological Anomalies," *Acta Chirurgiae Plasticae* 23 (1981): 139-51.

86. S. Elias and N.B. Esterly, "Prenatal Diagnosis of Hereditary Skin Disorders," *Clinical Obstetrics and Gynecology* 24 (1981): 1069-87.

87. R. Romero, J.C. Hobbins, and M.J. Mahoney, "Fetal Blood Sampling and Fetoscopy," in *Genetic Disorders and the Fetus: Diagnosis, Prevention, and Treatment*, 2d ed., ed. A. Milunsky (New York: Plenum Press, 1986).

88. Holzgreve and Golbus, "Prenatal Diagnosis of Ornithine Transcarbamylase Deficiency."

89. Hahnemann and Mohr, "Genetic Diagnosis in the Embryo."

90. Romero et al., "Fetal Blood Sampling and Fetoscopy."

91. Benzie, "Fetoscopy in Toronto."

92. Ibid.; Elias and Esterly, "Prenatal Diagnosis of Hereditary Skin Disorders"; Romero et al., "Fetal Blood Sampling and Fetoscopy."

93. Antsaklis et al., "Fetoscopy: Fetal Visualization and Blood Sampling."

94. Benzie, "Fetoscopy in Toronto"; Rodeck and Campbell, "Umbilical-Cord Insertion as Source of Pure Fetal Blood."

95. D.J.H. Brock and R.G. Sutcliffe, "Alpha-Fetoprotein in the Antenatal Diagnosis of Anencephaly and Spina Bifida," *Lancet* (29 July 1972): 197-99.

96. D.M. Main and M.T. Mennuti, "Neural Tube Defects: Issues in Prenatal Diagnosis and Counselling," *Obstetrics and Gynecology* 67 (1986): 1-16.

97. Ibid.

98. Ibid.

99. H. Foy, A. Kondi, and C.A. Linsell, "Fetoprotein in Pregnant African Women," *Lancet* (26 September 1970): 663-64; M. Seppälä and E. Ruoslahti, "α-Fetoprotein in Normal and Pregnancy Sera," *Lancet* (12 February 1972): 375-76.

100. Brock and Sutcliffe, "Alpha-Fetoprotein in the Antenatal Diagnosis of Anencephaly and Spina Bifida."

101. N.J. Wald and H.S. Cuckle, "Open Neural Tube Defects," in *Antenatal and Neonatal Screening*, ed. N.J. Wald (Oxford: Oxford University Press, 1984).

102. I.R. Merkatz et al., "An Association Between Low Maternal Serum α-Fetoprotein and Fetal Chromosomal Abnormalities," *American Journal of Obstetrics and Gynecology* 148 (1984): 886-94.

103. Ibid.; C.H. Miller et al., "Alteration in Age-Specific Risks for Chromosomal Trisomy by Maternal Serum Alpha-Fetoprotein and Human Chorionic Gonadotropin Screening," *Prenatal Diagnosis* 11 (1991): 153-58.

104. A. Lippman and J.A. Evans, "Screening for Maternal Serum α-Fetoprotein: What About the Low Side?" *Canadian Medical Association Journal* 136 (1987): 801-804.

105. F.W. Smith, A.H. Adam, and W.D.P. Phillips, "NMR Imaging in Pregnancy," *Lancet* (1 January 1983): 61-62.

106. F. Bloch, W.W. Hansen, and M. Packard, "Nuclear Induction," *Physical Review* 69 (1946): 127.

107. E. Odeblad and U. Bryhn, "Proton Magnetic Resonance of Human Cervical Mucus During the Menstrual Cycle," *Acta Radiologica* 47 (1957): 315-20; E. Odeblad and A. Ingelman-Sundberg, "Proton Magnetic Resonance Studies on the Structure of Water in the Myometrium," *Acta Obstetricia et Gynecologica Scandinavica* 44 (1965): 117-25.

108. J.S. Cohen et al., "Nuclear Magnetic Resonance in Biology and Medicine," *Life Chemistry Reports* 1 (1983): 281-457.

109. D.R. Mattison et al., "The Role of Magnetic Resonance Imaging and Spectroscopy in Clinical and Experimental Obstetrics," in *Magnetic Resonance of the Reproductive System*, ed. S. McCarthy and F. Haseltine (Thorofare: Slack, 1987).

110. D.H. Dinh, R.M. Wright, and W.C. Hanigan, "The Use of Magnetic Resonance Imaging for the Diagnosis of Fetal Intracranial Anomalies," *Child's Nervous System* 6 (1990): 212-15; W.C. Hanigan et al., "Medical Imaging of Fetal Ventriculomegaly," *Journal of Neurosurgery* 64 (1986): 575-80; M.C. Mintz et al., "MR Imaging of Fetal Brain," *Journal of Computer Assisted Tomography* 11 (1987): 120-23.

111. T.W. Lowe et al., "Magnetic Resonance Imaging in Human Pregnancy," *Obstetrics and Gynecology* 66 (1985): 629-33; S. McCarthy, "Magnetic Resonance Imaging in Obstetrics and Gynecology," *Magnetic Resonance Imaging* 4 (1986): 59-66.

112. Mattison et al., "The Role of Magnetic Resonance Imaging and Spectroscopy."

113. D.R. Mattison and T. Angtuaco, "Magnetic Resonance Imaging in Prenatal Diagnosis," *Clinical Obstetrics and Gynecology* 31 (1988): 353-89.

114. W.L. Heinrichs, "Biohazards of Magnetic Resonance to the Female Reproductive System," in *Magnetic Resonance of the Reproductive System*, ed. S. McCarthy and F. Haseltine (Thorofare: Slack, 1987); Mattison and Angtuaco, "Magnetic Resonance Imaging in Prenatal Diagnosis"; McRobbie and Foster, "Pulsed Magnetic Field Exposure During Pregnancy."

115. National Radiation Protection Board Ad Hoc Advisory Group on Nuclear Magnetic Resonance Clinical Imaging, "Revised Guidance on Acceptable Limits of Exposure During Nuclear Magnetic Resonance Clinical Imaging," *British Journal of Radiology* 56 (1983): 974-77.

116. A. McLaren, "Prenatal Diagnosis Before Implantation: Opportunities and Problems," *Prenatal Diagnosis* 5 (1985): 85-90.

117. K.B. Mullis and F.A. Faloona, "Specific Synthesis of DNA In Vitro via a Polymerase-Catalyzed Chain Reaction," *Methods in Enzymology* 155 (1987): 335-50.

118. R. Penketh and A. McLaren, "Prospects for Prenatal Diagnosis During Preimplantation Human Development," *Baillière's Clinical Obstetrics and Gynaecology* 1 (1987): 747-64.

119. McLaren, "Prenatal Diagnosis Before Implantation"; Y. Verlinsky, P. Zeunert, and E. Pergament, "Genetic Analysis of Abnormal Human Embryos: An Approach to Preimplantation Genetic Diagnosis," *American Journal of Human Genetics* 37 (1985) (Suppl. Abstract No. 675): A227.

120. Penketh and McLaren, "Prospects for Prenatal Diagnosis During Preimplantation Human Development."

121. B. Brambati and L. Tului, "Preimplantation Genetic Diagnosis: A New Simple Uterine Washing System," *Human Reproduction* 5 (1990): 448-50.

122. Medical Research Council, *Diagnosis of Genetic Disease by Amniocentesis*.

123. NICHD National Registry for Amniocentesis, "Midtrimester Amniocentesis for Prenatal Diagnosis"; Medical Research Council (U.K.), "An Assessment of the Hazards of Amniocentesis."

124. Genetics Society of Canada, Canadian Paediatrics Society, and Society of Obstetricians and Gynaecologists of Canada, "Canadian Guidelines for Antenatal Diagnosis of Genetic Disease: A Joint Statement," *Canadian Medical Association Journal* 111 (1974): 180-83.

125. Canada, Health and Welfare Canada, Environmental Health Directorate, Health Protection Branch, *Guidelines for the Safe Use of Ultrasound. Part I: Medical and Paramedical Applications*, Safety Code 23 (Ottawa: Minister of Supply and Services Canada, 1989).

126. J. Evans, personal communication.

127. "Canadian Recommendations for Prenatal Diagnosis of Genetic Disorders," *Bulletin of the Society of Obstetricians and Gynaecologists of Canada* 5 (November-December 1983).

128. J.L. Hamerton, "Introduction: Prenatal Diagnosis — Past, Present and Future," Report of an International Workshop held at Val David, Quebec, 4-8 November 1979, *Prenatal Diagnosis* (Special Issue) (1980): 3-4.

129. Canadian Collaborative CVS-Amniocentesis Clinical Trial Group, "Multicentre Randomised Clinical Trial."

130. Rhoads et al., "The Safety and Efficacy of Chorionic Villus Sampling."

131. Firth et al., "Severe Limb Abnormalities After Chorion Villus Sampling."

132. Canadian College of Medical Geneticists et al., "Canadian Guidelines for Prenatal Diagnosis."

133. Canadian College of Medical Geneticists, "Professional and Ethical Guidelines for the Canadian College of Medical Geneticists" (1991 draft version currently under review), in *Code of Ethics* (Toronto: Hospital for Sick Children, Department of Bioethics, 1992).

134. A. Lippman, "Prenatal Diagnosis: Reproductive Choice? Reproductive Control?" in *The Future of Human Reproduction*, ed. C. Overall (Toronto: Women's Press, 1989).

135. D.C. Wertz and J.C. Fletcher, eds., *Ethics and Human Genetics: A Cross-Cultural Perspective* (New York: Springer-Verlag, 1989); R. Harris, "Genetic Services in Britain: A Strategy for Success After the National Health Service and Community Care Act 1990," *American Journal of Medical Genetics* 27 (1990): 711-14.

136. J. Redman, personal communication.

137. T. Knutsen, personal communication.

138. G. Neri, personal communication.

139. A.S. Chau, S.T.S. Lam, and A. Ghosh, "Genetic Services in Hong Kong," *Journal of Medical Genetics* 27 (1990): 380-83.

140. M.A. Angastiniotis and M.G. Hadjiminas, "Prevention of Thalassaemia in Cyprus," *Lancet* (14 February 1981): 369-70; A. Cao et al., "The Prevention of Thalassemia in Sardinia," *Clinical Genetics* 36 (1989): 277-85.

141. J.E. Bowman, "Invited Editorial: Prenatal Screening for Hemoglobinopathies," *American Journal of Human Genetics* 48 (1991): 433-38.

142. Lippman, "Prenatal Diagnosis."

143. Ibid.

144. Ibid.

145. M.S. Henifin, R. Hubbard, and J. Norsigian, "Prenatal Screening," in *Reproductive Laws for the 1990s*, ed. S. Cohen and N. Taub (Clifton: Humana Press, 1989).

146. A.G. Motulsky and J. Murray, "Will Prenatal Diagnosis with Selective Abortion Affect Society's Attitude Toward the Handicapped?" in *Research Ethics*, ed. K. Berg and K.E. Tranøy (New York: A.R. Liss, 1983).

147. B.K. Rothman, *The Tentative Pregnancy: Prenatal Diagnosis and the Future of Motherhood* (New York: Viking Press, 1986).

148. A. Lippman, "Prenatal Genetic Testing and Screening: Constructing Needs and Reinforcing Inequities," *American Journal of Law and Medicine* 17 (1991): 15-50.

149. Simpson et al., "Prenatal Diagnosis of Genetic Disease in Canada."

150. P. Bradish, "From Genetic Counseling and Genetic Analysis, to Genetic Ideal and Genetic Fate?" in *Made to Order: The Myth of Reproductive and Genetic Progress*, ed. P. Spallone and D.L. Steinberg (Toronto: Pergamon Press, 1987).

151. R.M. Fineman and D.M. Gordis, "Occasional Essay: Jewish Perspective on Prenatal Diagnosis and Selective Abortion of Affected Fetuses, Including Some Comparisons with Prevailing Catholic Beliefs," *American Journal of Medical Genetics* 12 (1982): 355-60.

152. Congregation for the Doctrine of the Faith, *Instruction on Respect for Human Life in Its Origin and on the Dignity of Procreation: Replies to Certain Questions of the Day* (Vatican City, 1987).

153. P.T. Menzel, *Strong Medicine: The Ethical Rationing of Health Care* (New York: Oxford University Press, 1990).

154. J. Chamberlain, "Human Benefits and Costs of a National Screening Programme for Neural-Tube Defects," *Lancet* (16 December 1978): 1293-96.

155. W. Farrant, "Who's for Amniocentesis? The Politics of Prenatal Screening," in *The Sexual Politics of Reproduction*, ed. H. Homans (Brookfield: Gower, 1985).

156. Lippman, "Prenatal Diagnosis."

157. S.H. Taplin, R.S. Thompson, and D.A. Conrad, "Cost-Justification Analysis of Prenatal Maternal Serum Alpha-Feto Protein Screening," *Medical Care* 26 (1988): 1185-1202; L.L. Tosi et al., "When Does Mass Screening for Open Neural Tube Defects in Low-Risk Pregnancies Result in Cost Savings?" *Canadian Medical Association Journal* 136 (1987): 255-65.

158. A. Asch, "Reproductive Technology and Disability," in *Reproductive Laws for the 1990s*, ed. S. Cohen and N. Taub (Clifton: Humana Press, 1989).

159. Henifin et al., "Prenatal Screening."

160. A. Etzioni, *Genetic Fix* (New York: Harper Colophon Books, 1973).

161. M.A. Warnock, *A Question of Life: The Warnock Report on Human Fertilisation and Embryology* (Oxford: Basil Blackwell, 1985).

162. E.O. Nightingale and M. Goodman, *Before Birth: Prenatal Testing for Genetic Disease* (Cambridge: Harvard University Press, 1990).

163. M.Z. Pelias, "Torts of Wrongful Birth and Wrongful Life: A Review," *American Journal of Medical Genetics* 25 (1986): 71-80.

164. J.R. Botkin, "The Legal Concept of Wrongful Life," *JAMA* 259 (1988): 1541-45.

165. T. Perry, personal communication.

166. Milunsky, *The Prenatal Diagnosis of Hereditary Disorders*.

167. H.L. Nadler, personal communication.

168. D.J.H. Brock, personal communication.

169. J.R. Miller, personal communication.

170. N. Rudd, personal communication.

# Bibliography

Aburel, M.E. "Le déclanchement du travail par injections intra-amniotiques de sérum salé hypertonique." *Gynécologie et obstétrique* 36 (1937): 398-99.

Allan, L.D., et al. "Echocardiographic and Anatomical Correlates in the Fetus." *British Heart Journal* 44 (1980): 444-51.

Angastiniotis, M.A., and M.G. Hadjiminas. "Prevention of Thalassaemia in Cyprus." *Lancet* (14 February 1981): 369-70.

Antsaklis, A.J., R.J. Benzie, and R.M. Hughes. "Fetoscopy: Fetal Visualization and Blood Sampling in Prenatal Diagnosis." In *Human Prenatal Diagnosis*, ed. K. Filkins and J.F. Russo. New York: Marcel Dekker, 1985.

Asch, A. "Reproductive Technology and Disability." In *Reproductive Laws for the 1990s*, ed. S. Cohen and N. Taub. Clifton: Humana Press, 1989.

Bang, J. "Intrauterine Needle Diagnosis." In *Interventional Ultrasound*, ed. H.H. Holm and J.K. Kristensen. Copenhagen: Munksgaard, 1985.

Bang, J., J.E. Bock, and D. Trolle. "Ultrasound-Guided Fetal Intravenous Transfusion for Severe Rhesus Haemolytic Disease." *British Medical Journal* (6 February 1982): 373-74.

Barr, M.L., and E.G. Bertram. "A Morphological Distinction Between Neurones of the Male and Female, and the Behaviour of the Nucleolar Satellite During Accelerated Nucleoprotein Synthesis." *Nature* 163 (1949): 676-77.

Barr, M.L., L.F. Bertram, and H.A. Lindsay. "The Morphology of the Nerve Cell Nucleus, According to Sex." *Anatomical Record* 107 (1950): 283-97.

Benacerraf, B.R., and F.D. Frigoletto. "Amniocentesis Under Continuous Ultrasound Guidance: A Series of 232 Cases." *Obstetrics and Gynecology* 62 (1983): 760-63.

Benzie, R.J. "Fetoscopy in Toronto." In *Fetoscopy*, ed. I. Rocker and K.M. Laurence. Amsterdam: Elsevier/North Holland Biomedical Press, 1981.

Bevis, D.C.A. "The Antenatal Prediction of Haemolytic Disease of the Newborn." *Lancet* (23 February 1952): 395-98.

Blakemore, K.J., and M.J. Mahoney. "Chorionic Villus Sampling." In *Genetic Disorders and the Fetus: Diagnosis, Prevention and Treatment.* 2d ed., ed. A. Milunsky. New York: Plenum Press, 1986.

Bloch, F., W.W. Hansen, and M. Packard. "Nuclear Induction." *Physical Review* 69 (1946): 127.

Botkin, J.R. "The Legal Concept of Wrongful Life." *JAMA* 259 (1988): 1541-45.

Bowman, J.E. "Invited Editorial: Prenatal Screening for Hemoglobinopathies." *American Journal of Human Genetics* 48 (1991): 433-38.

Bradish, P. "From Genetic Counseling and Genetic Analysis, to Genetic Ideal and Genetic Fate?" In *Made to Order: The Myth of Reproductive and Genetic Progress*, ed. P. Spallone and D.L. Steinberg. Toronto: Pergamon Press, 1987.

Brambati, B., and A. Oldrini. "Methods of Chorionic Villus Sampling." In *Chorionic Villus Sampling: Fetal Diagnosis of Genetic Diseases in the First Trimester*, ed. B. Brambati, G. Simoni, and S. Fabro. New York: Marcel Dekker, 1986.

Brambati, B., and L. Tului. "Preimplantation Genetic Diagnosis: A New Simple Uterine Washing System." *Human Reproduction* 5 (1990): 448-50.

Brambati, B., A. Lanzani, and L. Tului. "Transabdominal and Transcervical Chorionic Villus Sampling: Efficiency and Risk Evaluation of 2411 Cases." *American Journal of Medical Genetics* 35 (1990): 160-64.

Brandenburg, H., et al. "Fetal Loss Rate After Chorionic Villus Sampling and Subsequent Amniocentesis." *American Journal of Medical Genetics* 35 (1990): 178-80.

Bree, R.L., and C.S. Marn. "Transvaginal Sonography in the First Trimester: Embryology, Anatomy, and hCG Correlation." *Seminars in Ultrasound, CT and MR* 11 (1990): 12-21.

Brent, R.L., R.P. Jensh, and D.A. Beckman. "Medical Sonography: Reproductive Effects and Risks." *Teratology* 44 (1991): 123-46.

Brock, D.J.H., and R.G. Sutcliffe. "Alpha-Fetoprotein in the Antenatal Diagnosis of Anencephaly and Spina Bifida." *Lancet* (29 July 1972): 197-99.

Campbell, S., and J.M. Pearce. "Ultrasound Visualization of Congenital Malformations." *British Medical Bulletin* 39 (1983): 322-31.

Campbell, S., et al. "Anencephaly: Early Ultrasonic Diagnosis and Active Management." *Lancet* (9 December 1972): 1226-27.

Canada. Health and Welfare Canada. Environmental Health Directorate. Health Protection Branch. *Guidelines for the Safe Use of Ultrasound. Part I: Medical and Paramedical Applications.* Safety Code 23. Ottawa: Minister of Supply and Services Canada, 1989.

Canadian Collaborative CVS-Amniocentesis Clinical Trial Group. "Multicentre Randomised Clinical Trial of Chorion Villus Sampling and Amniocentesis." *Lancet* (7 January 1989): 1-6.

Canadian College of Medical Geneticists. "Professional and Ethical Guidelines for the Canadian College of Medical Geneticists." (1991 draft version currently under review.) In *Codes of Ethics*. Toronto: Hospital for Sick Children, Department of Bioethics, 1992.

Canadian College of Medical Geneticists and Society of Obstetricians and Gynaecologists of Canada. "Canadian Guidelines for Prenatal Diagnosis of Genetic Disorders: An Update." *Journal of the Society of Obstetricians and Gynaecologists of Canada* 13 (August 1991): 13-31.

"Canadian Recommendations for Prenatal Diagnosis of Genetic Disorders." *Bulletin of the Society of Obstetricians and Gynaecologists of Canada* 5 (November-December 1983).

Cao, A., et al. "The Prevention of Thalassemia in Sardinia." *Clinical Genetics* 36 (1989): 277-85.

Chamberlain, J. "Human Benefits and Costs of a National Screening Programme for Neural-Tube Defects." *Lancet* (16 December 1978): 1293-96.

Chau, A.S., S.T.S. Lam, and A. Ghosh. "Genetic Services in Hong Kong." *Journal of Medical Genetics* 27 (1990): 380-83.

Cohen, J.S., et al. "Nuclear Magnetic Resonance in Biology and Medicine." *Life Chemistry Reports* 1 (1983): 281-457.

Congregation for the Doctrine of the Faith. *Instruction on Respect for Human Life in Its Origin and on the Dignity of Procreation: Replies to Certain Questions of the Day*. Vatican City, 1987.

Crandon, A.J., and K.R. Peel. "Amniocentesis With and Without Ultrasound Guidance." *British Journal of Obstetrics and Gynaecology* 86 (1979): 1-3.

Curtis, J.D., et al. "The Importance of Placental Localization Preceding Amniocentesis." *Obstetrics and Gynecology* 40 (1972): 194-98.

Dinh, D.H., R.M. Wright, and W.C. Hanigan. "The Use of Magnetic Resonance Imaging for the Diagnosis of Fetal Intracranial Anomalies." *Child's Nervous System* 6 (1990): 212-15.

Donald, I., J. MacVicar, and T.G. Brown. "Investigation of Abdominal Masses by Pulsed Ultrasound." *Lancet* (7 June 1958): 1188-95.

Eady, R.A.J., and C.H. Rodeck. "Prenatal Diagnosis of Disorders of the Skin." In *Prenatal Diagnosis: Proceedings of the Eleventh Study Group of the Royal College of Obstetricians and Gynaecologists 1983*, ed. C.H. Rodeck and K.H. Nicolaides. Chichester: Royal College of Obstetricians and Gynaecologists and Wiley, 1984.

Elias, S., and N.B. Esterly. "Prenatal Diagnosis of Hereditary Skin Disorders." *Clinical Obstetrics and Gynecology* 24 (1981): 1069-87.

Elias, S., and J.L. Simpson. "Amniocentesis." In *Genetic Disorders and the Fetus: Diagnosis, Prevention, and Treatment*. 2d ed., ed. A. Milunsky. New York: Plenum Press, 1986.

Emery, A.E.H. "Antenatal Diagnosis of Genetic Disease." In *Modern Trends in Human Genetics I*. London: Butterworths, 1970.

Etzioni, A. *Genetic Fix*. New York: Harper Colophon Books, 1973.

Evans, M.I., et al. "Early Genetic Amniocentesis and Chorionic Villus Sampling: Expanding the Opportunities for Early Prenatal Diagnosis." *Journal of Reproductive Medicine* 33 (1988): 450-52.

Fairweather, D.V.I., R.H.T. Ward, and B. Modell. "Obstetric Aspects of Midtrimester Fetal Blood Sampling by Needling or Fetoscopy." *British Journal of Obstetrics and Gynaecology* 87 (1980): 87-99.

Farrant, W. "Who's for Amniocentesis? The Politics of Prenatal Screening." In *The Sexual Politics of Reproduction*, ed. H. Homans. Brookfield: Gower, 1985.

Fineman, R.M., and D.M. Gordis. "Occasional Essay: Jewish Perspective on Prenatal Diagnosis and Selective Abortion of Affected Fetuses, Including Some Comparisons with Prevailing Catholic Beliefs." *American Journal of Medical Genetics* 12 (1982): 355-60.

Finikiotis, G., and L. Gower. "Chorion Villus Sampling — Transcervical or Transabdominal?" *Australian and New Zealand Journal of Obstetrics and Gynaecology* 30 (1990): 63-65.

Firth, H.V., et al. "Severe Limb Abnormalities After Chorion Villus Sampling at 56-66 Days' Gestation." *Lancet* (30 March 1991): 762-63.

Foy, H., A. Kondi, and C.A. Linsell. "Fetoprotein in Pregnant African Women." *Lancet* (26 September 1970): 663-64.

Fuchs, F., and P. Riis. "Antenatal Sex Determination." *Nature* 177 (1956): 330.

Genetics Society of Canada, Canadian Paediatrics Society, and Society of Obstetricians and Gynaecologists of Canada. "Canadian Guidelines for Antenatal Diagnosis of Genetic Disease: A Joint Statement." *Canadian Medical Association Journal* 111 (1974): 180-83.

Grebner, E.E., et al. "Prenatal Tay-Sachs Diagnosis by Chorionic Villi Sampling." *Lancet* (30 July 1983): 286-87.

Hahnemann, N. "Early Prenatal Diagnosis: A Study of Biopsy Techniques and Cell Culturing from Extra Embryonic Membranes." *Clinical Genetics* 6 (1974): 294-306.

Hahnemann, N., and J. Mohr. "Antenatal Foetal Diagnosis in Genetic Disease." *Bulletin of the European Society of Human Genetics* 3 (1969): 47.

—. "Genetic Diagnosis in the Embryo by Means of Biopsy from Extra-Embryonic Membranes." *Bulletin of the European Society of Human Genetics* 2 (1968): 23-29.

Hamerton, J.L. "Introduction: Prenatal Diagnosis — Past, Present and Future." Report of an International Workshop held at Val David, Quebec, 4-8 November 1979. *Prenatal Diagnosis* (Special Issue) (1980): 3-4.

Hanigan, W.C., et al. "Medical Imaging of Fetal Ventriculomegaly." *Journal of Neurosurgery* 64 (1986): 575-80.

Harris, R. "Genetic Services in Britain: A Strategy for Success After the National Health Service and Community Care Act 1990." *American Journal of Medical Genetics* 27 (1990): 711-14.

Harrison, R., S. Campbell, and I. Craft. "Risks of Fetomaternal Hemorrhage Resulting from Amniocentesis With and Without Ultrasound Placental Localization." *Obstetrics and Gynecology* 46 (1975): 389-91.

Heinrichs, W.L. "Biohazards of Magnetic Resonance to the Female Reproductive System." In *Magnetic Resonance of the Reproductive System*, ed. S. McCarthy and F. Haseltine. Thorofare: Slack, 1987.

Henifin, M.S., R. Hubbard, and J. Norsigian. "Prenatal Screening." In *Reproductive Laws for the 1990s*, ed. S. Cohen and N. Taub. Clifton: Humana Press, 1989.

Hobbins, J.C., and M.J. Mahoney. "*In Utero* Diagnosis of Hemoglobinopathies: Technics for Obtaining Fetal Blood." *New England Journal of Medicine* 290 (1974): 1065-67.

Holzgreve, W., and M.S. Golbus. "Prenatal Diagnosis of Ornithine Transcarbamylase Deficiency Utilizing Fetal Liver Biopsy." *American Journal of Human Genetics* 36 (1984): 320-28.

Horwell, D.H., F.E. Loeffler, and D.V. Coleman. "Assessment of a Transcervical Aspiration Technique for Chorionic Villus Biopsy in the First Trimester of Pregnancy." *British Journal of Obstetrics and Gynaecology* 90 (1983): 196-98.

Hsu, W.Y.F. "Prenatal Diagnosis of Chromosome Abnormalities." In *Genetic Disorders and the Fetus: Diagnosis, Prevention and Treatment.* 2d ed., ed. A. Milunsky. New York: Plenum Press, 1986.

Jacobson, C.B., and R.H. Barter. "Intrauterine Diagnosis and Management of Genetic Defects." *American Journal of Obstetrics and Gynecology* 99 (1967): 796-807.

Jeanty, P., et al. "Ultrasonic Evaluation of Fetal Limb Growth: Part I." *Radiology* 140 (1981): 165-68.

—. "Ultrasonic Evaluation of Fetal Limb Growth: Part II." *Radiology* 143 (1982): 751-54.

Kan, Y.W., and A.M. Dozy. "Antenatal Diagnosis of Sickle-Cell Anaemia by D.N.A. Analysis of Amniotic-Fluid Cells." *Lancet* (28 October 1978): 910-11.

—. "Polymorphism of DNA Sequence Adjacent to Human β-Globin Structural Gene: Relationship to Sickle Mutation." *Proceedings of the National Academy of Sciences* 75 (1978): 5631-35.

Kan, Y.W., M.S. Golbus, and A.M. Dozy. "Prenatal Diagnosis of α-Thalassemia: Clinical Application of Molecular Hybridization." *New England Journal of Medicine* 295 (1976): 1165-67.

Kazy, Z., I.S. Rozovsky, and V.A. Bacharev. "Chorion Biopsy in Early Pregnancy: A Method of Early Prenatal Diagnosis for Inherited Disorders." *Prenatal Diagnosis* 2 (1982): 39-45.

Kazy, Z., A.M. Stigár, and V.A. Bacharev. ["Chorionic Biopsy Under Immediate Real-Time (Ultrasound) Control."] *Orvosi Hetilap* 121 (1980): 2765-66.

Kerenyi, T.D., and B. Walker. "The Preventability of 'Bloody Taps' in Second Trimester Amniocentesis by Ultrasound Scanning." *Obstetrics and Gynecology* 50 (1977): 61-64.

Kullander, S., and B. Sandahl. "Fetal Chromosome Analysis After Transcervical Placental Biopsies During Early Pregnancy." *Acta Obstetricia et Gynecologica Scandinavica* 52 (1973): 355-59.

Lambl, D. "Ein seltener Fall von Hydramnios." *Centralblatt für Gynäkologie* 5 (1881): 329-34.

Lejeune, J., M. Gautier, and R. Turpin. "Étude des chromosomes somatiques de neuf enfants mongoliens." *Comptes rendus hebdomadaires des séances de l'Académie des Sciences* (Paris) 248 (1959): 1721-22.

Lippman, A. "Prenatal Diagnosis: Reproductive Choice? Reproductive Control?" In *The Future of Human Reproduction*, ed. C. Overall. Toronto: Women's Press, 1989.

—. "Prenatal Genetic Testing and Screening: Constructing Needs and Reinforcing Inequities." *American Journal of Law and Medicine* 17 (1991): 15-50.

Lippman, A., and J.A. Evans. "Screening for Maternal Serum α-Fetoprotein: What About the Low Side?" *Canadian Medical Association Journal* 136 (1987): 801-804.

Lowe, T.W., et al. "Magnetic Resonance Imaging in Human Pregnancy." *Obstetrics and Gynecology* 66 (1985): 629-33.

McCarthy, S. "Magnetic Resonance Imaging in Obstetrics and Gynecology." *Magnetic Resonance Imaging* 4 (1986): 59-66.

McKusick, V.A. "Mendelian Inheritance in Man." In *Catalogs of Autosomal Dominant, Autosomal Recessive, and X-Linked Phenotypes*. 8th ed. Baltimore: Johns Hopkins University Press, 1988.

McLaren, A. "Prenatal Diagnosis Before Implantation: Opportunities and Problems." *Prenatal Diagnosis* 5 (1985): 85-90.

McRobbie, D., and M.A. Foster. "Pulsed Magnetic Field Exposure During Pregnancy and Implications for NMR Foetal Imaging: A Study with Mice." *Magnetic Resonance Imaging* 3 (1985): 231-34.

Main, D., and M.T. Mennuti. "Neural Tube Defects: Issues in Prenatal Diagnosis and Counselling." *Obstetrics and Gynecology* 67 (1986): 1-16.

Mandelbaum, B., D.A. Pontarelli, and A. Brushenko. "Amnioscopy for Prenatal Transfusion." *American Journal of Obstetrics and Gynecology* 98 (1967): 1140-43.

Mattison, D.R., and T. Angtuaco. "Magnetic Resonance Imaging in Prenatal Diagnosis." *Clinical Obstetrics and Gynecology* 31 (1988): 353-89.

Mattison, D.R., et al. "The Role of Magnetic Resonance Imaging and Spectroscopy in Clinical and Experimental Obstetrics." In *Magnetic Resonance of the Reproductive System*, ed. S. McCarthy and F. Haseltine. Thorofare: Slack, 1987.

Matturri, M., B.E. Peters, and J.A. Kedziora. "Prenatal and Postnatal Sonographic Demonstration of Bilateral Ureteropelvic Junction Obstruction." *Medical Ultrasound* 4 (1980): 94-96.

Medical Research Council of Canada. *Diagnosis of Genetic Disease by Amniocentesis During the Second Trimester of Pregnancy: A Canadian Study.* Ottawa: Minister of Supply and Services Canada, 1977.

Medical Research Council (U.K.). Working Party on Amniocentesis. "An Assessment of the Hazards of Amniocentesis." *British Journal of Obstetrics and Gynaecology* 85 (Suppl. 2) (1978).

Meire, H.B. "The Safety of Diagnostic Ultrasound." *British Journal of Obstetrics and Gynaecology* 94 (1987): 1121-22.

Mendelson, E.B., M. Bohm-Velez, and M. Saker. "Transvaginal Sonography in the Abnormal First Trimester." *Seminars in Ultrasound, CT and MR* 11 (1990): 34-43.

Menees, T.O., J.D. Miller, and L.E. Holly. "Amniography: Preliminary Report." *American Journal of Roentgenology and Radium Therapy* 24 (1930): 363-66.

Menzel, P.T. *Strong Medicine: The Ethical Rationing of Health Care.* New York: Oxford University Press, 1990.

Merkatz, I.R., et al. "An Association Between Low Maternal Serum α-Fetoprotein and Fetal Chromosomal Abnormalities." *American Journal of Obstetrics and Gynecology* 148 (1984): 886-94.

Miller, C.H., et al. "Alteration in Age-Specific Risks for Chromosomal Trisomy by Maternal Serum Alpha-Fetoprotein and Human Chorionic Gonadotropin Screening." *Prenatal Diagnosis* 11 (1991): 153-58.

Milunsky, A. *The Prenatal Diagnosis of Hereditary Disorders.* Illinois: Charles C. Thomas, 1973.

Mintz, M.C., et al. "MR Imaging of Fetal Brain." *Journal of Computer Assisted Tomography* 11 (1987): 120-23.

Miskin, M., et al. "Use of Ultrasound for Placental Localization in Genetic Amniocentesis." *Obstetrics and Gynecology* 43 (1974): 872-77.

Mohr, J. "Foetal Genetic Diagnosis: Development of Techniques for Early Sampling of Foetal Cells." *Acta Pathologica et Microbiologica Scandinavica* 73 (1968): 73-77.

Moore, K.L., and M.L. Barr. "Smears from the Oral Mucosa in the Detection of Chromosomal Sex." *Lancet* (9 July 1955): 57-58.

Motulsky, A., and J. Murray. "Will Prenatal Diagnosis with Selective Abortion Affect Society's Attitude Toward the Handicapped?" In *Research Ethics*, ed. K. Berg and K.E. Tranøy. New York: A.R. Liss, 1983.

Mullis, K.B., and F.A. Faloona. "Specific Synthesis of DNA *In Vitro* via a Polymerase-Catalyzed Chain Reaction." *Methods in Enzymology* 155 (1987): 335-50.

Nadler, H.L. "Antenatal Detection of Hereditary Disorders." *Pediatrics* 42 (1968): 912-18.

—. "Newer Procedures in the Preconceptional, Prenatal and Early Postnatal Diagnosis of Birth Defects." *Birth Defects: Original Article Series* 6 (1)(1970): 26-31.

—. "Patterns of Enzyme Development Utilizing Cultivated Human Fetal Cells Derived from Amniotic Fluid." *Biochemical Genetics* 2 (1968): 119-26.

National Radiation Protection Board Ad Hoc Advisory Group on Nuclear Magnetic Resonance Clinical Imaging. "Revised Guidance on Acceptable Limits of Exposure During Nuclear Magnetic Resonance Clinical Imaging." *British Journal of Radiology* 56 (1983): 974-77.

NICHD National Registry for Amniocentesis Study Group. "Midtrimester Amniocentesis for Prenatal Diagnosis: Safety and Accuracy." *JAMA* 236 (1976): 1471-76.

Nicolaides, K.H., and S. Campbell. "Diagnosis of Fetal Abnormalities by Ultrasound." In *Genetic Disorders and the Fetus: Diagnosis, Prevention and Treatment.* 2d ed., ed. A. Milunsky. New York: Plenum Press, 1986.

Nightingale, E.O., and M. Goodman. *Before Birth: Prenatal Testing for Genetic Disease.* Cambridge: Harvard University Press, 1990.

Odeblad, E., and U. Bryhn. "Proton Magnetic Resonance of Human Cervical Mucus During the Menstrual Cycle." *Acta Radiologica* 47 (1957): 315-20.

Odeblad, E., and A. Ingelman-Sundberg. "Proton Magnetic Resonance Studies on the Structure of Water in the Myometrium." *Acta Obstetricia et Gynecologica Scandinavica* 44 (1965): 117-25.

Patrick, J.E., T.B. Perry, and R.A.H. Kinch. "Fetoscopy and Fetal Blood Sampling: A Percutaneous Approach." *American Journal of Obstetrics and Gynecology* 119 (1974): 539-42.

Pelias, M.Z. "Torts of Wrongful Birth and Wrongful Life: A Review." *American Journal of Medical Genetics* 25 (1986): 71-80.

Penketh, R., and A. McLaren. "Prospects for Prenatal Diagnosis During Preimplantation Human Development." *Baillière's Clinical Obstetrics and Gynaecology* 1 (1987): 747-64.

Pergament, E., et al. "Prenatal Tay-Sachs Diagnosis by Chorionic Villi Sampling." *Lancet* (30 July 1983): 286.

Rhine, S.A., C.G. Palmer, and J.F. Thompson. "A Simple Alternative to Amniocentesis for First Trimester Prenatal Diagnosis." *Birth Defects: Original Article Series* 12 (3D)(1977): 231-47.

Rhine, S.A., et al. "Prenatal Sex Detection with Endocervical Smears: Successful Results Utilizing Y-Body Fluorescence." *American Journal of Obstetrics and Gynecology* 122 (1975): 155-60.

Rhoads, G.G., et al. "The Safety and Efficacy of Chorionic Villus Sampling for Early Prenatal Diagnosis of Cytogenetic Abnormalities." *New England Journal of Medicine* 320 (1989): 609-17.

Rodeck, C.H., and S. Campbell. "Umbilical-Cord Insertion as Source of Pure Fetal Blood for Prenatal Diagnosis." *Lancet* (9 June 1979): 1244-45.

Romero, R., J.C. Hobbins, and M.J. Mahoney. "Fetal Blood Sampling and Fetoscopy." In *Genetic Disorders and the Fetus: Diagnosis, Prevention, and Treatment.* 2d ed., ed. A. Milunsky. New York: Plenum Press, 1986.

Rothman, B.K. *The Tentative Pregnancy: Prenatal Diagnosis and the Future of Motherhood.* New York: Viking Press, 1986.

Rumack, C., M.L. Johnson, and D. Zunkel. "Antenatal Diagnosis." *Clinics in Diagnostic Ultrasound* 8 (1981): 210-30.

Schatz, F. "Eine besondere Art von einseitiger Polyhydramnie mit anderseitiger Oligohydramnie bei eineiigen Zwillingen." *Archiv für Gynäkologie* 19 (1882): 329-69.

Scrimgeour, J.B. "Other Techniques for Antenatal Diagnosis." In *Antenatal Diagnosis of Genetic Disease*, ed. A.E.H. Emery. Edinburgh: Churchill Livingstone, 1973.

Seppälä, M., and E. Ruoslahti. "α-Fetoprotein in Normal and Pregnancy Sera." *Lancet* (12 February 1972): 375-76.

Serr, D.M., and E. Margolis. "Diagnosis of Fetal Sex in a Sex-Linked Hereditary Disorder." *American Journal of Obstetrics and Gynecology* 88 (1964): 230-32.

Serr, D.M., L. Sachs, and M. Danon. "The Diagnosis of Sex Before Birth Using Cells from the Amniotic Fluid (A Preliminary Report)." *Bulletin of the Research Council of Israel* 5B (1955): 137-38.

Simoni, G., et al. "Efficient Direct Chromosome Analyses and Enzyme Determinations from Chorionic Villi Samples in the First Trimester of Pregnancy." *Human Genetics* 63 (1983): 349-57.

Simpson, N.E., et al. "Prenatal Diagnosis of Genetic Disease in Canada: Report of a Collaborative Study." *Canadian Medical Association Journal* 115 (1976): 739-48.

Smith, F.W., A.H. Adam, and W.D.P. Phillips. "NMR Imaging in Pregnancy." *Lancet* (1 January 1983): 61-62.

Steele, M.W., and W.R. Breg, Jr. "Chromosome Analysis of Human Amniotic-Fluid Cells." *Lancet* (19 February 1966): 383-85.

Taplin, S.H., R.S. Thompson, and D.A. Conrad. "Cost-Justification Analysis of Prenatal Maternal Serum Alpha-Feto Protein Screening." *Medical Care* 26 (1988): 1185-1202.

Tietung Hospital of Anshan Iron and Steel Co., Anshan, China. Department of Obstetrics and Gynecology. "Fetal Sex Prediction by Sex Chromatin of Chorionic Villi Cells During Early Pregnancy." *Chinese Medical Journal* 1 (1975): 117-26.

Tolarová, M., and A. Zwinger. "The Use of Fetoscopy by Inborn Morphological Anomalies." *Acta Chirurgiae Plasticae* 23 (1981): 139-51.

Tosi, L.L., et al. "When Does Mass Screening for Open Neural Tube Defects in Low-Risk Pregnancies Result in Cost Savings?" *Canadian Medical Association Journal* 136 (1987): 255-65.

United States. Food and Drug Administration (FDA). *An Overview of Ultrasound: Theory, Measurement, Medical Applications, and Biological Effects.* Washington, DC: Food and Drug Administration, Bureau of Radiological Health, 1982.

United States. National Institutes of Health (NIH). *Diagnostic Ultrasound Imaging in Pregnancy. Consensus Statement.* Consensus Development Conference, Vol. 5 (1). Bethesda: NIH, 1984.

Valenti, C. "Antenatal Detection of Hemoglobinopathies: A Preliminary Report." *American Journal of Obstetrics and Gynecology* 115 (1973): 851-53.

—. "Endoamnioscopy and Fetal Biopsy: A New Technique." *American Journal of Obstetrics and Gynecology* 114 (1972): 561-64.

Verlinsky, Y., P. Zeunert, and E. Pergament. "Genetic Analysis of Abnormal Human Embryos: An Approach to Preimplantation Genetic Diagnosis." *American Journal of Human Genetics* 37 (1985) (Suppl. Abstract No. 675): A227.

Verp, M.S., and J.L. Simpson. "Amniocentesis for Prenatal Genetic Diagnosis." In *Human Prenatal Diagnosis.* 2d ed., ed. K. Filkins and J.F. Russo. New York: Marcel Dekker, 1990.

Wald, N.J., and H.S. Cuckle. "Open Neural Tube Defects." In *Antenatal and Neonatal Screening*, ed. N.J. Wald. Oxford: Oxford University Press, 1984.

Walker, A.H.C. "Liquor Amnii Studies in the Prediction of Haemolytic Disease of the Newborn." *British Medical Journal* (17 August 1957): 376-78.

Wapner, R.J., and L. Jackson. "Chorionic Villus Sampling." *Clinical Obstetrics and Gynecology* 31 (1988): 328-44.

Warnock, M.A. *A Question of Life: The Warnock Report on Human Fertilisation and Embryology.* Oxford: Basil Blackwell, 1985.

Weaver, D.D. "A Survey of Prenatally Diagnosed Disorders." *Clinics in Obstetrics and Gynecology* 31 (1988): 253-69.

Wells, P.N.T., ed. "The Safety of Diagnostic Ultrasound: Report of a British Institute of Radiology Working Group." *British Journal of Radiology* (Suppl. 20) (1987).

Wertz, D., and J.C. Fletcher, eds. *Ethics and Human Genetics: A Cross-Cultural Perspective.* New York: Springer-Verlag, 1989.

Westin, B. "Hysteroscopy in Early Pregnancy." *Lancet* (23 October 1954): 872.

Wladimiroff, J.W., P.A. Stewart, and H.M. Tonge. "The Role of Diagnostic Ultrasound in the Study of Fetal Cardiac Abnormalities." *Ultrasound in Medicine and Biology* 10 (1984): 457-63.

World Health Organization (WHO). "Ultrasound." In *Non-Ionizing Radiation Protection.* 2d ed., ed. M.J. Suess and D.A. Benwell-Morison. Copenhagen: WHO Regional Office for Europe, 1989.

Zimmerman, H.B. "Prenatal Demonstration of Gastric and Duodenal Obstruction by Ultrasound." *Journal of the Canadian Association of Radiologists* 29 (1978): 138-41.

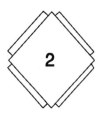

# Risk Assessment of Prenatal Diagnostic Techniques

## RCNRT Staff

**Executive Summary**

In its three decades of development, prenatal diagnosis (PND) has shown remarkable growth in numbers of available techniques, their sophistication, and their public acceptance. Amniocentesis is a well-established, invasive technique, available during the second trimester. Ultrasound scanning is routinely offered to pregnant women in many parts of the country.

Because many techniques currently under consideration are invasive procedures, with associated risks, a review of the safety of these techniques is appropriate. The invasive techniques include amniocentesis, chorionic villus sampling (CVS), fetoscopy, and embryoscopy. In addition, non-invasive techniques, such as ultrasound scanning, must be subject to stringent review ensuring that levels of exposure are well within the safety limits.

Considerable research, ranging from case studies and smaller projects to large multicentre cooperative efforts, has been reported. Differences in findings reflect variation in administration of the technologies as well as improvements that have occurred with experience and development. In general, safety is best assessed by large randomized studies that also include assessment of the normative data

---

This paper was completed for the Royal Commission on New Reproductive Technologies in December 1993.

indicating the rate of similar problems when no technological assessments are involved.

In the present review, complications were found to be of three types — procedural complications (including direct results such as bleeding), which may affect fetal growth or maternal well-being; uncertainties (related to the particular technology and abilities to predict); and human error.

Amniocentesis, still the most commonly used invasive PND procedure, is virtually without maternal risk, though some complications may be observed. Fetal injuries are rare, and fetal loss as a result of the procedure is in the order of 1 in 250. Magnetic resonance imaging is a non-invasive technique now under consideration that may in future be complementary to ultrasonography. Early amniocentesis is being considered as an alternative to CVS because of problems associated with CVS as the current major early diagnostic technique. Newer techniques, such as embryoscopy, are also being tested.

## Introduction

Prenatal diagnosis (PND) has seen remarkable growth since its beginnings only three decades ago. Its growth can be measured in terms of both the number of techniques available and their organized and widespread use in Canada and throughout the world.

Many of the techniques currently being used in clinical practice are invasive procedures and, consequently, are associated with complications and measurable risks to both the mother and fetus. Others, such as ultrasound, are non-invasive but data on their safety as used in practice should be reviewed.

Many questions and concerns about the safety, accuracy, and efficacy of these technologies have been raised. These questions come not only from people who seek PND, but also from people who have concerns over the wider implications of the technology.

As with all other medical tests and procedures, individuals who consent to PND do so with the understanding that in order to gain some benefit, they must accept a certain amount of risk. In fact, the explanation and discussion of risks and benefits of PND are a central aim of counselling.

The complications and risks of the procedures can be of three types: procedural complications that are a direct result of the technique and that can pose risks to the mother and fetus; uncertainties arising from the fact that diagnosis must sometimes be stated in terms of probabilities rather than certainties; and complications resulting from human error in laboratory analysis and interpretation.

In the early days of PND, experimental and clinical trials emphasized development and practice of techniques. Later, as techniques were perfected, the focus of much research shifted to the risks and complications. Today, there is consideration of both the techniques and risks of each procedure.

Much of the most recent and reliable information regarding the risks of PND comes from large randomized studies, which typically span a number of years and collect data from many centres. One such study, recently published by the Canadian Collaborative CVS-Amniocentesis Clinical Trial Group (1989), was one of the first to quantify, prospectively, the risks associated with chorionic villus sampling (CVS) relative to those associated with amniocentesis. Since that publication, similar studies have been carried out in other countries (Rhoads et al. 1989; Medical Research Council 1991). Case reports and small studies are also important in any assessment of risk, because they reflect the day-to-day experience of diagnostic centres and variations in quality of service.

## Risk Assessment

The assessment of risks is a complex exercise that aims to (1) identify the possible outcomes of a particular medical procedure, both good and bad; (2) estimate the magnitude of adverse consequences; and (3) estimate the probability that these adverse outcomes will occur. More recently, risk assessment has come to include an evaluation of how individuals perceive and act on risk information (O'Brien 1989).

Any assessment of the risks of PND procedures includes study of both tangible and intangible risks and complications. Tangible risks include fetal loss or damage and maternal complications such as infection and bleeding. These are relatively easy to quantify by collecting data through retrospective or prospective studies. Intangible risks, such as the experience of claustrophobia during magnetic resonance imaging (MRI) or the anxiety that couples face as they await a diagnosis following a test, are more difficult to define and measure, but are an important factor in the overall assessment of risk and safety of prenatal diagnostic techniques.

### Amniocentesis

Amniocentesis is the most commonly used invasive PND procedure. It is used to obtain amniotic fluid and fetal cells for the detection of biochemical and metabolic disorders, molecular genetic disease, and major malformations (Wilson 1991) in women at identified higher risk.

Amniocentesis for genetic purposes is usually performed by an obstetrician skilled in the technique and with ultrasound guidance. Under continuous ultrasound guidance and strict aseptic conditions, a spinal needle is introduced through the abdomen into the uterus and amniotic sac. An adequate sample is obtained on a first attempt in more than 99 percent of cases. A second attempt is made if no fluid is obtained in a first tap or if a tap is bloody, but multiple needle insertion is extremely rare and not recommended because of its association with higher rates of fetal loss (Andreasen and Kristoffersen 1989).

Fetal cells are separated from the amniotic fluid, cultured in the laboratory, and analyzed. The concentrations of various hormones and enzymes contained in the fluid can also be measured, the most notable of which are alpha-fetoprotein and acetylcholinesterase. Elevated concentrations of these proteins are a strong indication that a pregnancy may be affected with a neural tube defect or other malformation.

### Safety

Since its introduction in the early 1970s, the safety of second-trimester amniocentesis has been studied extensively. During the 1970s, three major studies conducted in the United States (National Institute of Child Health and Human Development 1976), Canada (Simpson et al. 1976), and Great Britain (Medical Research Council 1978) reported on the safety of amniocentesis. There have been numerous reports since their publication, but few contribute more understanding than these studies, which remain the definitive studies of mid-trimester amniocentesis.

### Maternal Risks

Infections have occasionally been reported and, at worst, can lead to fetal loss; however, they generally do not affect the mother significantly. Life-threatening maternal risks due to amniocentesis are virtually non-existent. Minor maternal problems are less rare. Approximately 3 percent of women undergoing amniocentesis experience leakage of amniotic fluid, transient vaginal spotting, and uterine contractions (cramping). Only persistent amniotic fluid leakage can lead to pregnancy loss, but this is rare and difficult to measure (Wilson 1991).

### Fetal Risks

The major risk of amniocentesis is fetal loss. On average, the risk of fetal loss as the result of the procedure is in the order of 1 in 250. At approximately 17 weeks, the spontaneous abortion rate is about 2 percent, and estimates of the procedural loss rate may range from 0.2 percent to 0.5 percent above this (Medical Research Council 1978; Wilson 1990). Other fetal risks include needle puncture, umbilical cord hematoma, placental separation, chorioamnionitis, premature labour, and amniotic band syndrome (Broome et al. 1976; Karp and Hayden 1977; Isenberg and Heckenlively 1985; Moessinger et al. 1981). These events are extremely rare, and recent reports indicate that they are virtually non-existent now that techniques have been improved and ultrasound guidance is used.

Only a few studies have dealt with the risk of fetal loss resulting from placental perforation (which is revealed by a blood-stained sample of amniotic fluid) since this occurs only rarely. Abortion may occur as the result of a subplacental hematoma caused by puncture of the placenta by the needle. A placenta covering the whole anterior wall (so that perforation of the placenta could not be avoided) and more than one needle insertion were associated with a fourfold to fivefold increase in spontaneous abortions (Andreasen and Kristoffersen 1989). Such findings reinforce the recommendation that the needle must be inserted with ultrasound guidance to avoid piercing the placenta.

## Diagnostic Complications

In addition to the maternal and fetal risks, a variety of things can go wrong after a successful sample of amniotic fluid is taken. These include (1) human and clerical errors, (2) laboratory and analytic errors, and (3) misinterpretation of laboratory results. Any one of these problems can have significant consequences because of the effect on parents' decisions regarding pregnancy termination. In cases for which a test must be repeated, mother and fetus are subjected to procedural and other risks once again.

Many of those laboratory errors involving mix-ups and misdiagnoses occur at the beginning of the testing procedure, when a sample may be incorrectly labelled or the paperwork may be separated from the sample or culture. These occurrences are rare, however, and can be eliminated with careful handling and checking procedures. The practice of setting up multiple cultures is common, if not mandatory, in most centres, which reduces the chance of mix-up, in addition to providing backup in cases of culture failure.

Methods used to analyze amniotic fluid have greatly improved over the last 15 years, reducing the likelihood of culture loss to a minimum. One centre, for instance, reports an overall success rate in obtaining a diagnosis of 99.5 percent, with a repeat amniocentesis required in 1.9 percent of cases (Benn et al. 1985).

## Early Amniocentesis

Medical and laboratory problems associated with the alternative, CVS, and the lack of diagnostic options between the 12th and 15th weeks of gestation have encouraged development of early amniocentesis (Aymé 1990; Neilson and Gosden 1991; Nevin et al. 1990; Penso et al. 1990). Despite its advantages, diagnosis using early amniocentesis, which can require a wait for results of more than four weeks, does not permit cytogenetic and biochemical studies to be performed as quickly as they can be done after CVS, though the results are more reliable. Furthermore, CVS provides more fetal material for the performance of biochemical and molecular testing.

Several recent studies, however, address concerns about the risks and complications of early amniocentesis compared to those of traditional second-trimester amniocentesis or CVS. Early amniocentesis is associated with slightly higher rates of fetal loss and amniotic fluid leakage than second-trimester amniocentesis (Elejalde et al. 1990), but the differences in risks are not significant (Choo 1991), and the risks are lower than those associated with CVS (Elejalde and Elejalde 1988; Godmilow et al. 1988; Hanson et al. 1987; Nevin et al. 1990).

One study, involving 222 samples taken between 11 and 14 weeks of gestation at two Belfast hospitals that have been performing early amniocentesis routinely since 1987, reported a 1.4 percent spontaneous abortion rate (Nevin et al. 1990). A larger study from Boston, of 407 cases, reported a 2.3 percent rate of post-procedural fetal loss, a 5.4 percent rate of maternal bleeding, 2.6 percent leakage of amniotic fluid, 1.8 percent cramping, and 0.3 percent uterine infection (Penso et al. 1990).

There is concern over the possibility that removal of amniotic fluid at less than 14 weeks of gestation might cause congenital respiratory or orthopaedic complications. Not only does early amniocentesis take place at an early phase of fetal growth, but the proportion of amniotic fluid withdrawn is greater than for mid-trimester amniocentesis, with a possibility of a pressure drop in the amniotic cavity after the puncture (Choo 1991). The Belfast study compared the pregnancy outcomes of 85 women who had had early amniocentesis (at or before 13 weeks) and 86 who had had mid-trimester amniocentesis (at or after 16 weeks), with no increased incidence in these complications reported among children exposed to early amniocentesis (Magee et al. 1991). The Boston group reported a 6.1 percent frequency of pulmonary complications that did not appear to be related to either post-procedural leakage or bleeding; however, the study did reveal a 1.4 percent incidence of orthopaedic deformities thought to be associated with post-procedural amniotic fluid loss (Penso et al. 1990).

Although early amniocentesis requires a cell culture and a waiting period before results are available, it is performed early enough to compensate for the needed laboratory time while remaining within the 14-week limit for an elective pregnancy termination if that option is chosen. Some researchers believe that if its safety can be shown, early amniocentesis may remove the need for CVS (Neilson and Gosden 1991). Further evaluation, by means of a large multicentre randomized controlled trial, is needed to compare first-trimester amniocentesis and CVS with mid-trimester amniocentesis (Evans et al. 1988; Neilson and Gosden 1991; Rooney et al. 1989).

## CVS

CVS, performed between 8 and 11 weeks of gestation, involves taking a small biopsy of the chorionic tissue (which is fetal in origin) and examining it to detect disorders at the chromosomal, metabolic, or DNA (deoxyribonucleic acid) level. The earlier diagnosis that it provides, compared to mid-trimester amniocentesis, is one of its advantages and is part of the reason CVS has become an increasingly popular method of PND. (It has been available for about 15 years, but has been used in Canada for only about five years on a limited basis.) CVS may be done by a transcervical or transabdominal approach; the latter is becoming the more commonly used method.

Because cells extracted using CVS are actively dividing, they can be examined immediately after sampling, without the need to culture, which can take between two and four weeks to complete (as is the case with amniocentesis). The diagnostic capabilities of CVS are similar to those of amniocentesis. It permits prenatal diagnosis of the same genetic disorders and abnormalities, with the exception of neural tube defects. It is believed that early diagnosis provided by CVS reduces the psychological stress experienced by the mother (Tunis et al. 1990), especially if she elects to terminate her pregnancy based on test results.

### Safety

The safety of CVS has undergone closer scrutiny than that of other techniques, because its more recent development has coincided with increased awareness of implications for women of the new reproductive technologies. Also, because amniocentesis was established as the foremost PND technique, many investigators felt that the safety of any newer technique should at least approximate the safety of amniocentesis. Many centres refrained from widespread offering of CVS until its safety was rigorously assessed by a number of large randomized studies.

As with other invasive procedures, CVS has risks associated with its use; some difficulties pertaining to accurate diagnosis are associated with the analysis of tissue and the interpretation of laboratory results. To date, however, four large prospective studies from Canada (Canadian Collaborative CVS-Amniocentesis Clinical Trial Group 1989), the United States (Rhoads et al. 1989), Britain (Medical Research Council 1991), and Denmark (Smidt-Jensen et al. 1992) have reported on the benefits and safety of CVS compared to amniocentesis, reporting very similar findings among thousands of pregnancies with regard to fetal risks, maternal complications, and diagnostic accuracy. In addition, many case studies that yield a wide range of results have been documented, but many of these are fraught with methodological problems that prevent any credible and useful interpretation of data.

### Maternal Risks

Maternal risks and complications associated with transcervical CVS include vaginal bleeding, intrauterine cramping, and infection. One author reports that mild to moderate bleeding occurs in 10 percent to 20 percent of transcervical cases (Wilson 1990). Although no fetal losses have been directly correlated with post-procedural bleeding, some reports suggest that losses may be linked to maternal bleeding. Transabdominal CVS is associated with a lower rate of bleeding (4.7 percent) than the transcervical approach (8.6 percent) (Smidt-Jensen et al. 1992).

Cramping is common in many cases, particularly with the use of a tenaculum, a pinching device used to support and manipulate the cervix during transcervical introduction of the sampling instruments. Many operators avoid the use of this instrument, though no relationship between cramping and malformations has been found (Silverman and Wapner 1990).

Multiple transcervical insertions increase the risk of intrauterine infection, but serious maternal infections occur in very few cases (0.2-0.3 percent) (Brambati et al. 1987a, 1990; Elejalde et al. 1990). The main advantage of transabdominal CVS is its lower risk of maternal complications and infection (Bovicelli et al. 1988) and of fetal loss (Smidt-Jensen et al. 1992).

## Fetal Risks

The major risk of CVS is miscarriage. Otherwise considered a relatively safe method of PND, CVS has a 4 percent average rate of procedure-related miscarriage (the range is 0.6 percent to 5.1 percent) (Bovicelli et al. 1988; Brambati et al. 1987c; Crane et al. 1988; Green et al. 1988; Hogge et al. 1986; Hunter et al. 1986; Jahoda et al. 1989; Ledbetter et al. 1990; Lilford et al. 1987; Rhoads et al. 1989; Silverman and Wapner 1990; WHO Consultation 1986; Zwinger 1988).

Factors contributing to fetal loss after CVS are bacterial colonization of the cervix and fetal membranes, mid-position or retroverted uterus, pre-procedural vaginal bleeding, and a previous spontaneous abortion. It also depends on the quality of the ultrasound guidance, the experience of the obstetrician or team performing the procedure, the technique used, and the number of catheter insertions (Green et al. 1988; Hunter et al. 1986; Keene and Saller 1989; Wade and Young 1989; Ward et al. 1988).

Transcervical CVS carries a higher risk of fetal loss than does the transabdominal approach (Hammarstrom and Marsk 1990; Wade and Young 1989), though not significantly so in some studies (Brambati et al. 1990; O'Brien 1991). In the Danish study (Smidt-Jensen et al. 1992) the rate of unintentional loss was 7.7 percent for transcervical and 3.7 percent for transabdominal CVS. Most reports cite that in 95 percent of cases sufficient villi are obtained with a single transcervical insertion (Brambati et al. 1990), but in cases that require more than one sampling attempt, the risk of fetal loss increases with each additional instrument insertion (Brambati et al. 1990; Muggah et al. 1987).

No difference has been found between CVS and amniocentesis for reduced birth weight, head circumference, body length (Crane et al. 1988), or frequency of intrauterine growth retardation (Canadian Collaborative CVS-Amniocentesis Clinical Trial Group 1989; Rhoads et al. 1989). CVS does not stimulate movements of the fetus or alter the intrauterine environment in a way that compromises normal fetal movement (Boogert et al. 1987).

It is known that fetal-maternal transfusion can occur after CVS, particularly after multiple catheter insertions, resulting in a rise in maternal serum alpha-fetoprotein (AFP) after the procedure. The potential risk is that maternal serum AFP values may be artificially raised without the presence of any abnormality. Such a false positive result, however, would presumably be corrected with further testing. Recent evidence suggests that the rise is transient and would not confound the results of maternal serum AFP screening for neural tube defects in the second trimester (O'Brien 1991; Shulman et al. 1990).

There is very little information regarding post-natal problems that may be associated with CVS, but recently there have been reports suggesting a link between its early use (between 56 and 66 days of gestation) and congenital limb deformities (Firth et al. 1991). These reports caused considerable concern, and many centres retrospectively examined their outcome data to see if they differed significantly from the normal expectation. Data from most centres did not show an increase in limb deformities; of the centres that did report an increase, the frequencies of the limb abnormalities, even though elevated above the norm, were low in absolute terms, ranging from 0.01 percent to 2.5 percent (Boyd et al. 1990; Christiaens et al. 1989; Firth et al. 1991; Hsieh et al. 1991; Jackson et al. 1991; Mahoney 1991; Mastroiacovo and Cavalcanti 1991; Miny et al. 1991; Monni et al. 1991; Planteydt et al. 1986). The possibility of selection bias must, therefore, be considered. A recent conference to review the problem recommended that CVS should not be done before 9 1/2 weeks' gestation, and that CVS at 10 weeks or more is extremely unlikely to cause developmental abnormalities and should be available to patients requesting PND (Rodeck 1993).

### *Diagnostic Complications*

The early embryo has an inner cell mass that becomes the embryo proper, and an outer surrounding layer that contributes to the chorion. The chorion consists of two tissues, the cytotrophoblast and the mesodermal core. The cytotrophoblast cells, which are dividing rapidly, are the ones examined directly, whereas the mesodermal cells are examined after being cultured. If results show mosaicism, two or more chromosomally different cell lines, amniocentesis is sometimes done for clarification (O'Brien 1991). Whereas true mosaicism is a rare phenomenon, occurring in approximately 1 in 1 000 pregnancies, CVS detects many more cases (up to 5 percent of cases). About three-quarters of the cases of mosaicism found by CVS are proven to have normal karyotypes in follow-up tests (either amniocentesis or fetal blood sampling). These require another three to four weeks' wait, meaning that a diagnosis may not be made until well into the second trimester (Canadian Collaborative CVS-Amniocentesis Clinical Trial Group 1989; Gosden 1991; Rhoads et al. 1989; Shulman et al. 1990; Silverman and Wapner 1990).

False negative results are relatively rare, in the order of 1 in 1 000. These can occur as the result of a discrepancy between fetal and placental karyotypes, where the fetus is abnormal and the placenta is normal (Gosden 1991). The accidental contamination of CVS tissue with maternal cells (and hence a different karyotype) is another possible source of error in the cytogenetic analysis using CVS that may occur in about 4 percent to

18 percent of cases (O'Brien 1991), and will require further testing. Almost all of these occur in cultured, rather than direct, preparations (Gosden 1991).

To reduce the risk of false or ambiguous diagnosis, many centres wait for results from the analysis of cultured cells, which can take up to four weeks. Because waiting reduces the practical advantage of CVS, some centres are phasing it out for cytogenetic indications, concentrating instead on the potential of early amniocentesis. To provide results within the first trimester, and without delay, adjunct tests that offer definitive and rapid confirmation of karyotypes are required. A number of possibilities are currently being explored, including the use of DNA probes to assist with cytogenetic work (Silverman and Wapner 1990).

## Ultrasound Scanning

The development of ultrasonography during the last 40 years has revolutionized diagnostic medicine and, in particular, obstetrics. It is now a routinely offered part of obstetric care, and at least 80 percent of all pregnant women have diagnostic ultrasound scanning in much of the Western world (Canada, Health and Welfare Canada 1989; Salvesen et al. 1992).

At present, three modes of ultrasound scanning are used for prenatal screening, monitoring, and diagnosis: traditional transabdominal and transvaginal, which employ continuous wave energy, and Doppler ultrasonography, which uses both continuous and pulsed wave energy. Each of these is a variation of the same technology that uses high-frequency sound waves, yet each has unique advantages. But transabdominal is, and will likely remain, the most popular mode.

Diagnostic ultrasonography may be used to detect and assess developmental abnormalities, multiple pregnancies, fetal size and gestational age, and placental position, and to determine fetal sex. It is easy to use, inexpensive, and, most important, non-invasive, using invisible energy to visualize the fetus *in utero*. Another attractive feature is its apparent safety. Reports of the safety of ultrasound are numerous (U.S. National Institutes of Health 1984) and show no confirmed deleterious effects from low-intensity diagnostic ultrasound. Over 50 million pregnant women have had diagnostic ultrasound, but there is no epidemiological evidence of increased fetal death, abnormality, or intrauterine growth retardation. Many studies have sought to study the bioeffects of ultrasonic energy and ultrasound technology, and while it is not possible to prove the safety of diagnostic ultrasound, few of the very many studies done have identified any measurable bioeffects at diagnostic levels. Although the great majority of proponents of diagnostic ultrasonography judge that it is completely safe, it is important to note that safety has only been shown at certain levels of exposure. Critics question the quality of some studies, and note that, because there is no single exposure parameter that can be used to measure all possible bioeffects, it is difficult to compare the many studies that have been published and draw credible conclusions from them (British Institute of Radiology Working Group 1987). Despite such questions about its safety, the numbers of pregnant women who request ultrasound and the numbers of physicians who recommend or perform it continue to grow.

The literature on ultrasound exposure and its safety is voluminous, including a range from epidemiologic studies (Lyons 1986; Mukubo 1986) to *in vitro* tissue experiments and animal studies (Miller 1985; Williams 1986; Maeda 1986). In 1984, a report published by the U.S. National Institutes of Health (NIH) concluded that there was no convincing evidence of any adverse effects, such as fetal complications or genetic abnormalities, of diagnostic ultrasound exposure. However, the NIH also warned of the possibility that as yet undetected effects may occur, and concluded that further study was needed. A more recent review (Brent et al. 1991) concludes from human epidemiological studies, animal studies, and secular trend data that ultrasonography as usually used in PND presents no measurable risk. Nevertheless, standards and guidelines to ensure higher levels of ultrasound are not inadvertently given are required.

## Bioeffects

Experiments in which animals are intentionally overexposed to high levels of ultrasound energy provide convincing evidence that ultrasound scanning could produce fetal growth retardation and congenital malformations. But this kind of exposure does not reflect normal human diagnostic exposures, and extrapolating conclusions from *in vitro* animal studies and even *in vitro* primate studies to humans is difficult at best (Sikov 1986).

### Cavitation

Ultrasound exposure in a sufficient dose has been shown to cause gaseous bubbles in tissues. Tissues fluctuate in size, and movement causes heat generation, which may in turn cause cytoplasmic microstreaming, macromolecular fragmentation, and platelet agglutination. These bubbles may also increase in size and implode, releasing concentrated heat and pressure, and inducing cavitation (i.e., formation of cavities). This is particularly associated with high intensities and is not a problem with high-frequency, low-intensity exposures. Since the latter types of exposure are used in diagnostic ultrasound, cavitation is unlikely to be an adverse bioeffect of its use (British Institute of Radiology Working Group 1987; Carstensen 1986; Williams 1986).

### Hyperthermia

Hyperthermia has been described as the predominant risk associated with ultrasound exposure. Many studies have shown that hyperthermia can have teratogenic effects (i.e., may produce anomalies). Studies pertaining to ultrasound have focussed on two areas, the effects of localized heating in fetal tissues and the duration of exposure. Many researchers conclude that even if localized temperatures were permitted to rise to 39°C in fetal tissues, exposure would not present any measurable risk. Effects below 39°C are non-existent or so small as to be unmeasurable (Angles et al. 1990; Miller and Ziskin 1989).

*Genetic Bioeffects*

Many studies have examined the possibility that ultrasonic energy as used in diagnostic ultrasonography can affect the nuclei of fetal cells and induce subtle chromosomal or genetic rearrangements, including sister chromatid exchanges and point mutations. *In vitro* mammalian cell studies using very high levels of ultrasound have produced a significant increase in mutation frequency, but it is difficult to relate these findings to human diagnostic exposure, because of the extraordinarily high intensities used. One study, for instance, used intensities that were approximately 1 000 times greater than those used for diagnostic purposes. The evidence thus far strongly suggests that diagnostic ultrasound scanning has little, if any, potential to cause chromosomal rearrangements or point mutations (British Institute of Radiology Working Group 1987; Doida et al. 1990).

The increased use of Doppler ultrasonography to study fetal circulation has provided new information about prenatal physiology and pathophysiology. Because Doppler ultrasound scanning involves high-pulse repetition frequencies and intensities, there have been concerns over its safety, but as yet no substantial studies have reported on its possible risks. However, considering that the real increase in intensity is not significantly higher than that of continuous wave ultrasound and dramatically less than that known to induce genetic and other bioeffects, Doppler ultrasonography is probably as safe as traditional ultrasound (Miller 1985).

After a comprehensive examination of the literature on ultrasound, Brent et al. (1991) conclude that much of the literature on diagnostic ultrasound scanning tends to be inconsistent, methodologically unsound, and in many cases not applicable to human exposure concerns. Because there is evidence that greatly elevated intensities of ultrasound can induce physical and physiological damage to human tissue, they recommended that ultrasound equipment for diagnostic and obstetric use be manufactured with controls to prevent any purposeful or accidental high-intensity scanning (at present, no such controls exist). However, this study by Brent and associates confirmed the general belief that diagnostic ultrasound scanning, with reasonable technological and clinical restrictions, is safe.

## Fetoscopy and Embryoscopy

In the 1970s and early 1980s, fetoscopy was used in the second trimester for direct viewing of the fetal surface through an endoscope, and to sample fetal blood through the umbilical cord. Its use was limited, however, because the risk of inducing an abortion was high (around 5 percent). The development of high-resolution ultrasound imaging has made fetoscopy obsolete, and it is no longer used in the second trimester (Pennehouat et al. 1992). There are, however, preliminary reports of its use in the first trimester, where it is referred to as embryoscopy.

Embryoscopy involves a rigid endoscope, inserted through the cervix and chorion into the extra-amniotic space, or transabdominally into the amniotic cavity. Insertion into the cavity is guided by ultrasound imaging, and the embryo can be visualized directly through the endoscope, or with a video camera and monitor. Embryoscopy could be used for the early diagnosis of major morphological defects of the head, neck, torso, and limbs at a time in gestation when ultrasound scanning has limited use (Pennehouat et al. 1992). First-trimester diagnosis of genetic diseases by organ tissue retrieval and blood sampling may also be feasible (Reece et al. 1991).

Because the technology is relatively new, there are no data on its safety. From the few reports that are available, it is impossible to evaluate the risks of embryoscopy. The most significant risk is thought to be rupture of the amnion by the endoscope. However, because the chorion and amnion do not fuse until the eleventh week of gestation and because embryoscopy will be performed before then, it is thought that there is a greater chance of amnion injury occurring during invasive, mid-trimester techniques, namely fetoscopy, CVS, and amniocentesis (Reece et al. 1991).

Whether or not the risks of an invasive technique such as embryoscopy are worth the early diagnosis it provides will continue to be debated. Recent developments in PND favour minimal or non-invasive techniques, and the future use of embryoscopy will depend ultimately on how its risks compare with those of other techniques. At present it should be regarded as a research procedure. It is not currently being done in Canada.

## Magnetic Resonance Imaging

Ultrasound scanning and MRI are both non-invasive procedures, capable of providing good tissue definition, and relatively safe. One major difference is that MRI is very expensive and not widely available (Mattison and Angtuaco 1988).

Although ultrasonography is likely to remain the foremost imaging technique for obstetrics, recent advances in MRI have cleared the way for its use. At present, it is considered to have the potential for a role complementary to that of ultrasonography, in that an ambiguous ultrasound finding could be clarified (Mattison and Angtuaco 1988).

Until recently, long exposure times limited the application of MRI in obstetrics because fetal movement produced imaging artifacts. Although this could be overcome by administering a sedative to the fetus, physicians were reluctant to do this in an otherwise non-invasive technique. Now, fast-scan MRI requires only a few seconds' exposure, which reduces the time during which the fetus could move. This development still does not permit real-time imaging, and the equipment is not portable (Garden et al. 1991).

### *Safety*

The safety of MRI has been studied by using bacteria cell cultures, *in vivo* animal studies, *in vitro* animal studies, and retrospective clinical follow-up studies of patients. These studies have failed to detect any measurable adverse effects of MRI at levels used for diagnostic purposes, but the potential biological effects on the fetus have not yet been sufficiently examined to justify a recommendation of its routine use (Dinh et al. 1990).

One large study examined three areas of potential hazards: (1) the effects of a static magnetic field; (2) the effects of a time-varying magnetic field, which may induce electrical currents; and (3) the effects of radio frequency magnetic fields, which may produce heat. Despite a lack of any evidence of biomedical effects of MRI, at least one safety board has recommended guidelines to prevent these potential hazards. One strong guideline is to not use MRI in the first trimester (during organogenesis) unless pregnancy is being terminated. Although more long-term studies are required to evaluate fully the effect of MRI on the fetus, it is currently permitted during pregnancy, but only during the second and third trimesters, and with limited magnetic field strengths (National Radiological Protection Board 1983).

Although MRI has never been demonstrated to cause any harm to the fetus, or indeed to any adult patient, it is difficult to be sure it will not cause some subtle abnormality to the fetus, as long-term follow-up studies do not exist. Newer, echo-planar imaging shows much promise, and experiments are currently under way to study its effects on the growth of fetal organs and determine whether it has any association with congenital abnormalities.

## Conclusions

- Much of the most recent and reliable information regarding the risks of prenatal diagnostic procedures comes from large randomized studies that typically span a number of years and collect data from many centres. Case studies are also important because they reflect the day-to-day experience of diagnostic centres and also variations in quality of service.
- The complications and risks of PND procedures fall into three categories: (1) procedural complications — those that are a direct result of the technique and that can cause harm to the mother and fetus; (2) uncertainties arising from the fact that diagnosis must

sometimes be stated in terms of probabilities rather than certainties; and (3) complications resulting from human error in laboratory analysis and interpretation.

- Amniocentesis is the most commonly used invasive PND procedure in the second trimester. Life-threatening maternal risks are virtually non-existent. Maternal complications include leakage of amniotic fluid, transient vaginal spotting, and uterine contractions. Fetal loss as a result of the procedure is in the order of 1 in 250. Fetal injuries are rare.

- CVS is a common first-trimester procedure because it permits early diagnosis and allows for an early decision regarding pregnancy termination. Maternal complications include bleeding, cramping, and infection. The transabdominal approach has fewer complications than the transcervical approach. Fetal loss rates as a result of CVS are comparable to, but slightly higher than, those associated with amniocentesis. No study has examined long-term effects of CVS. There may be a risk of limb defects if done before 9 1/2 weeks.

- Diagnostic complications are more common in CVS than in amniocentesis. Many of the problems with CVS stem from inability to distinguish confined placental mosaicism from true mosaicism in the fetus. In these cases mosaicism is confirmed with culture results or with amniocentesis.

- Early amniocentesis, which is performed before 15 weeks of gestation, is a recent development that is gaining popularity as an alternative to CVS. Although its safety has yet to be definitively established, a number of reports suggest that the risks are not significantly different from either second-trimester amniocentesis or first-trimester transabdominal CVS.

- Ultrasound examination is now a routinely offered part of obstetric care. Many reports have sought to assess specific risks and biological consequences of ultrasound. The evidence considered collectively leads to the conclusion that diagnostic medical sonography at the low intensities usually used has no measurable effect on the human fetus.

- MRI is considered to have the potential for a complementary role to that of ultrasound in being able to clarify an ambiguous ultrasound finding. Thus far, studies on the safety of MRI fail to report any measurable adverse effects at levels used for diagnostic purposes, but it has not been sufficiently examined to allow routine use in pregnancy.

- Embryoscopy is a very new technique still under development. Few data are available on risks associated with embryoscopy, which is still a research procedure.

- In small, independent studies, it is often difficult to differentiate between background spontaneous abortion rates and procedure-related abortion. Because the normative spontaneous abortion rate changes with the time of gestation, it is difficult to compare the safety of techniques performed at different times in pregnancy. Generally, only large randomized prospective studies can provide reliable information, with minimal biases, from which credible conclusions can be drawn.

## Bibliography

American Institute of Ultrasound in Medicine. Bioeffects Committee. 1988. "Bioeffects Considerations for the Safety of Diagnostic Ultrasound." *Journal of Ultrasound in Medicine* 7 (Suppl.): S1-S38.

Andreasen, E., and K. Kristoffersen. 1989. "Incidence of Spontaneous Abortion After Amniocentesis: Influence of Placental Localization and Past Obstetric and Gynecologic History." *American Journal of Perinatology* 6: 268-73.

Angles, J.M., et al. 1990. "Effects of Pulsed Ultrasound and Temperature on the Development of Rat Embryos in Culture." *Teratology* 42: 285-93.

Aymé, S. 1990. "New Trends in Prenatal Diagnosis of Genetic Disorders." *Current Opinion in Pediatrics* 2: 1161-67.

Benn, P.A., et al. 1985. "The Centralized Prenatal Genetics Screening Program of New York City III: The First 7,000 Cases." *American Journal of Medical Genetics* 20: 369-84.

Boogert, A., A. Mantingh, and G.H.A. Visser. 1987. "The Immediate Effects of Chorionic Villus Sampling on Fetal Movements." *American Journal of Obstetrics and Gynecology* 157: 137-39.

Bovicelli, L., et al. 1988. "Transabdominal Chorionic Villus Sampling: Analysis of 350 Consecutive Cases." *Prenatal Diagnosis* 8: 495-500.

Boyd, P.A., et al. 1990. "Limb Reduction and Chorion Villus Sampling." *Prenatal Diagnosis* 10: 437-41.

Brambati B., A. Lanzani, and A. Oldrini. 1988. "Transabdominal Chorionic Villus Sampling: Clinical Experience of 1159 Cases." *Prenatal Diagnosis* 8: 609-17.

Brambati, B., A. Lanzani, and L. Tului. 1990. "Transabdominal and Transcervical Chorionic Villus Sampling: Efficiency and Risk Evaluation of 2,411 Cases." *American Journal of Medical Genetics* 35: 160-64.

Brambati, B., M. Matarrelli, and F. Varotto. 1987a. "Septic Complications After Chorionic Villus Sampling." *Lancet* (23 May): 1212-13.

Brambati, B., A. Oldrini, and A. Lanzani. 1987b. "Transabdominal Chorionic Villus Sampling: A Freehand Ultrasound-Guided Technique." *American Journal of Obstetrics and Gynecology* 157: 134-37.

Brambati, B., et al. 1987c. "Chorionic Villus Sampling: An Analysis of the Obstetric Experience of 1000 Cases." *Prenatal Diagnosis* 7: 157-69.

—. 1991. "Genetic Diagnosis Before the Eighth Gestational Week." *Obstetrics and Gynecology* 77: 318-21.

Brent, R.L., R.P. Jensh, and D.A. Beckman. 1991. "Medical Sonography: Reproductive Effects and Risks." *Teratology* 44: 123-46.

British Institute of Radiology Working Group. 1987. "The Safety of Diagnostic Ultrasound." *British Journal of Radiology* (Suppl. 20): 1-43.

Broome, D., et al. 1976. "Needle Puncture of Fetus: A Complication of Second-Trimester Amniocentesis." *American Journal of Obstetrics and Gynecology* 126: 247-52.

Canada. Health and Welfare Canada. Environmental Health Directorate. Health Protection Branch. 1989. *Guidelines for the Safe Use of Ultrasound. Part I: Medical and Paramedical Applications.* Safety Code 23. Ottawa: Minister of Supply and Services Canada.

Canadian Collaborative Chorionic Villus Sampling-Amniocentesis Clinical Trial Group. 1989. "Multicentre Randomised Clinical Trial of Chorion Villus Sampling and Amniocentesis: First Report." *Lancet* (7 January): 1-6.

Carstensen, E.L. 1986. "Biological Effects of Acoustic Cavitation." *Ultrasound in Medicine and Biology* 12 (9): 703-704.

Choo, V. 1991. "Early Amniocentesis." *Lancet* (21 September): 750-51.

Christiaens, G.C.M.L., et al. 1989. "Fetal Limb Constriction: A Possible Complication of Chorionic Villus Sampling." *Prenatal Diagnosis* 9: 67-71.

Copeland, K.L., et al. 1989. "Integration of the Transabdominal Technique into an Ongoing Chorionic Villus Sampling Program." *American Journal of Obstetrics and Gynecology* 161: 1289-94.

Crane, J.P., H.A. Beaver, and S.W. Cheung. 1988. "First Trimester Chorionic Villus Sampling Versus Mid-Trimester Genetic Amniocentesis — Preliminary Results of a Controlled Prospective Trial." *Prenatal Diagnosis* 8: 355-66.

Dinh, D.H., R.M. Wright, and W.C. Hanigan. 1990. "The Use of Magnetic Resonance Imaging for the Diagnosis of Fetal Intracranial Anomalies." *Child's Nervous System* 6: 212-15.

Doida, Y., et al. 1990. "Confirmation of an Ultrasound-Induced Mutation in Two In-Vitro Mammalian Cell Lines." *Ultrasound in Medicine and Biology* 16: 699-705.

Elejalde, B.R., and M.M. Elejalde. 1988. "Early Genetic Amniocentesis, Safety, Complications, Time to Obtain Results and Contraindications." *American Journal of Human Genetics* 43 (Suppl. 3): A232.

Elejalde, B.R., et al. 1990. "Prospective Study of Amniocentesis Performed Between Weeks 9 and 16 of Gestation: Its Feasibility, Risks, Complications and Use in Early Genetic Prenatal Diagnosis." *American Journal of Medical Genetics* 35: 188-96.

Elias, S. 1987. "Use of Fetoscopy for the Prenatal Diagnosis of Hereditary Skin Disorders." *Current Problems in Dermatology* 16: 1-13.

Evans, M.I., et al. 1988. "Early Genetic Amniocentesis and Chorionic Villus Sampling: Expanding the Opportunities for Early Prenatal Diagnosis." *Journal of Reproductive Medicine* 33: 450-52.

Firth, H.V., et al. 1991. "Severe Limb Abnormalities After Chorion Villus Sampling at 56-66 Days' Gestation." *Lancet* (30 March): 762-63.

Garden, A.S., et al. 1991. "Fast-Scan Magnetic Resonance Imaging in Fetal Visualization." *American Journal of Obstetrics and Gynecology* 164: 1190-96.

Godmilow, L., S. Weiner, and L.K. Dunn. 1988. "Early Genetic Amniocentesis: Experience with 600 Consecutive Procedures and Comparison with Chorion Villus Sampling." *American Journal of Human Genetics* 43 (Suppl. 3): A234.

Gosden, C.M. 1991. "Fetal Karyotyping Using Chorionic Villus Samples." In *Antenatal Diagnosis of Fetal Abnormalities*, ed. J.O. Drife and D. Donnai. New York: Springer-Verlag.

Green, J.E., et al. 1988. "Chorionic Villus Sampling: Experience with an Initial 940 Cases." *Obstetrics and Gynecology* 71: 208-12.

Hammarstrom, M., and L. Marsk. 1990. "First Trimester Live Pregnancy and Subsequent Fetal Loss: Impact of Transcervical Chorionic Villus Sampling and Colonization of the Cervix." *Gynecologic and Obstetric Investigation* 30: 19-22.

Hanson, F.W., et al. 1987. "Amniocentesis Before 15 Weeks' Gestation: Outcome, Risks, and Technical Problems." *American Journal of Obstetrics and Gynecology* 156: 1524-31.

Hogge, W.A., S.A. Schonberg, and M.S. Golbus. 1986. "Chorionic Villus Sampling: Experience of the First 1000 Cases." *American Journal of Obstetrics and Gynecology* 154: 1249-52.

Hsieh, F.-J., et al. 1991. "Limb-Reduction Defects and Chorionic Villus Sampling." *Lancet* (4 May): 1091-92.

Hunter, A., et al. 1986. "Assessment of the Early Risks of Chorionic Villus Sampling." *Canadian Medical Association Journal* 134: 753-56.

Isenberg, S.J., and J.R. Heckenlively. 1985. "Traumatized Eye with Retinal Damage from Amniocentesis." *Journal of Pediatric Ophthalmology and Strabismus* 22: 65-67.

Jackson, L.G., R.J. Wapner, and B. Brambati. 1991. "Limb Abnormalities and Chorionic Villus Sampling." *Lancet* (8 June): 1423.

Jahoda, M.G.J., et al. 1989. "Evaluation of Transcervical Chorionic Villus Sampling with a Completed Follow-Up of 1550 Consecutive Pregnancies." *Prenatal Diagnosis* 9: 621-28.

Karp, L.E., and P.W. Hayden. 1977. "Fetal Puncture During Midtrimester Amniocentesis." *Obstetrics and Gynecology* 49: 115-17.

Keene, C.L., and D.N. Saller, Jr. 1989. "Prenatal Genetic Concerns." *Maryland Medical Journal* 38: 939-43.

Ledbetter, D.H., et al. 1990. "Cytogenetic Results of Chorionic Villus Sampling: High Success Rate and Diagnostic Accuracy in the United States Collaborative Study." *American Journal of Obstetrics and Gynecology* 162: 495-501.

Lilford, R.J., et al. 1987. "Transabdominal Chorion Villus Biopsy: 100 Consecutive Cases." *Lancet* (20 June): 1415-17.

Lyons, E.A. 1986. "Exposure of Human Fetus to Diagnostic Ultrasound: Human Epidemiological Studies." *Ultrasound in Medicine and Biology* 12: 689-91.

Maeda, K. 1986. "Studies on Safety of Diagnostic Ultrasound." *Ultrasound in Medicine and Biology* 12: 693-94.

Magee, A.C., et al. 1991. "Early and Conventional Amniocentesis: A Comparison of Pregnancy Outcome." *Journal of Medical Genetics* 28: 570-71.

Mahoney, M.J. 1991. "Limb Abnormalities and Chorionic Villus Sampling." *Lancet* (8 June): 1422-23.

Mastroiacovo, P., and D.P. Cavalcanti. 1991. "Limb-Reduction Defects and Chorion Villus Sampling." *Lancet* (4 May): 1091.

Mattison, D.R., and T. Angtuaco. 1988. "Magnetic Resonance Imaging in Prenatal Diagnosis." *Clinical Obstetrics and Gynecology* 31: 353-89.

Medical Research Council (U.K.). Working Party on Amniocentesis. 1978. "An Assessment of the Hazards of Amniocentesis." *British Journal of Obstetrics and Gynaecology* 85 (Suppl. 2).

Medical Research Council (U.K.). Working Party on the Evaluation of Chorion Villus Sampling. 1991. "Medical Research Council European Trial of Chorion Villus Sampling." *Lancet* (22 June): 1491-99.

Meire, H.B. 1987. "The Safety of Diagnostic Ultrasound." *British Journal of Obstetrics and Gynaecology* 94: 1121-22.

Miller, M.W. 1985. "Does Ultrasound Induce Sister Chromatid Exchanges?" *Ultrasound in Medicine and Biology* 11: 561-70.

—. 1986. "Influence of *In Vitro* Experimental Design." *Ultrasound in Medicine and Biology* 12: 682-83.

Miller, M.W., and M.C. Ziskin. 1989. "Biological Consequences of Hyperthermia." *Ultrasound in Medicine and Biology* 15: 707-22.

Miny, P., et al. 1991. "Limb Abnormalities and Chorionic Villus Sampling." *Lancet* (8 June): 1423-24.

Moessinger, A.C., et al. 1981. "Amniotic Band Syndrome Associated with Amniocentesis." *American Journal of Obstetrics and Gynecology* 141: 588-91.

Monni, G., et al. 1991. "Limb-Reduction Defects and Chorionic Villus Sampling." *Lancet* (4 May): 1091.

Muggah, H.F., M.E. D'Alton, and A.G.W. Hunter. 1987. "Chorionic Villus Sampling Followed by Genetic Amniocentesis and Septic Shock." *Lancet* (11 April): 867-68.

Mukubo, M. 1986. "Epidemiological Study: Safety of Diagnostic Ultrasound During Pregnancy on Fetus and Child Development." *Ultrasound in Medicine and Biology* 12: 691-93.

National Institute of Child Health and Human Development. National Registry for Amniocentesis Study Group. 1976. "Midtrimester Amniocentesis for Prenatal Diagnosis: Safety and Accuracy." *JAMA* 236: 1471-76.

National Radiological Protection Board. Ad Hoc Advisory Group on Nuclear Magnetic Resonance Clinical Imaging. 1983. "Revised Guidance on Acceptable Limits of Exposure During Nuclear Magnetic Resonance Clinical Imaging." *British Journal of Radiology* 56: 974-77.

Neilson, J.P., and C.M. Gosden. 1991. "First Trimester Prenatal Diagnosis: Chorionic Villus Sampling or Amniocentesis?" *British Journal of Obstetrics and Gynaecology* 98: 849-52.

Nevin, J., et al. 1990. "Early Amniocentesis: Experience of 222 Consecutive Patients, 1987-1988." *Prenatal Diagnosis* 10: 79-83.

O'Brien, B. 1989. "An Overview of the Estimation and Evaluation of Clinical Risks." In *Risk and Consent to Risk in Medicine*, ed. R.D. Mann. Carnforth: Parthenon.

O'Brien, W.D., Jr. 1991. "Ultrasound Bioeffects Related to Obstetric Sonography." In *The Principles and Practice of Ultrasonography in Obstetrics and Gynecology*. 4th ed., ed. A.C. Fleischer et al. Norwalk: Appleton & Lange.

Pennehouat, G.H., et al. 1992. "First-Trimester Transabdominal Fetoscopy." *Lancet* (15 August): 429.

Penso, C.A., et al. 1990. "Early Amniocentesis: Report of 407 Cases with Neonatal Follow-Up." *Obstetrics and Gynecology* 76: 1032-36.

Planteydt, H.T., M.J. van de Vooren, and H. Verweij. 1986. "Amniotic Bands and Malformations in Child Born After Pregnancy Screened by Chorionic Villus Biopsy." *Lancet* (27 September): 756-57.

Reece, E.A., et al. 1991. "A Viewpoint of Future Prenatal Diagnosis." *Prenatal Diagnosis* 11: 125-28.

Rhoads, G.G., et al. 1989. "The Safety and Efficacy of Chorionic Villus Sampling for Early Prenatal Diagnosis of Cytogenetic Abnormalities." *New England Journal of Medicine* 320: 609-17.

Rodeck, C.H. 1993. "Fetal Development After Chorionic Villus Sampling." *Lancet* (20 February): 468-69.

Rooney, D.E., et al. 1989. "Early Amniocentesis: A Cytogenetic Evaluation." *British Medical Journal* (1 July): 25.

Salvesen, K.A., et al. 1992. "Routine Ultrasonography *In Utero* and School Performance at Age 8-9 Years." *Lancet* (11 January): 85-89.

Shulman, L.P., et al. 1990. "Fetomaternal Transfusion Depends on Amount of Chorionic Villi Aspirated but Not on Method of Chorionic Villus Sampling." *American Journal of Obstetrics and Gynecology* 162: 1185-88.

Sikov, M.R. 1986. "Developmental Effects of Ultrasound Exposure in Mammals." *Ultrasound in Medicine and Biology* 12: 686-88.

Silverman, N.S., and R.J. Wapner. 1990. "Chorionic Villus Sampling and Amniocentesis." *Current Opinion in Obstetrics and Gynecology* 2: 258-64.

Simpson, N.E., et al. 1976. "Prenatal Diagnosis of Genetic Disease in Canada: Report of a Collaborative Study." *Canadian Medical Association Journal* 115: 739-46.

Smidt-Jensen, S., et al. 1992. "Randomized Comparison of Amniocentesis and Transabdominal and Transcervical Chorionic Villus Sampling." *Lancet* (21 November): 1237-44.

St. John Brown, B. 1984. "How Safe Is Diagnostic Ultrasonography?" *Canadian Medical Association Journal* 131: 307-11.

Tunis, S.L., et al. 1990. "Patterns of Mood States in Pregnant Women Undergoing Chorionic Villus Sampling or Amniocentesis." *American Journal of Medical Genetics* 37: 191-99.

United States. National Institutes of Health. 1984. *Diagnostic Ultrasound Imaging in Pregnancy. Consensus Statement.* Consensus Development Conference, Vol. 5 (1). Bethesda: NIH.

Wade, R.V., and S.R. Young. 1989. "Analysis of Fetal Loss After Transcervical Chorionic Villus Sampling — A Review of 719 Patients." *American Journal of Obstetrics and Gynecology* 161: 513-18; discussion 518-19.

Wapner, R.J., and L. Jackson. 1988. "Chorionic Villus Sampling." *Clinical Obstetrics and Gynecology* 31: 328-44.

Ward, R.H.T., et al. 1988. "Chorionic Villus Sampling in a High-Risk Population — 4 Years' Experience." *British Journal of Obstetrics and Gynaecology* 95: 1030-35.

WHO Consultation on First Trimester Fetal Diagnosis. 1986. "Risk Evaluation in Chorionic Villus Sampling." *Prenatal Diagnosis* 6: 451-56.

Williams, A.R. 1986. "*In Vitro* Biological Effects of Ultrasound." *Ultrasound in Medicine and Biology* 12: 685-86.

Wilson, R.D. 1990. "Prenatal Diagnosis by Invasive Techniques: Amniocentesis and Chorionic Villus Sampling." *Journal of the Society of Obstetricians and Gynaecologists of Canada* 12 (August): 27-28.

—. 1991. "How to Perform Genetic Amniocentesis." *Journal of the Society of Obstetricians and Gynaecologists of Canada* 13 (February-March): 61-63.

Zwinger, A. 1988. "Fetoscopy and Chorionic Villi Sampling in Prenatal Diagnosis of Genetic Disorders." In *The Genetics of Mental Retardation: Biomedical, Psychosocial and Ethical Issues*, ed. E.K. Hicks and J.M. Berg. Boston: Kluwer Academic.

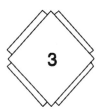

# A Survey of Research on Post-Natal Medical and Psychological Effects of Prenatal Diagnosis on Offspring

## Julie Beck

**Executive Summary**

This paper addresses the question of potential post-natal effects on offspring, both medical and psychological, of the three most prevalent prenatal diagnostic (PND) procedures: amniocentesis, chorionic villus sampling (CVS), and diagnostic ultrasound.

With regard to amniocentesis, studies to date indicate that this procedure carries only a very small risk, if any, of post-natal medical or psychological damage to offspring. However, little research is being done in the area of longer-term neurological effects, and much of what has been done has been judged to be insufficiently rigorous in methodology — specifically, most studies have not been large, randomized, or prospective. The most rigorous study on the long-term effects of amniocentesis on offspring is still under way by Canadian researchers. Until now, it has not revealed any obvious detrimental effects on physical or neurobehavioural development in children up to four years of age; its final results are expected to be published within the next two years.

No long-term studies have been done on the medical and neurobehavioural status of children exposed to CVS. With respect to

---

This paper was completed for the Royal Commission on New Reproductive Technologies in April 1992.

infants exposed *in utero* to CVS, there have been no reports of physical injury caused by the procedure. Diagnostic ultrasound during pregnancy has not been associated with any physical, neurologic, or cognitive problems in children up to nine years of age.

## Introduction

This paper documents the research that has been done on post-natal effects of the three most prevalent prenatal diagnostic (PND) techniques: amniocentesis, chorionic villus sampling (CVS), and diagnostic ultrasound. The safety of these techniques has been studied extensively with respect to the risks of fetal loss and maternal complications, but the question of any subtle long-term effects on offspring remains largely uninvestigated; only a few retrospective studies and small prospective follow-up studies have been done on the subject. Because it is theoretically possible that certain injuries caused to the fetus by PND might become evident only when language, perception, and other complex cognitive functions develop (Finegan et al. 1985; Hunt 1979), only longitudinal studies can give definitive answers as to whether or not a particular PND technique is hazardous to offspring.

## Amniocentesis

More is known of the immediate risks of amniocentesis on the fetus than of its long-term effects. It is generally agreed, on the basis of large and well-controlled studies, that the risk of fetal loss due to amniocentesis is about 1 percent or less (Canadian Collaborative CVS-Amniocentesis Clinical Trial Group 1989; Golbus et al. 1979; Hanson et al. 1987; Leschot et al. 1985; Manganiello et al. 1979; Medical Research Council 1978).

### Orthopaedic Abnormalities and Respiratory Problems

Experimental and clinical evidence shows that prolonged reduction in amniotic fluid volume (oligohydramnios) can compress the fetus, leading to pulmonary and orthopaedic problems (Jones 1988). This raises the question of whether the transient reduction in fluid volume at amniocentesis could have significant effects of this kind. Reports differ somewhat on the frequency of orthopaedic congenital anomalies and respiratory distress syndrome associated with amniocentesis, as do the sizes and rigour of the studies designed to investigate them.

No significant increases in orthopaedic postural anomalies among newborn infants who had been exposed to amniocentesis were reported in two studies conducted in England (n = 1 342, controlled, Wald et al. 1983; n = 1 750, uncontrolled, Davison et al. 1987). Similarly, no evidence of an association between exposure to amniocentesis and adverse physical or motor problems in the first year of life has been reported in several U.S. studies (n = 2 032, controlled, U.S. National Institute of Child Health 1978; n = 214, controlled, Howard and Crandall 1979; n = 22, uncontrolled, Robinson et al. 1975) and one study in England (n = 20, controlled, Vyas et al. 1982). In Sweden, a study of children between five and seven years of age who had been exposed to amniocentesis (n = 122, controlled) reported that no evidence had been found of an association between the procedure and an increase in orthopaedic abnormalities or respiratory problems (Gillberg et al. 1982).

In contrast, a statistically significant, though small (about 1 percent), increase in orthopaedic postural anomalies and respiratory difficulties among newborn infants who had been exposed to amniocentesis was reported in several studies conducted in England (n = 4 856, controlled, Medical Research Council 1978), Denmark (n = 4 606, controlled, Tabor et al. 1986), and the United States (n = 407, uncontrolled, Cruikshank et al. 1983; n = 884, uncontrolled, Penso et al. 1990). In England, a study of newborns also reported a statistically significant increase of about 1 percent in congenital abnormalities associated with amniocentesis (n = 578, controlled, Sant-Cassia et al. 1984). Different conclusions regarding increases in orthopaedic and respiratory problems associated with amniocentesis probably result because the increases, if real, are small and require very large samples to demonstrate them.

Only one group (Finegan et al. 1984, 1985, 1990) has conducted a prospective long-term study on the medical effects of amniocentesis that might appear only after the neonatal or infant stage; this study meets a comprehensive set of design recommendations that previous studies on long-term effects of PND have not (J.-A.K. Finegan, personal communication 1991; Finegan et al. 1985). Beginning in 1980, mothers were recruited from the Antenatal Genetic Clinic at the Toronto General Hospital, where they were undergoing PND because of late maternal age. The original experimental group consisted of 100 women who had chosen to have amniocentesis and the control group of 56 women who had declined it. The children of these women were assessed for physical and neurobehavioural status at birth, and at six months and four years of age. Annual contact, kept by sending each child a birthday card, has maintained an extremely low attrition rate. The most recent phase of the study included 88 of the original 100 women in the experimental group and 46 of the original 56 in the control group.

In their follow-up study of the infants at six months of age, Finegan et al. (1985) found no differences in physical growth or risk of orthopaedic abnormalities between the infants whose mothers had had amniocentesis (n = 91) and the control subjects (n = 53). These children were examined again at age four, and it was found that the mothers who had undergone amniocentesis were more likely to report a history of ear infections in their child (an increase from 58 percent to 75 percent; p = 0.04). This finding was interpreted as a possible indication of effects of amniocentesis on the upper respiratory system. However, since this was only one finding among many physical variables studied, including respiratory and orthopaedic status, physical growth, and the possibility that the mothers' information may not have been medically defensible, it needs to be replicated before being generalized. All children in this study will be examined for upper respiratory function in the subsequent follow-up at age seven.

## Psychomotor and Neurobehavioural Status

Between 10 and 18 weeks' gestation, there is rapid growth of fetal neuroblasts, the precursors of adult neuronal cells, and at this time the developing brain is vulnerable to damage (e.g., from malnutrition or endocrine imbalance) (Dobbing and Sands 1973). Because PND tests are performed during this time, their possible effect on the neurologic development of the exposed child is of interest; however, only a few follow-up studies have been conducted to examine the psychomotor and neurodevelopmental status of children exposed to amniocentesis.

The results of two previously mentioned studies in the United States revealed no evidence of neurodevelopmental harm caused to the fetus by amniocentesis. One, an uncontrolled study of 22 one-year-old infants who had been exposed to amniocentesis, reported no deviations from normal mental or motor development (Robinson et al. 1975). The larger, controlled study of 214 children between the ages of eight and thirty-seven months found no statistically significant differences between the exposed and control groups in the areas of fine and gross motor, language, and personal-social skills (Howard and Crandall 1979). Also, the previously mentioned controlled study in Sweden of 62 children between five and seven years of age reported no evidence of amniocentesis having caused any neurodevelopmental disabilities as tested by fine and gross motor skills, visual perception, speech, and attention (Gillberg et al. 1982).

The most recent and comprehensive follow-up of the neurodevelopment of children exposed to amniocentesis is the previously mentioned prospective study by Finegan et al. (1984, 1985, 1990), who assessed the neurobehavioural status of newborns and reassessed these children at six months and four years of age. The newborns were tested with a battery of 44 behavioural and orientation items, which can be grouped into the following characteristics: range of state (state changes and irritability), regulation of state (self-quieting activity), motor ability, autonomic stability (tremulousness), response decrement (habituation to repeated stimuli), reflexes, and alertness. The conditions examined at birth were chosen more for the purpose of assessing central nervous system dysfunction than for assessing behavioural status. No differences in neurobehavioural status were found between the infants whose mothers had had amniocentesis (n = 100) and the control subjects (n = 56). At the age of six months, the infants were reassessed for the same variables, with the addition of temperament. The results showed that the experimental (n = 91) and control (n = 53) groups were similar in mental and motor development, as well as in temperament, as rated by their mothers using a standard questionnaire. At age four, the neurobehavioural development of these children (88 exposed, 46 unexposed) was assessed in the areas of intelligence, visual-motor coordination and perception, language, behaviour, social competence, and temperament. After considering the influence of environmental factors on all variables, the researchers reported that they had failed to find any evidence of adverse effects of amniocentesis on cognition or behaviour. However, they noted that because only a narrow range of cognitive and motor abilities can be assessed during infancy, and because damage caused by amniocentesis might not become evident until later childhood, it is important to conduct longitudinal studies. The children, who were about seven years of age in 1992, are being reassessed, and the results will be published within two years (Finegan, personal communication 1991).

## Chorionic Villus Sampling

Canadian researchers were the first to study the long-term effects of CVS. A sample of children whose mothers had been part of the Canadian Collaborative Randomized Trial — a study that assessed the safety of CVS as compared to amniocentesis — were examined for any physical abnormalities in their first year of life (Canadian Collaborative CVS-Amniocentesis Clinical Trial Group 1989). Similar frequencies of malformations and minor anomalies were found among the children who had been exposed to either procedure. The authors suggested that a larger sample was needed to rule out small differences. One difference was a higher frequency of superficial cavernous haemangiomas (strawberry marks) among the 95 children in the CVS group than among the 87 children in the amniocentesis group (12.6 percent vs. 3.4 percent), although this was not statistically significant, and neither group had a significantly higher frequency than is found in the general population (Kaplan et al. 1990).

There is little information regarding adverse post-natal effects that may be associated with CVS, but recently there have been reports suggesting a link between its early use (between 56 and 66 days of gestation) and congenital limb deformities (Firth et al. 1991). Outcome data (examined retrospectively) from most genetics centres did not show an increase in limb deformities. Of those that did report an increase, the frequencies of the limb abnormalities, even though elevated above the norm, were low in absolute terms, ranging from 0.01 percent to 2.5 percent. The possibility of selection bias must, therefore, be considered.

A recent National Institutes of Health (NIH) Workshop on CVS and Limb and Other Defects found that the available data are inconclusive regarding a possible relationship between early CVS and limb defects. The NIH has recommended further studies to determine whether CVS-associated limb defects correlate with the level of experience of the person who performs the procedure or with the technique used, and more thorough evaluation of the prevalence of all types of limb deficiencies in unexposed and CVS-exposed infants. They have also recommended that women being offered CVS as an option be made aware of the current concerns about the possible association of CVS with an increased risk of limb and other defects (U.S. National Institutes of Health 1992).

No studies were found that examined either the medical status or the psychomotor and neurobehavioural development of older children who had been exposed to CVS.

## Diagnostic Ultrasound

Since the introduction of prenatal diagnostic ultrasound in the early 1970s, it has become an increasingly routine procedure in obstetric care. Most fetuses in developed countries (up to 80 percent) are exposed to diagnostic ultrasound (Canada, Health and Welfare Canada 1989; Salvesen et al. 1992).

Despite the clinical benefits of diagnostic ultrasound, including a trend toward a reduction of perinatal mortality and morbidity instead of an increase (Saari-Kemppainen et al. 1990), the medical community has not yet reached complete agreement on questions regarding the value of routine mid-trimester ultrasound screening. Although no clinical evidence points to diagnostic ultrasound causing damage to the fetus, there is concern that it might cause as yet unrecognized harm in a small proportion of children (Canada, Health and Welfare Canada 1989; Jack et al. 1987). Very few post-natal follow-up studies have been conducted to assess the long-term effects of diagnostic ultrasound (Salvesen et al. 1992), and several reviewers have found fault with these studies, stating that many were not large or rigorous enough to provide substantial answers regarding the benefits or harm of its routine use (Bracken 1987; De Crespigny et al. 1989; Grant 1986; Waldenstrom et al. 1988). It has also been noted that it is difficult to compare the many studies on ultrasound because results come out of clinical settings in which exposure conditions differ substantially. The frequency, intensity, duration, and repetition of pulses of energy vary greatly from one apparatus to another, as does the way in which the pulses are scanned through the tissue (Meire 1987). Large samples would be required to demonstrate potential small increases in damage, but, as was noted by one Canadian research team, with the rapid expansion in the use of diagnostic ultrasound, "it is becoming difficult to find children who were not exposed to ultrasound at some time during pregnancy" (Lyons et al. 1988), and thus it may become increasingly difficult to find a control group.

The results of a U.S. case-control study involving an examination of hearing, vision, cognition, behaviour, and neurologic status in 806 children, both at birth and between the ages of seven and twelve, showed that exposure to diagnostic ultrasound carried "little risk for subtle or long-term damage to the fetus" (Stark et al. 1984). Similarly, a Canadian study involving a six-year follow-up of 149 sibling pairs, where one member of each pair had been exposed to diagnostic ultrasound, reported in 1988 that no statistically significant differences were found in height or weight, at birth or up to six years of age, between the exposed and unexposed siblings (Lyons et al. 1988).

Recently, the results of a randomized controlled study in Norway indicated no association between exposure to diagnostic ultrasound and teacher-reported school performance (reading and writing skills) among 2 011 children of eight or nine years of age, and no evidence of an increased prevalence of dyslexia among these children (Salvesen et al. 1992).

A few studies on the effects of ultrasound that have reported significant findings regarding birth weight have attributed these findings to factors other than the ultrasound exposure. An association between more than one exposure of the fetus to ultrasound and reduced birth weight was reported in a U.S. retrospective study that compared the birth weights of 1 598 exposed and 944 unexposed newborns. The authors noted that the low birth weights were more consistently associated with the indication that led to the ultrasound examination than with the procedure (Moore et al. 1988). In Sweden, a large, randomized controlled trial examined the effectiveness of diagnostic ultrasound screening in women who had no particular indication for the procedure. The researchers reported that they found a higher mean birth weight among the screened babies, and suggested that this might be attributable to reduction in smoking among the women as a result of watching their fetus on the screen (Waldenstrom et al. 1988).

Ultrasound can cause biological damage if the intensity is sufficiently high. There are three mechanisms by which ultrasound can have biological effects on tissue: thermal heating, cavitation, and radiation. Experiments on animals and cells have demonstrated risks, but they are associated with heating caused by ultrasound at levels of intensity much higher than those used clinically for diagnostic ultrasound (McLeod and Fowlow 1989).

The American Institute of Ultrasound in Medicine (AIUM) recommended that diagnostic ultrasound be used without hesitation as long as appropriate equipment and procedures are used. It pointed to the "excellent safety record" of diagnostic ultrasound, made on the basis of decades of clinical use with no known instance of human injury. However, caution was expressed: "since evidence exists to believe that at least a hypothetical risk for clinical diagnostic ultrasound must be presumed, the

AIUM feels that the user should be properly informed about issues related to risk in order to ensure an effective decision-making process that can best serve to enhance patient care" (American Institute of Ultrasound in Medicine 1988).

An authoritative and topical review of the fetal effects of diagnostic ultrasound assessed its risks using five criteria: human epidemiology, secular trend data, animal experiments, dose-response relationship, and biologic plausibility (Brent et al. 1991). The report concluded that diagnostic levels of ultrasound were safe and did not pose a measurable risk to the developing embryo or fetus, but included some cautions:

> Guidelines should be established, limiting the number of sonograms and the length of a particular study for each patient. It may even be advisable to have timers on machines (governors) to record the length of each procedure ... Designers of equipment will have to be cognizant of the exposures that have the potential for producing reproductive effects. It would appear that if the embryonic temperature never exceeds 39° C then there is no risk. Equipment should be designed so that these temperatures are never even approached. (Brent et al. 1991, 141)

## Conclusions

Some equivocal evidence suggests that unexplained respiratory difficulties and orthopaedic postural deformities might result from amniotic fluid loss at amniocentesis. The likelihood of this occurring (if it is a real effect) is very small. There have been few serious attempts to identify possible effects of amniocentesis on post-natal neurologic development. So far, no neurobehavioural problems have been found in children up to four years of age who have been exposed to amniocentesis.

The results of a Canadian study of infants exposed to CVS showed no evidence of its causing harm to the developing fetus, but no long-term studies of older children exposed to the procedure were found. Although the routine use of diagnostic ultrasound in obstetric care has not been universally approved, follow-up studies of children, epidemiologic studies, animal studies, and an absence of reported injuries suggest that it is not harmful to the developing fetus.

These three PND procedures are considered to carry only a very small risk of harm to offspring, but more longitudinal research, in the form of large, randomized, prospective studies, is needed to fill gaps in information.

# Bibliography

American Institute of Ultrasound in Medicine (AIUM). Bioeffects Committee. 1988. "Bioeffects Considerations for the Safety of Diagnostic Ultrasound." *Journal of Ultrasound in Medicine* 7 (Suppl.): S1-S38.

Bracken, M.B. 1987. "Ultrasonography in Antenatal Management: Should It Be a Routine Procedure?" *Fetal Therapy* 2: 2-6.

Brent, R.L., R.P. Jensh, and D.A. Beckman. 1991. "Medical Sonography: Reproductive Effects and Risks." *Teratology* 44: 123-46.

Canada. Health and Welfare Canada. Environmental Health Directorate. Health Protection Branch. 1989. *Guidelines for the Safe Use of Ultrasound. Part I: Medical and Paramedical Applications.* Safety Code 23. Ottawa: Minister of Supply and Services Canada.

Canadian Collaborative CVS-Amniocentesis Clinical Trial Group. 1989. "Multicentre Randomised Clinical Trial of Chorion Villus Sampling and Amniocentesis. First Report." *Lancet* (7 January): 1-6.

Cruikshank, D.P., et al. 1983. "Midtrimester Amniocentesis. An Analysis of 923 Cases with Neonatal Follow-Up." *American Journal of Obstetrics and Gynecology* 146: 204-11.

Davison, E.V., A.S. McIntosh, and D.F. Roberts. 1987. "Effects of Amniocentesis for Genetic Purposes on the Pregnancy and Its Outcome." *Journal of Biosocial Science* 19: 295-304.

De Crespigny, L.C., P. Warren, and B. Buttery. 1989. "Should All Pregnant Women Be Offered an Ultrasound Examination?" *Medical Journal of Australia* (4-18 December): 613-15.

Dobbing, J., and J. Sands. 1973. "Quantitative Growth and Development of Human Brain." *Archives of Disease in Childhood* 48: 757-67.

Finegan, J.-A.K., et al. 1984. "Midtrimester Amniocentesis: Obstetric Outcome and Neonatal Neurobehavioral Status." *American Journal of Obstetrics and Gynecology* 150: 989-97.

—. 1985. "Infant Outcome Following Mid-Trimester Amniocentesis: Development and Physical Status at Age Six Months." *British Journal of Obstetrics and Gynaecology* 92: 1015-23.

—. 1990. "Child Outcome Following Mid-Trimester Amniocentesis: Development, Behaviour, and Physical Status at Age 4 Years." *British Journal of Obstetrics and Gynaecology* 97: 32-40.

Firth, H.V., et al. 1991. "Severe Limb Abnormalities After Chorion Villus Sampling at 55-60 Days' Gestation." *Lancet* (30 March): 762-63.

Gillberg, C., P. Rasmussen, and J. Wahlstrom. 1982. "Long-Term Follow-Up of Children Born After Amniocentesis." *Clinical Genetics* 21: 69-73.

Golbus, M.S., et al. 1979. "Prenatal Genetic Diagnosis in 3000 Amniocenteses." *New England Journal of Medicine* 300: 157-63.

Grant, A. 1986. "Controlled Trials of Routine Ultrasound in Pregnancy." *Birth* 13: 22-28.

Hanson, F.W., et al. 1987. "Amniocentesis Before 15 Weeks' Gestation: Outcome, Risks, and Technical Problems." *American Journal of Obstetrics and Gynecology* 156: 1524-31.

Howard, J.A., and B.F. Crandall. 1979. "Amniocentesis Follow-Up: Infant Developmental Evaluation." *Obstetrics and Gynecology* 53: 599-601.

Hunt, J.V. 1979. "Longitudinal Research: A Method for Studying the Intellectual Development of High-Risk Pre-Term Infants." In *Infants Born at Risk: Behavior and Development*, ed. T.M. Fiel et al. New York: SP Medical & Scientific Books.

Jack, B.W., T.M. Empkie, and R.B. Kates. 1987. "Routine Obstetric Ultrasound." *American Family Physician* 35 (5)(May): 173-82.

Jones, K.L. 1988. *Smith's Recognizable Patterns of Human Malformation*. 4th ed. Philadelphia: W.B. Saunders.

Kaplan, P., et al. 1990. "Malformations and Minor Anomalies in Children Whose Mothers Had Prenatal Diagnosis: Comparison Between CVS and Amniocentesis." *American Journal of Medical Genetics* 37: 366-70.

Leschot, N.J., M. Verjaal, and P.E. Treffers. 1985. "Risks of Midtrimester Amniocentesis: Assessment in 3000 Pregnancies." *British Journal of Obstetrics and Gynaecology* 92: 804-807.

Lyons, E.A., et al. 1988. "*In Utero* Exposure to Diagnostic Ultrasound: A 6-Year Follow-Up." *Radiology* 166: 687-90.

McLeod, D.R., and S.B. Fowlow. 1989. "Multiple Malformations and Exposure to Therapeutic Ultrasound During Organogenesis." *American Journal of Medical Genetics* 34: 317-19.

Manganiello, P.D., et al. 1979. "A Report of the Safety and Accuracy of Midtrimester Amniocentesis at the Medical College of Georgia: Eight and One Half Years' Experience." *American Journal of Obstetrics and Gynecology* 134: 911-16.

Medical Research Council (U.K.). Working Party on Amniocentesis. 1978. "An Assessment of the Hazards of Amniocentesis." *British Journal of Obstetrics and Gynaecology* 85 (Suppl. 2).

Meire, H.B. 1987. "The Safety of Diagnostic Ultrasound." *British Journal of Obstetrics and Gynaecology* 94: 1121-22.

Moore, R.M., Jr., E.L. Diamond, and R.L. Cavalieri. 1988. "The Relationship of Birth Weight and Intrauterine Diagnostic Ultrasound Exposure." *Obstetrics and Gynecology* 71: 513-17.

Penso, C.A., et al. 1990. "Early Amniocentesis: Report of 407 Cases with Neonatal Follow-Up." *Obstetrics and Gynecology* 76: 1032-36.

Robinson, J., K. Tennes, and A. Robinson. 1975. "Amniocentesis: Its Impact on Mothers and Infants. A 1-Year Follow-Up Study." *Clinical Genetics* 8: 97-106.

Saari-Kemppainen, A., et al. 1990. "Ultrasound Screening and Perinatal Mortality: Controlled Trial of Systematic One-Stage Screening in Pregnancy." *Lancet* (18 August): 387-91.

Salvesen, K.Å., et al. 1992. "Routine Ultrasonography In Utero and School Performance at Age 8-9 Years." *Lancet* (11 January): 85-89.

Sant-Cassia, L.J., M.B.A. MacPherson, and A.J. Tyack. 1984. "Midtrimester Amniocentesis: Is It Safe? A Single Centre Controlled Prospective Study of 517 Consecutive Amniocenteses." *British Journal of Obstetrics and Gynaecology* 91: 736-44.

Stark, C.R., et al. 1984. "Short- and Long-Term Risks After Exposure to Diagnostic Ultrasound In Utero." *Obstetrics and Gynecology* 63: 194-200.

Tabor, A., et al. 1986. "Randomised Controlled Trial of Genetic Amniocentesis in 4 606 Low-Risk Women." *Lancet* (7 June): 1287-93.

United States. National Institute of Child Health and Human Development. 1978. "The Safety and Accuracy of Mid-Trimester Amniocentesis: The NICHD Amniocentesis Registry." Washington, DC: U.S. Dept. of Health, Education, and Welfare.

United States. National Institutes of Health. 1992. "Workshop on CVS and Limb and Other Defects." Bethesda: NIH.

Vyas, H., A.D. Milner, and I.E. Hopkin. 1982. "Amniocentesis and Fetal Lung Development." *Archives of Disease in Childhood* 57: 627-28.

Wald, N.J., et al. 1983. "Congenital Talipes and Hip Malformation in Relation to Amniocentesis: A Case-Control Study." *Lancet* (30 July): 246-49.

Waldenstrom, U., et al. 1988. "Effects of Routine One-Stage Ultrasound Screening in Pregnancy: A Randomised Controlled Trial." *Lancet* (10 September): 585-88.

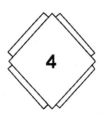

# A Demographic and Geographic Analysis of the Users of Prenatal Diagnostic Services in Canada

Patrick M. MacLeod,
Mark W. Rosenberg,
Michael H. Butler,
and
Susan J. Koval

**Executive Summary**

Prenatal diagnosis was introduced in Canada in the 1970s, and since then its use has become widespread. These services are obtainable, however, only in certain locations. Using data on users from the 21 genetics centres across the country and a data base on obstetricians/gynaecologists and general practitioners with an interest in obstetrics, the authors of this study demonstrate that utilization of these services is not uniform across the country.

After reviewing the literature on the subject, the authors outline their methodology, including a definition of "expected" use or referral for services. The authors map and analyze the expected and observed utilization of prenatal diagnostic services among women of different ages

---

This paper was completed for the Royal Commission on New Reproductive Technologies in August 1992.

and the expected and observed referrals for these services by physicians. The data are given by five regions of Canada — the Atlantic provinces, Quebec, Ontario, the Prairie provinces, and British Columbia — and also presented for Canada as a whole. Data are further arranged by province and census division, in a considerable amount of detail. They examine the effect of distance from services, income, education, the levels of employment and unemployment, and the number of physicians on utilization of prenatal diagnosis.

Lower than expected utilization rates occur in rural and northern areas of every region, but they are as expected or higher than expected in predominantly urban areas. Physicians play a key role in determining utilization patterns, and distance from prenatal diagnostic centres, women's educational attainment, levels of unemployment among women, and rural residence appear to be important variables in explaining utilization rates in particular regions.

## Introduction

One of the many topics the Royal Commission on New Reproductive Technologies needed information on was whether accessibility to new reproductive technologies varies as a result of socioeconomic status and location. This study focusses on women who utilized prenatal diagnostic services (chorionic villus sampling or genetic amniocentesis) in Canada in 1990. Fewer women than expected by our definition utilized prenatal diagnostic services. This is partly explained by differences in women's socioeconomic status (closely linked to education), the physician's role as the referral agent, and the geography of prenatal diagnostic services in Canada. Also part of the explanation is that some women and their families do not wish to take advantage of the service and that some women are not aware that these services exist. Our research is not designed to examine these last two factors.

First we briefly review the literature on prenatal services and access to medical care. We then outline the data and methodologies used in this study. The results of our analysis are presented for the five major regions of Canada — the Atlantic provinces, Quebec, Ontario, the Prairie provinces, and British Columbia — and for Canada as a whole. Finally, we summarize our major findings and conclusions.

## Literature Review

### Genetic Testing in Canada

Second-trimester prenatal diagnosis by genetic amniocentesis was introduced in Canada in the early 1970s. With its recognition as a safe, ethically acceptable procedure for the detection of birth defects, its utilization has grown rapidly (Baird et al. 1985).

The indications for prenatal diagnosis were initially established in 1974. These guidelines have been recently updated to reflect the explosive development of new technologies, including chorionic villus sampling and molecular diagnostic techniques, which have allowed a more sophisticated evaluation and understanding of the fetus and genetic diseases (Wilson and Rudd 1991).

Approximately 85% of amniocenteses are conducted for chromosomal evaluation. Of these, about three-quarters are on women over 35 years of age (Lippman-Hand and Cohen 1980; Verp and Simpson 1990). Furhmann, by comparing the number of cytogenetic tests in amniotic fluid reported by an international survey of laboratories with the number of births to women aged 35 years and over in those same areas, calculates a utilization rate by eligible women of approximately 47% (Furhmann 1989). This figure is very close to the predictions of a decade ago (Hook and Schreinemachers 1983; Adams et al. 1981). A number of authors felt that utilization rates are unlikely to greatly exceed an average of 60% because of ethnic, religious, educational, and socioeconomic factors. However, this increasing number of women below the age of 34 who are now eligible for prenatal diagnosis (currently 11% of all pregnancies) as a result of the availability of rapid, early, and accurate diagnostic tests for such conditions as cystic fibrosis, Duchenne muscular dystrophy, fragile X syndrome, and an increasing number of inborn errors of metabolism may increase the eventual percentage of women utilizing the service.

Attempts are being made to improve the efficiency with which limited laboratory capacity is used by evaluating the indications for prenatal diagnosis and screening based on the aggregate values of maternal age, alpha-fetoprotein, and two other fetal-placental products — human chorionic gonadotropins (hCG) and unconjugated estriol (so-called triple screening) (Wald et al. 1988).

Relatively little research has been published on the many factors that contribute to access to and utilization of prenatal diagnosis (Selle et al. 1979; Marion et al. 1980; Bernhardt and Bannerman 1982; Roghmann et al. 1983; Naber et al. 1987; Goodwin and Huether 1987; Crandall et al. 1986; Knutson et al. 1989). Still less has been written from the perspective of Canada, whose universal medicare system essentially gives all women equal financial access to these services (Baird et al. 1985; Lippman 1986; Davies and Doran 1982; Hunter et al. 1987; McDonough 1990).

The diffusion, adoption, and utilization of amniocentesis were initially slow and limited, but there has been a substantial increase in its use as centres across Canada have increasingly begun offering it. Provincial fiscal and planning policies play a role in determining the availability of new technologies (McDonough 1990). The reasons women decide not to have a genetic amniocentesis (or chorionic villus sampling) include a lack of information, the perception that they are at low risk, and fear of fetal loss or injury (Davies and Doran 1982). Under-utilization does not distinguish between informed decisions not to have amniocentesis, lack of opportunity to make an informed decision, or lack of provision of a service by the health care system (McDonough 1990).

The standard procedure, used in most studies, to calculate utilization rates is to divide the number of amniocenteses performed by the number of live births (sometimes including stillbirths) in the same area and during the same period. Such studies rarely examine the distance of the patient's residence from a prenatal diagnostic centre (Baird et al. 1985).

Approximately 8% of women are 35 years or older at the time of delivery (Canada, Statistics Canada 1992). Adams et al. (1981) predict that this percentage will increase by nearly 4% per year and that demand for prenatal diagnostic services will therefore continue to increase for advanced maternal age (Adams et al. 1982).

Impressionistic evidence indicates that the patterns observed in Canada are broadly similar to those in the United States; however, a recent report on the diffusion of amniocentesis in Ontario raises questions about applying the U.S. model describing widespread and rapid diffusion of medical innovations to the Canadian context (McDonough 1990). More information and analysis are needed on the Canadian context so that health care policy decisions can be based on a more accurate picture (Feeny 1986).

## Factors Affecting Women's Attendance for Screening Services[1]

Since little is known about factors affecting women's attendance for prenatal diagnostic services, we turned to the literature on barriers to women's attendance for screening services as a guide to the factors that might be included in this study. The literature suggesting that geographical factors influence the uptake of screening services is limited; that emphasizing the contribution of socioeconomic characteristics is somewhat larger.

Senior and Williamson's study, which is an investigation into the influence of geographical factors on attendance for cervical cytology screening in Salford, England, is perhaps the most closely related to the research presented here (Senior and Williamson 1990). Cervical screening programs are directed at asymptomatic women. Senior and Williamson suggest that one clear role of analysis of this type is to thoroughly investigate the significance of logistic or practical problems affecting attendance for cervical screening. Different socioeconomic groups experience different problems that affect their attendance at health care facilities, so the key to understanding variations in attendance may not be just the problems themselves but also the lack of resources to overcome them. Lack of local availability of a service may be a problem, but some are able to overcome the geographic barrier because they have access to a private automobile.

Senior and Williamson hypothesize that geographic constraints assume greater importance with preventive as opposed to curative medical services. If the client is not motivated by pain or illness there is likely to be less incentive to overcome the practical obstacles. One could conjecture, furthermore, that the tendency to procrastinate in making an initial appointment may be stronger among clients for screening services, since they are healthy. They conclude that their study of women who do, and do not, attend cervical screening services does not "offer any convincing support for the belief that geographic accessibility and geographic mobility are significant influences on women's decisions whether or not to make and attend smear test appointments" (Senior and Williamson 1990, 430-31). However, their study area consisted only of urban and suburban Salford. It could not offer any insight into geographical factors influencing uptake on a regional scale, where issues of rural access come into relief and distance is more of a barrier.

Hayward et al. examine attendance at breast cancer screening facilities but do not emphasize geographical barriers (Hayward et al. 1988). They analyze data from an extensive telephone survey in the United States (n = 4 659) to evaluate trends in the provision of cancer screening preventive care. Their objectives were to determine (1) what proportion of American women received recommended cervical and breast cancer screening, and (2) which groups were less likely to receive this type of preventive care. They find generally that the proportion of women who did receive preventive care was below American guidelines, and that older women, women of lower socioeconomic status, and women who live in rural areas are less likely than the general population to receive either breast or cervical cancer screening.

Vernon et al. (1990) review the literature on participation in breast screening programs. They find that variables associated with attendance could be grouped into six categories: (1) sociodemographic characteristics; (2) medical history and health status, including risk factors for breast cancer; (3) use of medical services and other health behaviour; (4) logistical barriers; (5) beliefs, attitudes, and knowledge about cancer and health care; and (6) intentions. Most of the studies they examine do not include all of the factors but are more narrowly focussed. Eight of the 10 studies they review find an inverse association between age and attendance at a screening program. Education was positively associated with attendance, and one study reports a positive association between occupational status and attendance among women employed by a university (Rutledge et al. 1988). The relationship between marital status and participation was ambiguous, with three studies finding that married women were more likely to attend screening, two finding no association between marital status and attendance, and one finding that single women were more likely to complete screening than married or ever-married women (especially those with large families).

Studies reviewed by Vernon et al. that examine health status factors look at the relationship between a reported family history of breast cancer and breast disease, and attendance for screening. Two studies find no association between family history and compliance, and one finds a positive association between attendance and having a mother with breast cancer, but no association when the relative was a sister (de Waard et al. 1984).

Another study finds that women who had benign breast symptoms were more likely to complete screening and that attenders were more than twice as likely than non-attenders to have seen a physician during the year prior to screening (Fink et al. 1968). Five other studies show completion of breast screening to be positively associated with regular dental check-ups and compliance with cervical screening guidelines.

Very few studies examine logistical barriers to attendance for screening; the only study that considers distance as a barrier shows no association between travel time and attendance (Fink et al. 1968). An American study finds that cost was a factor in non-attendance (Rutledge et al. 1988).

Beliefs, attitudes, and knowledge are explored in detail in four studies. Two show a positive association between the belief that it is better to know if one has cancer, and going for mammography. Four find that non-attenders were more likely to believe that X-rays, check-ups, and mammograms are only needed when one is ill or symptomatic.

Only one study examines a client's intentions and her actual completion of breast screening; it finds, not surprisingly, that there was a strong positive association between intention to attend and attendance for screening (Calnan 1984).

Since Vernon and her colleagues completed their review in 1990, there has been further research into the factors associated with compliance for breast screening. The study by Burg et al. (1990) of women aged between 50 and 75 years on Long Island, New York, makes important connections between age, education and income, use of other health services, and uptake of screening. While they find screening rates that are higher than those found in previous studies, they also find that women over 50 were underusing screening, with women over 65 the least likely to have had a recent screening. They find that patterns of usual health care are more directly related to the use of breast screening than is income level or education. That is, women who routinely visit an obstetrician/gynaecologist are more likely to make use of breast screening than women who routinely visit general practitioners. Younger women and those with higher incomes are more likely to be seeing an obstetrician. Burg et al. suggest that older women might view routine obstetrical/gynaecological care as a "luxury," particularly as earned income declines and other health problems take precedence over preventive health care in a country where there is no universal health insurance. Their findings show the importance of the primary care physician to participation in a breast screening program.

They suggest that women's age and socioeconomic status affect the type of primary care received and are thus important factors in attendance.

Kreitler et al. focus on the psychological factors associated with attendance (Kreitler et al. 1990). They attempt to determine why many women who have full information about the availability and importance of screening programs choose not to attend or discontinue a regimen of periodic screening. They suggest that personality and motivational factors play a role in attendance at mammography examinations. Their study compares several psychological variables of those who do and do not attend free breast screening clinics operated by the Israeli National Cancer Association. Those who attended differed from those who did not attend on several of the psychological variables, which suggests that there is a psychological profile that characterizes those who attend clinics.

An extensive telephone survey of 802 women of screening age in Los Angeles County lends support to many of the previous findings on factors affecting attendance for screening (Bastani et al. 1991). The cost of the procedure appeared to be the strongest factor, whereas concern about radiation proved to be a moderate factor. With respect to demographic and social variables, younger women and married women and those with high incomes and education were more likely to have had a mammogram. Consistent with other literature, a large majority of their sample reported that "the chances were very high that they would get a mammogram if their doctor recommended it" (ibid., 360). Again, the importance of primary source of care and the referral system in influencing the use of screening services is emphasized.

However, it is of interest in this regard that Lane et al. (1992) find that women with lower income and/or education who attend publicly funded health centres for primary care achieve screening rates comparable with those in the general population. This is because lower-income women receive regular, free care from health centre physicians who explain and promote the benefits and importance of early detection of breast cancer through mammographic screening. Thus, access to primary care proved to be a critical factor in affecting the rate of attendance for screening among socioeconomically disadvantaged women in Suffolk County, New York.

## Summary

Prenatal diagnosis by genetic amniocentesis is a service that has developed in the last 20 years in Canada. Estimates of utilization of prenatal diagnosis vary from one jurisdiction to another, with ethnic, religious, educational, and socioeconomic factors partially explaining the differences in utilization.

An analogy can be drawn between access to prenatal diagnostic services and access to other screening services for women. The literature on screening services indicates that in addition to ethnic, religious, educational, and socioeconomic factors, the roles of physicians, rural/

urban distance, and psychological factors need to be examined in order to increase our understanding of access to health services for women.

## Methodology

### Introduction

In this study, prenatal diagnostic services are defined as services received at one of the 21 regional medical genetics centres providing such services in Canada that participated in the study. Services might include one or several of counselling, amniocentesis, ultrasound, and chorionic villus sampling. Women who only made inquiries or who received counselling over the telephone are not included in the data bases described below.

Canada is divided into five regions: the Atlantic provinces (Newfoundland, Nova Scotia, Prince Edward Island, and New Brunswick), Quebec, Ontario, the Prairies (Manitoba, Saskatchewan, and Alberta), and British Columbia.[2] Five key measures are used: (1) the observed geographic distribution of women who received prenatal diagnostic services; (2) the expected geographic distribution of women who were projected by our formula (see "Calculation of 'Expected' Utilization," below) to receive prenatal diagnostic services; (3) the geographic distribution of physicians who potentially might make referrals for prenatal diagnostic services; (4) the geographic distribution of physicians who actually do make referrals; and (5) the sites where prenatal diagnostic services are offered.

We then use *ecological* models to examine the geographic distribution of women who receive prenatal diagnostic services as a function of the socioeconomic features of the areas in which women live, the geographic distribution of physicians who potentially might make referrals, and measures of rural/urban and geographic access to the nearest prenatal diagnostic centre.

Four aspects are assessed: (1) the difference between the observed and the expected patterns of prenatal diagnostic service utilization; (2) the difference between the observed physician referral patterns and potential physician referral patterns; (3) the difference between referral patterns based on the location of the physician and those based on the location of the patient's residence; and (4) the observed pattern of utilization as explained by the socioeconomic characteristics of the population, the distribution of physicians who potentially might make referrals, and measures of rural/urban and geographic access to prenatal diagnostic centres.

## Data Sources

To determine the geographic distribution of women who received prenatal diagnostic services and of physicians who made referrals, demographic data on every woman who had received a prenatal diagnostic consultation in 1990 were requested of the 21 prenatal diagnostic centres across Canada (see Appendix 1). The information included the patient's residential postal code and date of birth, the name of the referring physician, and the reason for the referral. These data were kept confidential, in very secure conditions, with access only by investigators, and they will be destroyed at the completion of the study. Only the centres at Wellesley Hospital in Toronto and the Alberta Children's Hospital in Calgary failed to provide data on women who had received a prenatal diagnostic procedure; all of the maps of prenatal service utilization are therefore reasonably accurate. For Metropolitan Toronto and its surrounding census divisions, the values might be slight underestimates, but there are four other prenatal diagnostic centres in the area providing services. For southern Alberta the values are likely significant underestimates, because the only other prenatal diagnostic centre is located in Edmonton.

To determine the number of physicians who potentially might make referrals, a data base of every family physician and general practitioner who indicated an interest in obstetrics and all obstetricians/gynaecologists in Canada was purchased from Southam Direct Marketing Services. For all physicians, the name, specialty code, and postal code of the practice are listed. In this study the term "family/general practitioner" refers *only* to family physicians and general practitioners with a declared interest in obstetrics, unless otherwise indicated. Socioeconomic data are taken from the 1986 census.

There was some variation in the quality and detail of the data provided by the prenatal diagnostic centres (Table 1). There are two general problems (region-specific problems are noted at the beginning of the discussion of each region). First, in some cases either the names of the referring physicians were missing or there were difficulties in matching them to the physician data base file to identify a postal code because of the way they were recorded. Second, some referring family/general practitioners were not captured because their interest in obstetrics was not indicated on the Southam data base.

In Table 1 the number of referring physicians is the number of physicians whose names were provided by the prenatal diagnostic centres. The centres at Hôpital Ste-Justine in Montreal and Shaughnessy-Grace hospitals in Vancouver provided postal codes for the women who received services but not the names of the physicians who made the referrals. For the data on referrals made, only those from the Wellesley and the Alberta Children's hospitals are missing. The unmatched physicians are those whose names could not be matched with the Southam data base. The maps of family physicians and general practitioners, obstetricians/ gynaecologists, and the total number of physicians making referrals compared with physicians who potentially might make referrals therefore underestimate the values of the ratios, but the geographic patterns are likely reasonable approximations of the relative distributions. The maps of the total number of referrals per 100 physicians overestimate the values of the ratios, but again the geographical patterns are likely reasonable approximations of the relative distributions of referrals. Nevertheless, particular care should be taken in interpreting the analysis of the geographic distribution of referrals and referring physicians.

**Table 1. Summary of Referrals and Physicians Making Referrals to Prenatal Diagnostic Centres, by Region, Canada, 1990**

| Region | Referring physicians* | Referrals made | Unmatched referring physicians** | Unmatched referrals |
|---|---|---|---|---|
| Atlantic provinces | 48 | 606 | 14 | 168 |
| Quebec | 387 | 3 758 | 311 | 807 |
| Ontario | 1 189 | 6 073 | 703 | 1 207 |
| Prairie provinces | 233 | 1 460 | 144 | 257 |
| British Columbia | 45 | 79 | 97 | 167 |

\* Provided by participating centres.
\*\* Referring physicians who could not be matched with the Southam data base.

In all provinces except Quebec, census divisions are used as the geographic unit of measurement. In Quebec the cantons are aggregated in health regions. In Nova Scotia, Prince Edward Island, and New Brunswick, census divisions are the equivalents of counties. In Ontario, census divisions are the equivalent of Metropolitan Toronto, regional municipalities, counties, or districts. In British Columbia, they are the equivalent of regional districts. In the remaining provinces, census divisions are identified only with numbers.

## Key Measures

To determine the geographic distribution of women who received prenatal diagnostic services from data provided by the prenatal diagnostic centres, the patient's residential postal code was matched with the census division where she lived at the time, using Census of Canada Postal Code Conversion Tapes. In a small number of cases there were multiple locations for one postal code. This sometimes occurs where a postal code crosses the boundary of two census divisions. Since the data did not contain the patients' names, it was not possible to check back with the centre to obtain the actual address. Instead, because virtually all of the multiple locations were in rural areas, the individuals concerned were assigned a census division by means of a rural location population-weighted variable on the Postal Code Conversion Tapes, which estimates the most likely township for the rural postal station.

We distinguished between women aged between 15 and 34 years (young women) and those aged 35 years and over (older women) who utilized prenatal diagnostic services. For ease of presentation and because of small numbers in many census divisions, the observations are converted to a rate per 100 000 in the two age groups for each census division. The observed rates are mapped for each age group and for both age groups combined for each region. In the legends, "No services" means that no woman in that census division utilized a prenatal diagnostic service in 1990. For ease of presentation, only the figures showing observed utilization by all women are presented.

## Calculation of "Expected" Utilization

How to calculate the expected utilization of prenatal diagnostic services per census division is difficult. Based on the literature we concluded that a conservative estimate of the number of young women who might be eligible for prenatal diagnostic services because of an indication other than maternal age was approximately 109 per 1 000 young, pregnant women (see Appendix 2). Since biochemical markers such as maternal serum alpha-fetoprotein were not generally available across Canada during the survey year, we reduced the anticipated rate of utilization to 36 out of 1 000 women. It was then assumed that utilization rates were unlikely to exceed an average of 60%, because of ethnic, religious, and social factors. Therefore, we decided on an expected utilization figure of 2% of pregnant women under 35. By multiplying this rate by the average number of births for the period 1987-89 to young women per census division, we arrived at an estimate of the number of younger women per census division who might be expected to utilize prenatal diagnostic services. In the case of older women, 100% are eligible for prenatal diagnostic services. Therefore the average number of births for the period 1987-89 among older women, per census division, was multiplied by 60% to provide an estimate of the number of older women who might be expected to utilize prenatal diagnostic services.

Expected rates of utilization were mapped for each age group and for both age groups combined. Only the figures for expected utilization by all women are presented. The "No services" category should be interpreted in the same way as for the observed utilization rates.

The difference between observed and expected rates is also calculated and mapped as "utilization much less than expected" (< −499), "utilization less than expected" (–499 to –100), "utilization as expected" (–99 to 99), "utilization more than expected" (100 to 499), and "utilization much more than expected" (> 499). Note that the range for utilization as expected is very broad. Our approach is to err on the conservative side in identifying the differences between observed and expected utilization patterns.

To determine geographic patterns of physicians making referrals, for each patient the name of the referring physician was cross-checked against the Southam data base to obtain the postal code and specialty of the referring physician. Following a procedure similar to the one outlined above, each postal code was then allocated to a specific census division to determine the number of family/general practitioners and obstetricians/gynaecologists making referrals per census division.

The geographical distributions of family/general practitioners, obstetricians/gynaecologists, and all physicians who made referrals in 1990, respectively, were analyzed. Only the figures showing the geographic distributions of obstetricians/gynaecologists and family/general practitioners are presented. In the legends, "No physicians" means that no physician made a referral in these census divisions in 1990. It does *not* mean that these census divisions contain no physicians. (There may, however, be census divisions where there are no obstetricians/gynaecologists.)

Using the data provided by Southam, we also determined the number of family/general practitioners and obstetricians/gynaecologists within each census division who potentially might make referrals. The ratio of physicians who did make referrals to the number of physicians who potentially might make referrals in a census division was calculated and mapped in a fashion similar to the observed number of physicians making referrals for each region. In the legends, "No physicians" should be interpreted as described above except in census divisions where the number of referrals made is "0 to 0.1." Here it is possible that no referrals were made in 1990 but that there were family/general practitioners who expressed an interest in obstetrics and/or obstetricians/gynaecologists.

It is important to determine whether the referrals are evenly distributed among the physicians who make referrals or whether the pattern of referrals is somehow skewed. To summarize the distribution, tables are constructed that show the number of physicians who potentially might make referrals, the number who actually made referrals, and the number of referrals actually carried out.

Two types of ranges are used in the map legends. On the maps of observed and expected utilization the numbers of family/general practitioners and of obstetricians/gynaecologists are shown, and on the maps of referral patterns the ranges in the legends reflect the distribution of values and breakpoints in those distributions. This means that the ranges can vary from map to map, so care must be taken in making comparisons between regions. For the maps of observed compared with expected utilization, all of the values for the country were examined and the ranges chosen to allow comparisons between regions.

The final step in the analysis is the development of a set of ecological models to explain the geographic distribution of women who received prenatal diagnostic services. The number of women per census division who received prenatal diagnostic services is modelled in the form of multiple regression equations as a function of the socioeconomic characteristics of the people in the census division, the number of referring physicians, and measures of rurality and distance from the services.

The underlying assumption is that the aggregate characteristics of the people in an area explain the pattern of results, but do *not* explain individual behaviour. While it would be preferable to explain the utilization of prenatal diagnostic services as a function of specific characteristics of the individuals who are known to have used the services, data of this nature do not exist for all centres, either because the same information is not gathered or the data that are gathered are not relevant to this study. Such data are collected in a survey of users and published in another study for the Royal Commission on New Reproductive Technologies (Grant 1993).

Ecological models are relatively inexpensive to design because they employ secondary data collected by Statistics Canada for the census or data that can be constructed from other data sources without surveying individuals. It bears repeating, however, that they are not models of individual behaviour.

With stepwise regression procedures, the dependent variable ($Y_i$) is the number of women who received prenatal services in census division i. The independent variables entered are the straightline distance from the geographic centre of a census division to the nearest centre where prenatal diagnostic services are offered ($X_{1i}$), the median income of women in census division i ($X_{2i}$), the number of women with more than a high school education in census division i ($X_{3i}$), the number of people employed in primary sector activities in census division i ($X_{4i}$), the number of women unemployed in census division i ($X_{5i}$), and the number of family/general practitioners and obstetricians/gynaecologists who potentially might make referrals in census division i ($X_{6i}$). With the exceptions of the distance and the median income variables, the dependent and independent variables are converted to rates per 100 000 women aged 15 and over. The theoretical equations for the regional models take the following form:

$$Y_i = \beta_0 + \beta_1 X_{1i} + \beta_2 X_{2i} + \beta_3 X_{3i} + \beta_4 X_{4i} + \beta_5 X_{5i} + \beta_6 X_{6i} + u_i \qquad (1)$$

In all of the statistical models, distance is converted into common logarithms because the relationship between the dependent variable and distance is more curvilinear than linear. In the national model, an additional adaptation is the creation of a set of dummy variables to take into account the regional structure of the data. Results of the stepwise regression procedures are presented for each region and the country as a whole.

The following hypotheses are tested:

1. The number of women per census division who utilize prenatal diagnostic services declines with distance from the nearest centre (DIST);
2. The number of women per census division who utilize prenatal diagnostic services increases with median female income (INC);
3. The number of women per census division who utilize prenatal diagnostic services increases with the number of women with more than a high school education (EDUC);
4. The number of women per census division who utilize prenatal diagnostic services decreases as employment in the primary sector increases (RURAL);
5. The number of women per census division who utilize prenatal diagnostic services decreases as unemployment increases (UNEMP); and
6. The number of women per census division who utilize prenatal diagnostic services increases with the number of family/general practitioners and obstetricians/gynaecologists (MDS).

The choice of the variables included in the ecological models results directly from the lessons learned by other researchers who have examined access to other health services for women. Decreasing utilization as a function of distance from the nearest prenatal diagnostic centre has been widely cited in other studies of access to medical services (Girt 1973; Ingram et al. 1978; Jones and Moon 1987; Joseph 1979; Joseph and Phillips 1984; Meade et al. 1988; Thouez 1987). It is hypothesized that, for a variety of reasons — including access to better information, more time to seek services, and delayed childbearing — utilization will increase with women's relative wealth. Closely related to the income hypothesis is the hypothesis that better-educated women are more likely to utilize prenatal services than poorly educated women. The number of people employed in primary sector industries is a measure of rurality. As rurality increases, utilization decreases, according to many studies of access to other health care services. Unemployment is also often cited as negatively affecting utilization, the rationale being the obverse of the arguments made for the relationship between utilization and income. Recognizing the importance of physicians as referral agents is the rationale for the final hypothesis — where there are more physicians, there are more physicians who are likely to make referrals and therefore more women who are likely to utilize prenatal diagnostic services.

What is missing are measures of religion, ethnicity, values, attitudes, and perceptions. While the census provides measures of religion and ethnicity by census division, they are at best poor measures of values, attitudes, and perceptions because they do not distinguish between people born into a religion who do not practise and people who are strictly observant, or how deep people's ethnic roots are.

Neither the census nor ecological modelling is designed to measure how values, attitudes, or perceptions affect a woman's utilization of prenatal diagnostic services; this would require a totally different approach. As a complement to this study, however, interested readers should see the study by Grant that appears in this volume (Grant 1993).

# Results of the Analysis

## The Atlantic Provinces

### Introduction

There are prenatal diagnostic centres in St. John's, Newfoundland, and Halifax, Nova Scotia (Appendix 1). There are no centres in Prince Edward Island or New Brunswick. This means that women in these two provinces must seek prenatal diagnostic services elsewhere.

### Utilization of Prenatal Diagnostic Services

For both young and older women the geographic pattern of utilization is complex. Higher utilization rates tend to be in more urban census divisions and lower utilization rates tend to be in more rural census divisions. Even when the two age groups are combined, there are some census divisions where the utilization rate was 0 (Figure 1), even though there were older women who had children in every census division in 1990.

There is no census division in the Atlantic provinces with an expected utilization rate of 0 (Figure 2). Among young women in the Atlantic provinces, when observed rates are subtracted from expected rates, there is less than expected utilization in most census divisions. Only in 12 census divisions out of 45 did observed minus expected utilization rates fall into the utilization as expected range. Among older women in the Atlantic provinces the pattern of less than expected utilization is even more stark. There is one census division in Nova Scotia that falls into the much less than expected utilization range; all the census divisions in Newfoundland and Prince Edward Island fall into the less than expected utilization range; and most of the census divisions in New Brunswick and Nova Scotia fall into the less than expected utilization range. Only 7 census divisions out of 187 fall into the utilization as expected range. When both age groups are combined (Figure 3), the pattern of utilization is virtually identical to that of the over-34 age group.

### Physician Location

The distributions of family/general practitioners and obstetricians/gynaecologists are similar in pattern but different in magnitude. Far fewer obstetricians/gynaecologists than family/general practitioners made referrals in 1990. What is perhaps most noteworthy is that there are some census divisions where there were no family/general practitioners who indicated an interest in obstetrics and there were no obstetricians/gynaecologists. Even when the two groups of physicians are combined (Figure 4), there are five census divisions where there were no physicians — generalists or specialists — with an indicated interest in obstetrics.

### Referral Behaviour

In census divisions where there were family/general practitioners with an expressed interest in obstetrics, many made no or very few referrals for prenatal diagnostic services in 1990. Even within the areas where the centres are located, fewer than 20% of family/general practitioners referred women in 1990. What may be even more surprising is that in some of the census divisions where there were obstetricians/gynaecologists in 1990, no referrals were made. When the total number of physicians making referrals is compared with the total number of physicians who potentially might make referrals, the ratios are very small for most census divisions in the Atlantic provinces (Figure 5).

Another way of looking at referral behaviour is to calculate the observed referrals per 100 physicians who potentially might make referrals (Figure 6). Of those census divisions where the number of referrals per 100 physicians is 101 or greater, three out of four contain major urban centres. If we look at Table 2, however, it is clear that Figure 6 provides only a partial view of referral behaviour in the Atlantic provinces. In Newfoundland 88 out of 101 referrals in 1990 were made in the census division containing St. John's. In Nova Scotia 385 out of 396 referrals were made in Halifax County, which contains the city of Halifax. In Prince Edward Island no referrals were made in 1990, and in New Brunswick 44, 21, and 36 out of 109 referrals were made in the census divisions containing Saint John, Moncton, and Fredericton, respectively. Put another way, most referrals are done by a small number of obstetricians and gynaecologists, mainly in the major urban centres.

### An Ecological Model of the Geographic Distribution of Utilization

A stepwise regression for the Atlantic provinces yields the following model:

$$Y_i = -11.44569062 - 26.46532341 \text{ DIST} + 0.01702095 \text{ INC} \qquad (2)$$
$$\qquad\qquad\qquad (8.76299946) \qquad (0.00803947)$$

where
$F = 12.40$ (d.f.=2,42), and
$R^2 = 0.37120588$.

Consistent with the hypotheses outlined earlier, as distance from the nearest prenatal diagnostic centre increases, utilization declines, and as the median income of census divisions increases, utilization increases. The model explains about 37% of the variation in utilization rates in the Atlantic provinces. The independent variables are statistically significant at the 0.05 level or better, and the overall equation is statistically significant at the 0.0001 level.

### *Summary*

Utilization rates are highest in urban areas and appear to decline with distance from the prenatal diagnostic centres in the more rural census divisions. When the pattern of physician location is examined, what is most striking is the largely urban bias of family/general practitioners and obstetricians/gynaecologists. There are rural census divisions where there are no physicians with an indicated interest in obstetrics. Even in urban centres, the number of physicians making referrals is small compared with the number of physicians who potentially might make referrals. When the data are modelled in the form of a multiple regression equation, hypotheses about distance to the nearest prenatal diagnostic centre and median income of census divisions are statistically supported, indicating that as distance increases, utilization decreases, and as the median income of a census division increases, utilization increases. Whether one examines referral patterns from a population- or physician-based perspective or using an ecological model, the results support the view that prenatal diagnostic services in Atlantic Canada are essentially services for urban women and women in areas with higher incomes.

## Quebec

### *Introduction*

One of the Quebec prenatal diagnostic centres sent their data organized by the system of administrative health regions used in that province to plan health services. Therefore all the data used in the analysis of Quebec had to be matched with the health regions.[3] There is one prenatal diagnostic centre in Quebec City and there are two in Montreal (Appendix 1). One centre provided data only on women who received prenatal diagnostic services, and therefore some values in the analysis of physician patterns and referral behaviour are either overestimates or underestimates of the true values.

### *Utilization of Prenatal Diagnostic Services*

Although the magnitude of utilization in Quebec varies by age group, the rates are high in Montreal (health region 6) and the communities surrounding it, and low in the health regions on the periphery of the province (Figure 7).

Among women aged 15-34, expected prenatal service utilization is high in health regions 1, 5-8, 11, 16, and 26. Among women aged 35 and over, only health regions 6, 7, 11, and 26 stand out compared with the other health regions. Expected utilization rates for both age groups combined fall into three distinct groups (Figure 8). In health region 3, containing

122 PND: Background and Impact on Individuals

Table 2. Number of Referrals to Prenatal Diagnostic Centres, by Province and Census Division, Atlantic Provinces, 1990

| Census division | FPs/GPs | OBs/GYNs | Total physicians | FPs/GPs making referrals | OBs/GYNs making referrals | Total making referrals | Referrals by FPs/GPs | Referrals by OBs/GYNs | Total referrals |
|---|---|---|---|---|---|---|---|---|---|
| **Newfoundland** | | | | | | | | | |
| 1 | 48 | 19 | 67 | 4 | 8 | 12 | 5 | 83 | 88 |
| 2 | 2 | 3 | 5 | 0 | 0 | 0 | 0 | 0 | 0 |
| 3 | 0 | 0 | 0 | 0 | 0 | 0 | 0 | 0 | 0 |
| 4 | 1 | 2 | 3 | 0 | 0 | 0 | 0 | 0 | 0 |
| 5 | 7 | 3 | 10 | 1 | 3 | 4 | 3 | 8 | 11 |
| 6 | 7 | 3 | 10 | 0 | 0 | 0 | 0 | 0 | 0 |
| 7 | 3 | 1 | 4 | 1 | 0 | 1 | 1 | 0 | 1 |
| 8 | 8 | 2 | 10 | 1 | 0 | 1 | 1 | 0 | 1 |
| 9 | 1 | 0 | 1 | 0 | 0 | 0 | 0 | 0 | 0 |
| 10 | 6 | 0 | 6 | 0 | 0 | 0 | 0 | 0 | 0 |
| Total | 83 | 33 | 116 | 7 | 11 | 18 | 10 | 91 | 101 |
| **New Brunswick** | | | | | | | | | |
| 1 | 22 | 10 | 32 | 0 | 2 | 2 | 0 | 44 | 44 |
| 2 | 3 | 0 | 3 | 0 | 0 | 0 | 0 | 0 | 0 |
| 3 | 1 | 0 | 1 | 0 | 0 | 0 | 0 | 0 | 0 |
| 4 | 0 | 0 | 0 | 0 | 0 | 0 | 0 | 0 | 0 |
| 5 | 4 | 1 | 5 | 0 | 0 | 0 | 0 | 0 | 0 |
| 6 | 8 | 1 | 9 | 0 | 0 | 0 | 0 | 0 | 0 |
| 7 | 38 | 11 | 49 | 0 | 5 | 5 | 0 | 21 | 21 |
| 8 | 2 | 0 | 2 | 0 | 0 | 0 | 0 | 0 | 0 |
| 9 | 5 | 3 | 8 | 0 | 1 | 1 | 0 | 1 | 1 |

# A Demographic and Geographic Analysis of Users of PND Services

|  | | | | | | | | |
|---|---|---|---|---|---|---|---|---|
| 11 | 6 | 0 | 6 | 0 | 0 | 0 | 0 | 0 |
| 12 | 3 | 1 | 4 | 0 | 0 | 0 | 0 | 0 |
| 13 | 7 | 2 | 9 | 0 | 1 | 1 | 7 | 7 |
| 14 | 5 | 0 | 5 | 0 | 0 | 0 | 0 | 0 |
| 15 | 10 | 3 | 13 | 0 | 0 | 0 | 0 | 0 |
| Total | 137 | 39 | 176 | 0 | 15 | 15 | 109 | 109 |

## Nova Scotia

|  | | | | | | | | |
|---|---|---|---|---|---|---|---|---|
| 1 | 0 | 0 | 0 | 0 | 0 | 0 | 0 | 0 |
| 2 | 0 | 2 | 2 | 0 | 1 | 1 | 2 | 2 |
| 3 | 0 | 0 | 0 | 0 | 0 | 0 | 0 | 0 |
| 4 | 2 | 0 | 2 | 0 | 0 | 0 | 0 | 0 |
| 5 | 3 | 0 | 3 | 0 | 0 | 0 | 0 | 0 |
| 6 | 9 | 1 | 10 | 0 | 0 | 0 | 0 | 0 |
| 7 | 12 | 6 | 18 | 0 | 0 | 0 | 0 | 0 |
| 8 | 5 | 2 | 7 | 0 | 0 | 0 | 0 | 0 |
| 9 | 94 | 39 | 133 | 0 | 10 | 10 | 385 | 385 |
| 10 | 5 | 3 | 8 | 0 | 2 | 2 | 5 | 5 |
| 11 | 0 | 1 | 1 | 0 | 0 | 0 | 0 | 0 |
| 12 | 8 | 4 | 12 | 1 | 1 | 2 | 3 | 4 |
| 13 | 1 | 0 | 1 | 0 | 0 | 0 | 0 | 0 |
| 14 | 2 | 4 | 6 | 0 | 0 | 0 | 0 | 0 |
| 15 | 0 | 0 | 0 | 0 | 0 | 0 | 0 | 0 |
| 16 | 1 | 0 | 1 | 0 | 0 | 0 | 0 | 0 |
| 17 | 8 | 5 | 13 | 0 | 0 | 0 | 0 | 0 |
| 18 | 2 | 0 | 2 | 0 | 0 | 0 | 0 | 0 |
| Total | 152 | 67 | 219 | 1 | 14 | 15 | 395 | 396 |

Table 2. (cont'd)

| Census division | FPs/GPs | OBs/GYNs | Total physicians | FPs/GPs making referrals | OBs/GYNs making referrals | Total making referrals | Referrals by FPs/GPs | Referrals by OBs/GYNs | Total referrals |
|---|---|---|---|---|---|---|---|---|---|
| | | | | Prince Edward Island | | | | | |
| 1 | 3 | 0 | 3 | 0 | 0 | 0 | 0 | 0 | 0 |
| 2 | 12 | 10 | 22 | 0 | 0 | 0 | 0 | 0 | 0 |
| 3 | 7 | 2 | 9 | 0 | 0 | 0 | 0 | 0 | 0 |
| Total | 22 | 12 | 34 | 0 | 0 | 0 | 0 | 0 | 0 |
| Regional total | 394 | 151 | 545 | 8 | 40 | 48 | 11 | 595 | 606 |

Trois-Rivières, the expected rate of utilization is relatively low; in health regions 6 and 11 the expected rate of utilization is very high; and in the remaining health regions expected utilization falls into the middle range. Health regions 6 and 11 are, however, very different from each other. Health region 6 is Montreal, whereas health region 11 is mainly a northern landscape dotted with isolated communities of Native peoples.

When observed utilization is compared with expected utilization, there is a strong contrast between the health regions along the Ottawa River and the far north, and those in southern and eastern Quebec (Figure 9). Health regions 7 and 11 fall within the less than expected utilization range, but likely for very different reasons. Health region 7 contains Hull and many other communities where women live who are employed and receive their health care in Ottawa. This would lower the observed utilization rates, leading to a greater than expected difference between the observed and the expected utilization rates. Health region 11, which has a small population of mostly Native peoples living in isolated communities, had less than expected utilization, which is likely indicative of real differences between observed and expected utilization. Fertility behaviour there is significantly different from that in the southern, urbanized parts of the province; Native peoples have among the highest fertility rates in Canada, whereas the population of the south has among the lowest.

### Physician Location

The largest number of family/general practitioners with an expressed interest in obstetrics is in Montreal (health region 6) and the health regions surrounding it. Obstetricians/gynaecologists are even more concentrated in health regions 3, 6, and 26 — the health regions of Montreal, Quebec City, and Sherbrooke, the three largest cities in the province. When the total number of physicians is considered, the urban concentration is also pronounced (Figure 10).

### Referral Behaviour

Given the strong urban bias in the geographic distribution of physicians, it should not be surprising that the physicians making referrals are heavily concentrated in Montreal and the health regions surrounding it (Figure 11). This urban bias in the Quebec data would have been even greater except for the lack of referral data from the prenatal diagnostic centre in Quebec City.

When the number of referrals per 100 physicians is considered (Figure 12), only Montreal and health region 11 have rates above 200, but for very different reasons. In Montreal, 679 physicians made 2 998 referrals (Table 3). In contrast, in health region 11, where there are only 10 family/general practitioners with an expressed interest in obstetrics and no obstetricians/gynaecologists, only one physician made any referrals (27).

### An Ecological Model of the Geographic Distribution of Utilization

Extreme caution should be exercised in drawing inferences from a multiple regression model based on only 13 observations. Nevertheless, stepwise regression yielded a model that supports what has been described. The equation for the model is

$$Y_1 = 327.51463173 - 40.1830426 \text{ DIST} \qquad (3)$$
$$(13.9391193)$$

where
$F$ = 8.31 (d.f.=1,10), and
$R^2$ = 0.45385831.

Consistent with the distance hypothesis, the equation indicates that as distance from the nearest prenatal diagnostic centre increases, utilization decreases. The model explains about 45% of the variation in utilization rates in Quebec. The independent variable is statistically significant at better than the 0.05 level, and the overall equation is statistically significant at better than the 0.01 level.

### Summary

There are clearly two Quebecs where the utilization of prenatal diagnostic services is concerned. There is urban southern Quebec, where observed and expected utilization rates are not far apart, where most of the referring physicians are concentrated in Montreal, Sherbrooke, and Quebec City, and where most of the referrals are in Montreal and to a lesser extent in Quebec City (although this can only be surmised, given the reporting problems there). The other Quebec consists of the scattered and isolated communities of mainly Native peoples in the north, where the number of women who utilized prenatal diagnostic services is very small, and where there are few physicians and even fewer who are likely to refer someone to travel to Montreal or Quebec City for prenatal diagnostic services. These findings are given greater currency by the ecological model, which supports the distance hypothesis (i.e., utilization rates decline with increasing distance from the nearest prenatal diagnostic centre).

## Ontario

### Introduction

Ontario is made up of Metropolitan Toronto, regional municipalities such as Ottawa-Carleton, counties such as Middlesex, which contains London, and districts such as Kenora. It is the only province with a network of prenatal diagnostic centres (Appendix 1); there are nine of them spread from London in the southwest to Ottawa in the east.

Table 3. Referrals to Prenatal Diagnostic Centres, by Health Region, Quebec, 1990

| Health region | FPs/GPs | OBs/GYNs | Total physicians | FPs/GPs making referrals | OBs/GYNs making referrals | Total making referrals | Referrals by FPs/GPs | Referrals by OBs/GYNs | Total referrals |
|---|---|---|---|---|---|---|---|---|---|
| 1 | 41 | 18 | 59 | 1 | 4 | 5 | 2 | 8 | 10 |
| 2 | 25 | 19 | 44 | 0 | 1 | 1 | 1 | 1 | 2 |
| 3 | 147 | 112 | 259 | 10 | 2 | 12 | 13 | 2 | 15 |
| 4 | 62 | 26 | 88 | 14 | 15 | 29 | 34 | 48 | 82 |
| 5 | 121 | 23 | 144 | 14 | 16 | 30 | 36 | 92 | 128 |
| 6 | 415 | 264 | 679 | 33 | 183 | 216 | 180 | 2 818 | 2 998 |
| 7 | 55 | 9 | 64 | 3 | 1 | 4 | 3 | 1 | 4 |
| 8 | 37 | 10 | 47 | 7 | 2 | 9 | 13 | 11 | 24 |
| 9 | 19 | 3 | 22 | 2 | 1 | 3 | 4 | 1 | 5 |
| 11 | 10 | 0 | 10 | 1 | 0 | 1 | 27 | 0 | 27 |
| 16 | 58 | 25 | 83 | 17 | 13 | 30 | 48 | 92 | 140 |
| 26 | 129 | 52 | 181 | 9 | 38 | 47 | 18 | 306 | 324 |
| Total | 1 119 | 561 | 1 680 | 111 | 276 | 387 | 379 | 3 380 | 3 759 |

## Utilization of Prenatal Diagnostic Services

The observed rates of utilization of prenatal diagnostic services by women aged 15-34 in the census divisions surrounding Metropolitan Toronto are relatively high. They are also high in a small number of rural counties such as Prince Edward, Northumberland, Victoria, and Haliburton and Bruce. Elsewhere, rates are fairly uniform at 1-150 per 100 000 women in the 15-34 age group. For women aged 35 or more, again the census divisions surrounding Metropolitan Toronto stand out, as do Prince Edward County, Frontenac County, and the Regional Municipality of Ottawa-Carleton. When the two age groups are combined (Figure 13), the geographic pattern of the rates resembles that among women aged 15-34.

In contrast, the expected utilization rates among women aged 15-34 are uniformly high for most of the province. For women aged 35 and over expected rates are high in Metropolitan Toronto and the surrounding census divisions, in the larger urban centres of southern Ontario (the census divisions containing London, Kitchener-Waterloo, and Hamilton), in Frontenac County, and in the Regional Municipality of Ottawa-Carleton. Also striking are the high expected rates in the Regional Municipality of Sudbury and in Kenora. With slightly lower expected utilization rates, the geographic distribution for all women (Figure 14) is similar to that for women aged 35 and over.

When the observed and expected utilization rates among women aged 15-34 are compared, there is, as one might anticipate, less than expected utilization in most of the census divisions in northern Ontario and rural southern Ontario. Utilization is as expected in the Thunder Bay census division in northern Ontario, in a string of counties along the shores of Lake Huron, and in most of the heavily populated census divisions in southern Ontario, including Metropolitan Toronto, Hamilton, Kingston, and Ottawa. The census divisions directly to the east and west of Metropolitan Toronto and Prince Edward County stand out as falling into the more than expected utilization range. For women aged 35 and over, all of the census divisions in northern Ontario fall into the less than expected utilization range. Most of the census divisions in southern Ontario fall into the range of utilization as expected, except for a block in the southwest, Metropolitan Toronto, and the Regional Municipality of York, which fall into the less than expected utilization range. Only Prince Edward County and the Regional Municipality of Ottawa-Carleton fall into the more than expected utilization and much more than expected utilization ranges, respectively. When total observed and expected utilization are compared (Figure 15), the geographic distributions are much the same as those for women aged 35 and over.

## Physician Location

The geographic distribution of family/general practitioners with an expressed interest in obstetrics correlates with the geographical distribution of the population. The census divisions with the largest populations, such as Metropolitan Toronto, the Regional Municipality of Ottawa-Carleton, the

Regional Municipality of Hamilton-Wentworth, and Middlesex County (where London is located), have the largest number of family/general practitioners with an expressed interest in obstetrics. It is also interesting to note that there is at least one in each of these census divisions. The geographic distribution of obstetricians/gynaecologists is much more concentrated in the largest urban centres of Ontario. Even in Ontario, however, there are some census divisions with no obstetricians/gynaecologists. When the two groups of physicians are combined, the correlation between the geographic distribution of physicians and that of the population is clearly evident (Figure 16).

## *Referral Behaviour*

Referrals to prenatal diagnostic centres among family/general practitioners in Ontario fall into three groups. First, in the north and in rural southern Ontario the ratios of physicians making referrals to the total number of physicians in the census division are relatively high. This is because these census divisions have only a small number of family/general practitioners, more than 40% of whom make referrals, and each makes only a small number of referrals. Algoma District and Haldimand-Norfolk are the two most notable examples of this pattern. Second, there are the census divisions with the largest populations in Ontario, where many family/general practitioners have an expressed interest in obstetrics and over 20% are making referrals. This pattern occurs in the regional municipalities of Peel and Halton. Third, there is another group of census divisions in rural southern Ontario and in northern Ontario where the number of family physicians and general practitioners making referrals is very small, even compared with the small total number of family/general practitioners.

The referral behaviour of obstetricians/gynaecologists is equally complex. In many of the census divisions from Sudbury to Windsor, whether there are a few or many obstetricians/gynaecologists in a census division, more than half of them are making referrals to prenatal diagnostic centres. But there is also a small number of mainly rural census divisions in southern Ontario and the remainder of northern Ontario where the number of obstetricians/gynaecologists is small and there is little referral.

When the two groups of physicians are combined, the ratios of physicians making referrals to the total number of physicians who potentially might make referrals is relatively high and widespread throughout southern Ontario in comparison with other regions of Canada (Figure 17). The highest number of referrals per 100 physicians is found in the census divisions surrounding Metropolitan Toronto, the Regional Municipality of Ottawa-Carleton, Essex County (including Windsor), and Lambton County (Figure 18). The high rate in Lambton County reflects the relatively small number of physicians who are making referrals. For most of the remainder of the province the referral rate per 100 physicians is fairly uniform.

In Table 4 one can see even more clearly how the referral patterns in Ontario are skewed in the direction of urban centres, but also how a small number of physicians can have a disproportionate impact. For example, in Lambton County (census division 38) there are nine obstetricians/ gynaecologists. Six of these made referrals in 1990, and these six physicians made 57 out of the total of 58 referrals made by all physicians in the county in 1990.

## An Ecological Model of the Geographic Distribution of Utilization

For the Ontario data, the fitted multiple regression model takes the following form:

$$Y_i = -178.76974885 + 0.02459397 \text{ EDUC} - 0.06282288 \text{ UNEMP} \quad (4)$$
$$\phantom{Y_i = -178.76974885 + } (0.00343456) \phantom{\text{ EDUC}} (0.01069051)$$

where
$F = 30.64$ (d.f.=2,45), and
$R^2 = 0.57656996$.

In this case the number of women who receive prenatal diagnostic services per census division increases as the number with more than a high school education increases, and decreases in census divisions where female unemployment increases. The signs on the parameter estimates are consistent with the hypotheses. The model explains almost 58% of the variance in the dependent variable. The equation is statistically significant at the 0.0001 level, and the parameter estimates are statistically significant at the 0.0001 level as well.

## Summary

Ontario has the most developed system of prenatal diagnostic centres in the country. In southern Ontario they are spread from London in the southwest to Ottawa in the east. There are therefore higher rates of utilization of prenatal diagnostic services, because there is a greater number of physicians making referrals. The geographic distribution of utilization and referrals appears to correlate with the geographic distribution of the population to a very great extent. There are, however, anomalous rural regions where an individual physician or a small number of physicians can make a substantial difference in utilization or referral rates.

Unlike most other provinces, where prenatal diagnostic centres can be found only in one or two locations, in southern Ontario distance is not likely to be a great barrier to access to prenatal diagnostic services. Support for this view can be found in the ecological model, where the distance variable did not enter the final equation. The socioeconomic condition of women appears to be a better predictor of utilization.

## Table 4. Referrals to Prenatal Diagnostic Centres, by Census Division, Ontario, 1990

| Census division | FPs/GPs | OBs/GYNs | Total physicians | FPs/GPs making referrals | OBs/GYNs making referrals | Total making referrals | Referrals by FPs/GPs | Referrals by OBs/GYNs | Total referrals |
|---|---|---|---|---|---|---|---|---|---|
| 1 | 2 | 6 | 28 | 3 | 4 | 7 | 3 | 15 | 18 |
| 2 | 13 | 1 | 14 | 2 | 1 | 3 | 2 | 8 | 10 |
| 6 | 331 | 88 | 419 | 73 | 55 | 128 | 178 | 654 | 832 |
| 7 | 14 | 3 | 17 | 1 | 2 | 3 | 1 | 4 | 5 |
| 9 | 18 | 1 | 19 | 8 | 1 | 9 | 12 | 1 | 13 |
| 10 | 107 | 23 | 130 | 18 | 11 | 29 | 41 | 136 | 177 |
| 11 | 12 | 0 | 12 | 2 | 0 | 2 | 3 | 0 | 3 |
| 12 | 30 | 12 | 42 | 8 | 5 | 13 | 12 | 34 | 46 |
| 13 | 9 | 0 | 9 | 1 | 0 | 1 | 1 | 0 | 1 |
| 14 | 12 | 2 | 14 | 2 | 1 | 3 | 4 | 4 | 8 |
| 15 | 54 | 9 | 63 | 9 | 7 | 16 | 18 | 23 | 41 |
| 16 | 5 | 0 | 5 | 1 | 0 | 1 | 1 | 0 | 1 |
| 18 | 63 | 14 | 77 | 25 | 12 | 37 | 76 | 170 | 246 |
| 19 | 134 | 22 | 156 | 27 | 17 | 44 | 41 | 242 | 283 |
| 20 | 718 | 259 | 977 | 143 | 177 | 320 | 375 | 1 645 | 2 020 |
| 21 | 143 | 34 | 177 | 65 | 28 | 93 | 194 | 499 | 693 |
| 22 | 7 | 2 | 9 | 2 | 2 | 4 | 2 | 7 | 9 |
| 23 | 55 | 14 | 69 | 12 | 9 | 21 | 18 | 26 | 44 |
| 24 | 125 | 24 | 149 | 57 | 21 | 78 | 38 | 214 | 352 |
| 25 | 220 | 43 | 263 | 54 | 22 | 76 | 110 | 148 | 258 |

132  PND: Background and Impact on Individuals

Table 4. (cont'd)

| Census division | FPs/GPs | OBs/GYNs | Total physicians | FPs/GPs making referrals | OBs/GYNs making referrals | Total making referrals | Referrals by FPs/GPs | Referrals by OBs/GYNs | Total referrals |
|---|---|---|---|---|---|---|---|---|---|
| 26 | 85  | 30 | 115 | 11 | 18 | 29 | 40  | 94  | 134 |
| 28 | 9   | 0  | 9   | 4  | 0  | 4  | 8   | 0   | 8   |
| 29 | 30  | 10 | 40  | 5  | 5  | 10 | 6   | 16  | 22  |
| 30 | 117 | 23 | 140 | 28 | 16 | 44 | 53  | 69  | 122 |
| 31 | 24  | 2  | 26  | 5  | 0  | 5  | 7   | 0   | 7   |
| 32 | 22  | 2  | 24  | 2  | 2  | 4  | 3   | 10  | 13  |
| 34 | 22  | 0  | 22  | 4  | 0  | 4  | 0   | 0   | 0   |
| 36 | 19  | 4  | 23  | 7  | 2  | 9  | 7   | 10  | 17  |
| 37 | 36  | 20 | 56  | 5  | 13 | 18 | 13  | 105 | 118 |
| 38 | 14  | 9  | 23  | 1  | 6  | 7  | 1   | 57  | 58  |
| 39 | 175 | 36 | 211 | 48 | 22 | 70 | 127 | 188 | 315 |
| 40 | 17  | 1  | 18  | 2  | 1  | 3  | 5   | 3   | 8   |
| 41 | 17  | 1  | 18  | 3  | 1  | 4  | 4   | 3   | 7   |
| 42 | 35  | 4  | 39  | 8  | 3  | 11 | 9   | 10  | 19  |
| 43 | 69  | 10 | 79  | 23 | 8  | 31 | 32  | 34  | 66  |
| 44 | 12  | 1  | 13  | 1  | 1  | 2  | 2   | 5   | 7   |
| 46 | 3   | 0  | 3   | 1  | 0  | 1  | 1   | 0   | 1   |
| 47 | 19  | 4  | 23  | 3  | 3  | 6  | 4   | 5   | 9   |
| 51 | 6   | 0  | 6   | 2  | 0  | 2  | 3   | 0   | 3   |
| 52 | 32  | 9  | 41  | 4  | 5  | 9  | 4   | 15  | 19  |
| 54 | 17  | 0  | 17  | 1  | 0  | 1  | 1   | 0   | 1   |
| 56 | 27  | 4  | 31  | 2  | 0  | 2  | 2   | 0   | 2   |
| 57 | 5   | 10 | 15  | 3  | 3  | 6  | 3   | 8   | 11  |
| 58 | 44  | 13 | 57  | 7  | 2  | 9  | 11  | 11  | 22  |

|  |  |  |  |  |  |  |  |  |  |
|---|---|---|---|---|---|---|---|---|---|
| 59 | 14 | 0 | 14 | 1 | 1 | 2 | 1 | 4 | 5 |
| 60 | 34 | 2 | 36 | 2 | 0 | 2 | 3 | 0 | 3 |
| Total | 3 020 | 757 | 3 784 | 698 | 491 | 1 189 | 1 583 | 4 490 | 6 073 |

## The Prairie Provinces

### Introduction

There are five prenatal diagnostic centres in the Prairie provinces, one each in Winnipeg, Regina, Saskatoon, Edmonton, and Calgary (Appendix 1). Because the Calgary prenatal diagnostic centre did not provide any data, women who utilized prenatal diagnostic services and physicians who made referrals in southern Alberta in 1990 are underrepresented in our analysis.

### Utilization of Prenatal Diagnostic Services

In Manitoba, women aged 15-34 have high rates of utilization of prenatal diagnostic services. One cluster of high rates centres on Winnipeg and the other centres on Brandon. Utilization rates are also relatively high in northern Manitoba. Across Saskatchewan and central and northern Alberta, utilization rates are fairly uniform. For women aged 35 and over, utilization rates are high in Winnipeg in southern Manitoba and in northern Manitoba. In Saskatchewan, the higher rates are in the census divisions containing Regina (S6) and Saskatoon (S11). In Alberta, the rates are high in the census division containing Edmonton. When the two age groups are combined (Figure 19), the geographic distribution is similar to the geographic distribution of women aged 35 and over.

When expected rates of prenatal service utilization are calculated for women aged 15-34, the rates are higher mainly in the census divisions in the north of each province. This can be partly explained by the relative concentrations there of Native peoples, whose age structure is younger and fertility rates are higher compared with those in the south. For women aged 35 and over there is a crescent of census divisions in the south with relatively low expected utilization rates. In contrast, in the remaining census divisions, which include the major population centres, the rates of expected utilization are relatively high. The low rates are found mainly in census divisions that are almost totally rural and whose populations have been declining during the 1980s. When the two age groups are combined, the rates in this cluster of census divisions are still low, but most of the census divisions in the three provinces have relatively high utilization rates (Figure 20).

When the observed and expected utilization rates among women aged 15-34 are compared, only in southern Manitoba and in the census divisions containing Regina and Saskatoon are they as expected or more than expected. Virtually all of the remaining census divisions in the three provinces fall into the less than expected range, although in southern Alberta this may be because of reporting problems.

There are even fewer census divisions where utilization is as expected among women aged 35 and over, and all of them are in southern Manitoba and Saskatchewan. The rest fall within the less than expected range, and two northern census divisions in Saskatchewan and Alberta fall within the much less than expected range.

When the two age groups are combined, there are only 11 census divisions where utilization is as expected (Figure 21), all of them in southern Manitoba and Saskatchewan. The rest fall into the less than expected utilization range, and census division S18 falls into the much less than expected utilization range.

## Physician Location

The distribution of family/general practitioners with an expressed interest in obstetrics is concentrated in the major urban centres of the Prairie provinces. The five census divisions that fall into the high ranges are those containing Winnipeg, Regina, Saskatoon, Calgary, and Edmonton. There is also a small number of census divisions where there are no family/general practitioners with an expressed interest in obstetrics.

Obstetricians/gynaecologists are even more concentrated in the census divisions containing Winnipeg, Calgary, and Edmonton. What is perhaps more striking is that in every province there are several census divisions with no obstetricians/gynaecologists. Even when the two groups of physicians are combined, there are five census divisions in Manitoba, three in Saskatchewan, and one in Alberta where there are no physicians with an expressed interest in obstetrics (Figure 22).

## Referral Behaviour

The referral behaviour of family/general practitioners making referrals compared with that of family/general practitioners with an expressed interest in obstetrics is complex. For the most part, the census divisions where more than 20% of family/general practitioners made referrals are in the south of all three provinces. With two exceptions in Manitoba, the census divisions where more than 20% of the obstetricians/gynaecologists made referrals either contain or are adjacent to a major urban centre. When the two groups of physicians are combined, the census divisions where more than 40% of physicians made referrals are all in the south of the three provinces (Figure 23). With the exception of one census division in Manitoba and one in Saskatchewan, the only other census divisions where referrals per 100 physicians were above 100 are the census divisions containing Winnipeg, Regina, Saskatoon, and Edmonton (Figure 24).

The dominance of physicians making referrals in Winnipeg, Regina, Saskatoon, and Edmonton cannot be understated (Table 5). In Manitoba, 92% of the referrals were made by physicians in Winnipeg. In Saskatchewan, physicians in Regina and Saskatoon accounted for almost 97% of referrals to prenatal diagnostic centres. Of the referrals to the Edmonton prenatal diagnostic centre, 83% were by physicians in Edmonton.

## Table 5. Referrals to Prenatal Diagnostic Centres, by Province and Census Division, Prairie Provinces, 1990

| Census division | FPs/GPs | OBs/GYNs | Total physicians | FPs/GPs making referrals | OBs/GYNs making referrals | Total making referrals | Referrals by FPs/GPs | Referrals by OBs/GYNs | Total referrals |
|---|---|---|---|---|---|---|---|---|---|
| Manitoba | | | | | | | | | |
| 1 | 6 | 1 | 7 | 1 | 0 | 1 | 1 | 0 | 1 |
| 2 | 2 | 0 | 2 | 0 | 0 | 0 | 0 | 0 | 0 |
| 3 | 19 | 0 | 19 | 3 | 0 | 3 | 7 | 0 | 7 |
| 4 | 2 | 0 | 2 | 1 | 0 | 1 | 1 | 0 | 1 |
| 5 | 4 | 0 | 4 | 1 | 0 | 1 | 1 | 0 | 1 |
| 6 | 0 | 0 | 0 | 0 | 0 | 0 | 0 | 0 | 0 |
| 7 | 8 | 6 | 14 | 4 | 4 | 8 | 10 | 25 | 35 |
| 8 | 0 | 0 | 0 | 0 | 0 | 0 | 0 | 0 | 0 |
| 9 | 4 | 0 | 4 | 3 | 0 | 3 | 3 | 0 | 3 |
| 10 | 0 | 0 | 0 | 0 | 0 | 0 | 0 | 0 | 0 |
| 11 | 169 | 57 | 226 | 48 | 35 | 83 | 90 | 534 | 624 |
| 12 | 0 | 0 | 0 | 0 | 0 | 0 | 0 | 0 | 0 |
| 13 | 3 | 1 | 4 | 1 | 0 | 1 | 2 | 0 | 2 |
| 14 | 1 | 0 | 1 | 0 | 0 | 0 | 0 | 0 | 0 |
| 15 | 3 | 0 | 3 | 0 | 0 | 0 | 0 | 0 | 0 |
| 16 | 0 | 0 | 0 | 0 | 0 | 0 | 0 | 0 | 0 |
| 17 | 8 | 0 | 8 | 1 | 0 | 1 | 1 | 0 | 1 |
| 18 | 1 | 1 | 2 | 0 | 0 | 0 | 0 | 0 | 0 |
| 19 | 0 | 0 | 0 | 0 | 0 | 0 | 0 | 0 | 0 |
| 20 | 1 | 0 | 1 | 1 | 0 | 1 | 1 | 0 | 1 |
| 21 | 3 | 1 | 4 | 0 | 1 | 1 | 0 | 4 | 4 |
| 22 | 1 | 1 | 2 | 0 | 0 | 0 | 0 | 0 | 0 |
| 23 | 1 | 0 | 1 | 0 | 0 | 0 | 0 | 0 | 0 |
| Total | 236 | 68 | 304 | 64 | 40 | 104 | 117 | 563 | 680 |

| | Saskatchewan | | | | | | | | |
|---|---|---|---|---|---|---|---|---|---|
| 1 | 0 | 1 | 1 | 0 | 0 | 0 | 0 | 0 | 0 |
| 2 | 1 | 0 | 1 | 0 | 0 | 0 | 0 | 0 | 0 |
| 3 | 1 | 0 | 1 | 0 | 0 | 0 | 0 | 0 | 0 |
| 4 | 0 | 0 | 0 | 0 | 0 | 0 | 0 | 0 | 0 |
| 5 | 0 | 0 | 0 | 0 | 0 | 0 | 0 | 0 | 0 |
| 6 | 56 | 15 | 71 | 5 | 9 | 14 | 35 | 138 | 173 |
| 7 | 5 | 2 | 7 | 0 | 0 | 0 | 0 | 0 | 0 |
| 8 | 2 | 4 | 6 | 0 | 0 | 0 | 0 | 0 | 0 |
| 9 | 0 | 3 | 3 | 0 | 1 | 0 | 0 | 2 | 2 |
| 10 | 0 | 0 | 0 | 0 | 0 | 1 | 0 | 0 | 0 |
| 11 | 65 | 23 | 88 | 4 | 15 | 19 | 6 | 120 | 126 |
| 12 | 1 | 0 | 1 | 0 | 0 | 0 | 0 | 0 | 0 |
| 13 | 1 | 1 | 1 | 1 | 0 | 1 | 2 | 0 | 0 |
| 14 | 8 | 3 | 9 | 0 | 0 | 0 | 0 | 0 | 6 |
| 15 | 8 | 1 | 11 | 0 | 2 | 2 | 0 | 6 | 0 |
| 16 | 3 | 1 | 4 | 0 | 0 | 0 | 0 | 0 | 0 |
| 17 | 1 | 1 | 2 | 0 | 0 | 0 | 0 | 0 | 0 |
| 18 | 5 | 0 | 5 | 0 | 0 | 0 | 0 | 0 | 0 |
| Total | 157 | 54 | 211 | 10 | 27 | 37 | 43 | 266 | 309 |
| | Alberta | | | | | | | | |
| 1 | 22 | 4 | 26 | 1 | 0 | 1 | 2 | 0 | 2 |
| 2 | 43 | 6 | 49 | 2 | 0 | 2 | 3 | 0 | 3 |
| 3 | 7 | 1 | 8 | 1 | 0 | 1 | 1 | 0 | 1 |
| 4 | 2 | 0 | 2 | 0 | 0 | 0 | 0 | 0 | 0 |
| 5 | 11 | 3 | 14 | 0 | 0 | 0 | 0 | 1 | 0 |
| 6 | 361 | 53 | 414 | 9 | 1 | 10 | 35 | 1 | 36 |
| 7 | 4 | 1 | 5 | 0 | 1 | 1 | 0 | 2 | 2 |

Table 5. (cont'd)

| Census division | FPs/GPs | OBs/GYNs | Total physicians | FPs/GPs making referrals | OBs/GYNs making referrals | Total making referrals | Referrals by FPs/GPs | Referrals by OBs/GYNs | Total referrals |
|---|---|---|---|---|---|---|---|---|---|
| | | | | | Alberta | | | | |
| 8 | 28 | 8 | 36 | 2 | 0 | 2 | 18 | 0 | 18 |
| 9 | 3 | 0 | 3 | 2 | 0 | 2 | 2 | 0 | 2 |
| 10 | 3 | 2 | 5 | 0 | 1 | 1 | 0 | 4 | 4 |
| 11 | 246 | 78 | 324 | 26 | 39 | 65 | 43 | 347 | 390 |
| 12 | 5 | 1 | 6 | 1 | 0 | 1 | 2 | 0 | 2 |
| 13 | 3 | 0 | 3 | 0 | 0 | 0 | 0 | 0 | 0 |
| 14 | 3 | 0 | 3 | 1 | 0 | 1 | 1 | 0 | 1 |
| 15 | 15 | 0 | 15 | 3 | 0 | 3 | 8 | 0 | 8 |
| 16 | 9 | 2 | 11 | 0 | 0 | 0 | 0 | 0 | 0 |
| 17 | 7 | 3 | 10 | 0 | 0 | 0 | 0 | 0 | 0 |
| 18 | 0 | 0 | 0 | 0 | 0 | 0 | 0 | 0 | 0 |
| 19 | 12 | 1 | 13 | 2 | 0 | 2 | 2 | 0 | 2 |
| Total | 784 | 163 | 947 | 50 | 42 | 92 | 117 | 354 | 471 |
| Regional total | 1 177 | 285 | 1 462 | 124 | 109 | 233 | 277 | 1 183 | 1 460 |

## An Ecological Model of the Geographic Distribution of Utilization

Fitting a model for the Prairie provinces is problematic because of the lack of data on utilization in southern Alberta. To gauge the impact of this lack of data, two models are fitted. In the first all of the census divisions in Alberta are included, and in the second census divisions A1-A7 and A15 are deleted, leaving only those census divisions that are adjacent to the census division containing Edmonton or north of Edmonton.

The form of the equation of the first model is

$$Y_1 = 316.85688537 - 46.32911691 \text{ DIST} \tag{5}$$
$$(12.21708674)$$

where
$F$ = 14.38 (d.f.=1,58), and
$R^2$ = 0.19867874.

In this case, only about 20% of the variance in the geographic distribution of utilization of prenatal diagnostic services is accounted for by the independent variable, distance. The model and the parameter estimates are, however, statistically significant at the 0.0004 level, and the distance hypothesis is again supported (e.g., as distance from the nearest prenatal diagnostic centre increases, utilization decreases).

When the census divisions of southern Alberta are deleted, the regression equation takes the following form:

$$Y_1 = 307.41913048 - 0.00170300 \text{ AGR} - 30.55297663 \text{ DIST} \tag{6}$$
$$(0.0007016) \quad\quad (13.49762531)$$

where
$F$ = 7.80 (d.f.=2,49), and
$R^2$ = 0.24152882.

Here the amount of variance in utilization explained increases to slightly over 24% and, interestingly, the rurality hypothesis (as rurality increases, utilization decreases) and distance hypothesis are supported. The parameters are statistically significant at the 0.05 level, and the overall equation is statistically significant at the 0.01 level.

## Summary

The patterns of utilization of prenatal diagnostic services and referrals made by physicians in the Prairie provinces are dominated by the four largest urban centres: Winnipeg, Regina, Saskatoon, and Edmonton. In the census divisions containing Winnipeg and those south of it, utilization rates are relatively high compared with most other census divisions in the three provinces. Although utilization rates tend to be lower in the north of the three provinces, expected utilization in these areas tends to be higher than in the southern census divisions of the provinces. These northern census divisions have relatively larger populations of Native peoples compared with most southern census divisions. What is also unique to the Prairie provinces is the pattern in the census divisions mainly in southern Saskatchewan but also stretching into Manitoba and Alberta. Here the populations are mainly rural and on the decline, and because of this unique demographic trend, not only is utilization low but expected utilization is also low.

The four major urban centres include most of the family/general practitioners with an expressed interest in obstetrics and most obstetricians/gynaecologists. Needless to say, these physicians make most of the referrals to prenatal diagnostic centres in the three provinces.

Taken together, these observations suggest that women living outside the four major centres who need prenatal diagnostic services are at a severe disadvantage and very unlikely to get referral. This view is lent support by the ecological model that includes all the census divisions, indicating that as distance from the nearest prenatal diagnostic centre increases, utilization rates decline.

## British Columbia

### *Introduction*
British Columbia has two prenatal diagnostic centres, one in Vancouver and one in Victoria (Appendix 1). Unfortunately, the Vancouver centre at the Grace Hospital was not able to provide physician referral data, so the physician referral data should be interpreted with great caution.

### *Utilization of Prenatal Diagnostic Services*
The highest utilization rates among women aged 15-34 are in the census divisions of Greater Vancouver and those adjacent to it. Although there are several census divisions with high rates dotted around the province, the other dominant pattern is the low rates of utilization in census divisions running from south to north in the interior. Utilization rates are high among women aged 35 and over in three distinct groupings of census divisions. First, they are high in all of the census divisions of Vancouver Island, with the exception of census division 23. Second, they are high in an extended cluster of census divisions around Greater Vancouver and following the coast as far as census division 25. The third cluster of census divisions with high rates is along the Canada-U.S. border in the interior of the province. The geographic pattern of utilization among both age groups combined (Figure 25) is very similar to that among women aged 35 and over.

Among women aged 15-34 the highest rates of expected utilization of prenatal services are in two census divisions adjacent to Greater Vancouver and in all of the census divisions in the northwest of the province. These are also census divisions where Native peoples make up a relatively large proportion of the population. In the remaining census divisions the expected utilization rates among younger women fall within a range of 151-200 per 100 000 women. Among women aged 35 and over, the expected utilization rates are lowest in a band of census divisions along the Canada-U.S. border and then increase farther north. Among the two age groups combined, the geographic pattern of expected utilization is more complex because the rates are high in both southern and northern British Columbia (Figure 26).

In a comparison of observed and expected rates among women aged 15-34, prenatal diagnostic services are under-utilized in most census divisions. Only four census divisions, including Greater Vancouver, fall into the range of utilization as expected. For women aged 35 and over the geographic pattern is virtually the same, except for two notable differences — a cluster of census divisions in the interior near the Canada-U.S. border and census division 57, where values fall into the utilization as expected category. When the total observed and expected rates of utilization of prenatal diagnostic services are compared (Figure 27), only the southern end of Vancouver Island (including Victoria), Greater Vancouver and one census division adjacent to it, and a cluster of three census divisions along the Canada-U.S. border fall into the utilization as expected range. The remainder of the province falls into the under-utilization range, and one census division actually falls into the extreme under-utilization range.

### Physician Location

The three census divisions with the highest number of family/general practitioners with an expressed interest in obstetrics are Greater Vancouver, Victoria, and the Central Okanagan, which contains Kelowna. In the rest of the province the number decreases farther north and in the interior. The geographic distribution of obstetricians/gynaecologists is even more concentrated in Greater Vancouver than is the geographic distribution of family/general practitioners. When the two groups of physicians are combined, the dominance of Greater Vancouver and Victoria with respect to physician supply is evident (Figure 28).

### Referral Behaviour

It bears repeating that because the Vancouver prenatal diagnostic centres did not provide physician referral data, the values presented in Figures 29 and 30 grossly underestimate the actual values, and the geographic patterns are not representative of the actual provincial patterns. There are, however, two interesting points to be made. First, the impact of the Victoria prenatal diagnostic centre must be highly localized. Second, the relatively high ratio for census division 41 is a function of the lack of sensitivity of these ratios to very small numbers. In this case there is only one obstetrician/gynaecologist in the region, and he or she made one referral to the Victoria prenatal diagnostic centre (Table 6).

### An Ecological Model of the Geographic Distribution of Utilization

For British Columbia the regression model yielded an equation of the following form:

$$Y_i = 338.39051179 - 44.22674254 \text{ DIST} \quad (7)$$
$$(12.00909326)$$

where
$F = 13.56$ (d.f.=1,27), and
$R^2 = 0.33436554$.

The equation indicates that the variation in the geographic distribution of the utilization of prenatal diagnostic services by women aged 15 and over declines as distance from the nearest prenatal diagnostic centre increases. Again, this is consistent with the hypothesis. In this case the model accounts for just over 33% of the variation in the geographic distribution of the utilization of prenatal diagnostic services by women of all ages. The model and the distance variables are statistically significant at the 0.001 level.

### *Summary*

The analysis of observed and expected utilization indicates that to a very large extent women living in Greater Vancouver and Victoria and in a small number of census divisions in southern British Columbia are receiving a reasonable level of service. For women in the interior and the far north of the province utilization appears to be substantially less than expected. These findings are not surprising, given the concentration of physicians who potentially might make referrals in Greater Vancouver and Victoria, but even the impact of the Victoria prenatal diagnostic centre appears to be geographically constrained. These observations are supported by the regression analysis, which indicates that as distance from the nearest prenatal diagnostic centre increases, utilization rates per census division decline.

## Canada

### *Introduction*

There are 21 prenatal diagnostic centres in Canada. In two provinces (Prince Edward Island and New Brunswick) there is no centre; in Newfoundland, Nova Scotia, and Manitoba there is one centre; in Saskatchewan, Alberta, and British Columbia there are two centres; in Quebec there are three centres, although they are in two locations; and the rest are in Ontario.

### *Utilization of Prenatal Diagnostic Services*

According to the data provided by the prenatal diagnostic centres, 18 169 women utilized prenatal diagnostic services in 1990. This is a slight underestimate because of the missing data from Toronto's Wellesley Hospital and Calgary's Alberta Children's Hospital. The actual number is likely still below 20 000. The utilization rate per 100 000 women aged between 15 and 34 is 100 (1 in 1 000), for women aged 35 and over it is 236.1 (1 in 424), and for all women it is 141.7 (1 in 706), in Canada.

Table 6. Referrals to Prenatal Diagnostic Centres, by Census Division, British Columbia, 1990

| Census division | FPs/GPs | OBs/GYNs | Total physicians | FPs/GPs making referrals | OBs/GYNs making referrals | Total making referrals | Referrals by FPs/GPs | Referrals by OBs/GYNs | Total referrals |
|---|---|---|---|---|---|---|---|---|---|
| 1 | 11 | 1 | 12 | 0 | 0 | 0 | 0 | 0 | 0 |
| 3 | 18 | 4 | 22 | 0 | 0 | 0 | 0 | 0 | 0 |
| 5 | 9 | 2 | 11 | 0 | 0 | 0 | 0 | 0 | 0 |
| 7 | 12 | 3 | 15 | 0 | 0 | 0 | 0 | 0 | 0 |
| 9 | 8 | 2 | 10 | 0 | 0 | 0 | 0 | 0 | 0 |
| 11 | 35 | 7 | 42 | 0 | 0 | 0 | 0 | 0 | 0 |
| 13 | 22 | 3 | 25 | 0 | 0 | 0 | 0 | 0 | 0 |
| 15 | 404 | 129 | 533 | 5 | 1 | 6 | 7 | 1 | 8 |
| 17 | 76 | 22 | 98 | 19 | 6 | 25 | 34 | 15 | 49 |
| 19 | 15 | 4 | 19 | 3 | 1 | 4 | 7 | 2 | 9 |
| 21 | 21 | 5 | 26 | 3 | 1 | 4 | 5 | 1 | 6 |
| 23 | 8 | 1 | 9 | 1 | 0 | 1 | 1 | 0 | 1 |
| 25 | 13 | 6 | 19 | 0 | 2 | 2 | 0 | 2 | 2 |
| 27 | 2 | 1 | 3 | 0 | 0 | 0 | 0 | 0 | 0 |
| 29 | 9 | 2 | 11 | 0 | 0 | 0 | 0 | 0 | 0 |
| 31 | 4 | 0 | 4 | 0 | 0 | 0 | 0 | 0 | 0 |
| 33 | 17 | 7 | 24 | 0 | 0 | 0 | 0 | 0 | 0 |
| 35 | 31 | 4 | 35 | 1 | 0 | 1 | 1 | 0 | 1 |
| 37 | 22 | 3 | 12 | 0 | 0 | 0 | 0 | 0 | 0 |
| 39 | 5 | 1 | 22 | 0 | 0 | 0 | 0 | 0 | 0 |
| 41 | 4 | 1 | 5 | 0 | 1 | 1 | 0 | 1 | 1 |
| 43 | 4 | 0 | 4 | 0 | 0 | 0 | 0 | 0 | 0 |

**Table 6.** (cont'd)

| Census division | FPs/GPs | OBs/GYNs | Total physicians | FPs/GPs making referrals | OBs/GYNs making referrals | Total making referrals | Referrals by FPs/GPs | Referrals by OBs/GYNs | Total referrals |
|---|---|---|---|---|---|---|---|---|---|
| 45 | 3 | 1 | 4 | 0 | 0 | 0 | 0 | 0 | 0 |
| 47 | 10 | 1 | 11 | 0 | 0 | 0 | 0 | 0 | 0 |
| 49 | 9 | 2 | 11 | 0 | 0 | 0 | 0 | 0 | 0 |
| 51 | 4 | 0 | 4 | 0 | 0 | 0 | 0 | 0 | 0 |
| 53 | 22 | 6 | 28 | 1 | 0 | 1 | 0 | 0 | 2 |
| 55 | 4 | 2 | 6 | 0 | 0 | 0 | 0 | 0 | 0 |
| 57 | 0 | 0 | 0 | 0 | 0 | 0 | 0 | 0 | 0 |
| Total | 802 | 220 | 1 022 | 33 | 12 | 45 | 57 | 22 | 79 |

Utilization rates vary tremendously within and between regions among both age groups. Compared with expected utilization rates, most census divisions in Canada have less than expected utilization. In some areas of rural and northern Canada utilization is much less than expected. In the major urban areas (where many prenatal diagnostic centres are located) and adjacent areas utilization is as expected.

## *Physician Location and Referral Behaviour*

It is well known in Canada that all provinces have difficulty in finding physicians to practise in rural and northern communities. Obstetricians/ gynaecologists who potentially might make referrals are almost all located in major urban areas across the country. This has an impact on access to prenatal diagnosis for women, given that they are much more likely to make referrals than family/general practitioners.

## *An Ecological Model of the Geographic Distribution of Utilization*

The ecological models developed for all the regions except Ontario consistently identify the relationship between utilization rates and the distance from the nearest prenatal diagnostic centre. Utilization rates per census division decline as the distance between the census division and the nearest prenatal diagnostic centre increases. The income hypothesis was also supported (i.e., utilization rates per census division increase as women's median income increases) in Atlantic Canada and in the Prairie provinces. When the southern Alberta census divisions were removed from the data on the Prairie provinces, the rurality hypothesis was supported (i.e., utilization rates per census division decline as the level of rurality increases).

Only for Ontario, with its much larger network of prenatal diagnostic centres, does distance not enter the regression model. The Ontario model supported the education hypothesis (i.e., utilization rates per census division increase as the rate of women with post-secondary education increases) and the unemployment hypothesis (i.e., utilization rates per census division decrease as female unemployment increases). The models were able to explain from a low of 24% of the variance in utilization in the Prairie provinces to a high of 57% in Ontario.

Given the regional nature of the findings, a multiple regression model was developed for the country as a whole and a set of dummy variables included. The data used were from all census divisions in nine of the provinces and the health regions in Quebec.

The estimated model takes the following form:

$$Y_i = 384.07992454 - 0.00136647 \text{ AGR} - 48.79556541 \text{ DIST} \quad (8)$$
$$(0.00042062) \quad (6.83807826)$$
$$- 179.85005165 \text{ ATL}$$
$$(19.71457144)$$

where
F = 36.72 (d.f.=3,190), and
$R^2$ = 0.36698955.

The model for the country as a whole supports the rurality and distance hypotheses. In addition, living in the Atlantic provinces (ATL) decreases the utilization rate. The model accounts for almost 37% of the variance in utilization rates across the country. The equation and all of the parameters are statistically significant at better than the 0.001 level.

## Conclusions

This study is a demographic and geographic analysis of the utilization of prenatal diagnostic services by women aged 15-34, 35 and over, and both age groups combined. The chief source of data was the 1990 records of prenatal diagnostic centres across Canada, which provided the ages and places of residence of women who utilized prenatal diagnostic services and in most cases the names of referring physicians. With this information, expected and observed rates of utilization were calculated and examined for differences between them. By matching the physician's name with a data base from Southam that provided their addresses, referral patterns could be determined. All of these measures were presented at the census division level, except for the data from Quebec, which were presented at the level of that province's administrative health regions.

In all instances the most conservative assumptions were chosen. Except where there were problems because some prenatal diagnostic centres did not provide some or all of the data requested, if errors have been made they likely understate the magnitude of under-utilization. In addition to examining utilization and referral behaviour of physicians, we created a set of ecological models using regression techniques. Employing utilization rates as the dependent variable and distance and socioeconomic measures as the independent variables, we tested hypotheses that were based on research into access to other health services for women in each region and in the country as a whole.

In every province women who live in rural and northern communities utilize prenatal diagnostic services at rates that are lower than expected. This is because in most provinces prenatal diagnostic centres are located in the largest urban centres. This means that usually they are only in one or two places in a province. There are no prenatal diagnostic centres in Prince Edward Island or New Brunswick, at one end of the spectrum, and at the other end Ontario has a network of centres stretching across the southern half of the province.

The geographic distribution of family/general practitioners with an expressed interest in obstetrics and obstetricians/gynaecologists is a factor also affecting utilization. Fewer than expected family/general practitioners are referring women for prenatal diagnostic services, a problem that is magnified in rural and northern areas because they are usually the only physicians practising. The obverse of this is that the vast majority of obstetricians/gynaecologists (who make most of the referrals) are concentrated in the largest urban centres in every province. The implication is that women living in rural or northern communities who want prenatal diagnostic services may have to travel to an urban location just to get a referral. They will also have to travel to yet another urban location for the prenatal diagnostic service itself.

The ecological models for the regions and the country lend support to these observations. With the exception of Ontario with its more developed network of prenatal diagnostic centres, the distance hypothesis (e.g., utilization rates per census division decline with distance from the nearest prenatal diagnostic centre) was consistently supported in the regional and national models. In the regional models for the Atlantic provinces and Ontario, other hypotheses based on the socioeconomic conditions of women were supported. In the Prairie provinces model and the national model the rurality hypothesis was supported, and the national model also indicated that utilization rates for women in Atlantic Canada are lower than those in the rest of the country. The models accounted for anywhere from a quarter to more than half of the variation in utilization rates.

A necessary step in evaluating access to prenatal diagnosis services is to examine if and how utilization differs across Canada. Only then is it possible to look for explanations for such differences. This study documents utilization in this country and reminds us that the geography of services and physicians plays a significant part in women's access to prenatal diagnostic services.

## Appendix 1. Medical Genetics Centres in Canada Providing Prenatal Diagnosis

**ATLANTIC PROVINCES**
Medical Genetics Clinic
Atlantic Research Centre
Halifax, Nova Scotia

Janeway Medical Genetics Program
St. John's, Newfoundland

**QUEBEC**
Hôpital Ste-Justine
Montreal, Quebec

Montreal Children's Hospital
Montreal, Quebec

Génétique Humaine
Centre Hospitalier de
l'Université Laval
Quebec City, Quebec

**ONTARIO**
Chedoke-McMaster Hospital
Hamilton, Ontario

Kingston General Hospital
Kingston, Ontario

Children's Hospital of
Western Ontario
London, Ontario

Credit Valley Hospital
Mississauga, Ontario

North York General Hospital
North York, Ontario

Oshawa General Hospital
Oshawa, Ontario

Children's Hospital of
Eastern Ontario
Ottawa, Ontario

Toronto General Hospital
University of Toronto Centre
Toronto, Ontario

Wellesley Hospital
Toronto, Ontario

**PRAIRIE PROVINCES**
Alberta Children's Hospital
Calgary, Alberta

University Hospital
Edmonton, Alberta Genetics Clinic
Regina, Saskatchewan

University Hospital
Saskatoon, Saskatchewan

Health Sciences Centre
Winnipeg, Manitoba

**BRITISH COLUMBIA**
Shaughnessy-Grace Hospitals
Vancouver, British Columbia

Medical Genetics Clinic
Victoria General Hospital
Victoria, British Columbia

# Appendix 2. Genetic Indications for Prenatal Diagnosis and the Expected Demand for Services

### Table 2A. Genetic Indications for Prenatal Diagnosis and the Expected Demand for Services

|  | Occurrence per 1 000 established pregnancies | Minimum estimate of utilization |
|---|---|---|
| **A. Increased risk for chromosomal abnormalities** | | |
| 1. Advanced maternal age | 77.8 | 46.7* |
| 2. Biochemical markers (maternal serum AFP) | 73.0 | 48.0** |
| 3. Family history | | |
|    a. previously affected child | ? | 24.0 |
|    b. parent with a rearrangement | | |
|    c. relative with a trisomy | | |
|    d. other cytogenetic marker | | |
|       i   fragile X | | |
|       ii  chromosomal breakage | | |
|       iii fetal sexing | | |
|       iv parental radiation exposure | | |
| 4. Abnormal ultrasound | | |
|    a. polyhydramnios | 13.0 | 8.4*** |
|    b. fetal anomaly | 3.0 | 2.0*** |
| **B. Morphological abnormalities** | | |
| 1. Neural tube defect | | |
|    a. elevated maternal serum AFP | 12.0 | 8.0** |
| 2. Positive family history | 4.2 | 2.7*** |
| **C. Biochemical/molecular disorder** | | |
| 1. Haemoglobinopathies | 1.8 | 1.2** |
|    a. thalassaemia | | |
|    b. sickle cell | | |
| **D. Carrier screening** | | |
| 1. Tay-Sachs | 1.5 | 1.0** |
| 2. Cystic fibrosis | | |
| **TOTAL** | 186.3 | 142.0 |

\* We estimate that only 60% of the eligible women would wish to have amniocentesis/CVS.
\*\* We estimate that only 65% of women would wish to have screening.
\*\*\* We estimate that only 65% of women with this indication would wish to proceed to genetic amniocentesis.

150 PND: Background and Impact on Individuals

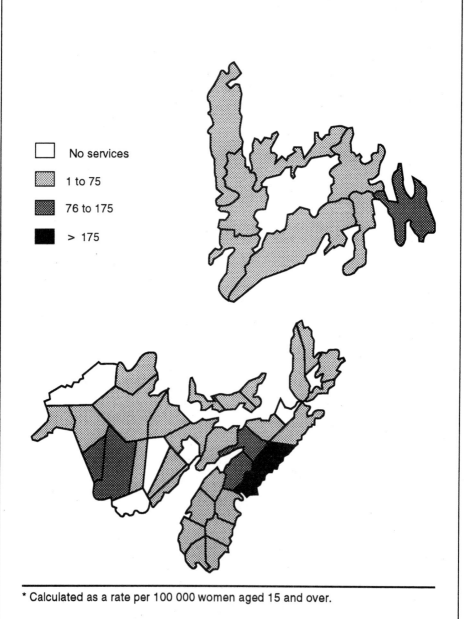

Figure 1. Observed Utilization of Prenatal Diagnostic Services*
by All Women, Atlantic Provinces, 1990

☐ No services
▨ 1 to 75
▦ 76 to 175
■ > 175

* Calculated as a rate per 100 000 women aged 15 and over.

A Demographic and Geographic Analysis of Users of PND Services 151

**Figure 2.** Expected Utilization of Prenatal Diagnostic Services*
by All Women, Atlantic Provinces, 1990

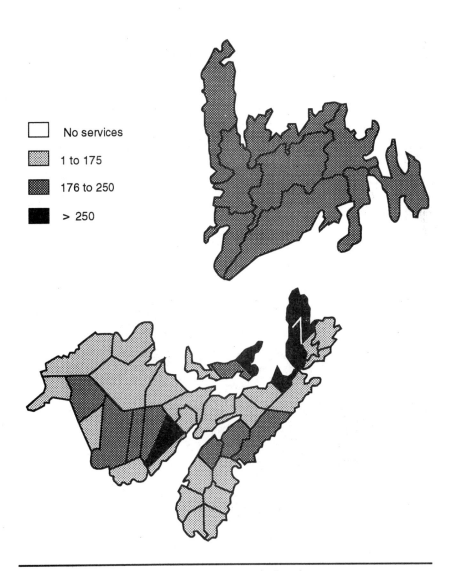

* Calculated as a rate per 100 000 women aged 15 and over.

**Figure 3. Observed Compared with Expected Utilization of Prenatal Diagnostic Services\* by All Women, Atlantic Provinces, 1990**

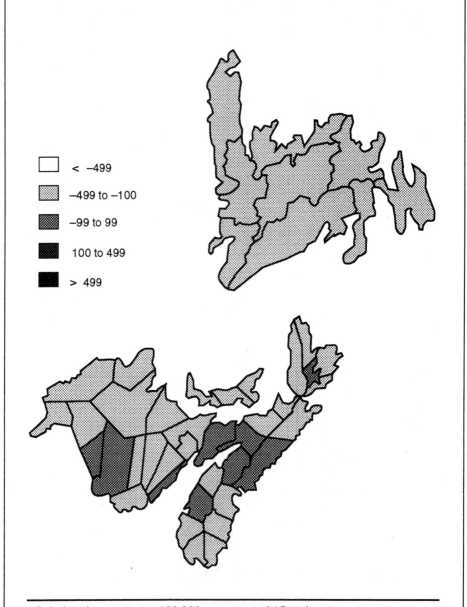

\* Calculated as a rate per 100 000 women aged 15 and over.

**Figure 4. Obstetricians/Gynaecologists and Family/General Practitioners,\* Atlantic Provinces, 1990**

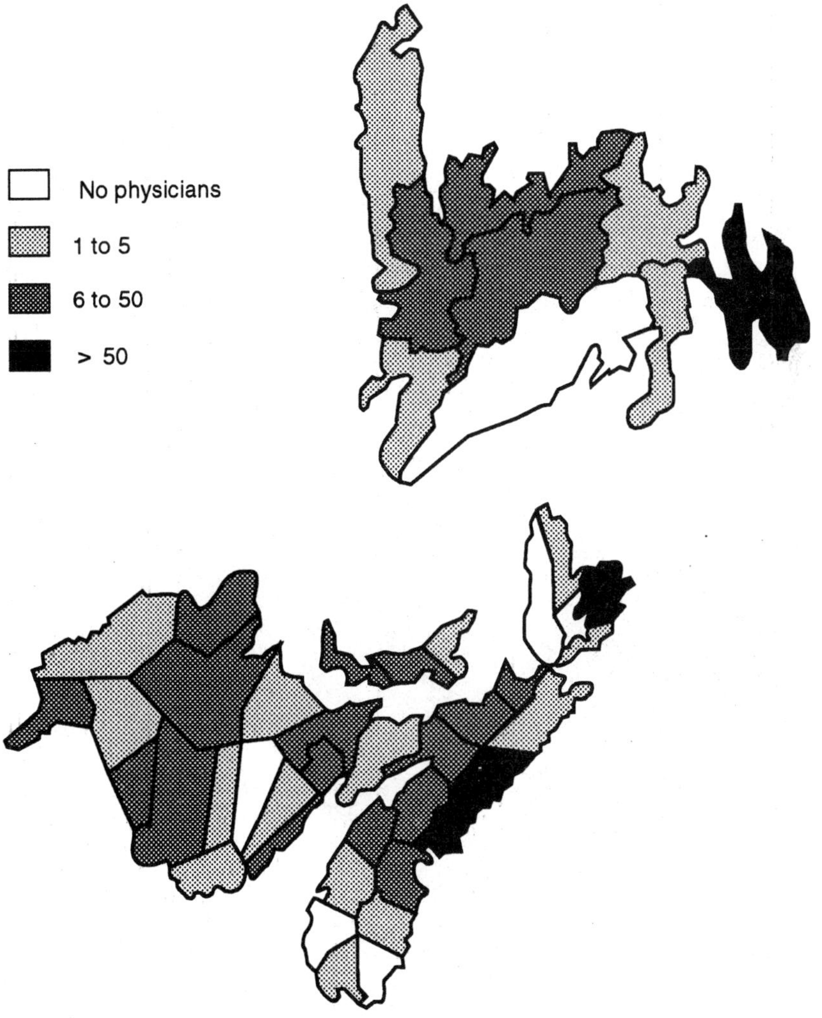

☐ No physicians
▨ 1 to 5
▨ 6 to 50
■ > 50

\* With an expressed interest in obstetrics.

154 PND: Background and Impact on Individuals

**Figure 5. All Physicians* Making Referrals to Prenatal Diagnostic Centres Compared with Total Physicians, Atlantic Provinces, 1990**

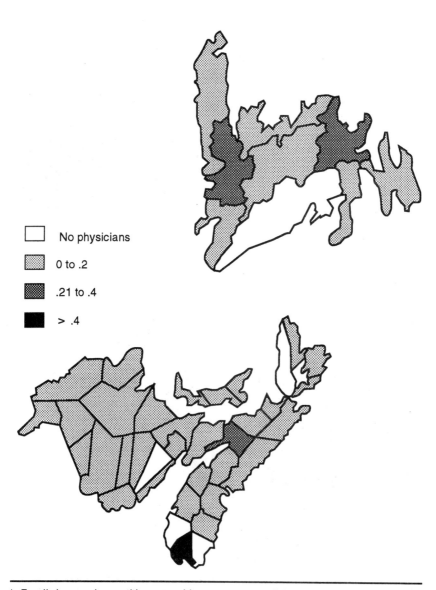

- ☐ No physicians
- 0 to .2
- .21 to .4
- \> .4

* Family/general practitioners with an expressed interest in obstetrics and obstetricians/gynaecologists.

A Demographic and Geographic Analysis of Users of PND Services 155

**Figure 6. Total Referrals to Prenatal Diagnostic Centres per 100 Physicians,* Atlantic Provinces, 1990**

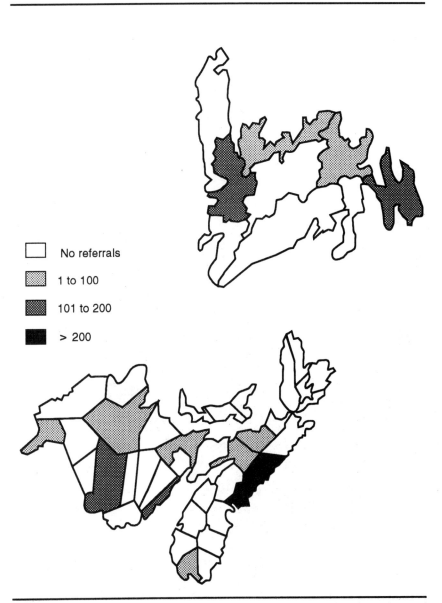

* Family/general practitioners with an expressed interest in obstetrics and obstetricians/gynaecologists.

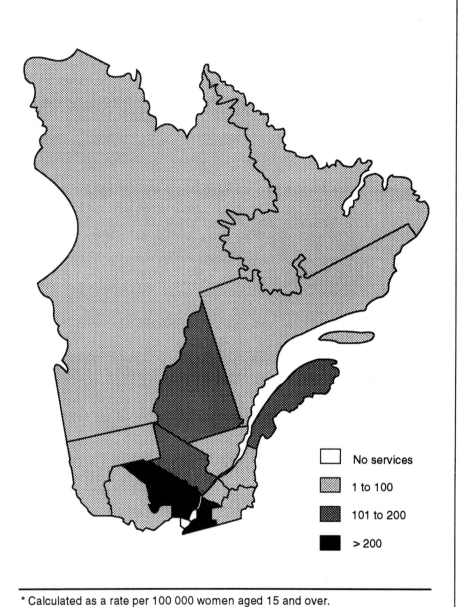

**Figure 7. Observed Utilization of Prenatal Diagnostic Services\* by All Women, Quebec and Labrador, 1990**

Legend:
- ☐ No services
- 1 to 100
- 101 to 200
- ■ > 200

\* Calculated as a rate per 100 000 women aged 15 and over.

A Demographic and Geographic Analysis of Users of PND Services 157

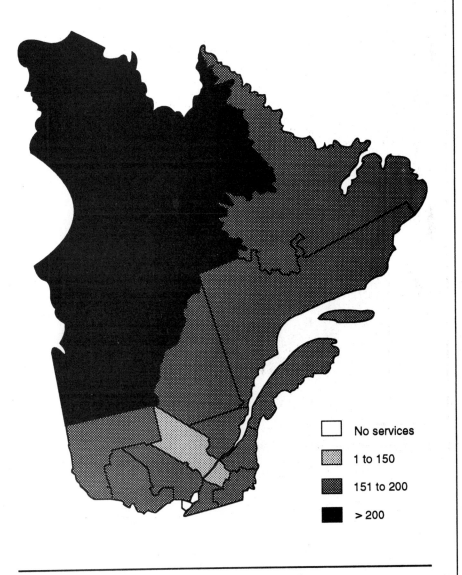

Figure 8. Expected Utilization of Prenatal Diagnostic Services* by All Women, Quebec and Labrador, 1990

Legend:
- No services
- 1 to 150
- 151 to 200
- > 200

* Calculated as a rate per 100 000 women aged 15 and over.

**Figure 9. Observed Compared with Expected Utilization of Prenatal Diagnostic Services\* by All Women, Quebec and Labrador, 1990**

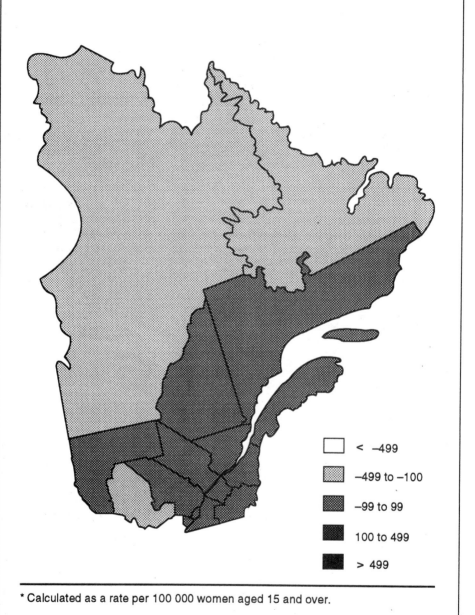

\* Calculated as a rate per 100 000 women aged 15 and over.

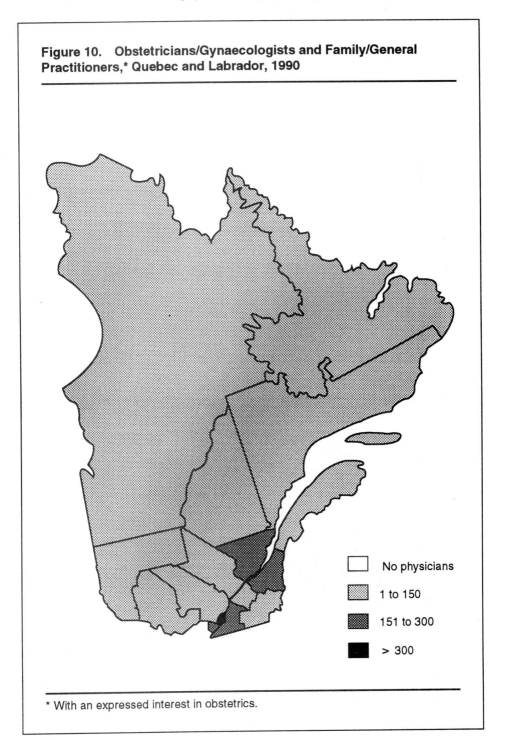

Figure 10. Obstetricians/Gynaecologists and Family/General Practitioners,* Quebec and Labrador, 1990

* With an expressed interest in obstetrics.

**Figure 11. All Physicians* Making Referrals to Prenatal Diagnostic Centres Compared with Total Physicians, Quebec and Labrador, 1990**

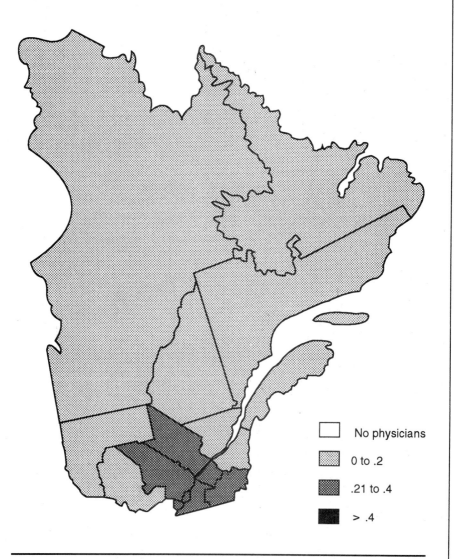

* Family/general practitioners with an expressed interest in obstetrics and obstetricians/gynaecologists.

**Figure 12. Total Referrals to Prenatal Diagnostic Centres per 100 Physicians,\* Quebec and Labrador, 1990**

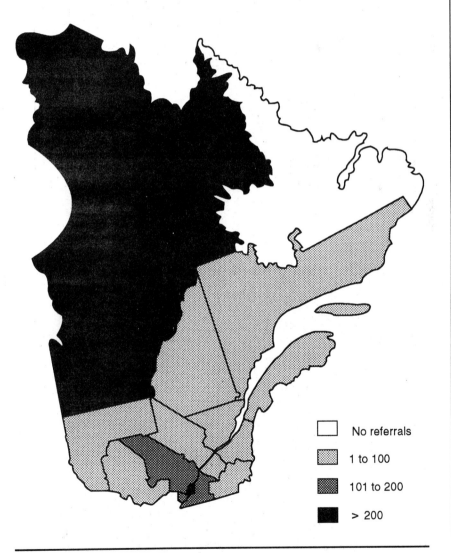

- ☐ No referrals
- 1 to 100
- 101 to 200
- \> 200

\* Family/general practitioners with an expressed interest in obstetrics and obstetricians/gynaecologists.

**Figure 13. Observed Utilization of Prenatal Diagnostic Services\* by All Women, Ontario, 1990**

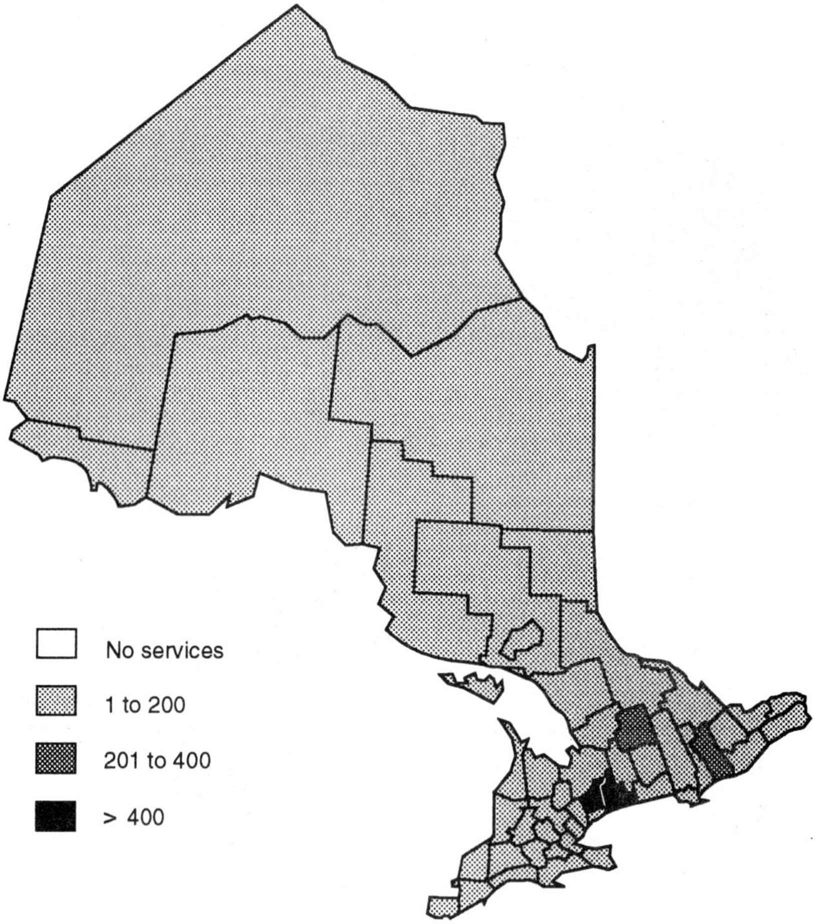

- ☐ No services
- ▒ 1 to 200
- ▓ 201 to 400
- ■ > 400

\* Calculated as a rate per 100 000 women aged 15 and over.

A Demographic and Geographic Analysis of Users of PND Services 163

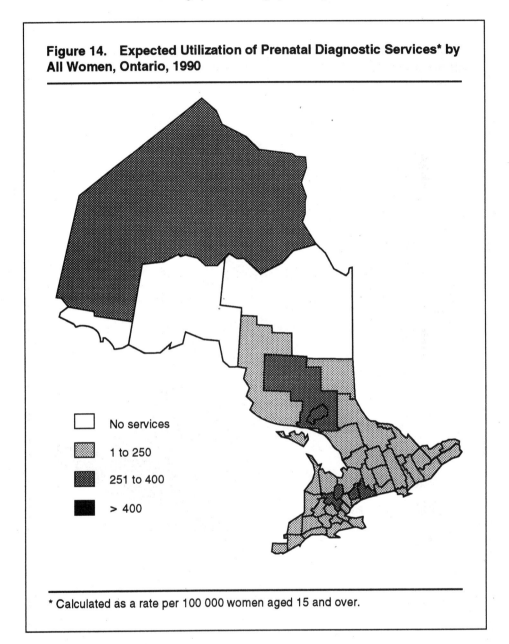

Figure 14. Expected Utilization of Prenatal Diagnostic Services* by All Women, Ontario, 1990

* Calculated as a rate per 100 000 women aged 15 and over.

**Figure 15. Observed Compared with Expected Utilization of Prenatal Diagnostic Services\* by All Women, Ontario, 1990**

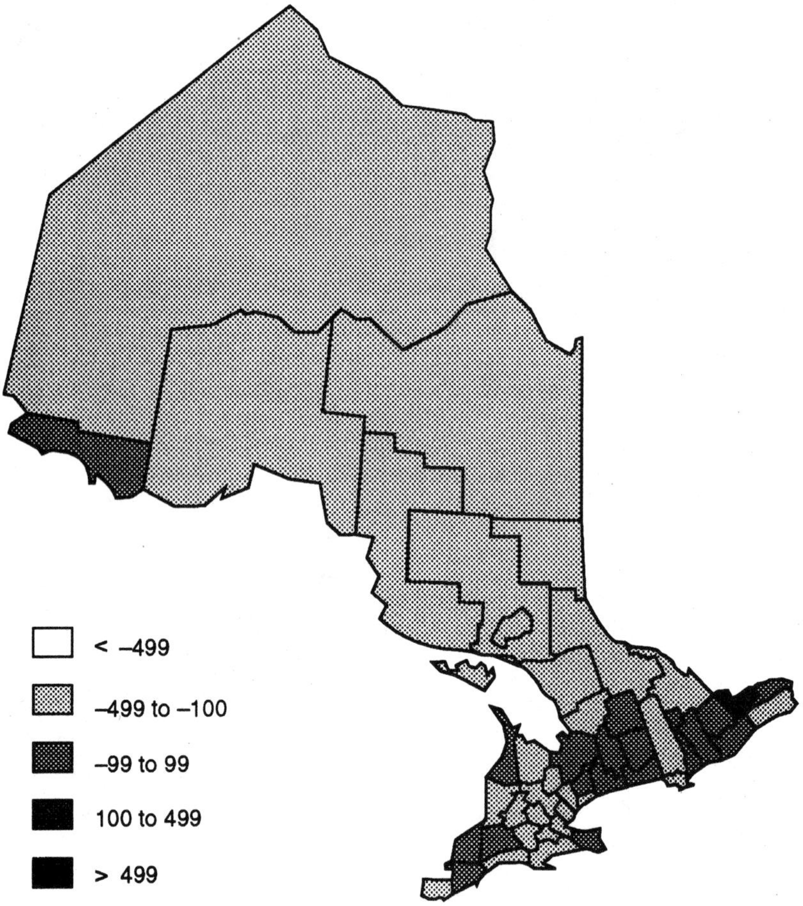

- ☐ < –499
- –499 to –100
- –99 to 99
- 100 to 499
- ■ > 499

\* Calculated as a rate per 100 000 women aged 15 and over.

A Demographic and Geographic Analysis of Users of PND Services 165

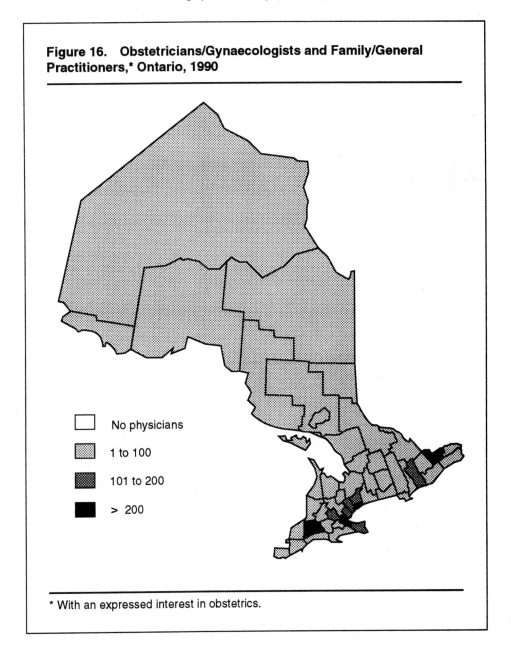

Figure 16. Obstetricians/Gynaecologists and Family/General Practitioners,* Ontario, 1990

Legend:
- No physicians
- 1 to 100
- 101 to 200
- > 200

* With an expressed interest in obstetrics.

166 PND: Background and Impact on Individuals

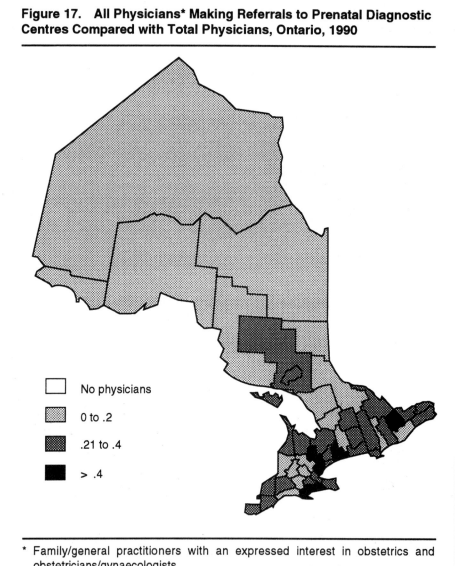

Figure 17. All Physicians* Making Referrals to Prenatal Diagnostic Centres Compared with Total Physicians, Ontario, 1990

- No physicians
- 0 to .2
- .21 to .4
- > .4

* Family/general practitioners with an expressed interest in obstetrics and obstetricians/gynaecologists.

A Demographic and Geographic Analysis of Users of PND Services 167

**Figure 18. Total Referrals to Prenatal Diagnostic Centres per 100 Physicians,* Ontario, 1990**

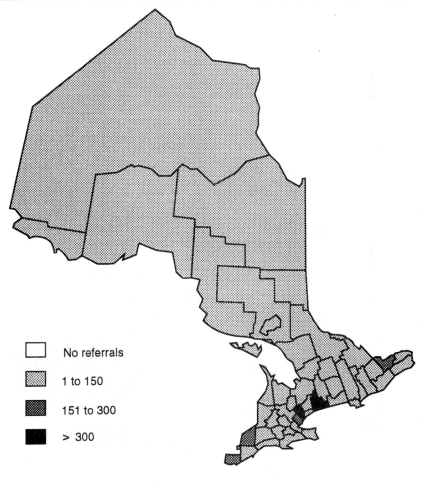

* Family/general practitioners with an expressed interest in obstetrics and obstetricians/gynaecologists.

168  PND: Background and Impact on Individuals

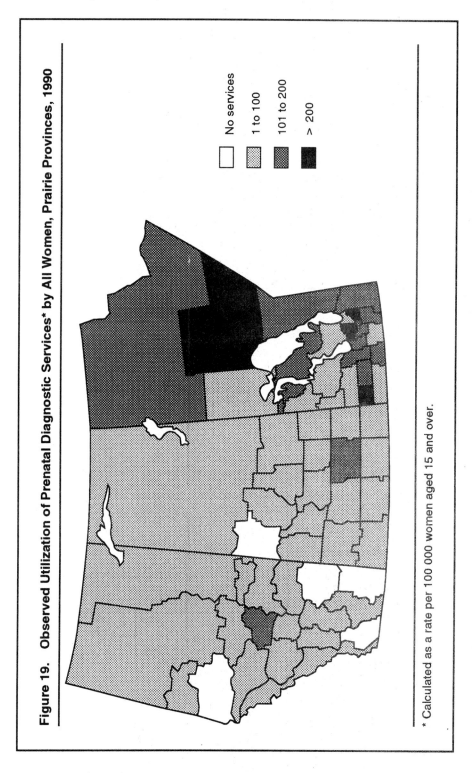

Figure 19. Observed Utilization of Prenatal Diagnostic Services* by All Women, Prairie Provinces, 1990

No services
1 to 100
101 to 200
> 200

* Calculated as a rate per 100 000 women aged 15 and over.

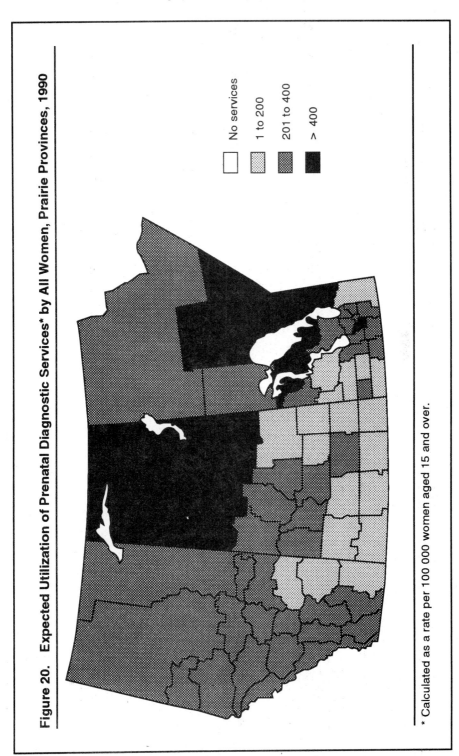

Figure 20. Expected Utilization of Prenatal Diagnostic Services* by All Women, Prairie Provinces, 1990

* Calculated as a rate per 100 000 women aged 15 and over.

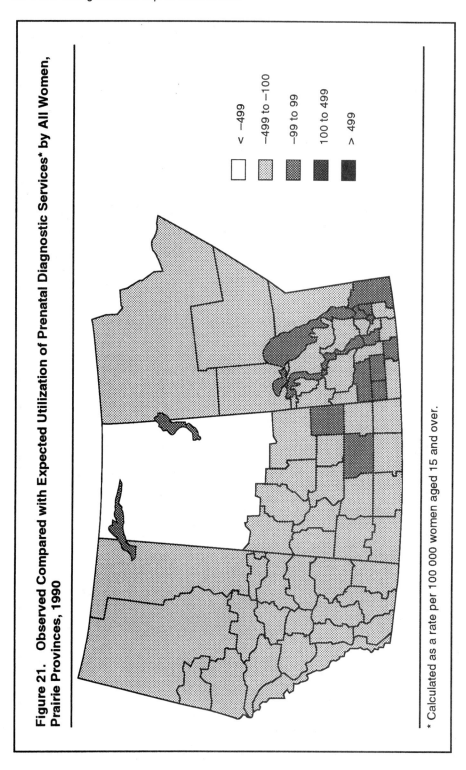

Figure 21. Observed Compared with Expected Utilization of Prenatal Diagnostic Services* by All Women, Prairie Provinces, 1990

* Calculated as a rate per 100 000 women aged 15 and over.

A Demographic and Geographic Analysis of Users of PND Services 171

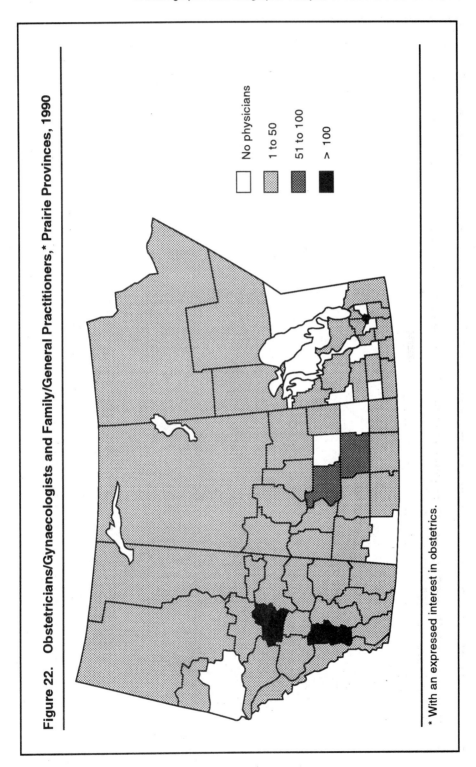

Figure 22. Obstetricians/Gynaecologists and Family/General Practitioners,* Prairie Provinces, 1990

* With an expressed interest in obstetrics.

172  PND: Background and Impact on Individuals

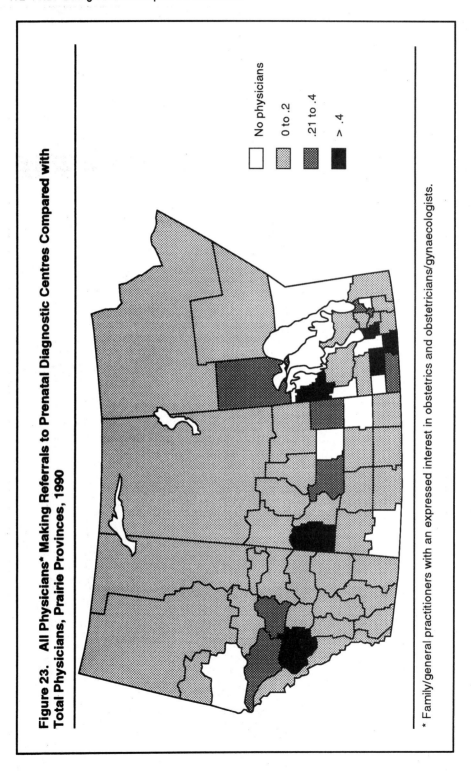

Figure 23. All Physicians* Making Referrals to Prenatal Diagnostic Centres Compared with Total Physicians, Prairie Provinces, 1990

* Family/general practitioners with an expressed interest in obstetrics and obstetricians/gynaecologists.

A Demographic and Geographic Analysis of Users of PND Services 173

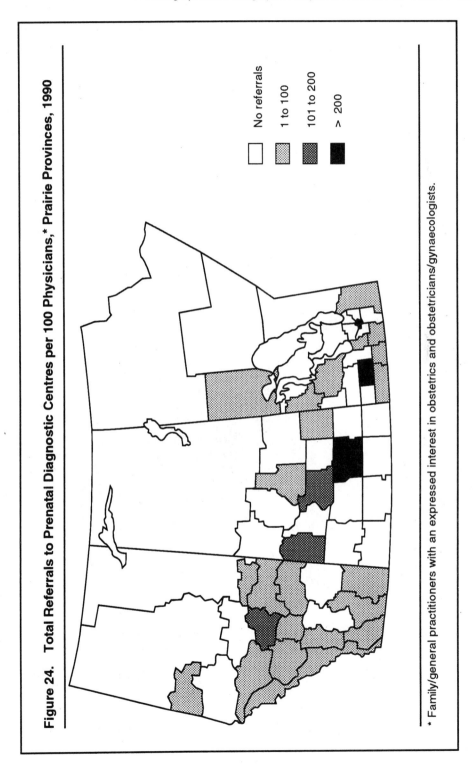

Figure 24. Total Referrals to Prenatal Diagnostic Centres per 100 Physicians,* Prairie Provinces, 1990

* Family/general practitioners with an expressed interest in obstetrics and obstetricians/gynaecologists.

**Figure 25. Observed Utilization of Prenatal Diagnostic Services\* by All Women, British Columbia, 1990**

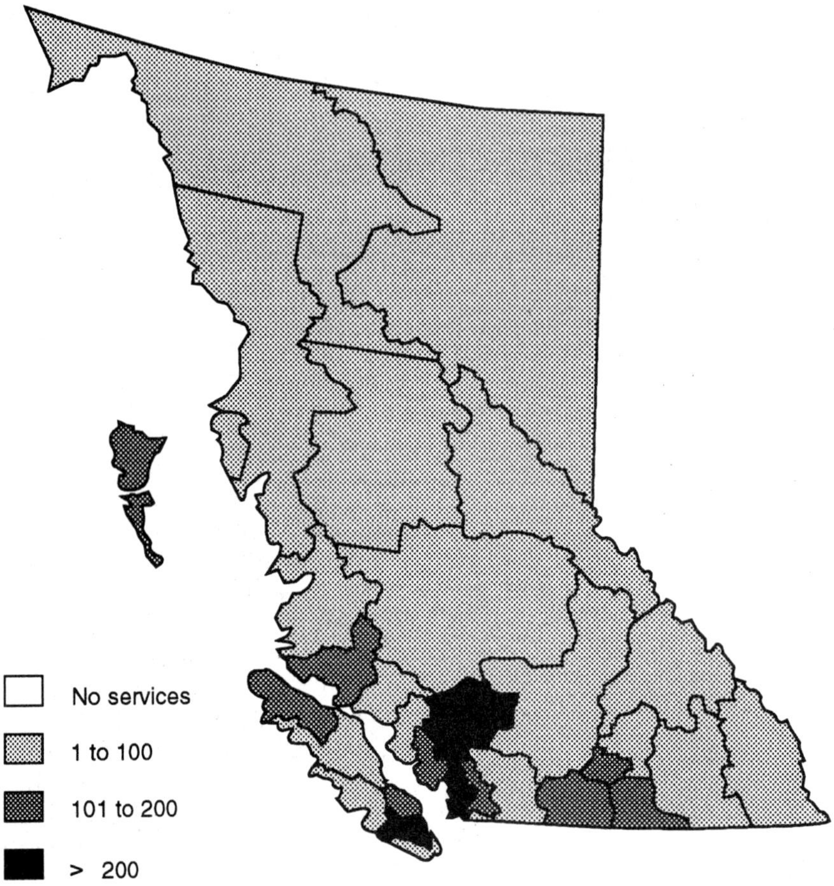

- ☐ No services
- 1 to 100
- 101 to 200
- \> 200

\* Calculated as a rate per 100 000 women aged 15 and over.

**Figure 26. Expected Utilization of Prenatal Diagnostic Services\* by All Women, British Columbia, 1990**

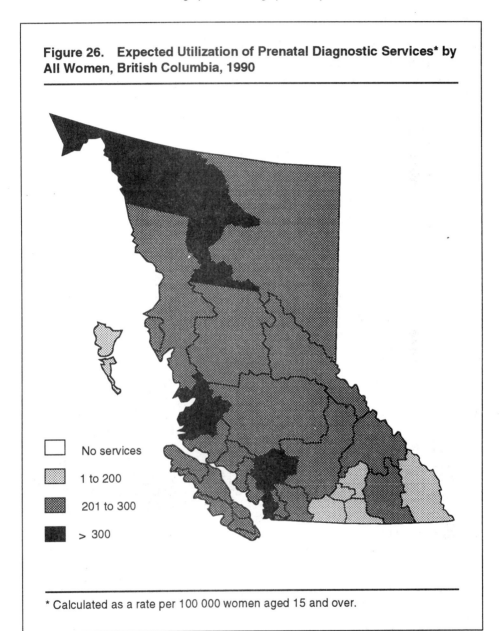

\* Calculated as a rate per 100 000 women aged 15 and over.

**Figure 27. Observed Compared with Expected Utilization of Prenatal Diagnostic Services\* by All Women, British Columbia, 1990**

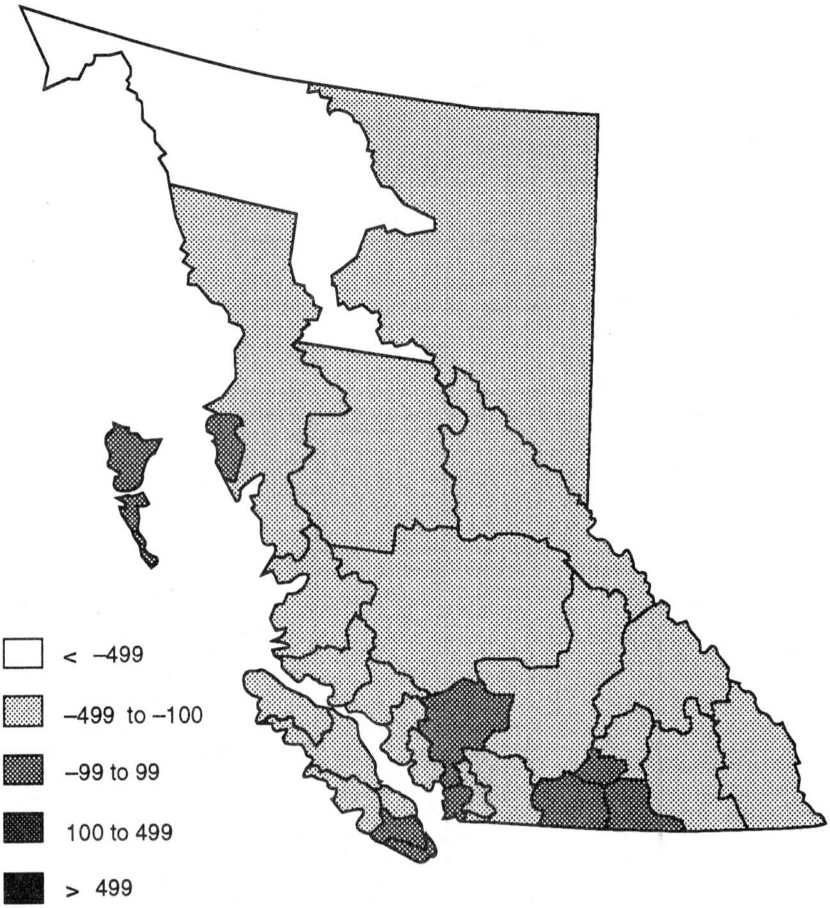

- ☐ < −499
- −499 to −100
- −99 to 99
- 100 to 499
- \> 499

\* Calculated as a rate per 100 000 women aged 15 and over.

A Demographic and Geographic Analysis of Users of PND Services 177

**Figure 28. Obstetricians/Gynaecologists and Family/General Practitioners,* British Columbia, 1990**

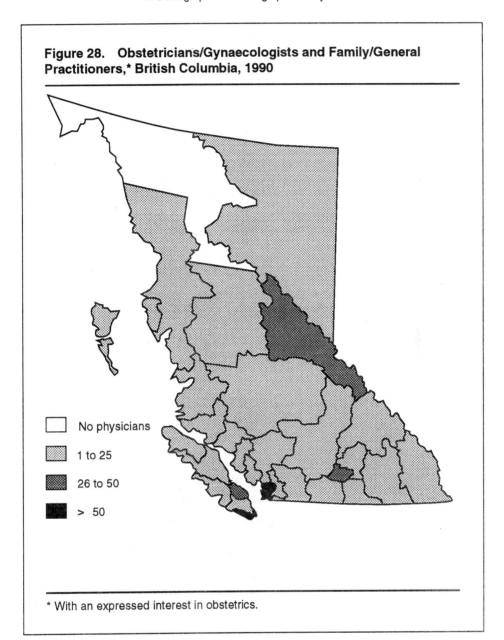

* With an expressed interest in obstetrics.

**Figure 29. All Physicians\* Making Referrals to Prenatal Diagnostic Centres Compared with Total Physicians, British Columbia, 1990**

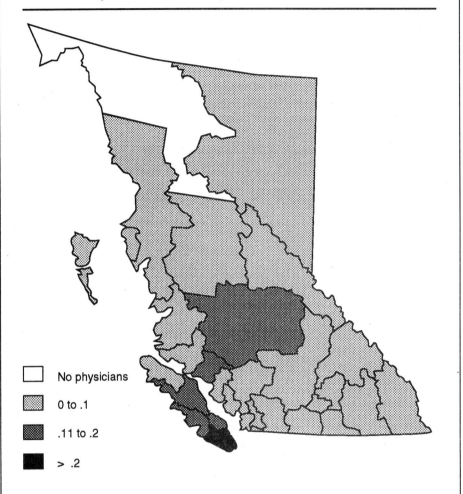

\* Family/general practitioners with an expressed interest in obstetrics and obstetricians/gynaecologists.

**Figure 30. Total Referrals to Prenatal Diagnostic Centres per 100 Physicians,\* British Columbia, 1990**

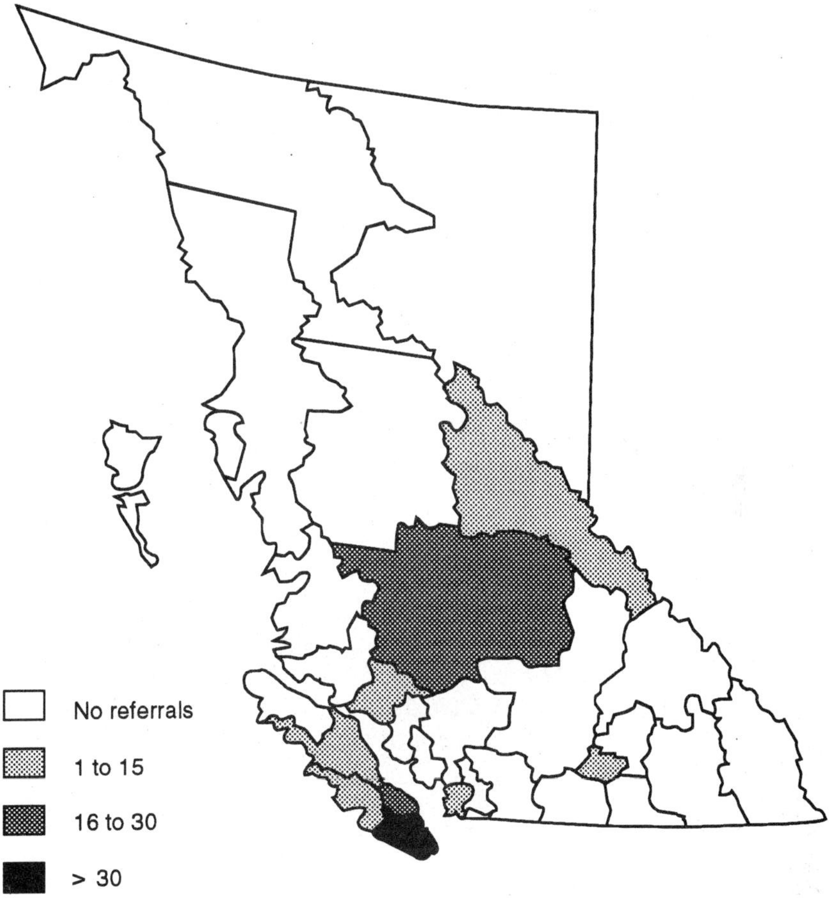

- ☐ No referrals
- ▨ 1 to 15
- ▩ 16 to 30
- ■ > 30

\* Family/general practitioners with an expressed interest in obstetrics and obstetricians/gynaecologists.

## Notes

1. This section is adapted from N.A. Ross, "Women's Access to Health Care. A Case Study of the Ontario Breast Screening Program, Kingston, Ontario" (M.A. thesis, Queen's University, 1992), 17-24, by permission of the author.

2. The Yukon and Northwest Territories are excluded from the analysis because there are no prenatal diagnostic services offered in either territory, and therefore women who need these services must travel to a centre in southern Canada. By definition, then, prenatal diagnostic services are inaccessible to all women in northern Canada. In southern Canada, on the other hand, the issue is one of relative accessibility.

3. Labrador (N10) has been included in the maps of Quebec for purely cartographic reasons. It is, however, recognized as part of Atlantic Canada for analytical purposes (e.g., see Table 2).

## Bibliography

Adams, M.M., G.P. Oakley, Jr., and J.S. Marks. 1982. "Maternal Age and Births in the 1980s." *JAMA* 247: 493-94.

Adams, M.M., et al. 1981. "Utilization of Prenatal Genetic Diagnosis in Women 35 Years of Age and Older in the United States, 1977 to 1978." *American Journal of Obstetrics and Gynecology* 139: 673-77.

Baird, P.A., A.D. Sadovnick, and B.C. McGillivray. 1985. "Temporal Changes in the Utilization of Amniocentesis for Prenatal Diagnosis by Women of Advanced Maternal Age, 1976-1983." *Prenatal Diagnosis* 5: 191-98.

Bastani, R., A.C. Marcus, and A. Hollatz-Brown. 1991. "Screening Mammography Rates and Barriers to Use: A Los Angeles County Survey." *Preventive Medicine* 20: 350-63.

Bernhardt, B.A., and R.M. Bannerman. 1982. "The Influence of Obstetricians on the Utilization of Amniocentesis." *Prenatal Diagnosis* 2: 115-21.

Burg, M.A., D.S. Lane, and A. Polednak. 1990. "Age Group Differences in the Use of Breast Cancer Screening Tests. The Effects of Health Care Utilization and Socioeconomic Variables." *Journal of Aging and Health* 2: 514-30.

Calnan, M. 1984. "The Health Belief Model and Participation in Programmes for the Early Detection of Breast Cancer: A Comparative Analysis." *Social Science and Medicine* 19 (8): 823-30.

Canada. Statistics Canada. 1992. *Health Reports: Births 1990.* Suppl. 14, Vol. 4. Cat. 82-003S14. Ottawa: Statistics Canada.

"Canadian Guidelines for Antenatal Diagnosis of Genetic Disease: A Joint Statement." 1974. *Canadian Medical Association Journal* 111: 180-83.

"Canadian Guidelines for Prenatal Diagnosis of Genetic Disorders: An Update. A Joint Document of the Canadian College of Medical Geneticists and the

Society of Obstetricians and Gynaecologists of Canada." 1991. *Journal of the Society of Obstetricians and Gynaecologists of Canada* 13 (August): 13-31.

Crandall, B.F., T.B. Lebherz, and K. Tabsh. 1986. "Maternal Age and Amniocentesis: Should This Be Lowered to 30 Years?" *Prenatal Diagnosis* 6: 237-42.

Crandall, B.F., L. Robinson, and P. Grau. 1991. "Risks Associated with an Elevated Maternal Serum Alpha-Fetoprotein Level." *American Journal of Obstetrics and Gynecology* 165: 581-86.

Davies, B.L., and T.A. Doran. 1982. "Factors in a Woman's Decision to Undergo Genetic Amniocentesis for Advanced Maternal Age." *Nursing Research* 31: 56-59.

de Waard, F., et al. 1984. "The DOM Project for the Early Detection of Breast Cancer, Utrecht, The Netherlands." *Journal of Chronic Diseases* 37: 1-44.

Feeny, D. 1986. "The Diffusion of New Health Care Technologies." In *Health Care Technology: Effectiveness, Efficiency, and Public Policy*, ed. D. Feeny, G. Guyatt, and P. Tugwell. Montreal: Institute for Research on Public Policy.

Fink, R., S. Shapiro, and J. Lewison. 1968. "The Reluctant Participation in a Breast Screening Program." *Public Health Reports* 83: 479-90.

Furhmann, W. 1989. "Impact, Logistics, and Prospects of Traditional Prenatal Diagnosis." *Clinical Genetics* 36: 378-85.

Girt, J.L. 1973. "Distance to General Medical Practice and Its Effect on Revealed Ill-Health in a Rural Environment." *Canadian Geographer* 17: 154-66.

Goodwin, B.A., and C.A. Huether. 1987. "Revised Estimates and Projections of Down Syndrome Births in the United States, and the Effects of Prenatal Diagnosis Utilization, 1970-2002." *Prenatal Diagnosis* 7: 261-71.

Grant, K.R. 1993. "Perceptions, Attitudes, and Experiences of Prenatal Diagnosis: A Winnipeg Study of Women Over 35." In *Prenatal Diagnosis: Background and Impact on Individuals*. Vol. 12 of the research studies of the Royal Commission on New Reproductive Technologies. Ottawa: Minister of Supply and Services Canada.

Hamerton, J.L., J.A. Evans, and L. Stranc. 1993. "Prenatal Diagnosis in Canada — 1990: A Review of Genetics Centres." In *Current Practice of Prenatal Diagnosis in Canada*. Vol. 13 of the research studies of the Royal Commission on New Reproductive Technologies. Ottawa: Minister of Supply and Services Canada.

Hayward, R.A., et al. 1988. "Who Gets Screened for Cervical and Breast Cancer? Results from a New National Survey." *Archives of Internal Medicine* 148: 1177-81.

Hook, E.B., and D.M. Schreinemachers. 1983. "Trends in Utilization of Prenatal Cytogenetic Diagnosis by New York State Residents in 1979 and 1980." *American Journal of Public Health* 73: 198-202.

Hunter, A.G.W., D. Thompson, and M. Speevak. 1987. "Midtrimester Genetic Amniocentesis in Eastern Ontario: A Review from 1970 to 1985." *Journal of Medical Genetics* 24: 335-43.

Ingram, D.R., D.R. Clarke, and R.A. Murdie. 1978. "Distance and the Decision to Visit an Emergency Department." *Social Science and Medicine* 12 (1D): 55-62.

Jones, K., and G. Moon. 1987. *Health, Disease and Society: A Critical Medical Geography*. New York: Routledge and Kegan Paul.

Joseph, A.E. 1979. "The Referral System as a Modifier of Distance Decay Effects in the Utilization of Mental Health Care Services." *Canadian Geographer* 23: 159-69.

Joseph, A.E., and D.R. Phillips. 1984. *Accessibility and Utilization: Geographical Perspectives on Health Care Delivery*. New York: Harper and Row.

Kaffe, S., and L.Y. Hsu. 1992. "Maternal Serum Alpha-Fetoprotein Screening and Fetal Chromosome Anomalies: Is Lowering Maternal Age for Amniocentesis Preferable?" *American Journal of Medical Genetics* 42: 801-806.

Knutson, C., et al. 1989. "Utilization of Amniocentesis and Chorionic Villus Sampling by South Carolina Women 35 Years of Age and Older." *Journal of the South Carolina Medical Association* 85: 463-67.

Kreitler, S., S. Chaitchik, and H. Kreitler. 1990. "The Psychological Profile of Women Attending Breast-Screening Tests." *Social Science and Medicine* 31: 1177-85.

Lane, D.S., A.P. Polednak, and M.A. Burg. 1992. "Breast Cancer Screening Practices Among Users of County-Funded Health Centers vs. Women in the Entire Community." *American Journal of Public Health* 82: 199-203.

Lippman, A. 1986. "Access to Prenatal Screening Services: Who Decides?" *Canadian Journal of Women and the Law* 1: 434-45.

Lippman-Hand, A., and D.I. Cohen. 1980. "Influence of Obstetricians' Attitudes on Their Use of Prenatal Diagnosis for the Detection of Down's Syndrome." *Canadian Medical Association Journal* 122: 1381-86.

McDonough, P.A. 1990. "The Diffusion of Genetic Amniocentesis in Ontario: 1969-1987." *Canadian Journal of Public Health* 81: 431-35.

Marion, J.P., et al. 1980. "Acceptance of Amniocentesis by Low-Income Patients in an Urban Hospital." *American Journal of Obstetrics and Gynecology* 138: 11-15.

Meade, M.S., J.W. Florin, and W.M. Gesler. 1988. *Medical Geography*. New York: Guilford Press.

Modell, B. 1988. "Ethical and Social Aspects of Fetal Diagnosis of the Hemoglobinopathies: A Practical View." In *Prenatal Diagnosis of Thalassemia and the Hemoglobinopathies*, ed. D. Loukopoulos. Boca Raton: CRC Press.

Naber, J.M., C.A. Huether, and B.A. Goodwin. 1987. "Temporal Changes in Ohio Amniocentesis Utilization During the First Twelve Years (1972-1983), and Frequency of Chromosome Abnormalities Observed." *Prenatal Diagnosis* 7: 51-65.

Nelson, K., and L.B. Holmes. 1989. "Malformations Due to Presumed Spontaneous Mutations in Newborn Infants." *New England Journal of Medicine* 320: 19-23.

Norgaard-Pedersen, B., et al. 1990. "Maternal Serum Markers in Screening for Down Syndrome." *Clinical Genetics* 37: 35-43.

Roghmann, K.J., et al. 1983. "The Selective Utilization of Prenatal Genetic Diagnosis. Experiences of a Regional Program in Upstate New York During the 1970s." *Medical Care* 21: 1111-25.

Ross, N.A. 1992. "Women's Access to Health Care. A Case Study of the Ontario Breast Screening Program, Kingston, Ontario." M.A. thesis, Queen's University.

Rutledge, D.N., et al. 1988. "Exploration of Factors Affecting Mammography Behaviors." *Preventive Medicine* 17: 412-22.

Selle, H.F., D.W. Holmes, and M.L. Ingbar. 1979. "The Growing Demand for Mid-Trimester Amniocentesis: A Systems Approach to Forecasting the Need for Facilities." *American Journal of Public Health* 69: 574-80.

Senior, M.L., and S.M. Williamson. 1990. "An Investigation into the Influence of Geographical Factors on Attendance for Cervical Cytology Screening." *Transactions of the Institute of British Geographers* 15: 421-34.

Thouez, J-P. 1987. *Organisation spatiale des systèmes de soins*. Montreal: Les Presses de l'Université de Montréal.

Vernon, S.W., E.A. Laville, and G.L. Jackson. 1990. "Participation in Breast Screening Programs: A Review." *Social Science and Medicine* 30: 1107-18.

Verp, M.S., and J.L. Simpson. 1990. "Amniocentesis for Prenatal Diagnosis." In *Human Prenatal Diagnosis*, ed. K. Filkins and J.F. Russo. 2d ed., rev. New York: Marcel Dekker.

Wald, N.J., et al. 1988. "Maternal Serum Screening for Down's Syndrome in Early Pregnancy." *British Medical Journal* (8 October): 883-87.

Wilson, R.D., and N.L. Rudd. 1991. "Canadian Guidelines for Prenatal Diagnosis of Genetic Disorders: An Update." *Journal of the Society of Obstetricians and Gynaecologists of Canada* 5 (August): 5-6.

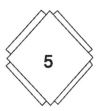

# Perceptions, Attitudes, and Experiences of Prenatal Diagnosis:
# A Winnipeg Study of Women Over 35

### Karen R. Grant

**Executive Summary**

This study explored the perceptions and attitudes of a sample of 122 women of advanced maternal age (over 35) toward prenatal diagnosis (PND). They had been referred to the Section of Clinical Genetics (Winnipeg) and completed a post-counselling questionnaire (91% response rate), with 70 also being interviewed before their counselling session.

The interviews showed that women have favourable views toward counselling; view it as informative, helpful, and not too stressful; and see the counsellors as professional. However, testing also evokes heightened concern about the procedures and possible outcomes. Although, with one possible exception, they experienced no direct persuasion to have testing, the women felt subtle pressures to ensure fetal health. Concerns about bearing and raising a disabled child were common because of the physical, intellectual, and social problems they face. Women worried about the effects a disabled child could have on themselves and on their family's lives. Few women take the testing process lightly; some minimize their attachment to the pregnancy until the results are known.

---

This paper was completed for the Royal Commission on New Reproductive Technologies in April 1992.

The quantitative analysis describes the users of counselling. Generally, more highly educated, affluent women are using PND. Approximately 75% of the sample found genetic counselling to be helpful; however, a few women would have preferred receiving more counselling, not only the presentation of medical facts. Attempts to explore the multivariate associations between women's satisfaction with genetic counselling yielded only tentative findings due to the high variable-to-sample-size ratio.

## Chapter 1. Introduction

The new reproductive technologies, including those used in the field of medical genetics, have had a dramatic impact on human reproduction (Arditti et al. 1989; Blank 1982; Bortner 1990; A.E. Clarke 1990; Corea 1985, 1991; Currie 1988; Duster 1990; Elias and Annas 1987; Lappe 1984; Overall 1987, 1989; St. Peter 1989; Sawicki 1991; Scutt 1988; Spallone 1989; Stanworth 1987; Tymstra 1991; Woliver 1989, 1991; Zimmerman 1981). Sophisticated technologies now make it possible to diagnose and treat various genetic abnormalities; thus, these technologies have given women (and their partners) the opportunity to make conscious and proactive decisions about reproduction, including whether to continue a pregnancy involving an affected fetus (Ajjimakorn et al. 1988; al-Jader et al. 1990; Antley 1979; Bundey and Broughton 1989; Clark and DeVore 1989; Elkins et al. 1986; Henifen et al. 1988; Holmes-Siedle et al. 1987; Hubbard 1986; G.E. Robinson et al. 1988, 1991; Tymstra et al. 1991; Verp et al. 1988; Yoxen 1982). However, it is alleged that prenatal diagnostic tests are being used not only to detect abnormalities, but for social reasons related to, among other things, sex selection and the preferred ordering of offspring (Corea 1985; Dickens 1986; Fletcher 1980; Parikh 1990; Saxton 1987b; Winestine 1989). Whether the reasons underlying the use of prenatal diagnostic services are, strictly speaking, medical or social, some authors feel these technologies may be changing the nature of human reproduction in profound ways (Rothman 1987; Tymstra 1991).

It has been suggested by some that the new reproductive technologies raise the spectre of creating a world of "perfect babies" (Chadwick 1987, 94). With declining fertility among the post-baby boom generation in the developed world, partly related to the changing status of women in these societies, ever more attention has been focussed on planned pregnancies and on having a healthy child. Often, concerns about the genetic health of a fetus centre on the impact an abnormality will have on the people and supports involved: (1) How will the child deal with the health and social effects of the abnormality? What about the stigma associated with some abnormalities? What will the survivability be? How will the abnormality affect autonomy?; (2) How will an affected child impact the marital relationship, parenting of other children, sibling relationships, the extended family? How will an affected child influence family and social life?; (3) What are the costs in social and economic terms of children born with genetic abnormalities? What institutional supports will be necessary to assist families with affected children?; and (4) Is the gene pool affected by "not exercising quality control over the species"? In other words, there are the questions raised concerning "genetic load" (Chadwick 1987, 95).

Prenatal screening has implications not only for the individuals using it, but also for the health care delivery system. Other ethical and legal questions arise, particularly in view of the increasingly litigious world in which we live, and the ominous spectre of "wrongful life" suits (Henifen et al. 1988), which clearly are a by-product of this technological development. The predictive capacity of medicine, which is currently being enhanced by the Humane Genome Initiative (Beckwith 1991), means that there will be increased capacity to detect genetic make-up and therefore the possibility of increased use of testing prenatally.

In light of these considerations, the significance of genetic screening and counselling in relation to reproductive decision making should not be underestimated. Given the greater availability of these technologies and the changed patterns of utilization (e.g., the increasing number of advanced maternal age [AMA] women) that have been noted in recent years, it seems timely to explore the nature and scope of women's perceptions of, attitudes toward, and experiences with genetic services.

Of the many studies in this area, Sorenson et al.'s (1981) research is likely the most comprehensive. However, these U.S. data are now more than 10 years old, and the sample included individuals seeking genetic testing for all reasons. It is widely recognized that genetic counselling for individuals with a family predisposition to genetic abnormality is quite different from the counselling that occurs with those whose only known risk is age. Recently, there are more older pregnant women in Canadian society and there has been a lowering of the risk barrier for genetic screening (from 40 to 35 years of age), meaning that this group is the largest having prenatal diagnosis (PND), although their risk is low. Generalizing from research on all users of prenatal testing and applying it to a group defined as at risk for age alone is inappropriate and potentially misleading. Understanding aspects of prenatal testing and its social and psychological dimensions in this large group is particularly important.

This study provides data on a group of women in Manitoba who were referred for genetic counselling (and testing) because of AMA (i.e., 35 years of age or older at the time of delivery). None of these women had a known family or medical history of genetic abnormalities. Like women in many parts of the world, they were referred for counselling as a routine part of ante-natal care, given that the incidence of chromosomal abnormalities such as Down syndrome tends to increase with maternal age. The juxtaposition of the risk of bearing a child with one of these conditions and the risk of miscarriage associated with testing procedures (approximately 1 in 300 to 1 in 350 pregnancies) has meant that this is considered to be an "optimal" age at which to perform genetic screening, using methods such as amniocentesis and chorionic villus sampling. Some would add as well that this is the age group for which service provision is the most economically efficient (Gill et al. 1987; Hook 1991; Swint and Greenberg 1988).

The overriding aim of this study was to conduct a sociological examination of these women's perceptions of, attitudes toward, and experiences with genetic screening services. Information was sought on why women were using PND and how they planned to use the information obtained through genetic counselling and screening. This study aimed to discover if there was any foundation to the allegations that women were either being pressured into having genetic testing or being told that they must be prepared to have an abortion to be considered for genetic testing (Farrant 1985; McDonnell 1988; Rothman 1987). Both of these issues were raised in the public hearing process of the Royal Commission and, if founded, could have implications on the organization and delivery of prenatal diagnostic services in Manitoba (and potentially in Canada). Moreover, such allegations, if founded, would suggest far-reaching implications in terms of the societal view toward the disabled (Asch 1989; Asch and Fine 1988; Finger 1989; Oliver 1990; Saxton 1987a, 1987b, 1989) and toward the use of genetic screening for social, instead of strictly medical, reasons. Finally, issues of reproductive choice are also relevant in this connection (Rapp 1984; Rowland 1987).

The specific research objectives addressed in this study were:

1. To determine patterns of utilization of, and referral to, PND. More specifically, this study explores: why women avail themselves of PND; the patterns of referral that lead women to PND; and whether there are any major sources of variation in referral patterns, on the basis of sociodemographic characteristics, medical characteristics, or both.

2. To determine women's perceptions, attitudes, and knowledge of PND. More specifically, this study identifies: what these women know about PND, a priori; what women know of the medical (and social) reasons for using PND during pregnancy; what women know of the risks and benefits associated with various PND tests; what women perceive their options to be upon learning of the outcome of genetic diagnoses; how women use genetic testing to influence their reproductive decisions; and what concerns women bring to genetic counselling sessions.

3. To determine whether women are satisfied with PND counselling services, in terms of information being provided that is accessible, understandable, relevant, and provided in a socially and psychologically supportive manner.

In brief, this study provides detailed information on who uses PND in Manitoba, and why. The study was conducted during the summer and autumn of 1991. The methodological strategy combined quantitative and qualitative data collection techniques.

The findings of this study indicate that many women were satisfied with the genetic counselling they received, and stated that they found it informative (85.7%) and helpful (75.2%). Yet, women's ambivalence about genetic counselling was evident when they were asked about the reassurance genetic counselling provided (43.2% found counselling to be reassuring, 12.7% did not find it reassuring at all, and 44.1% stated it was neither). Other measures detailed in the qualitative and quantitative analysis of this study show that the women who were studied are not generally of one voice on the use of procedures such as amniocentesis and chorionic villus sampling. In their experiences with these technologies, many women find they raise difficult ethical and moral questions. Concerns identified by some women include the eugenic context in which prenatal testing is seen to exist, and apprehensions about bearing and raising a child with a disability. The routinization of prenatal testing in pregnancy was identified by some women as an issue. This is consistent with the literature that documents the ways that technologies contribute to the medicalization of pregnancy and childbirth. All of these issues relate directly to the mandate of the Royal Commission on New Reproductive Technologies to provide recommendations regarding the uses to which such technologies are currently put in Canadian society.

There was a relatively high level of satisfaction in this sample regarding the counselling services they have received at the Section of Clinical Genetics. A few women volunteered that they were concerned that medical facts were emphasized over the social, emotional, and ethical dimensions of prenatal screening. At the same time, the view that counsellors were helpful and professional was widespread.

Organizationally, this report is divided into six chapters. Following a review of the literature on genetic counselling and genetic testing (Chapter 2), the methodology for this study is outlined (Chapter 3). Next, the study findings are presented (Chapters 4 and 5). The closing section includes a discussion of the study, in terms of its strengths and weaknesses, along with some consideration of directions for policy and for future research in this area (Chapter 6).

## Chapter 2. Prenatal Diagnosis in Ante-Natal Care

**Introduction**

PND has become a routinely offered part of ante-natal care for older women in Canadian society. Although not an "overnight" development, this has preceded, rather than followed, an in-depth and considered analysis or debate between the users of this type of reproductive technology, the providers of the service, and policy makers themselves. That such a debate is occurring now under the aegis of the Royal Commission on New Reproductive Technologies (and presumably will continue after its report to the Government of Canada) signifies the degree to which a need exists for an informed public policy in this area of health services.

PND has been only one of the many technological innovations that have been the hallmark of medicine in the latter decades of the twentieth century. The ethos of Western medicine seems to favour technology, such that care is heavily biased toward the use of technology for the detection, management, treatment, and prevention of disease and disability (Wright 1989). Fuchs (1968) has referred to this phenomenon as the technological imperative — that if something can be done, it will be done, using whatever technological means exist at the time. He tells us that, to a large degree, this imperative has been embraced enthusiastically by physicians and the public. Both of these groups have come to see technological means as more desirable and progressive, and as evidence of our mastery over perplexing health challenges. The technology of medicine makes possible what was at one time considered improbable, or even impossible. This is certainly true in reproductive medicine.

The proliferation of technology in medicine has not been without its critics both within and outside the profession. Researchers such as McKinlay (1982) and Cohen and Rothschild (1979) discussed the public policy implications of technological diffusion and the problems posed by technologies that have been poorly or inadequately evaluated (cf. Bunker 1985). Illich (1977) commented that many technologies are iatrogenic — that is, they introduce new problems while attempting to solve the old ones. Similarly, Gruenberg (1982) spoke of technologies that represent "the failures of success." Some medical technologies may prolong a disabled and diminished life, even though the goal was to improve diagnostic and treatment methods in medicine. Thomas (1979) noted that many technologies used in medicine are, at best, only "halfway" technologies, in that they fail to ameliorate the underlying problem, yet may offer some respite to individuals afflicted with various health conditions. Certainly many of the new reproductive technologies (e.g., *in vitro* fertilization [IVF]) could be classified as "halfway" technologies, to the extent that they fail to address the underlying causes of infertility, while making it possible for a small percentage of women to bear children.

Feminist critics have also voiced concerns regarding reproductive technologies that bear directly on the health and well-being of women. Criticism has focussed on the gender-biased values both of the technology and of the practitioners using it (Arditti et al. 1989; Hubbard 1990; Koch and Morgall 1987; Ratcliff 1989; Sandelowski et al. 1991; Scutt 1988; Spallone 1989; Stanworth 1987; Wajcman 1990). Also, these technologies have been seen as further evidence of the extent to which women's lives and their reproductive function have been medicalized (Rothman 1987).

In addition, feminist critics have challenged the use of many technologies because of the recognized harms and risks of use of drugs such as thalidomide, diethylstilbestrol, and Depo-Provera®, hormone replacement therapy, and surgical procedures such as episiotomy, Caesarian section, hysterectomy, and breast implantation. It has been argued that many of the technologies of medicine (and, in particular, those used in the field of reproductive and genetic engineering) can and do pose serious physical and psychological health threats to women (Corea 1985; Klein 1991). Yet, an examination of the discourse surrounding these (and other) technologies reveals an emphasis on the benefits, rather than the risks, associated with their use.

Some think that the dominance of technology in modern medicine virtually ensures that other alternatives will not be explored or even considered, given our tendency toward "technophilia" (Wright 1989, 13). They think that discourse of science is such that the underlying values of the technology are seldom explored and we continue on, with our "Western faith in the usefulness and benevolence of medical technology" (ibid.). In the opinion of some, it means that the consequences for women, collectively, of new reproductive technologies are minimized, even though many critics have pointed out that these technologies further fragment and objectify women's bodies (Klein 1991).

Feminist critiques of new reproductive technologies have also focussed on the fact that although most women have concerns about controlling reproduction, the emphasis of such technologies is primarily to enhance reproduction. Among other things, they think there is a gulf between what women want (or are concerned about) and what the health system is oriented to, illustrating that women have largely been absent from discussions of the impact of this medical technology on their lives (cf. Redman et al. 1988). In a small way, then, this research project provides women with an opportunity to offer their insights into one type of new reproductive technologies — prenatal testing.

## PND and the Social Construction of Risk

PND has introduced revolutionary changes to ante-natal care and the manner in which having children takes place today (Furhmann 1989). Not too long ago, a couple could judge its risk of conceiving a child with some genetic disease only on the basis of family history. Today, "with the analysis of amniotic fluid and cultured fetal cells, ultrasonography, analysis of maternal serum for alpha-fetoprotein and radiography, ... it is now possible to make a more accurate estimation of genetic risks" (Paez-Victor 1988, 3). PND, because it can predict with a knowable certainty whether a woman will bear an affected child, introduces a new level of decision making that has not existed before.

> The physical, social, psychological and moral dilemma then becomes: should this particular pregnancy be continued or should it be terminated? ... A "natural" risk has been transformed into a decision involving risks where the alternatives have to be decided upon in a deliberate manner. (Paez-Victor 1988, 4)

A critical element to the discussion of PND use among women 35 years of age or older is the notion of their "high risk" status (Ales et al. 1990). What exactly does it mean to be at high risk of bearing a child with a genetic abnormality? If one considers the actual probability of bearing a child with Down syndrome, for example, it must be realized that the risk increases gradually over the course of women's reproductive years; a sudden, dramatic increase in risk does not occur at age 35. The overall incidence of Down syndrome (in the United States) is 1 in 800 (Elias and Annas 1987). Although the risk of bearing a child with Down syndrome is 1 in 1 700 at age 20, it increases to 1 in 350 in women at age 35 and 1 in 100 at age 40 (Section of Clinical Genetics pamphlet, n.d.). The probability of bearing a child with a chromosome abnormality is higher: at age 35, the risk is 1 in 180, and at age 40, it is 1 in 80 (Section of Clinical Genetics pamphlet, n.d.).

The criterion for routine prenatal testing of women has fallen over the years from 40 years of age to 37 to 35. This drop reveals that factors other than the absolute probability of bearing a child with a genetic abnormality influence medical practice in this area. The arbitrariness of the definition of risk is self-evident. However, this definition and criterion have had immense power in the construction of the "at-risk" pregnancy. For some women, reaching the age of 35 is akin to passing through an invisible barrier that signifies pregnancy as immensely perilous.

Tymstra and his colleagues (Tymstra 1991; Tymstra et al. 1991) suggested that as technologies are discussed in terms of their possibilities, the ease with which they are diffused and accepted into standard medical practice is heightened. This seems to be so with the technologies of PND. Certainly, some studies have revealed that there is a high level of acceptability of various methods of PND (under certain conditions) within the population (Sjögren 1992; Tymstra et al. 1991). That in some countries amniocentesis is often performed to alleviate "maternal anxiety" is evidence of the power of technology, not only to shape demands for it but to reinforce the notion of pregnancy as a risk-laden state. (In Canada, it is rarely done for "maternal anxiety.") This is not a new idea; the social construction of pregnancy, as characterized by elevated risk, means that PND strengthens a definition of pregnancy as pathological, a point made extensively in the medicalization literature (Arditti et al. 1989; Corea 1985; Grant 1981; Overall 1989; Riessman 1983; Rothman 1987; Sjögren and Uddenberg 1990; Tymstra 1991; Wright 1989).

More than this, though, is the creation of an imperative for women to undergo testing as any "responsible" mother[1] would. The emergence of PND in modern obstetrics has occurred alongside a growing debate on whose rights should take precedence — those of the woman or those of the fetus (Bradish 1987; Fost 1989; Klein 1991; Laborie 1987; Maier 1989; Raymond 1987; Rose 1987; Scutt 1988; Stanworth 1987; Stein and Redman 1990).[2] This debate does not centre on PND, but it is certainly relevant. Women may not be told they must have testing; indeed, testing with amniocentesis and chorionic villus sampling is a voluntary decision in Western countries like Canada. But, a clear and powerful message that they ought to have testing resonates throughout our culture. As Rothman wrote:

> We are in little danger of the state sending cops to the doors of pregnant women and demanding prenatal diagnosis and selective abortion for eugenic reasons. That does not mean that women are not put under enormous pressures to undergo these procedures. The pressures here tend to be economic: by providing little — and ever less — support to families and to people with disabilities, women are made to feel little choice but to abort fetuses that would become children and adults whom the state would treat so badly. The pressures are also social: women are increasingly held responsible, not for the gene pool, but for the health of their children. Disabilities in children are increasingly seen less as the product of god or acts of fate, and more as the direct responsibilities of their mothers. (Rothman 1990, 81)

Similarly, Tymstra et al. concluded that "parents cannot permit themselves to ignore these types of technology which involve some degree of risk, because they would be guilty of inflicting illness and suffering on their child" (1991, 898). In a climate where risks can be known and where tests can be performed economically, the personal and social costs (monetary and otherwise) of not having testing are high. Those costs are usually borne most heavily by the women in our society.

## PND: The Technologies

At present, PND includes the use of several technologies, the most common being amniocentesis and chorionic villus sampling (Grant and Mohide 1982; Mohide and Grant 1989). These methods of PND are performed typically on AMA women who are thus identified by their age as being at risk; and on those whose risk is a function of a family or medical history of genetic abnormality. In addition, forms of prenatal screening such as the maternal serum alpha-fetoprotein (AFP) determination may be used to identify those at risk, who are then offered amniocentesis and chorionic villus sampling. The maternal serum AFP test was developed to detect neural tube defects (NTDs) such as spina bifida and anencephaly, but it can also be used to identify an increased risk of Down syndrome in the fetus. Maternal serum AFP testing is done routinely in some jurisdictions for women presenting themselves to ante-natal care (Greenberg 1988). Finally, ultrasound is now one of the most common forms of PND used in modern obstetrics. This technology was developed initially to monitor the development of the fetus *in utero* and now finds many other applications, from the identification of treatable kidney disease, to identification of fetal sex, to being used in conjunction with amniocentesis and chorionic villus sampling (Tymstra et al. 1991).

Daker and Bobrow (1989) estimated that at least 75% of all referrals for PND are women 35 years of age or older. Elias and Annas (1987) put the estimate at 85%. Lippman (1986) noted that 7 500 Canadian women use amniocentesis each year and that most of them have been referred for prenatal testing solely because of AMA. Even still, a significant number of women referred for prenatal testing decline it, for a variety of reasons (Lippman-Hand and Piper 1981). Although the research literature is not generally clear on the actual extent of the use of such technologies, it is generally agreed that their use (particularly ultrasound) has increased markedly in the decades since first being offered (Baird and Sadovnick 1988; Baird et al. 1985; Goodwin and Huether 1987; Holloway and Brock 1988; Knott et al. 1986).

Chodirker (1991), examining the use patterns in Manitoba, reported that in the five-year period between 1984 and 1989, maternal serum AFP testing doubled (from 5 000 to 10 000). In that same period, the number of amniocenteses nearly doubled (from 317 to 600) (Section of Clinical Genetics, Health Sciences Centre, Winnipeg, personal communication, 1992). While in 1986 12 chorionic villus sampling tests were performed on women in Manitoba, 75 such tests were done in 1989. In Manitoba, the proportion of pregnant women undergoing prenatal maternal serum screening is estimated to be approximately 50% (Chodirker 1991), which also represents a significant increase within the past decade.

## *Amniocentesis*

Amniocentesis was first developed in 1969 and is now the most widely used procedure for detecting fetal abnormalities. As noted in the literature, this method of genetic testing is considered safe, as established in various studies worldwide (Daker and Bobrow 1989). The procedure is usually performed between the 15th and 20th weeks of gestation, when there is sufficient amniotic fluid in the sac surrounding the fetus. A small sample of about 10 to 20 mL is withdrawn from the sac through a needle inserted into the woman's abdomen. Before withdrawing the amniotic fluid, an ultrasound is usually performed to check the location and viability of the fetus (a second ultrasound is performed during the procedure to check the indicators again). The amount of amniotic fluid removed during the procedure is quickly replenished naturally (usually within a few hours). The cells are cultured, a process that requires two to four weeks (depending on the cell specimen, laboratory conditions, and so on).

Amniocentesis is customarily performed for the identification of chromosomal abnormalities such as trisomies, the most common being Down syndrome. (The test also can detect certain structural abnormalities, although this is not why AMA women are referred for amniocentesis.)

Clinically, some of these chromosomal abnormalities vary in severity, and the degree of severity cannot be known from the chromosomal picture. This type of uncertainty is a built-in quality of this kind of genetic testing, but the range of severity is known for the most common chromosomal abnormalities.

Although widely used and hailed as an effective method of prenatal testing, amniocentesis has several drawbacks. The procedure carries a risk of miscarriage of approximately 1% (though different studies estimate the risk to be between 0.5% and 1.5%) (Daker and Bobrow 1989). It is customary in the management of pregnancies among AMA women to consider this risk to be "acceptable." The risk of fetal abnormality and the risk of miscarriage are approximately the same in women of this age group (Elias and Annas 1987). The test only reveals what it is designed to test for — namely, chromosomal abnormalities (Kolata 1983).

Two drawbacks associated with amniocentesis are the time needed to culture cells and the timing of the test. Cells require two to four weeks to be cultured and then karyotyped; the waiting period involves worry, distress, and anticipation for most women (Farrant 1985; Kolker and Burke 1987; Rothman 1987). Because the procedure is normally performed in the second trimester of a pregnancy (when sufficient amniotic fluid has accumulated),[3] if a decision is made to terminate the pregnancy, the woman will have to undergo a second-trimester abortion that is far more difficult physically (and usually psychologically) than if the procedure had been done in the first trimester. Normally, a second-trimester abortion requires the woman to have labour induced, and she will usually deliver a dead fetus (Rapp 1984, 1987, 1989; Rothman 1987).

An amniocentesis also may have to be repeated if an inadequate sample was extracted (Daker and Bobrow 1989). If the culture reveals mosaicism (a finding of the presence of both normal and abnormal cells), a repeat amniocentesis is usually indicated. Sometimes a cordocentesis is performed, which provides results more quickly. However, precautions are usually taken in laboratories to avoid the need for a repeat amniocentesis by testing two or more cultures from the same sample to see if mosaicism is genuine. Such technical problems make decision making at a later stage of a pregnancy precarious not only from the standpoint of the woman's health, but also because they may have serious legal implications in countries where abortion laws prohibit late termination of pregnancy.

Despite its various limitations, amniocentesis is widely used in ante-natal care for AMA women (Chodirker 1991; Kromberg et al. 1989). Its primary strength is the high level of accuracy in the detection of chromosomal abnormalities. Its limitations have contributed to the development of an alternative method of testing, namely, chorionic villus sampling (or biopsy).

## *Chorionic Villus Sampling*

In some instances, it is desirable to perform testing at an earlier stage of the pregnancy. One of the great advantages of chorionic villus sampling, a procedure developed in the mid-1980s, is that it can be safely performed in the first trimester, as early as the 8th week of a pregnancy. However, it is normally done between 11 and 13 weeks (the potential of an increased risk to the fetus has led to chorionic villus sampling being discouraged before 9 weeks' gestation). The test can be performed in one of two ways, with the sample being removed transabdominally (a method of extraction similar to that used in amniocentesis) or transcervically (a somewhat more invasive method thought to be more commonly associated with intrauterine infection) (Daker and Bobrow 1989). Chorionic villus sampling is done under direct ultrasound guidance (i.e., ultrasound is used throughout the procedure). A small sample or biopsy (10 to 40 mg) of villi of the chorion frondosum (what will later become the placenta) is removed, and is processed either directly (with results known within a few days) or by culturing the cells (which takes two to three weeks) (ibid.). Chorionic villus sampling is used primarily to detect chromosomal abnormalities, but provides fetal cells so that testing for metabolic or molecular disorders can also be conducted if needed. Like amniocentesis, although chromosomal abnormalities are identified, there is a range of severity. Several randomized clinical trials have been undertaken to ascertain whether it is a safe and effective method of PND (Canadian Collaborative CVS-Amniocentesis Clinical Trial Group 1989; Lippman et al. 1992), and all have concluded that it is.

Although chorionic villus sampling offers the possibility of earlier testing, it too has drawbacks. Foremost is the slightly higher risk (an extra 0.6% chance) of miscarriage from the procedure than for amniocentesis (Section of Clinical Genetics pamphlet, n.d.), although the difference in risk of miscarriage between the two is not statistically significant (Canadian Collaborative CVS-Amniocentesis Clinical Trial Group 1989). As well, and not insignificantly, if abnormal results are found, a woman may be referred for amniocentesis at 16 weeks, in which case the woman is subjected to another invasive procedure (Daker and Bobrow 1989). Under such circumstances, the benefits of early testing are more or less lost.

In addition, many pregnancies in which a fetal abnormality is detected through chorionic villus sampling could be destined to result in a miscarriage anyway. Thus, a proportion of women are undergoing testing and side-effects (i.e., uncertainty, worry, apprehension, a possible decision to terminate a pregnancy) that are unnecessary. Unfortunately, knowing which pregnancies would have spontaneously aborted is impossible. The bottom line is that the timing of chorionic villus sampling has both advantages and disadvantages.

Although the use of chorionic villus sampling has increased in recent years, it is performed less often than amniocentesis. Whether it replaces amniocentesis as the key diagnostic tool for the identification of fetal abnormalities remains to be seen (Brandenburg et al. 1991).

### *Genetic Counselling*

For many women the first step to obtaining PND is genetic counselling. Genetic counselling is usually provided by people trained as geneticists (with an M.D. or Ph.D. degree) or genetic counsellors (with either baccalaureate or master's level degrees). All of these people have had training in counselling, and some are trained in psychological counselling as well.

In 1974, the Ad Hoc Committee on Genetic Counseling (a committee of Canadian and American physicians and scientists) defined the purpose of genetic counselling as:

> ... a communication process which deals with the human problems associated with the occurrence, or the risk of occurrence, of a genetic disorder in a family. This process involves an attempt by one or more appropriately trained persons to help the individual or family (1) comprehend the medical facts, including the diagnosis, the probable course of the disorder, and the available management; (2) appreciate the way heredity contributes to the disorder, and the risk of recurrence in specified relatives; (3) understand the options for dealing with the risk of recurrence; (4) choose the course of action which seems appropriate to them in view of their risk and their family goals and act in accordance with that decision; and (5) make the best possible adjustment to the disorder in an affected family member and/or to the risk of recurrence of that disorder. (Fraser 1974, 637)

In most centres offering genetic counselling to AMA women, it is customary to verify that age is the only likely risk. To do this, a history is taken (referred to as a "pedigree"), detailing the pregnancies and live births for members of the woman's family and that of her partner (Stoeber et al. 1991). Then, the counsellor assesses the information provided to arrive at an estimate of risk of chromosomal abnormality in the pregnancy. Some explanation of the nature of the risk is provided, for example, as compared to women who are older or younger. It is usually left to the woman (and her partner, as relevant) to decide whether the risk is high or low. Research suggests that individuals judge the probability of having a child with Down syndrome in bipolar terms (either high or low) (d'Ydewalle and Evers-Kiebooms 1987; Evans et al. 1990; Evers-Kiebooms et al. 1987; Shiloh and Saxe 1989; Wertz et al. 1984, 1986). Obviously, this assessment is personal, influenced by social, moral, ethical, and religious considerations (Seals et al. 1985). Under varied circumstances, different individuals who are told that they stand the same numerical likelihood of having a Down syndrome child might judge their risk differently — one person opting to take the risk of carrying a pregnancy to term, while another might opt to terminate the pregnancy (Lippman-Hand and Fraser 1979).

Genetic counselling routinely provides clients with factual information about the probability of bearing an affected child and what this entails technically. In addition, genetic counsellors explain how the testing is performed, and what the woman can expect before, during, and after the procedure. The way in which genetic counselling is provided in most genetics centres across Canada (and in many other countries) is that the counsellor functions in a "non-directive" way; that is, the client is provided with the statistical information about the risk of genetic abnormalities, but no explicit direction is given as to how to act under the circumstances. This non-directive style is in contrast to the traditional doctor-patient relationship, which is much more directive (Clarke 1991; Elias and Annas 1987; Kessler 1979, 1989; Kessler and Levine 1987).

Genetic counselling has gone the non-directive route, on the argument that individuals should be given the information and then be allowed to make a choice freely about how to react (Antley 1979). The historical misuse of genetics in a coercive and discriminatory way (especially during the Nazi era) has likely reinforced the current orientation toward non-directive counselling.[4] It is hoped being non-directive makes it possible to minimize imposition of the counsellor's values in the process.

In theory, the idea of non-directive counselling is compelling but, in practice, it is recognized that it is not truly possible (Clarke 1991; Yarborough et al. 1989). The information counsellors provide is not neutral, and the structure of the relationship between counsellor and counsellee means that messages are transmitted about what the counsellor thinks (Hubbard 1989; Rapp 1989; Saxton 1989). The choices individuals are given during genetic counselling are not necessarily "free" — the ideal toward which the notion of non-directive counselling is directed (Brown 1989). As Rothman noted,

> For those whose choices meet the social expectations, for those who want what the society wants them to want, the experience of choice [through prenatal diagnosis] is very real. Perhaps what we should realize is that human beings living in society have precious little choice ever. There may really be no such thing as individual choice in a social structure, not in any absolute way. The social structure creates needs — the needs for women to be mothers, the needs for small families, the needs for 'perfect children' — and creates the technology that enables people to make the needed choices. The question is not whether choices are constructed, but *how* they are constructed. Society, in its ultimate meaning, may be nothing more and nothing less than the structuring of choices. (emphasis in original) (Rothman 1987, 14)

Similarly, Zola made the following observation:

> Bombarded on all sides by realistic concerns (the escalation of costs) and objective evidence (genetics) and techniques (genetic counsellors), the basic value issue at stake will be obfuscated. The freedom to choose will be illusory. Someone will already have set the limits of choice (cuts in medical care and social benefits but not in defense spending), the

dimensions of choice (if you do this then you will have an X probability of a defective child), and the outcomes of choice (you will have to endure the following social, political, legal and economic costs). (Zola 1983, 296)

Counselling and screening programs for common genetic disorders (e.g., Down syndrome, spina bifida) are influenced by, and influence, societal values regarding the role of science and technology in the management of pregnancy, and the attitudes and prejudices toward the people with disabilities in our society.

This issue is often disputed by some of those providing the service. In its own right, the issue is important, as it sets the context in which counselling is offered and in which individuals make decisions about how to use the information they obtain in counselling.

## Review of the Social and Psychological Literature on PND and Genetic Counselling

There has been an extensive body of research examining various aspects of prenatal diagnostic services (Capron et al. 1979; Milunsky 1975). Several studies conducted previously, such as Rothman's (1987), have influenced the research questions asked in this particular study and the methodology that was used. Although the present study considers only AMA women, many studies of PND have considered other risk groups. Some of the literature pertaining to the use of PND by AMA women and those with other known a priori risks is reviewed here, even if selectively.

A fair amount of research has been conducted into women's attitudes toward obstetric care (Garcia 1982; Hyde 1986; Reid 1988; Reid and Garcia 1989; Stewart 1986). The results of such studies have revealed the predominance of technology in this field of medicine, which has medicalized women's childbearing experience (Riessman 1983; Rothman 1987). Considering the issue of screening in pregnancy, Reid and Garcia (1989) noted that women seldom get the full complement of information they desire about testing and, consequently, women's anxiety tends to increase accordingly. Despite this, they noted that the findings of many studies have shown that women are, as a group, quite compliant when it comes to the use of screening tests.

Related to this line of research are studies on women's preferences or choices of different methods of prenatal testing (Abramsky and Rodeck 1991; Bryce et al. 1989; McGovern et al. 1986). A recent study on women's choices in PND showed that women's preference for amniocentesis often was because their referral had come too late to allow chorionic villus sampling (Brandenburg et al. 1991). This finding highlights that, once a woman has decided to undergo PND, her choices as to which technology to use depend on providers offering sufficient information to make an informed decision.

An important area of research has focussed on issues of access, utilization, and referral patterns (Crandall et al. 1986; Fahy and Lippman

1988; Hyde 1986; Jones 1991; Kyle et al. 1988; Macri 1986; Moatti et al. 1990; Reid 1988; Reid and Garcia 1989). For example, Lippman (1986, 1991) has shown that PND is used more by couples of a higher socioeconomic level, and that PND reinforces social inequities. At present, an AMA client (and her partner) are likely to fit into a certain demographic profile, not unlike the following:

> 56.2 per cent of the mothers and 78.6 per cent of their mates had some college education, including 25.9 per cent and 35.5 per cent, respectively, who had done graduate work. The average gross annual income for all families was $25 271. These statistics suggest that the lower socioeconomic groups have yet to use prenatal diagnosis facilities as fully as those in the higher socioeconomic groups. (Golbus et al. 1979, 158)

Research shows that individuals with less education and members of some ethnocultural communities may be somewhat less likely to use PND, although some of this variation depends on the reason for prenatal testing (Duster 1990). If this is so, and if higher socioeconomic groups are more inclined to have testing, a situation in which certain trisomies are reduced in some segments of the population and stay the same in others is not impossible. This raises the questions of whether service should be increased or decreased, for whom, and how? Lippman (1991) raised a significant public policy question in her insightful analysis, which deserves further consideration but cannot be addressed here.

Some studies have considered the effectiveness of genetic counselling (Frets et al. 1990a, 1990b; Loader et al. 1991; Somer et al. 1988; Sorenson and Wertz 1986) and the ways in which reproductive decisions are made as a result of PND services (Earley et al. 1991; Humphreys and Berkeley 1987; Laurence and Morris 1981; Pauker and Pauker 1987a, 1987b; Pitz 1987; Sjögren and Uddenberg 1988a; Sorenson et al. 1987; Swerts 1987; Vlek 1987; Zeitune et al. 1991). Some investigators have explored PND in the context of the educative aspects of counselling (Faden et al. 1985; Naylor 1975; Rice and Doherty 1982; Sanden and Bjurulf 1988a; Welshimer and Earp 1989) and the psychological sequelae associated with PND (Blumberg 1984; Blumberg et al. 1975; Campbell et al. 1982; Fletcher 1984; Fletcher et al. 1980; Gillot-de Vries 1988; Green and Malin 1988; Green 1990; Hunter et al. 1987; Keenan et al. 1991; Kessler 1989; Kessler and Levine 1987; Leff 1987; Marks et al. 1989; Marteau 1989; Marteau et al. 1988a, 1988b, 1989a, 1989b; Minogue and Reedy 1988; Phipps and Zinn 1986a, 1986b; Reading and Cox 1982; Robinson et al. 1984; Sjögren and Uddenberg 1990; Thomassen-Brepols 1987; Tsoi et al. 1987; Tunis et al. 1990a, 1990b; Villeneuve et al. 1988). Still others have looked at the effects of PND technology (including ultrasonography) on women's attachment to their pregnancy and to maternal-infant bonding (Heidrich and Cranley 1989; Sjögren and Uddenberg 1988b; Sparling et al. 1988). Studies have also examined women's attitudes toward abortion in relation to PND (Elder and Laurence 1991; Elkins et al. 1986; Faden et al. 1987; Fresco and Silvestre 1982; Jahoda et al. 1987; Landenburger and Delp 1987; Leschot et al. 1982; Magyari et al. 1987; Sjögren and Uddenberg 1987; Wertz et al. 1991), women's attitudes toward access to PND (Johnson and Caccia 1991; Reading et al. 1988; Sanden and Bjurulf 1988a, 1988b), and women's attitudes toward giving birth to an affected child (Ekwo et al. 1987; Evans et al. 1988; Young and Robinson 1984).

Not surprisingly, there has been considerable interest in PND and genetic counselling, in terms of the ethical and moral dimensions of this technology (McCance 1984; MacDiarmid 1991; Macklin 1977; Motulsky 1989; Pelosi and David 1989; Richards 1989; Roy 1986; Waltz and Thigpen 1973). Questions on the morality of selective eugenic abortion for congenital disease are common in this area of the literature (Beck 1990; Welch et al. 1991). Other studies in the bioethics literature have examined the moral basis of this technology, in terms of questions regarding the quality of life and what "the minimum requirements for a worthwhile life" mean in the context of our society (Ruse 1980).

Some interesting international (Kromberg et al. 1989; Papp 1989; Youings et al. 1991) and comparative studies have been done, most notably by Wertz and Fletcher (1988, 1989) and Wertz et al. (1990). This research clearly showed how the social and political context of a society, and of professional practice in the field of genetic counselling, influences the encounter between providers and consumers of this service. The authors showed that in countries where individual autonomy is valued counselling is less directive, while in countries where there is greater state control counsellors' practice tends to be more directive.

Of particular interest in this study are the limited number of sociological investigations of prenatal testing and screening. Black (1989) and Black and Furlong (1984) found that for most families, the testing experience is quite stressful. The results of their study suggested that adequate services must be available to ensure supports for families (especially those with young children) in dealing with difficulties related to PND testing. Rapp (1987) and Kolker and Burke (1987) have studied the social meanings surrounding PND and the ways in which PND socially constructs pregnancy.

Perhaps one of the most important sociological investigations into PND (and the one study most relevant to this research) is Rothman's (1986, 1987) work on the "tentative pregnancy." She interviewed 120 women (including genetic counsellors, women who had either opted for or declined amniocentesis, and a group of women who had received positive diagnoses). She used the term "tentative pregnancy" to describe the state of limbo that women experience as they undergo PND, when it remains uncertain whether they are "'mothers' or 'carriers of a defective fetus'" (Rothman 1987, 7). Rothman noted that it is not unusual for women to hide their pregnancies (i.e., deliberately limit who they told about their pregnancies, and thus shield children at home, family members, employers, and others from the knowledge that an abortion was performed). Her study revealed, among other things, that the new reproductive technologies raise new problems as they solve old ones. She believes they have a fundamental impact on our definition of motherhood. (Tymstra (1991) and Tymstra et al. (1991) have also done work on the concept of the tentative pregnancy.)

All of these studies and others reveal the array of complex issues in the area of PND and genetic counselling. It is worth noting that few of the aforementioned studies were conducted on Canadian women (and their partners). In this respect, the report on the study that follows provides an important set of data on the use of PND in one Canadian centre. Although it is clear that this study does not overcome the limitations that can be noted regarding prior studies (e.g., limited samples), it does have certain strengths worthy of note (e.g., the use of prospective and retrospective reports, the combination of qualitative data and survey data). In the next chapter, a detailed description of the methods used in the present study is given. Thereafter, the findings of the study are reported.

## Chapter 3. Methodology

### Introduction

This chapter outlines the methodology that was used in studying women's attitudes toward, and experiences with, PND. To reiterate, the study aims were:

1. to determine patterns of utilization of, and referral to, PND;
2. to determine women's perceptions, attitudes, and knowledge of PND; and
3. to determine whether women are satisfied with PND counselling services.

The following aspects of the methodology are detailed: the research design and study protocol, the sample and ascertainment protocol, the research model, and measurement and instrument design. Aspects of the analysis are discussed in Chapters 4 and 5 of this report.

At the outset, it is important to note that this study was somewhat exploratory, since relatively little of the extant (particularly Canadian) research on this topic has systematically examined women's attitudes and perceptions toward PND in the way that this study examined these issues. As already detailed, the existing research has a somewhat different focus. Lippman-Hand and Fraser (1979) suggested that, as a first step in understanding how women (and their partners) see their situations, one must begin the process by grounding their interpretations in terms of their everyday experiences. This recommendation was the basis for the methodology of this study.

## Study Design and Research Protocol

The design employed in this study involved the use of a multi-method strategy, incorporating both a qualitative and quantitative component. The combination of methodologies was used to ensure that sufficient and adequate data were obtained on the women's attitudes toward, perceptions of, and experiences with PND. Qualitative (inductive) methodologies are best used in circumstances in which relatively little is known about a topic, where there is an intrinsic value in getting at individuals' subjective experiences, and where data are not necessarily amenable to quantification (Babbie 1986; Glaser and Strauss 1967; Lofland 1984). Qualitative methods were used to explore women's reasons for obtaining PND and to ascertain their concerns about counselling and testing (primarily objectives 1 and 2).

By contrast, quantitative methodologies are suitable in circumstances in which researchers are testing specific hypotheses (derived from prior research and theory) and studying large samples (Babbie 1986). In this study, quantitative methods were used to gather data on women's attitudes and perceptions of PND and to measure the hypothesized psychosocial correlates of PND use (objectives 2 and 3).

The study was conducted over a 19-week period, 9 August through 13 December 1991, inclusive. In total, 28 clinics were attended by the research staff to secure the sample. Data collection followed a two-week pilot study in which both the instruments and the research protocol were fully pre-tested.

Through an arrangement with the Section of Clinical Genetics at the Health Sciences Centre in Winnipeg, all women defined as being at risk because of AMA (and with no other known family or genetic history), who had been referred for genetic counselling during the study period, were invited to participate in this study. The reason for restricting the study to AMA women was that women with a family history or other prior known risk of genetic problems undergo genetic counselling that is somewhat different and unique, and these differences would have confounded the analysis. Since it is recognized that age is an a priori risk (Elias and Annas 1987), AMA women were the group of interest in this research.

The Section of Clinical Genetics provides genetic counselling to women in a catchment area that includes all of Manitoba, northwestern Ontario, and part of the Northwest Territories (the area covered by the Northern Medical Unit). Counselling is provided to AMA women in two different sites — most are seen at The Women's Hospital (Friday clinics) and the remainder are seen at The Children's Hospital (Monday and Thursday clinics). The Section of Clinical Genetics is staffed by geneticists and genetic counsellors, some of whom have medical degrees, and others who have training in genetics (mostly at the master's or doctoral levels) or training in genetic counselling. During the study, six counsellors — three female, three male — provided service in the Section of Clinical Genetics.

In addition, three medical residents provided counselling cooperatively with the head of the Section of Clinical Genetics, but to a limited number of clients.

The study began with a letter being sent to physicians (general practitioners and obstetricians) in the catchment area who refer women to the Section of Clinical Genetics for prenatal counselling and testing. The study coordinator of the research project had contact weekly with the clinic coordinator of the Section of Clinical Genetics to obtain the list of AMA women who had been referred for counselling. Referred women were sent a letter explaining the study and their potential involvement. At least one week before their scheduled appointment at the clinic, women were contacted by telephone by the study coordinator and were invited to participate in the study. Women were initially invited to be interviewed, and if uninterested or unable to attend the clinic early enough to be interviewed, they were invited to complete a questionnaire on their attitudes and perceptions toward PND. This design allowed for some women to be interviewed and all participants to complete a post-counselling questionnaire. Participation was fully voluntary; no coercive methods were used to pressure women to participate. Women who agreed to the pre-counselling interview were asked to arrive at the clinic 15 to 30 minutes before their scheduled counselling appointment and, as compensation, each woman who was interviewed received a $5 cheque (reimbursement for the additional expense incurred for parking). All other study participants were asked to arrive at the clinic at the time of their scheduled counselling appointment.

When women arrived at the clinic, they were given an information sheet and consent form (different consent forms were prepared for those participating in the interview/questionnaire components and the questionnaire-only component of the study — see Appendix 1). If being interviewed, the woman was directed to a room in the clinic where the interview was conducted; if participating in the questionnaire component of the study only, she was asked to sit in the waiting area until her counselling appointment. After the interviews, the women were directed to the waiting area, pending their counselling appointment. When the women had received genetic counselling, they returned to the study coordinator who gave them a questionnaire in a self-addressed stamped envelope.

To maximize the response rate on the mail-in questionnaire, a modification of Dillman's Total Design Method (TDM) was used (Dillman 1978). This approach to such questionnaires has consistently produced response rates of 75% or better in general population studies. The TDM involves careful planning of follow-up mailings. At the end of the first week post-PND counselling, a postcard reminder was sent to everyone. For those who had already returned the questionnaire, the reminder served as a thank you for participation; for those who had not completed the survey, it was a friendly reminder to complete the questionnaire and return it to the investigator. At the end of three weeks, a letter with a replacement questionnaire was sent only to non-respondents. This letter included a brief statement of the study objectives, a reminder of how important their participation was, and that their questionnaire had not yet been received. An appeal for their participation in the study (through completion of the questionnaire) was also included.

Dillman (1978) recommended that, at the end of seven weeks, a final mailing be sent out (by certified mail) to non-respondents, with a replacement questionnaire. The third mailing, while somewhat costly, can increase response rates by as much as 13 percentage points and often results in responses from typically "hard-to-reach" individuals (e.g., less educated, lower income individuals). Due to time constraints, this third follow-up was not conducted. However, two follow-ups helped to foster a high response rate. Although a third follow-up reminder might have improved the response rate further, the cost would have been substantial without necessarily improving an already high response rate.

During the planning stages of the research, we were advised that, on average, approximately 10 to 20 AMA clients are normally seen weekly for counselling by the Section of Clinical Genetics. Of these, approximately 20% are clients referred for immediate counselling either because of late entry into ante-natal care or because they have also shown low maternal serum AFP. The remainder of clients seen are referred with ample time before counselling is to take place. The original design proposed that both of these kinds of referrals would be included in the study sample. In practice, making arrangements to interview women whose referral to genetic counselling came late often proved to be difficult or impossible. Without adequate notice to prospective participants, it was not always possible to arrange interviews and, consequently, the major effort was directed at securing participation of the women who had been referred during routine ante-natal care.

The original design was based on data collection over 22 weeks (1 July through 30 November 1991, inclusive). It was projected that during this period of time approximately 100 women would be interviewed and 50 to 75 others would complete the questionnaire-only component of the study. During the period of study (which was three weeks shorter than originally planned),[5] fewer referrals were received than had been projected based on past experience in the clinic and, accordingly, the total possible sample size was smaller than originally planned. Nonetheless, the study team was able to reach a substantial number of women referred for counselling during the data collection period.

## Sample and Ascertainment Protocol

In total, 267 women were referred to the Section of Clinical Genetics between 1 August and 31 December 1991. During the period of study (9 August through 13 December), 176 referrals came to the attention of the research team (Table 1). The discrepancy between the number of women seen in the Section of Clinical Genetics and those whose names were passed on to the research team is because some women did not satisfy the eligibility requirements of the study. A woman was deemed to be ineligible if she:

(a) had an indication for prenatal testing (e.g., a family or medical history of genetic abnormality) other than age alone;

(b) was unable to communicate effectively in English (or required a translator to participate);

(c) did not meet the age criterion of 35 years or older at the time of delivery; or

(d) was seen by staff in the Section of Clinical Genetics on days unscheduled for the study (data collection was confined to Mondays, Thursdays, and Fridays, the days on which most AMA women are seen in the clinic) or was missed in the clinic as a result of scheduling difficulties.

Of the 176 women referred to this study, 171 were classified as eligible participants. Of the referrals received by the study team, two women were defined as ineligible on the basis of language, one was defined as ineligible because of age, and two were missed as a result of scheduling problems. Of the remaining 171 women, 34 (19.8%) were subsequently lost as potential participants because of miscarriage (n = 9) or because they had pre-emptively declined genetic counselling and testing (n = 16). Another 9 did not appear at the clinic for their scheduled appointments or cancelled their appointments. Consequently, the effective population of AMA referrals was 137.

The number of women refusing to participate in this study was remarkably low; only 15 women refused (10.9% of the eligible study participants). The reasons offered related to a lack of interest in the study or lack of time to participate in the project (n = 11) and concerns that the research team had obtained the clients' names from the Health Sciences Centre (n = 4).

A total of 122 women participated in this study (representing 71.3% of the eligible referrals to the Section of Clinical Genetics and 89.0% of the women with whom this research team made contact). On the whole, the women who chose to participate in the study were enthusiastic to share their experiences, particularly given that the findings would be incorporated into the report of the Commission.

### Table 1. Referrals to the Study and Number of Participants

| | |
|---|---|
| Total number of referrals for all indications | 267 |
| Total number of AMA referrals to study | 176 |
|    Number of women who were ineligible | 5[1] |
| Total number of eligible referrals | 171 |
|    Number of women lost to the study | 34[2] |
| Effective study population (N) | 137 |
|    Number of women refusing to participate | 15[3] |
| Total sample size (n) | 122 |

[1] Ineligibles:
   Language (2)
   Scheduling difficulties (2)
   Age (1)
[2] Eligible participants lost to study:
   Number of women who miscarried (9)
   Number of women who declined counselling (16)
   Number of women who did not show at clinic (9)
[3] Refusals:
   Lack of interest/time in study (11)
   Concerns about confidentiality matters (4)

In terms of ascertaining the sample, the process of liaison between the study coordinator and the clinic coordinator has been noted previously. The research team was provided with the address, telephone number, date of birth, referring physician, time of counselling appointment, and, if prearranged, the scheduled date of prenatal testing[6] for all women referred to the Section of Clinical Genetics. The goal was to have a sample consisting of at least 50% who would be interviewed before the genetic counselling session, with all study participants completing a questionnaire after the counselling session.

Although the sampling design originally specified that interview participants would be selected randomly, in practice this was not feasible. To illustrate why, consider the routine clinic flow on Fridays (the day when most AMA women are seen in the Section of Clinical Genetics). There are usually three or four counsellors providing service to, on average, between 10 and 15 women (alone or with their partners or others). Appointments in the clinic are set up at four times: 1:00 p.m. (usually for chorionic villus sampling clients, who go directly into counselling), 1:15 p.m., 2:00 p.m., and 2:30 p.m. (usually for amniocentesis clients, who watch a 15-minute video on prenatal testing and are then counselled). Since each of the counsellors does not provide service at every clinic (some counsel part-time), and because several appointments are booked concurrently (usually three to four, depending on the number of referrals), it was impossible to assign women to "interview" and "non-interview" categories on a random basis.

In practice, the women with whom an interview was requested were selected on the basis of clinic appointment time. No systematic bias is known to have been introduced in this process of selection (no significant differences were found between the women who were interviewed and the women who participated only in the questionnaire). All of the women, regardless of where they lived, primiparous or multiparous women, older or younger AMA women, women considering amniocentesis or chorionic villus sampling, were invited to be interviewed, given only the constraints of clinic scheduling. Whether women were interviewed depended largely on their willingness to participate in this component of the study, and whether they were able to come to the clinic at least 15 (but preferably 30) minutes before their scheduled counselling appointment.

Table 2. Sample Distribution by Clinic Day of the Week

| Clinic day (no. of clinics) | No. of study participants | No. of interviews |
|---|---|---|
| Mondays (6) | 9 | 3 |
| Thursdays (5) | 8 | 5 |
| Fridays (17) | 105 | 62 |
| Total (28) | 122 | 70 |

The objective was to conduct as many interviews as possible without interrupting the flow of the clinic. On some clinic days, no women were interviewed; the most interviews conducted at any single clinic were seven. Both of these numbers represent the exception rather than the rule. On most clinic days, two to four interviews were conducted. Table 2 shows the breakdown of the sample by clinic day of the week.

## Research Model

The model guiding this research is shown in Figure 1. Corresponding to this model, numerous hypotheses were postulated. For instance, it was hypothesized that demographic variables such as pregnancy history (gravidity and parity), socioeconomic status (including education and income levels), religion and religiosity, to name a few, would influence women's perceptions of PND. Similarly, prior experience with PND was also hypothesized to be related to women's perceptions of PND. Women's access to information about PND, whether through health care personnel or through networks of affiliation, was expected to influence women's perceptions of PND. Women with high levels of psychosocial assets (e.g., high internal locus of control, access to information about reproductive health care and PND, high levels of social support) were expected to be more knowledgeable about PND and to hold attitudes more favourable toward PND.

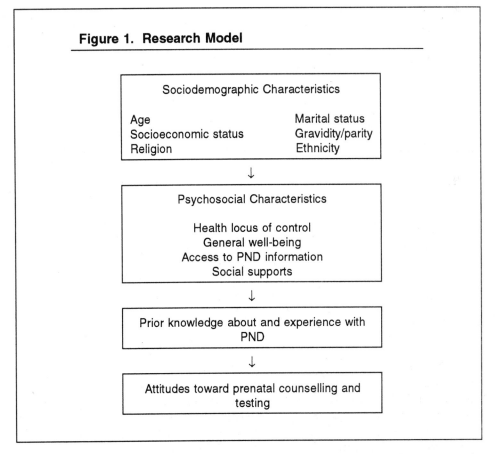

Figure 1. Research Model

A few points should be noted at this juncture. First, these are only selected hypotheses, and are offered to give the reader an idea of the direction that the current research took. I have, however, been deliberately circumspect here because the design of the study was exploratory. In addition, the one-time measurement, with no follow-up of the women, did not allow a clear statement of directionality on these or any other hypotheses. The research reported here is based on a correlational analysis and no causal associations are implied. Also, it is important to note that the design, in combining qualitative (hypothesis-generating) and quantitative (hypothesis-testing) methods, means that as many new questions have arisen out of this research endeavour as were contemplated at the start.

In the final chapter of this report, future directions for research in this area are detailed.

## Measurement and Instrument Design

As noted previously, two methodologies were employed in this study. The first was a pre-counselling interview, intended to gather in-depth qualitative data on the women's attitudes and perceptions regarding PND. The emphasis in this method of data collection was on gathering information about PND in women's own words (Anderson and Jack 1991; Gluck and Patai 1991; Minister 1991; Oakley 1981). The second method of data collection was a post-counselling mail-in questionnaire, which augmented the qualitative data and included discrete measurements of important sociodemographic, psychosocial, and related variables.

### *Pre-Counselling Interview*

Pre-counselling interviews, using a semi-structured interview guide, were conducted by a trained interviewer. The objective of the interview was to elicit women's perceptions and concerns regarding PND. Of particular interest was the woman's understanding of what brought her to PND counselling. The interview included questions on:

(a) why the woman had been referred to PND counselling;

(b) what her impression was of the purpose of the counselling (and testing); and

(c) what, if any, concerns she had about counselling (and testing).

The interview also sought to determine what women knew about PND counselling and the sources of such information (e.g., medical or lay sources of information). (See Appendix 2 for the Interview Guide.) The pre-counselling interview was developed largely to satisfy the first and second aims of this study, specified earlier.

Although a standardized set of questions was used in the interviews, time was available for women to provide detailed personal accounts of their experiences with, and perceptions of, PND. Philosophically, the interview was intended to provide women with an opportunity to tell in their own words about their experience in connection with PND. The only constraints expected were those created by clinic scheduling (i.e., the time available before being seen by the genetic counsellor). The interviews were admittedly brief. Optimally, it would have been desirable to conduct interviews without the time limitation, not only before counselling but also after counselling (and after testing), but this was not possible in this particular study. (Another study by the principal investigator, conducted in Australia in 1992, involved interviews with women regarding their experiences of PND testing. In that study, the duration of the interview was 60 to 90 minutes. Obviously, the time constraints imposed by clinic scheduling limited the range of topics that could be covered and the depth in which women could explore these topics.) Nonetheless, the pre-counselling interviews reveal much about the range of experiences women have in relation to PND.

The data from the interviews provide important information on why and how women come to prenatal counselling, the various pressures they feel in relation to testing (whether to have it or not and how to act in relation to the information from testing), and their perceptions of the place of testing in pregnancy management for older women. As will be detailed in Chapter 4, this interview was less informative in terms of men's views and experiences, since they were not a key focus of the study. Although decisions regarding PND testing are not restricted to women necessarily, and although it is important to learn about men's experiences with PND, this research has taken the view that it is a priority to learn about women's experiences, as they are the ones whose bodies and lives are most intimately affected by these technologies and by the decisions taken because of the testing.

The interviewer underwent an intensive training period before the initiation of data collection. In addition, regular interaction between the interviewer and the principal investigator ensured that problems could be remedied in the process of data collection. The interviewer was instructed to refer all client questions of a specific nature on PND and counselling directly to genetic counsellors, not only because the interviewer lacked expertise in the field of genetics, but also to ensure that the study was seen as distinct from the counselling program.

The interviews were audio-taped for later transcription. The interviewer took minimal notes during the interview but completed a brief form detailing any notable non-verbal behaviour of the women who were interviewed. This form also included an assessment of the quality of the interview and the interviewer's assessment of the general anxiety level of interviewees.

Although the primary focus of interest in the interview portion of this research was the women being counselled, it was expected that some male partners might be in attendance and want to be included in the interview. All questions were directed at the women, but their male partners' involvement in the interview process was noted (and assessed in the interview process form, as relevant). The interviewer took particular note of the dynamics between women and their partners, if both participated in the interview.

### *The Mail-In Questionnaire*

The post-counselling mail-in questionnaire was provided to all study participants upon leaving the clinic. (Identification numbers were synchronized for the study participants who were involved in both the pre-counselling interview and the mail-in questionnaire phases of the study.) The primary objective of this component of the research was to gather from clients relevant sociodemographic, psychosocial, and attitudinal information (including measures of satisfaction) on women's experiences with genetic counselling. The questionnaire was designed to satisfy the second and third objectives of the research, specified earlier. (See Appendix 3 for the questionnaire.)

The questionnaire included sociodemographic measures such as age, marital status, occupation (classified in terms of both Statistics Canada's Standard Occupational Classification and the Pineo-Porter McRoberts occupational classification), education level, income, religion, ethnic status, and other relevant variables. Standard measures of these variables were used. As discussed previously, many of these characteristics have been found to be predictive of attitudes in general, and in relation to PND in particular.

A set of questions measuring various psychosocial assets was also included. Psychosocial assets refer to all of the resources (intra- and inter-personally) the woman possesses that may have a direct or indirect bearing on decisions related to use of, and satisfaction with, PND. Examples of relevant indicators here include measures of health locus of control (HLOC), general well-being (GWB), and access to social support (from partner or lay others). There is extensive literature in the sociology of health and in health psychology that indicates such measures may be predictive of health attitudes and behaviours (Nuckolls et al. 1972). Several standard measures, with demonstrated validity and reliability, were employed.

Locus of control is defined as "the degree to which individuals perceive events in their lives as being a consequence of their own actions, and thereby controllable (internal control), or as being unrelated to their own behaviour, and therefore beyond personal control (external control)" (Lau and Ware 1981, 1147). A measure of HLOC considers specifically the ways in which individuals perceive that their health is the product of internal, external, or chance factors. Prior studies show that HLOC is a good predictor of health-related behaviours (Lau and Ware 1981). In the context of a study on women's attitudes toward PND, it was hypothesized that HLOC may be an important predictor of women's attitudes. Although the measure of HLOC used by Lau and Ware contained 27 items, an abbreviated version of this instrument (15 items) was used in the present study. In terms of measuring women's attitudes, standardized response categories ranging from "strongly agree" to "strongly disagree" (scores ranging between 1 and 5) were used. Figure 2 provides a listing of the indicators of HLOC used in this study, along with an identification of each

### Figure 2. List of Questionnaire Items Used to Define Health-Specific Locus of Control Scales

1. Staying well has little or nothing to do with chance. (CH)
2. Seeing a doctor for regular check-ups is a key factor in staying healthy. (PC)
3. People's ill health results from their own carelessness. (SC)
4. Doctors relieve or cure only a few of the medical problems their patients have. (PC)
5. There is little one can do to prevent illness. (SC)
6. Whether or not people get well is often a matter of chance. (CH)
7. I have a lot of confidence in my ability to cure myself once I get sick. (SC)
8. People who never get sick are just plain lucky. (CH)
9. Doctors can almost always help their patients feel better. (PC)
10. In the long run, people who take very good care of themselves stay healthy and get well quick. (SC)
11. Recovery from illness requires good medical care more than anything else. (PC)
12. Health-wise, there isn't much you can do for yourself when you get sick. (SC)
13. Doctors can do very little to prevent illness. (PC)
14. Recovery from illness has nothing to do with luck. (CH)
15. Good health is largely a matter of fortune. (CH)

Key: CH: Chance health outcomes scale item.
PC: Provider control scale item.
SC: Self-control scale item.

statement as part of the chance health outcomes (CH) scale, the provider control (PC) scale, or the self-control (SC) scale.

GWB was measured using an 18-item instrument designed by Dupuy (1978) for the U.S. National Health and Nutrition Examination Survey. GWB measures psychological well-being in terms of six major dimensions: anxiety, depression, general health, positive well-being, self-control, and vitality. Items and their dimensions are shown in Figure 3.

> **Figure 3. General Well-Being Schedule and Its Dimensions**
>
> 1. How have you been feeling in general? (P)
> 2. Have you been bothered by nervousness or your "nerves"? (A)
> 3. Have you been in firm control of your behaviour, thoughts, emotions, or feelings? (SC)
> 4. Have you felt so sad, discouraged, hopeless or had so many problems that you wondered if anything was worthwhile? (D)
> 5. Have you been under or felt you were under any strain, stress, or pressure? (A)
> 6. How happy, satisfied, or pleased have you been with your personal life? (P)
> 7. Have you had any reason to wonder if you were losing your mind, or losing control over the way you act, talk, think, feel or of your memory? (SC)
> 8. Have you been anxious, worried or upset? (A)
> 9. Have you been waking up fresh and rested? (V)
> 10. Have you been bothered by any illness, bodily disorder, pains or fears about your health? (GH)
> 11. Has your daily life been full of things that were interesting to you? (P)
> 12. Have you felt down-hearted and blue? (D)
> 13. Have you been feeling emotionally stable and sure of yourself? (SC)
> 14. Have you felt tired, worn out, used-up, or exhausted? (V)
> 15. How concerned or worried about your health have you been? (GH)
> 16. How relaxed or tense have you been? (A)
> 17. How much energy, pep, vitality have you felt? (V)
> 18. How depressed or cheerful have you been? (D)
>
> Key: A: Anxiety dimension.
> D: Depression dimension.
> P: Positive well-being dimension.
> SC: Self-control dimension.
> V: Vitality dimension.
> GH: General health dimension.

Social support has been extensively studied in sociology and psychology and has been found to influence health status and health-related behaviours and buffer stressful life events (Berkman and Syme 1979; House 1981). Numerous measures of this concept are available. The one chosen for this study was an abbreviated version of

Sarason's Social Support Questionnaire (SSQ), which quantifies the availability of, and satisfaction with, social support (Sarason 1983). During the pre-test phase of the study, the modified SSQ used 12 items, but the final instrument narrowed this to 7. The primary reason for using fewer questions here was because of the demands placed on respondents to answer detailed questions that summarized both the range of overall support and their satisfaction with that support. Rather than run the risk of respondent fatigue or disinterest, fewer questions were asked on general social support. The questions included are shown in Figure 4.

**Figure 4. Measures of Social Support**

1. Whom can you really count on to listen to you when you need to talk?
2. Whom could you really count on to help you out in a crisis situation, even though they would have to go out of their way to do so?
3. Whom can you really count on to distract you from your worries when you feel under stress?
4. Whom can you really count on to be dependable when you need help?
5. Whom do you feel would help if a family member very close to you died?
6. Whom do you feel truly loves you deeply?
7. Whom can you count on to console you when you are very upset?

In addition, it was considered important to ascertain the specific type of social support the women received. Accordingly, a set of four questions was developed to elicit information about decisions such as when to have children, how many children to have, whether to use PND, and how to use the information from PND. In each instance, the woman was asked to indicate who participated in the decision and whether she was satisfied with the process. The format of the questions was intended to provide a rough parallel to the kind of information obtained about general social support (as per the Sarason measure), but this time the focus was narrowed to the area of the present research.

The two major dependent variables of interest were women's level of knowledge concerning PND and their attitudes toward PND. In terms of women's knowledge of PND, information was obtained primarily through the qualitative interview. Presumably, their cognitive understanding of PND is essential to being able to formulate an attitude. No actual test of women's knowledge, per se, was included in this study, nor was there any measurement or assessment of whether the information women had (before genetic counselling) was factually correct.

To measure women's attitudes toward PND, an opportunity was provided during the interview to ascertain what women thought about the process. In the mail-in questionnaire, a series of questions was asked about the counselling that women had received. These questions concerned the quality and level of satisfaction women had regarding the counselling and counsellor (i.e., did women consider the session informative, stressful, helpful, and reassuring?). Questions such as these have been included in prior studies of genetic counselling, and this research has drawn heavily from the Sorenson et al. (1981) study. Although the same questions have been used, the sample reported here is different from that studied by Sorenson and colleagues, so a direct comparison cannot be made.

Although this research is about "women's perceptions and attitudes" toward PND, neither the interview nor the questionnaire specifically sought information on women's views of the appropriateness of PND in pregnancy management or their views as to whether PND should be used for medical or social reasons. As will be detailed in the next two chapters, some women did express views on these (and other) matters, but the research did not explicitly attempt to survey women's attitudes in this way. The focus of this research was somewhat more limited and provides information about a sample of women already in the system of service delivery who have impressions about the technology (and genetic counselling) and its impact on their pregnancies and their lives.

## Chapter 4. Presentation of Findings:
## Part 1. A Qualitative Study of Women's Perceptions of Prenatal Diagnosis

> No understanding of women will ever be possible until women themselves begin to tell what they know. (John Stuart Mill)

### Introduction

The above quotation from John Stuart Mill, a nineteenth-century philosopher, encapsulates the perspective that guided the research reported here. Unlike some of his contemporaries and many who have followed since, Mill believed that it was important to find out about women from women. The continuity between this statement by Mill and the guiding philosophy of feminist researchers today is quite remarkable. Yet, surprisingly, relatively few studies have been done in the area of PND that have afforded women an opportunity to speak, in their own words, about their experiences (Farrant (1985) and Rothman (1987) being the notable exceptions). Although survey research and other quantitative methods of data collection clearly provide important data about the various correlates and predictors of social behaviours and attitudes (as will be discussed in the next chapter), a fundamentally different kind of understanding of a phenomenon is possible when one is capturing women's lived experiences, subjectively understood and articulated, in the language of women themselves.

In this, the first of two chapters devoted to the research findings, women's narratives of their experiences with PND are presented. These accounts provide a glimpse at how women see prenatal testing and the concerns that they have about counselling and testing. The presentation of findings from the qualitative study draws extensively on women's articulation of the experience they are about to have. In the tradition of qualitative research, the tendency is to speak mostly about "many," "some," or "few" women as opposed to quantifying the range of experience. Quotations from the study participants form an integral part of the data presentation.[7] The analysis of this qualitative data was guided by a search for both the commonalities among the women participating in the study and the identification of the uniqueness of each woman.

To begin, a few preliminary details are provided about the sample of women who were interviewed and the interviewing process. Thereafter, the major thematic content of the interviews is presented and we learn what this sample of AMA women have to say about PND and genetic counselling.

## Interview Sample

In total, 70 interviews were conducted during the period of data collection.[8] Of these, 89.7% were conducted at The Women's Hospital, and 10.3% were conducted at The Children's Hospital. Corresponding to these proportions, most women were interviewed at the Friday afternoon clinics when most AMA women receive counselling in the Section of Clinical Genetics. On average, the interviews lasted 10.9 minutes (standard deviation [SD] = 4.2), although the range was between 5 and 22 minutes. It is worth noting that even in the short interviews all of the essential information was obtained. The variability in the length of interviews reflected how much women had to say about their experiences. At the same time, the relative brevity of the interviews was related to the fact that women were to be counselled directly after the interview session. In some cases, this did result in an interview being terminated at a stage earlier than it might have been had we not been pressed for time. The issue of the time and the timing of the interviews is a subject of discussion in the final chapter of this report.

A substantial number of interviews involved the woman alone (n = 50). When the woman was accompanied, that person was usually her partner or spouse (n = 16). One woman was accompanied by her partner and a child, and one was accompanied by her sister. Only rarely did the others participate in the interviews; all questions were directed to the women specifically.

Although a detailed analysis of the demographic characteristics of the entire sample is in the next chapter, it is important to identify some of the demographic characteristics of the interview sample alone. First, the average age was 36.4 years (SD = 2.0). Relatively few women in the interview sample were 40 years of age or older (10.2%) and a large proportion were at or approaching the 35-year mark, which automatically resulted in a referral (41.2%). The pregnancy was not the first for most of the women: 43% were in their second pregnancy, 22% were in their third, 13% were in their fourth, and some were in their fifth or sixth. Only seven women mentioned that the pregnancy was unplanned, but none specifically mentioned that the pregnancy was unwanted. Although most of the women had been pregnant before, only 8 (11.7%) had had previous experience with either genetic counselling, prenatal testing, or both.

Most of the women (94.1%) were married or living in a common-law relationship. Two identified themselves as single and two were either separated or divorced.

## Assessment of the Interviews

The interviewer evaluated the quality of the interview using a form employed by the principal investigator in a former study (see Appendix 2). Interviews were judged to be of high quality in 77.6% of cases and adequate in 22.4%. No interview was judged to be of questionable quality. Also, in keeping with the methodology used in the previous study by the principal investigator, the interviewer rated the level of cooperation of the interviewees; all participants but one were considered to be cooperative. The interview process form included a checklist of sources of interference during the interview. This checklist included language, noise, interference by spouse or partner, children, or others present, and other factors; few sources of interference were noted in the interviews. Few sources of interference contributed to a reduction in quality of the interviews, and few problems except limited time were encountered during the interviews. The participants were generally cooperative and interested.

One other set of criteria was judged by the interviewer about those participating in this component of the study. The interviewer, on the basis of her own subjective interpretation, assessed whether the woman (and, if relevant, her partner) was excited about the pregnancy, concerned about counselling, and concerned about testing. Each of these criteria was easier to assess for the women than for their partners because of the lack of the partners' participation. Most of the women were judged to be either excited (57.4%) or very excited (33.8%) about the pregnancy. In terms of concern evident to the interviewer, 16.1% of the sample were seen to be somewhat or very concerned about counselling and a larger proportion (42.1%) were seen to be somewhat or very concerned about testing.[9]

## Analysis of Women's Experiences of PND

What brings women to PND? What do they know about prenatal testing? What do they hope to learn from counselling? What are their concerns about counselling and testing? How do they experience being classified as "at risk"? These and many other questions provided the structure of the pre-counselling interview.

A brief methodological note is required as we begin to look at women's experiences with PND. The process of analyzing the interview data involved systematically reviewing the transcripts for common thematic content, first with QualPro, a software program for the analysis of qualitative data, and then manually. Transcripts were read and re-read to develop a set of coding categories. Broadly, these categories dealt with (1) aspects of the referral process; (2) sources of information on PND; (3) concerns about the testing process; (4) concerns about disability; and (5) aspects of the decision-making process. In addition, some attention was focussed on the language used by the women (e.g., references to fetus versus baby); however, this is an area not developed in this report.

In terms of the presentation of the data, direct quotations are used extensively to give voice to women's experiences and perceptions. Generally, these quotations are presented unedited, except that some expressions such as "um" and "uh" have been deleted, particularly when extensive. In no instance does the omission of such utterances alter the content or meaning of a woman's account. Identification of interview subjects by number only is provided at the end of quotations. Such identification is to protect the personal identity of the women who participated in the study.

Finally, one must be cautious in interpreting these data. The structure of the interview was broad, involving a limited number of questions (see Appendix 2). The exact content of any particular interview was largely dependent on the woman herself — what she chose to mention or emphasize or what she chose not to discuss. Consequently, when we look at any particular area explored in the interviews, it must be remembered that categories of analysis reflect what women had to say. All women did not necessarily comment on all areas. In addition, the analysis of interviews presented here offers a mere fragment of women's lived experiences of pregnancy and of PND.

### *Referral Patterns of Women Accessing Counselling*

Most of the women (n = 67) had come to the Section of Clinical Genetics because of a referral by their family physician or obstetrician. Some women said that they were surprised to have been referred (i.e., they had no idea of this service or of their apparent heightened risk), but many knew, expected, or had been told that their referral was "automatic" because of their age. Some of the women (n = 15) said that they had requested a referral for genetic testing or would have requested one had their doctors not made the referral. One woman indicated that she had contacted the Section of Clinical Genetics directly to have testing performed.

At the point of referral, there is the possibility to disseminate information to women about the testing process and about their risk status. However, most women stated that their doctors had told them very little about the process. For example, when asked what she perceived the purpose to be of the counselling session she was asked to attend, one woman responded:

> I have ... I have absolutely no idea. My doctor said "Look, go." He set up an appointment and that was it. I came to this thing absolutely, totally blind. You know, except for the little bit of ... the information that they mailed out to me. And in there they never really said exactly what they were going to be discussing. They just basically gave you the information on the procedures and that was it. (#158)

In reviewing the transcripts, one is struck by how little information physicians in the community provided to their patients. It is possible that referring physicians are making referrals on a pro forma basis and advising their patients that the genetic counsellors are better placed to provide detailed information about the testing process, the risks to pregnancy, and so on. On the one hand, deferring to one's specialist colleagues is a responsible way in which to practise medicine; on the other, a few of the women who were surprised by the referral said that they wished their doctor had told them more about why they were being sent for testing. The referral, in other words, may be experienced as somewhat stressful. The lack of information simply exacerbates this feeling. This is obviously not the intent, but it may be the consequence, of the manner in which referrals are made to the Section of Clinical Genetics.

Some women reported that their physicians did provide them with some information about PND. This information was usually cursory, outlining the process of counselling, the options available, and the expectation that all of this information would be elaborated by the counsellors at the Section of Clinical Genetics. A few women said that their doctors had specific ideas on the use of PND; these are cited because of the specific content of the messages received by women.

The first case is of a woman who, as has been alleged during the public hearings process of the Royal Commission on New Reproductive Technologies, had been told by her referring doctor that her choices are limited in relation to PND:

> Like, your doctor can tell you one thing and that's all he can tell you. He also told me that if I went through with the testing and then it turned out that the baby was Down syndrome, that I'd have no choice as to whether I wanted to carry the child or not. And I found out later on that, yes, I do have a choice. (#134)

This connection between prenatal testing and abortion is, of course, not uncommon, and the idea that PND is related to abortion has been discussed in the literature (Beck 1990). In addition, there has been the suggestion that PND is unnecessary if one would not be prepared to act on the results — action being defined as willingness to abort the fetus. One woman recounted the following:

> "My doctor said that ... you should go to this ... to the counselling session. It's important because if you're a person who wouldn't ever consider clinical abortion, for whatever reason, there's no point in having the amnio. But she said the counselling will help you decide that better. You know, if for ... if for religious or moral reasons you would never consider a clinical abortion ... um ... you shouldn't even take the test."
>
> *Interviewer:* "Do you agree with that?"
>
> "Not necessarily. But ... um ... you know, that was her opinion and ... and, you know, she's been my doctor for a long time. But I think it's probably good to be prepared either way." (#166)

In a similar respect, consider the following account of another woman:

> "So, that was what my doctor told us. There's only one reason to do this, and that is if you would make a decision one way or another. And if you're not going to make a decision if you find out there's a problem, then why bother going through the testing and risking the baby and everything, so ..."
>
> *Interviewer:* "And so you had the impression from your doctor that you would only ... go through it if you were going to abort if there was a problem?"
>
> "Yeah. Yeah, like what was the point if you're not, really? ... And I ... I still feel that way. Unless it's to prepare yourself, you know." (#140)

This woman later said that her doctor was clear in leaving the decision up to her. His intent, she recalled, was not to try to pressure her in one direction or another but to give her reason to think about why she would use the testing.

One woman said that her physician had actively encouraged her to have an abortion; however, this was the exception rather than the rule. (The full circumstances surrounding this recommendation are not entirely clear from the transcript.)

Looking at the interviews as a whole, few women indicated that their doctors were pressuring or influencing them to have or not to have PND. Instead, most women indicated that their doctors referred them for counselling as a part of routine care, and that their doctors left it to the women to decide whether to have the counselling and testing subsequent to the counselling.

It is interesting that there was a high level of acceptance of the referral process (cf. Reid and Garcia 1989); that is, the AMA women in the study seemed to see their referral as natural, normal, and even desirable. Most of the women said that they appreciated the opportunity that the referral presented in terms of learning more about their risks in pregnancy. At the same time, many women obviously experience the process of genetic counselling and the decision making related to it as troubling. This is a theme to which we will return later.

### What Do Women Know About PND?

The level of information about PND and about the risk of genetic abnormalities in AMA women varied considerably among the women who were interviewed. Most of the women (n = 43) said that the primary source of their information on prenatal testing and the risks associated with childbearing at their age came from the brochure provided by the Section of Clinical Genetics.[10] Only rarely did women say that their physician had been a primary source of information. As noted previously, this may reflect the fact that referring physicians depend upon the Section of Clinical Genetics to provide women with up-to-date information on genetic risks and PND.

A relatively small proportion of the sample indicated that they had read about PND in books. Some women with professional backgrounds as health care workers or personal contacts with health care professions indicated that they had access to information on PND. In other words, the level of information on PND that some women in the sample had was quite extensive, while for others, the primary (and perhaps only) source of information was that provided by the Section of Clinical Genetics.

The women stated that they were generally pleased with the written information that they had received from the Section of Clinical Genetics. They found the pamphlet to be comprehensive and informative. However, some women did express concern over how information was presented. One woman whose physician had not explained anything about PND or the counselling that she would receive stated:

> When they sent me that information on the prenatal diagnosis, they had a tendency to make you feel kind of upset. You start thinking, well ... like they tell all the things that could be wrong with it. (#157)

Other women were concerned about the presentation of statistical data in the pamphlets. One woman thought that the data might be "tainted," although the exact nature of the perceived bias cannot be discerned from her interview. The greatest concern among those mentioning the statistical information had to do with the meaning of the statistical risks presented. Women wanted to know whether the statistical risks were population-specific (for Manitoba? Canada? worldwide?) or if this made a difference in terms of their own risk. Also, several wanted to know how recent the data were. This was sometimes mentioned where, in a matter of a year, the woman was now defined as being at risk. Concerns such as these were paramount for the women as they tried to place themselves within the odds — that is, how they tried to apply the statistics to themselves as individuals. Before counselling, and as revealed in their interviews, the connection was not understood. Making the statistical probabilities relevant to women clearly requires that there be some context for them.

Some women did not find that the context was adequately explained in the brochure they received and they counted on the counsellors to provide this information.[11]

Another source of information to women was the experience of other women. In total, 19 women indicated that they knew other women who had had counselling, PND, or both.[12] The information that the women in the study gleaned from other women concerned what the test was "really like." These women seem to see a qualitative difference in the way they understand the process of PND as explained in books and brochures, as opposed to how other women actually experienced testing. Many of the women commented that knowing other women who had gone through this experience was helpful in knowing what to expect, during both the counselling and the testing process. Two women said that they knew of other women who had declined PND. One had known a woman who had had an abnormality on testing and another had known a woman with a false-positive result after testing.[13]

Although information was available, there is evidence of misinformation among some women. For example, some women thought that prenatal testing could determine whether their fetus was healthy in most every respect, yet the brochure indicated that testing was done only to identify the risk of certain genetic abnormalities. Also, two of the women thought that amniocentesis could reveal more than chorionic villus sampling, which may stem from the fact that the former is a more established technique and the latter is still somewhat experimental.

Most of the women understood that PND could reveal only the risks of certain abnormalities, with a few stating that they knew that the testing could not provide a guarantee of a healthy child. Women generally expected that the counsellors would tell them the probability of having a child with Down syndrome (the birth defect mentioned most), and about the other abnormalities (including neural tube defects, for which a test is available). For those who mentioned the issue of the severity of genetic abnormalities, there was a general understanding that the tests could not tell women how severe a birth defect might be, or whether the birth defect would manifest primarily physical, intellectual, or developmental problems. For those women concerned about bearing a disabled child, this was a worry that could not be easily reconciled.

> "If it's determined that the child is a Down's then, yes, we have decided to terminate the pregnancy. Not that I have a concern about having a retarded child. I am concerned about the physical defects that go along with it, and I'm not prepared to watch a child go through that ... the surgeries and the needles and ... ignorance would be bliss. But unfortunately my husband is also a nurse and we're just not prepared to ... to do that."
>
> *Interviewer:* "You know about all the things that can happen."

"I just couldn't watch a child go through that, so, um ... easy to say now. When we get the results we may change our mind but um, I don't have a religious feeling about it. I also don't think society needs the burden." (#119)

### *Age and the Experience of "Risk"*

Most women (n = 52) spoke of their age and about the connection between maternal age and the increased risk of genetic abnormalities. Twenty-six women specifically mentioned that they knew that maternal age was a contributing risk factor. (One woman specifically mentioned that she did not think that maternal age was a risk factor.) None of the women spoke of paternal age as a risk factor. Only 13 of these AMA women specifically mentioned family history as a risk factor. Almost all women mentioned family history in relation to how a family member's experience with Down syndrome or some other condition might influence their own risk of bearing an affected child. Very few women commented about occupational and environmental factors in connection with genetic abnormalities.

What exactly does it mean to these women to be of "advanced maternal age"? If we look at what women had to say about their age, there is an interesting, if sometimes disturbing, picture that emerges. References to being "old" and "elderly" were not uncommon in this sample. Several commented that 35 was a "magic age." One woman said that this meant not only amniocentesis but mammograms as well. Women said things like:

> 'Cause people say "oh, you're too old" or "it's dangerous" or, you know, things happen at a certain age. But I think a lot of times it's the individual and not necessarily your age. (#117)

As much as women talked about age — this age — being so precarious from the standpoint of the risk of bearing a child with a genetic abnormality, many women understand the arbitrary nature of the 35-year-old criterion for PND. Some were frustrated by it, as seen in the comments of the following two women:

> If nobody mentioned it, we just didn't think about it, or you know ... that there's something funny here too. You know, the magic number is 35, and if I'd been pregnant two months earlier or three months earlier ... it's not such an issue. All of a sudden, at 35, it's an issue ... it just makes you wonder why it becomes such an issue. (#160)

> I don't feel any different, I feel healthy, I feel kind of healthier than I did in my 20s, in some ways. 'Cause I try to look after myself, that it's just sort of, you know ... it's an artificial level in a way. And ... actually ... even the whole description... I think they still call it a geriatric pregnancy... you know, when somebody's over 35, and I sort of think, I don't really feel geriatric! (#137)

The experience of age as a risk factor seems to vary depending on a woman's prior experience both with pregnancy and with PND. Consider this account from one of the many women who had had a previous pregnancy, but who was going through counselling (and testing) for the first time.

> *Interviewer:* "How do you feel about being referred?"
>
> "I was a little surprised. I didn't know that this existed. Um ... it's ... um ... not scary ... but a little ... you feel a little bit different because all of a sudden I ... I think that people are looking at me differently because I'm older, I've reached this certain age that ... I've, you know, something might go wrong all of a sudden, whereas before, you know, it was ... it was very ... uh ... very healthy and sort of looked ... you know ... it's a little bit more negative than it was before."
>
> *Interviewer:* "Are ... do you get that sensation, that people are sort of ... why are you pregnant now or ...?"
>
> "Yeah. Yeah. Well, no, not ... not really, but just the way that your appointments are made for you and you come to this and you have the counselling and ... uh ... I ... none of that ever existed before, and ... I ... everything went smoothly before and I'm just assuming the same thing would happen now but there's ... there's something else in the background there, that all of a sudden, you know, there's this little bit of a ... of a doubt somehow. But I have friends that have ... a couple friends that have gone through this at the age of 36 and 38 and, you know, they're quite reassuring, saying how this ... nothing to worry about. So I'm okay with that. A little bit different somehow!" (#124)

Similarly, the following woman spoke of how her own concern has changed because of her referral, now that she is of advanced maternal age:

> I had ... uh ... my last baby eight years ago and ... um ... at that time it wasn't really a consideration. I wasn't overly concerned with genetic abnormalities. But ... uh ... at this point, it becomes a concern. (#129)

The number of pregnancies to older women has increased markedly in the past few decades. The women in this sample clearly knew that being older is associated with being at greater risk. Listening to these women gives the impression that too much is sometimes made of age or that some women do not necessarily think that what applies to "women" necessarily or inevitably applies to them as individuals. Perhaps this is a reflection of how individuals interpret their risk, a subject that will be discussed more fully in the next chapter.

### What Any Responsible Mother Would Do: The Pressure to Have Testing

Although the majority of women interviewed indicated that they felt no coercion to undergo testing, there is, at the same time, a sense that they should. The way in which women feel pressured to have testing seems to be quite subtle and is not tied to particular individuals. This pressure is expressed in different ways. For example, some spoke of the testing as offering a "comfort level." A few lamented that they wished that they didn't have to go through with this process, as illustrated by one woman:

> Part of me wishes I didn't have to go through this ... in a way. Like, really, I wish ... It's weird, like even a few months earlier this would not have been a concern. I mean, I don't turn 36 till April and my child will be born in January. And to me, I mean it's such a, you know ... part of me just doesn't want to go through it. (#101)

If there was a circumstance that women experienced as pressure, it was the scheduling of testing. When women are scheduled for counselling, an appointment is also routinely set for PND testing. The understanding is that the scheduling of the testing is tentative and subject to change or cancellation if the woman wishes. For women coming into Winnipeg from rural areas, testing is routinely set to occur directly after counselling to minimize the amount of travelling.

What the scheduling of the test means, however, is not necessarily taken as neutral. For example, one women stated:

> I'm going to ask ... why they kind of push the CVS test. Like, of all the information they sent me, it seemed like that's what they did. They kind of ... they've already set up a ... a date for me to have the chorionic villus sampling test without even asking me which one I wanted. (#106)

Another woman remarked "They gave me an hour [to decide] and ... it's a good thing I made up my mind ahead!" (#143).

### Women's Views of PND

To understand the "pressure" that women (or couples) feel to have testing performed, one must understand how they see this technology. The women tended to see the technology as good because it gave them options; 38 of the women interviewed said this was why they thought they had been referred for counselling. Another 24 commented that they saw this technology as desirable, as a service that was good to have available. But again, it is not without its problems. For example, one woman said that the "technology is too there!" Another remarked:

> I wish that none of this had to happen. I wish that there wasn't any because then you don't have any decision to make. But now that there is, you know ... you either choose to open your eyes to technology or you choose to close your eyes to technology. So ... that'll be a real ... you know ... I guess ... moral decision. (#122)

Another woman said:

> I'm not concerned about the test itself ... the procedure itself doesn't bother me at all. I guess I'm more concerned about the outcome, the possible ... and then dealing with the results should they be negative, and ... uh ... or should they show something. That concerns me more ... finding out the results. I think it will be tense probably for the next three to four weeks until we get the results from them. That's about all. (#129)

Another woman, in her third pregnancy, commented about the ambivalence she felt about the testing:

> I was kind of torn, like, do I want to do it, or, am I sure I'm ready for, if it turns out that the baby isn't right, am I ready for the consequences? And in the other way, I thought to myself, well, if I'm not, if something does happen, if something is wrong, I'm the one who has to live with it, not anybody else. (#134)

For some others, the technology is problematic because of how it can be used:

> "Well, I mean it's a ... I guess because it is such a new ... relatively new procedure and ... it does give people the option. But I'm just sort of wondering whether it's an option that we should be fooling around with so much ... You know? I mean, maybe 20 years ago or 50 years ago people didn't have that choice and ... um ... you know, you live with what you get sort of thing."
>
> *Interviewer:* "Mm hmm. And ... and how did this worry you ... that people have maybe too much of a choice?"
>
> "Well, it doesn't worry me that other people will ... I mean, that's great, if you want to take advantage of that. But for me, I ... I don't think it will really affect the way we live and what we decide for the pregnancy anyway." (#163)

Although none of the women interviewed said she thought this technology should be limited or restricted in any way, some were somewhat apprehensive about how it is used. (The current research did not include a survey of women's attitudes toward the availability of PND. This, in its own right, is an important area of research that should be investigated further.)

## Women's Concerns About PND: The Tentative Pregnancy Revisited

As already noted, most women taking advantage of genetic counselling and testing believed this technology to be an important resource, insofar as they believe it gives them greater choice about their reproductive futures. The choice, for many, centres on using the technology to decide how or whether to proceed with the pregnancy. Most of the women believed that this is the reason why the technology is used and why they are using the technology. However, few actually couched this belief explicitly in terms of the option to have a termination if the test showed an abnormal fetus. The women who contemplated using the technology carried the burden of their decision; not only their lives, but also those of their partners, spouses, and families, would be directly affected by the decision. Using PND is not a simple, open-and-shut matter; the consequences for some raise a wide variety of concerns.

In her book by the same name, Rothman (1987) described "the tentative pregnancy." When a pregnancy is tentative, she tells us, women are in a state of limbo, unsure whether to see themselves as mothers of a child, or carriers of a fetus — a potentially defective fetus that might be aborted. When a pregnancy is tentative, the reality of parenthood becomes obscured. When a pregnancy is tentative, the woman's relationship to the fetus she is carrying is very much mediated through technology. When a pregnancy is tentative, it is not necessarily safe to "go public" with the pregnancy. A level of secrecy is associated with this state until the technology makes it safe to announce the pregnancy. In short, much about the experience of pregnancy is changed, particularly the choices that are conferred upon women and the choices that are taken away from women.

If there was a theme heard repeatedly in the interviews, it was that women considered this technology had an impact on the pregnancy experience. Although most women did not speak specifically about their pregnancy being "tentative," a careful examination of the interviews reveals that aspects of their pregnancy experiences are seen as somewhat uncertain. The reasons why women say they are using the technology can be interpreted to indicate the tentativeness of pregnancy, and how integral the technology of PND has become in shaping the course of that experience. Consider this woman's experience of testing:

> I'll be 42 when I have this baby, so I have ... once this procedure's done and we get hopefully a ... a good result, then I can get on with enjoying my pregnancy. So that's ... yeah ... 'cause I've waited a long time to be pregnant, and so ... uh ... I want to get this out of the way because that's ... when I talked to my doctor last year about being pregnant, he said the greatest concern to the fetus ... is a much higher incidence of Down syndrome. There are problems with being an older mother that ... uh ... such as high blood pressure, and ... uh ... gestational diabetes. But I'm not really concerned about that, because I'm healthy and every woman in my family has had a healthy pregnancy, so ... the pregnancy itself I'm not really concerned with. I'm ... I'm concerned in a ... in a fairly normal way, I think ... more than I need to be concerned. But I get ... uh ... proper nutrition and take care of myself. But right now, the earlier part ... finding out that everything is okay, and ... and even then there's no guarantee that everything will be okay, I mean, there may be problems somewhere down the road. But I want to get this thing, the thing that's age related, the old age ... old aches, you know?! I want to get that out of the way and get on with it. (#168)

For most women in the sample, the purpose behind using genetic counselling was to gather additional information — to educate themselves about the testing process and to find out what it could tell about the genetic make-up of the fetus they are carrying.[14] Many women stated that they believed that the purpose behind counselling was to educate and inform, and to give women (or couples) options. For example, when asked what she thought the purpose of counselling was, one woman responded:

"Well, to make me probably feel more comfortable getting it done ... I mean, that's my perception of why they're counselling, so you don't go in ignorant. And then if something happens, for example, if you're one of the 3% of the people that miscarry, that you won't blame anybody for having this done. You know? So I think it's to cover their rear ends and to educate you so you feel more comfortable in having it done."

*Interviewer:* "Do you feel like you have a choice about whether or not to get the test done?"

"Well, I do have a choice. It just depends on, um ... you know, if I find out that this baby is not going to be a healthy, normal baby, if I'm actually going to do something about it. And if I'm going to do something about it, then I should have the testing." (#104)

Another woman said:

[It's a] means to an end. Uh, you know, I appreciate why they do it ... whether I will benefit from it directly, but I think you have to go ... sometimes you find out things that you don't know and ... uh ... it gives you an opportunity to ask any questions ... that you may not want to ask, or may not have the opportunity to ask your physician. And also to give you the time prior to the amnio to decide whether, one, you're, you know, at higher risk than you thought you were, or ... you know ... and ... other options or, you know, and the risk factors of each. (#119)

In connection with the genetic counselling session offering information and options, many women reduced the matter to making a decision about whether to maintain or terminate a pregnancy. Half of the sample specifically mentioned that they were seeking this information to make a decision on whether or not to continue their pregnancy; 31 of these women indicated that if they received positive (abnormal) results from testing, they would definitely terminate the pregnancy.

"I know my chances are not very high that ... that I'm going to have like, a mongoloid baby or if ... if there's Down's. That's the only concern I have, is if there's Down's. Then I have to go through, you know, an abortion at this point in time. I don't really look forward to that, but I'll do it. You know, 'cause ... I mean, it stands to reason. Why bother having this done ... you know, if you're not going to do anything about it, if ... if it happens."

*Interviewer:* "Mm hmm. Well, could you see the ... uh ... the purpose to having ... having the test done if you weren't going to go through with an abortion?"

"Well, maybe if you wanted to prepare yourself for something like that ... But, I don't think you can ever prepare yourself for something like that. I mean, I don't think you could ... I think it would just make you worry. I mean, if you're not going to do anything, you might as well just find out at the time of the birth. I don't know. Maybe other women feel differently, but the reason that I'm doing this is to avoid having a child that's retarded. And I know that I would have difficulty coping. I mean, I have a hard time coping with my son, who's perfectly normal. So, you know, to have a child like that, it's not ... it's not in my nature, and I know that. And it's a ... it's a tremendous burden to me and to society, I mean, somebody's got to look after this kid, if he lives to be older, even when I'm gone." (#149)

Another woman said:

So ... uh ... it would be far easier for me to do something like that now than ... well, I couldn't do anything later. Once the child is born and ... and if something was really, you know, really terrible, I mean ... okay, if the child is born, if it gets cancer or leukaemia, or something like that, that's what you have to go through. But, if you can prevent something at the beginning, I really feel that, for me it would ... it's ... uh ... it would be the aspect I would take. (#151)

In contrast, eight women said that they would definitely not abort the pregnancy, given a positive result. Although women's stated intentions to abort the fetus or carry it to term were often related to their views on abortion and reproductive choice, this was not always so. For instance, some women stated that although they believed it was every woman's choice as to whether to carry a pregnancy to term, for them, abortion simply was not an option. Also some women, opposed philosophically to abortion, believed that they could not continue a pregnancy where a positive (abnormal) result was reported:

You know, I don't really agree with abortions and stuff, but, at this point in my life, I'm not ready to have a Down syndrome child. (#152)

Another woman made the following comments:

"I do know it would be difficult to ... to raise a child that way. But ... you know ... when I said to my doctor, 'is ... is having a child with Down syndrome, if I find that out, is that any reason for ... uh ... I mean, that's not a lawful reason for a clinical abortion, is it?' And she said 'well, why not?' And she said 'you give it a lot of thought.' 'Cause I thought it had to be ... I don't know what I thought, but I didn't think that just 'cause a child had Down's that you could have a ... could even consider a legal clinical abortion."

*Interviewer:* "What are your feelings about abortion?"

"I ... don't believe in abortion just ... I guess if there's any ... health repercussions ... you know ... to the mother, I suppose ... you know ... that when the child is fated to be severely retarded or physically handicapped plus dangerous to the mother, I guess I could almost rationalize it. But otherwise, I can't. Not just 'cause you'd only ... you know ... not only just 'cause you want to have a ... get rid of a pregnancy 'cause it's inconvenient right at that moment ... I guess if I thought my life was on the line and I knew ... you know ... that the child just wouldn't have any health anyway, then I might be predetermined to ... to consider it. But I would never consider it ... uh ... just for ... you know ... convenience or it just doesn't fit in with your lifestyle or something like that." (#166)

For many women, the prospect of making a decision one way or another was daunting to contemplate. As useful as the information might be, the uncertainty surrounding the technology and having the information makes the experience of counselling and testing difficult.

> I don't know that I could terminate a pregnancy. It's hard to say until you're actually in that position ... You know, it's easy to ... you know, look at it in a very distant and objective way, and say ... "yes I would" or "no I wouldn't." Right now, I don't think I would. I don't think ... um ... given the timing of it, for one thing, 'cause it is amnio and by the time that happened I guess I would be close to 20 weeks by the time I found out. And also just generally, I don't know that I have the right to decide that one person has more right to live than another does ... I just ... I don't know if I could live with myself afterwards if I did terminate. I mean, it would be good to know in that you could prepare yourself and I think you make a more informed decision. (#142)

Thus far, the accounts of women in this study reveal the complex ways in which women encounter this technology. As mentioned previously, for some women the effects of PND on the pregnancy experience are quite profound — not how the technology makes decision making about continuing a pregnancy difficult, but how the technology alters the experience of pregnancy itself. Rothman's (1987) notion of a tentative pregnancy is a fitting characterization:

> *Interviewer:* "So you don't feel any sense of anxiety about the tests at all?"
>
> "Oh, yeah, yeah. There's anxiety that ... I think it's safer finding out."
>
> *Interviewer:* "You'd rather find out ..."
>
> "I'd rather know than go through nine months. At least if there is something wrong, I'd have time to prepare. And if there's nothing wrong, then I can just go ahead and ... 'cause I haven't uh ... I've told my parents, my husband knows, and that's it. And it's killing me not ... not telling anyone. It's hard."
>
> *Interviewer:* "Will you wait for the results before you ...?"
>
> "Yeah. And then once I find out the results, I'd tell them."
>
> *Interviewer:* "Just to be on the safe side? Don't want everyone to know what's going on?"
>
> "Uh-huh. They just think I'm getting fat. Now, that's all right. 'Cause I've put on about 10 pounds, and they kind of 'ummm ... getting kind of chunky, Susan,' and I can't tell them — or, I won't tell them."
>
> *Interviewer:* "Right, but if everything works out then they'll know the real reason."
>
> "Then they'll know soon enough. Yeah." (#113)[15]

Similarly, from another woman:

> You know, I've ... we haven't told anyone about ... well, we've told one or two people ... about myself being pregnant, and so I'm anxious to have the results as early as possible, because I know I'm starting to show and they're starting to wonder. Um ... you know, I'm anxious to find out about how they're going to inform me. (#129)

Another woman echoes the desire for testing as a guide to making the pregnancy public:

> I guess I'm paranoid in the fact that I don't want anything to be wrong with the baby. Nobody knows yet. I haven't told a single ... I haven't told my parents, I haven't told anybody yet. It's been really quiet. It's just my boyfriend and I know and that's it. And I want to keep it that way until I get the results of the chorionic villus sampling back.

She later added:

> I want to do this as soon as possible. Like I said, my parents ... nobody knows yet. So the sooner I can find out that everything is probably okay, the sooner I'll tell everybody. So, I don't want to wait for amnio. I mean, I haven't really checked into that but I know it ... you do it at a later date. And ... um ... I don't want to wait. I want to get this over with as quickly as possible. (#165)

Another woman said:

> Winnipeg is a really ... a ... a big little town and you don't ... you ... I know everybody here and so it was so much easier in Toronto where I could go and have the chorionic villus sampling and nobody knew about and ... and you know, effectively, nobody here except yourselves and my parents and ... uh ... know about the pregnancy. Like, I haven't told my ... uh ... superiors ... because, I don't know. I don't know what's going to happen. I mean if there is a problem, I don't want to say, "listen I can't do my rounds in April because I'm going to be pregnant," then find out that there is a problem and, maybe I won't be pregnant in April! (#120)

The tentative nature of pregnancy in relation to the technology goes beyond women making public announcements. Some women spoke of how glad they were not to have felt fetal movement yet as it would make deciding to terminate a pregnancy more difficult. One woman reported that she had already experienced fetal movement. She said:

> The sensation of the baby's starting to kick now ... or I can feel the flutters and stuff like that. But it's still really not ... not much to me right now. You know, it doesn't have a personality or anything like that. (#151)

Rothman (1987) also found women's experience of fetal movement and the meaning that they attached to it were profoundly influenced by the timing of testing.

Altogether, nine women explicitly defined their experiences of testing and pregnancy in terms that correspond to Rothman's characterization of the tentative pregnancy — that is, they said that they had not told anyone about their pregnancy or that they were waiting for the results of PND to feel attached to the pregnancy. Many more, in recounting their experiences of the technology, provided more subtle evidence that such technology influenced their definition of their pregnancies.

## What Do Women Want from PND? What Are They Concerned About?

The women were asked what concerns they brought to the counselling session and what they wanted from PND. Their concerns can be classified at two interrelated levels: first, concern about having and raising a child with a disability and, second, concern about the testing procedure.

### *Concern About Disability: The Reason They Have the Test*

There is a clear and pressing concern about giving birth to and raising a child with a disability. The concerns women expressed cover a wide range of issues, many of which have been explored in depth by previous researchers (Asch 1989; Asch and Fine 1988; Saxton 1987a, 1987b, 1989; Tait 1986); the concern mentioned most often in this study was Down syndrome.

Why exactly does having a Down syndrome baby concern women? This account of a nurse (which has been previously cited) captures the essence of what many women believed:

"If it's determined that the child is a Down's, then yes, we have decided to terminate the pregnancy. Not that I have a concern about having a retarded child. I am concerned about the physical defects that go along with it, and I'm not prepared to watch a child go through that ... the surgeries and the needles and ... ignorance would be bliss. But unfortunately my husband is also a nurse and we're just not prepared to ... uh ... to do that ... I just couldn't watch a child go through that, so, um ... easy to say now. When we get the results we may change our mind but um, I don't have a religious feeling about it. I also don't think society needs the burden. Plus, when you hit 35, when the child's 35, I'm 70. And who's going to look after, you know ... the extended family just isn't there. And um, you know, I don't have a younger brother or sister who could take over. And having had a 39-year-old lady come in who was raped, a mental age of four, I just can't, you know. I just see a little too much to, uh, to bring a child in ... there you are, 80 years old, trying to stay alive so that you can look after your child. Plus it means, you know, such a change in everybody's lifestyles. It um, you know, having a child who has an accident after birth, or something happens and you deal with it. But um, multiple surgeries are required for heart defect ... and ... everything else ... I'm just ... neither of us is really prepared to go through it, so, that's the reason for the amnio ... to allay those fears."

*Interviewer:* "Mm hmm. So, you think it's a good idea ... amnio?"

"Yeah. Um, I think if ... if I wasn't going to terminate the pregnancy I wouldn't have an amnio 'cause the risks are the same anyway. Um, the amnio is a risk itself so, uh ... anybody I've ever talked to who has strong religious — colleagues of mine, friends of mine — who said 'well I'm not sure, I definitely wouldn't terminate the pregnancy.' I said, 'well, don't have an amnio then!' Um, except for giving you some time to ... to go to support groups and things like that." (#119)

The issues discussed by women about having a child with Down syndrome fall into three areas: (1) concern over caring for the child, (2) concern over the implications of having a Down syndrome child for the woman, her partner, and her other children, and (3) concern over the physical, educational, and social problems of the child (including the stigma likely to be experienced by the child). In the previous quotation, each of these themes is mentioned directly.

Several women commented that they believed the current system does not adequately support families with disabled children and adults. Having decided that she would abort in the event of a positive (abnormal) result, this woman offered this as her reason:

I've made that ... that decision having been with a handicapped person, you know. Weighed that ... that all through because there aren't ... uh ... services available for ... special needs children. Um ... No, no there ... there aren't. I've had to go through the full gamut of ... um ... with the single mother, you know, finding a home ... I thought ... a special home for him would help him. It's not anything that I would wish upon someone who has an option ... if you have choices and there are alternatives. Because it isn't that easy. And there's no real respite for families that have to deal with severely handicapped people. (#144)

Several women also expressed concern about their ability to care for someone with Down syndrome. Comments such as "I don't know that I have what it takes" or "I'm not ready to have a Down syndrome child" were not uncommon. Typically, such comments would be made apologetically, and disclaimers were not uncommon, as illustrated by the following woman:

"I don't really agree with abortions and stuff, but, at this point in my life, I'm not ready to have a Down syndrome child. You know, if it would be my first, I would never have hesitated. You know, they're very loving, but they take a lot of time, a lot of patience, and I don't have that now. You know? I had it 10 years ago when I had my first, but ... uh ... it could be harder now."

*Interviewer:* "'Cause of the structure of your life and ...?"

"That's right. Two little kids that demand a lot, and I just don't think I could handle it." (#152)

For many women who had concerns about raising a Down syndrome child, the issue focussed primarily on the fact that they would have the major responsibility for caregiving. Some women said that they doubted that their husbands or partners would be very involved in the care of such a child, and some said that they expected that they would have to give up paid employment and their lifestyle, both being seen as major sacrifices.

> It is such a hard world, and ... um ... for both the child and for myself, to be quite honest. Could I ... could I do it, because as much as my husband may love that child and be involved with it, I ... good thing he's not here, he would shoot me if I said this ... but the bottom line is I think the mother. And ... uh ... as much as fathers are participating, I ... I still think, bottom line, it comes down to the mothering. And, I don't know whether I could give that child the support that it needs, and I don't know what impact it would have on my other child. (#131)

Another said:

> I'm just not um ... maybe it's selfish ... but I'm just not prepared to ... to give up my whole life for a child that will be suffering. (#119)

Clearly for some women, contemplating the birth of a disabled child is painful:

> "Maybe other women feel differently, but the reason that I'm doing this is to avoid having a child that's retarded. And I know that I would have difficulty coping. I mean, I have a hard time coping with my son, who's perfectly normal. So, you know, to have a child like that, it's not ... it's not in my nature, and I know that. And it's a ... it's a tremendous burden to me and to society, I mean, somebody's got to look after this kid, if he lives to be older, even when I'm gone. So ... no, it's just not worth it to me. So ...."
>
> *Interviewer:* "Do you feel like the main burden of care would fall on to you?"
>
> "Yeah, I think so. I mean it's my responsibility. It's my child. And I ... I think I would ... I mean, some people wouldn't, but I would feel resentful and, you know, I'd feel disappointed, and all those things that people feel when they know that their child isn't going to have the potential that they think it's going to have. So ... that's the scary part for me." (#149)

Some women were particularly concerned about the impact a Down syndrome child would have on their family, and a few were concerned about its effect on their marital relationship:

> I guess I want somebody to tell me that ... the tests aren't positive ... that there is no Down syndrome ... and that there is no birth ... any type of genetic defect. Okay? I mean, nothing is for sure, nothing is 100 percent guaranteed, okay. But my understanding of this test, the test will tell me whether or not there is Down syndrome. Um, and I guess that's about my biggest concern ... because of my age. Okay? This wasn't a planned pregnancy. This was not planned. So, it was kind of like ... you know, you kind of have to step back. I have an eight-year-old and now I'm carrying another one and I ... I don't know how I feel about it I guess. I'm very cautious. I'm just waiting for the test ... to see what the test will tell.

She subsequently added:

> I also think that every child that's brought into this world should be a child that is ... I guess, loved, healthy ... I think bringing in a child that has any type of birth defect or Down syndrome ... I mean, I think it would be a tremendous strain on our marriage. And ... I don't think I could take care of it, myself. So we'd have to rely on, you know, the public purse, institutions and that to take care of it. I just don't think that's right, and I ... if I have a choice, I want to make the choice that I think is the right one and I will live with my conscience and, you know ... so that we've ... we've discussed it and I'm hoping that, uh, you know, the tests come back that show that there isn't anything and we have a healthy baby. But if it comes back (otherwise) we've decided I would have an abortion. (#115)

Another woman said:

> Uh ... I don't wish to bring a child into this world disadvantaged. And ... uh ... I also don't wish to be ... I guess disadvantaged myself in a way. And ... and that would mean I don't wish to be ... um ... parenting a ... a child that is handicapped when I could have had the option not to. Um ... I don't think it's fair to the child or to me or to my husband. And I think that having the option to terminate is ... uh ... is ideal as far as my feelings go. (#167)

Some women were also concerned about the effect having a disabled child would have on other children, particularly in the years to come.

> I have a ... a very well daughter ... I mean, she's good and she's healthy and she's ... she's bright and ... the concern for me is ... is not so much during my time on this earth dealing with a Down's that may or may not require a lot of care, but what's going to happen to her if we ... you know ... if we have a Down syndrome and now she's burdened with that child after we're gone. And that's not fair to her, I don't think and so ... you know, particularly if it's a severe Down's, and ... and I've seen that so many times, you know, where ... uh ... you know, friend ... a good friend of mine ... uh ... her brother was a Down's, it was the first of two pregnancies, and so the elder brother was a Down's and then they had this girl. And she's just taken off ... you know ... she's gone and she's moved elsewhere and now he's with elderly parents, you know, who are into their seventies and having problems coping with him and, 'cause she just wants nothing to do with him, I mean ... I don't know where he's going to end up once they pass on and ... so it's a really sad story. So, those are the kind of considerations that one has to make, you know, I'm an elderly parent and I may not be around for much more than 30 or 40 years of my child's life and if I'm going to burden my eldest daughter with this kind of a child ... um ... to care for, and then that puts any kind of family life she might have at risk. So I think, I would probably opt for termination of the pregnancy. (#120)

Concern over their own aging was a paramount issue for some, who realized that someone would eventually have to care for the disabled child they might bring into the world:

> First of all, being older parents. Um ... we have a concern that with a Down syndrome child ... eventually that child would have to be institutionalized because we may not live long enough to look after it. And the other concern is ... um ... to be really realistic, I think a Down syndrome child is born with the world against it to start off with. The world is not open towards ... to that kind of child or human being or adult. And he's going to have a rough, rough life. And it's unfair to the child. And seriously I don't really know how well I could cope, or my husband, with ... um ... that kind of child. I don't know if I have what it takes. (#156)

This quotation draws attention to another set of concerns that women voiced — the array of physical, educational, and social problems that people with disabilities face. Some spoke of the stigma that disabled people experience and of how difficult life is for those not fitting into the mould of being "normal." One woman, who had worked with the intellectually disabled, mentioned that there is still intolerance and a lack of understanding about the disabled. Further, she worried that PND testing might actually exacerbate this situation, considering the predictive ability of PND technologies at present and in the future. There is considerable discussion of this point in the literature (Asch 1989; Bell et al. 1986; Boss 1990). Although PND with selective abortion might alter the incidence of some forms of disability, it is not clear that the overall result would actually be a reduction in the prevalence of disability in the population. This is because a significant amount of disability occurs after birth. The question that arises in this discussion is whether the use of PND with selective abortion to eliminate certain kinds of disability might lead to greater prejudice or discrimination against the disabled. However, one can only speculate, as the interviews did not specifically address this question.

### Concern About the Testing Procedure

The other major area of concern to women was the testing process. Several issues were raised by women, such as the safety, accuracy, and invasiveness of the technique (n = 12), the skill of the technicians performing the procedure (n = 7), and the pain associated with the technique (n = 11). However, the issue that most worried women was the risk of miscarriage or of harm to the fetus (n = 38).[16] For women seeing this as a "last chance" pregnancy, the worry about miscarriage was quite profound:

> The only thing I'm concerned about is the ... the percentage of miscarriage. This is my last shot ... I'll never get pregnant again, I'll never be able to persuade my husband to do it again! And that concerns me, 'cause I don't want to lose this baby. (#146)

Another said:

> Well, the only thing I'm concerned about is ... uh ... I hope that a very trained doctor is doing the test ... because I'm too old to have a ... [I don't have] much time left to keep on trying to get pregnant. (#156)

Women often remarked that they worried about the fetus being hit by the needle, although most were comforted knowing that the procedures are guided by ultrasound. The technical skill of the physician performing the procedure was typically mentioned as a safeguard against miscarriage, and most women saw the staff as being skilled, intelligent, and competent. A few women worried that inexperienced (student) physicians might perform the procedure and that this might increase the risk of miscarriage.

Many of the women who were worried about the risk of miscarriage said they would feel guilt or remorse if they miscarried subsequent to testing. Particularly if the fetus was determined to be normal, women worried that a miscarriage would weigh heavily on their consciences:

> I guess mostly the test has ... the actual test kind of concerns me, you know. I hate the thought of it, actually. I'm most concerned because a very low percentage of cases will miscarry. So I'm a little concerned about that. I mean, if the baby's perfectly normal, which I'm hoping that it is, that you could, you know, miscarry. So that's kind of something I'm not too thrilled about. (#101)

Another stated:

> I would hate to think that, you know, I would have this healthy kid and I went through with this and miscarried, and ... you know what I mean? That would make me feel sort of ... stressed, probably, for the rest of my life. (#104)

And this from another woman:

> For me the thought of having a test and miscarrying because of the test is probably the grossest thing I could imagine. I mean I ... that just is such a waste of life ... (#122)

For some, the real dilemma is that having the testing is an option, and by virtue of taking advantage of that option, one might actually lose a pregnancy. Several women thought that this would be a high price to pay for the sake of getting information about the genetic health of their fetuses.

Another area of concern was the anxiety over the results of the procedure. One woman wondered if she might be better off not knowing the information that PND could reveal. Others spoke of the weight of this information in terms of making a decision about the continuation of a pregnancy. The issue mentioned most often was women's concern over the waiting period for the results of PND (n = 18). Some women said that they were opting for chorionic villus sampling simply because the results of amniocentesis come too late in the pregnancy (i.e., when making a decision about abortion becomes more difficult in many different respects — medically and personally). For example:

> I see the advantage of the chorionic villus sampling as being earlier in the pregnancy, so that if there is a severe problem, we will be able to terminate it more easily because it would be before feeling your baby move. The last time I had to wait ... doing the amnio and then waiting another ... I think it was three weeks before they called me. I had already felt the baby. I knew that there was something in there. So it would have been a very difficult decision. (#164)

Another woman who had said she worried about the reported higher risk of miscarriage associated with chorionic villus sampling said:

> I don't know if I'll get any information that will ease my mind because if we have a Down syndrome fetus we are pretty sure that we'd probably want an abortion. And I do not want to have an abortion later on. I ... if it's got to happen I want to have it as early as possible. As soon as I ... apparently the amniocentesis is done later, and the ... results take longer to come in. So by the time we got the results and I had to make ... we had to make a decision, I might already be feeling fetal movement, and I ... I'm going to have a really ... I'm going to have a tough time anyway, making a decision to abort if I have to. I'd rather make it sooner than later. (#168)

These kinds of concerns are not unique to this sample; other qualitative studies have reported similar kinds of experiences (Rothman 1987). Some of the research on women declining PND suggests that concerns such as these are critical to women's decision to refuse amniocentesis or chorionic villus sampling (Farrant 1985).

## To Test or Not to Test: That Is the Question

Women were asked, during the interviews, about their intentions with respect to testing. As already noted, many of the women used the counselling session to help them decide whether to undergo testing. At the time of the pre-counselling interviews, some women remained undecided; others had already decided well before they arrived for counselling. Why are some women so clear and others not? This is a difficult question to answer, given the extent of the qualitative data. One can only make assumptions on the basis of what some women said. For example, some women believe that the effectiveness of the technology is such that they would not want to decline the opportunity to have testing; these women were usually clear also on their intention to abort a pregnancy in the event of a positive finding.

Other women needed to be convinced of the benefits of testing — that is, they needed some kind of reassurance that the benefits of testing were substantially greater than the risks. Several women said that they would reserve judgment until they had had genetic counselling. Were some women expecting to be told about testing (in a directive manner) by the genetic counsellors? Some were counting on receiving counselling — that is, help with their feelings about their situation and not just the medical facts. As is noted in the following chapter, some women were clearly disappointed when they did not get the kind of counselling and direction they thought would be helpful.

Whatever their own personal decision with regard to testing, many women said that they believed counselling and the option to test were desirable. Even women steadfastly opposed to abortion said that prenatal screening should not be restricted or eliminated. The interview did not specifically examine whether women thought PND was desirable or not, whether they believed such programs should be made available for all or some, or whether testing should be voluntary or mandatory. Some women offered their insights into these matters, particularly on whether testing was desirable. The following quotation seems to capture the ambivalence that many women expressed:

> *Interviewer:* "Do you feel that it's sort of become necessary to have the testing ... um ... sort of as if because it's available you have to do it?"
>
> "Well, I think that ... I mean ... we do that in everyday life, you know, we do it because it's there. Right? I mean that's just the way we use technology, because it's there. I mean, you go when you get ... you know ... health check-ups, which are far more in-depth now than they used to be 20 years ago, just general health ... you know ... heart and blood and all that stuff. So, it's there. It's there for pregnancy as well so ... you uh ... if you do choose to use it then you're opening a door that maybe you don't want to open! But, I think ... yeah ... because it's there."
>
> *Interviewer:* "Mm hmm. So just sort of ends up being used and people say ... technology! Let's use it!"
>
> "Well, yeah. I mean, there's a lot ... there are important things ... if ... if someone really can see themselves going through if ... I mean nowadays with the ... um ... if they were going to lose the child anyway in six or seven months or something because it didn't have a brain or ... you know ... didn't have the spinal thing ... whatever that is ... then I think it would make it certainly a lot easier on the parents and the family not to have to go through so many months of pregnancy ... I mean if it's inevitable ... you know ... I mean ... I think certainly technology's a good thing. It just ... it makes decisions more difficult in certain circumstances. And then you have to ... you have to choose how to use it ... it's like the H-bomb, too, I don't know. It's there, but you have to choose how to use it."
>
> *Interviewer:* "Or to use it at all, God help us!"
>
> "Exactly, you know, like ... but once it's there then you have to make decisions that other people didn't have to make." (#122)

Even with all of the dilemmas that testing presented, the women in this study seemed to think the program they had come to was good. It would be worthwhile to find out, from the women who declined counselling (and testing) when offered it by the referring doctors, if they shared this view, but this was beyond the scope of the study.

## Conclusions

It is difficult to summarize briefly the wealth of experience and feeling that has been documented in this chapter. In part, it is because to do so is to subvert the very intention of a qualitative study; to do so trivializes the range of experiences of the women in the study. This chapter provides a record of women's encounters with genetic counselling, and their anticipated experiences with PND.

For the women whose accounts are documented here, this technological development is both a blessing and a curse; it gives them choice, but restricts their choice as well. In almost every respect, this technology is somewhat paradoxical. But, it is there to be used. And women do feel, even if subtly, the compulsion to use this technology "for their own good." For many, their use of this technology is a response to a society that is biased toward the able-bodied (Asch 1989; Oliver 1990). Women's perception of this ableism is that it will be manifest in terms of little support for families with a disabled person, and even less support for them, the women, who will be expected to assume a primary role in caregiving.

As conflicted as some women are about making a decision to use PND — and there were many such women in this sample — it is almost as if using PND is the path of least resistance. It is, as Rothman (1987) found, a choice between what is bad and what is worse. One woman asked:

> "Are you better [off] not knowing, or ... what are you going to do should you know?" (#131)

And another said, almost in response:

> "It's like telling a child you got to take medicine and they say 'yuck, I don't like it,' but it's better for you, it'll make you feel better ... and ... you pick ... "
>
> *Interviewer:* "Mm hmm. You have to go through whatever to ..."
>
> "Yeah. Whatever it is that will make you feel better, and whatever it is that will help you feel better or make you feel more comfortable, why not do it?" (#134)

As this chapter has shown, for a variety of reasons, PND is a bitter — but for some women, necessary — pill to swallow.

## Chapter 5. Presentation of Findings:
## Part 2. A Survey of Women's Attitudes Toward, and Perceptions of, Prenatal Diagnosis

### Introduction

The findings from the questionnaire are presented in this chapter. The questionnaire was developed to measure the aspects of women's PND experience that were quantifiable. In addition, this survey measured the psychosocial variables thought to be predictive of women's PND experience, and, more generally, reproductive decision making. (See Appendix 3 for the questionnaire.)

The response rate on the questionnaire was very high. Other researchers[17] have suggested that because of the relevance of the subject matter, there is a high level of motivation to participate in research of this type among those referred for PND; this seems to have been so in this study. Also, it is likely that the effectiveness of the total design method (TDM) advocated by Dillman (1978) in improving response rates contributed to the high rate of completion in this study. Only one follow-up reminder was necessary to encourage most study participants to return the questionnaire. A second follow-up reminder (with a second questionnaire included in the mailing) was sent to only a few.

As was noted in Chapter 3, 122 women agreed to participate in this study. Seventy (57.4%) were interviewed and took questionnaires to complete after counselling; and 52 (42.6%) were in the questionnaire-only segment of the study. A total of 111 questionnaires were returned, producing an overall response rate of 90.9%. The response rate was slightly higher for those in the interview-questionnaire sample (68 of 70 questionnaires were returned, or 97.1%), compared to the questionnaire-only sample (43 of 52 questionnaires were returned, or 82.6%).[18] The higher completion rate among interview-questionnaire sample participants may show that the women who were interviewed had a somewhat greater commitment to the project.

Since so little information is available on non-respondents, it is difficult to know with certainty whether they were different from the respondents of the survey. The only demographic characteristic known to the research team for all referrals was the woman's date of birth. The average age of respondents was 36.5 years, while the average age of non-respondents was 38.3 years. Comparisons on the variable age were also tabulated for the women completing the survey with those who declined counselling (mean = 36.7 years), those who miscarried (mean = 37.2 years), those who did not arrive at the clinic (mean = 37.4 years), and those who refused to participate in the study (mean = 37.7 years). (No tests of statistical difference were calculated here.)

It is important to note that the sample used in this research is not random. Also, because of the way in which utilization data are kept at the

Section of Clinical Genetics, there is no exact way of ascertaining whether this sample is representative of all women seen in the 1991 calendar year. The Section of Clinical Genetics only keeps records of all women seen and does not separate those seen only because of AMA. It is also worth remembering that with data collection over a four-month period only, if there are seasonal factors operating they cannot be discerned. Consequently, the findings reported here reflect the experiences of the AMA women participating and should be generalized beyond this group with caution.

## Sample Characteristics

The characteristics of the study participants are detailed in Table 3. The sample ranged between the ages of 34 and 42 years, with an average age of 36.5 years (SD = 2.0). Most participants in the study were either married or living common-law (95.4%). Only two women were single and had never been married. Most (77.6%) women had been pregnant at least one time before the current pregnancy. The average number of pregnancies (gravidity) in this sample was 2.5 (SD = 1.2). In terms of parity (number of children born), the mean was 1.0 (SD = 0.9), with a range between zero and four children born.

The socioeconomic profile of the sample is of particular interest because it has been noted in the literature that it is highly educated, economically advantaged individuals who are more likely to use PND (Golbus et al. 1979); this seems true in the present study as well. A sizable proportion of the sample had at least some undergraduate university education (56.2%), and many of these women had obtained a university certificate, diploma, or degree (48.6%). Eleven women in the sample (10.5%) had a master's degree. Women's partners were also highly educated, with 45.1% having some undergraduate university education, and 12.7% having either a master's or doctoral degree. The partners of the participants were somewhat more likely to have technical/vocational training (18.7% of partners compared to 12.4% of the women).

Most of the women were employed outside the home, with 59.3% employed full time and 26.9% employed part time; 13% were not employed outside the home. The occupations of participants (and their partners) have been coded by both the Standard Occupational Classification developed by Statistics Canada and the revised Pineo-Porter McRoberts (PPM) occupational classification (Pineo 1985). Using the PPM classification, 29% of the sample were employed in professional occupations and 40.9% in supervisory and managerial positions. The two most common occupational classifications for the women in the sample were employed professional and semi-professional (each with 23.7% of the sample). Women's partners' occupational classifications were similarly weighted in

### Table 3. Distribution of Study Participants by Selected Sample Characteristics

| Age (n = 109) | % |
|---|---|
| 34 | 7.3 |
| 35 | 33.0 |
| 36 | 22.9 |
| 37 | 11.9 |
| 38 | 9.2 |
| 39 | 5.5 |
| 40 | 3.7 |
| 41 | 2.8 |
| 42 | 3.7 |

| Marital status (n = 109) | % |
|---|---|
| Married/common-law | 95.4 |
| Never married | 1.8 |
| Divorced/separated | 2.8 |

| Gravidity (total pregnancies) (n = 107) | % |
|---|---|
| 1 | 22.4 |
| 2 | 36.4 |
| 3 or more | 41.1 |

| Parity (total children born) (n = 108) | % |
|---|---|
| 0 | 32.4 |
| 1 | 38.9 |
| 2 | 21.3 |
| 3 or more | 7.4 |

| Education level (n = 105) | % |
|---|---|
| Junior high or less | 1.0 |
| High school | 20.0 |
| Technical/vocational | 12.4 |
| Undergrad university | 56.2 |
| Post-grad university | 10.5 |

| Employment status (n = 108) | % |
|---|---|
| Full-time | 59.3 |
| Part-time | 26.9 |
| Full- and part-time | 0.9 |
| Not employed outside home | 13.0 |

## Table 3. (cont'd)

| Occupation (Pineo-Porter McRoberts classification) | Respondents (n = 93) % | Partners (n = 95) % |
|---|---|---|
| Self-employed professional | 5.4 | 6.3 |
| Employed professional | 23.7 | 13.7 |
| High-level management | 6.5 | 7.4 |
| Semi-professional | 23.7 | 9.5 |
| Technician | 0.0 | 4.2 |
| Middle-management | 7.5 | 14.7 |
| Supervisor | 3.2 | 4.2 |
| Foremen/women | 0.0 | 6.3 |
| Skilled clerical/sales/service | 12.9 | 7.4 |
| Skilled crafts/tradesperson | 0.0 | 8.4 |
| Semi-skilled clerical/sales/service | 9.7 | 1.1 |
| Semi-skilled manual | 2.2 | 8.4 |
| Unskilled clerical/sales/service | 2.2 | 2.1 |
| Unskilled manual | 2.2 | 2.1 |
| Farm labourer | 1.1 | 4.2 |

| Personal income (n = 92) | % |
|---|---|
| No income | 3.3 |
| Under $20 000 | 28.3 |
| $20 000-29 999 | 20.7 |
| $30 000-39 999 | 17.4 |
| $40 000-49 999 | 17.4 |
| $50 000-59 999 | 3.3 |
| $60 000-69 999 | 4.3 |
| $70 000-79 999 | 2.2 |
| $80 000-89 999 | 1.1 |
| $90 000-99 999 | 1.1 |
| $100 000 and over | 1.1 |

**Table 3.** (cont'd)

| Household income (n = 94) | % |
|---|---|
| No income | 1.1 |
| Under $20 000 | 4.3 |
| $20 000-29 999 | 3.2 |
| $30 000-39 999 | 16.0 |
| $40 000-49 999 | 9.6 |
| $50 000-59 999 | 10.6 |
| $60 000-69 999 | 13.8 |
| $70 000-79 999 | 10.6 |
| $80 000-89 999 | 10.6 |
| $90 000-99 999 | 7.4 |
| $100 000 and over | 12.8 |

| Religion | Respondents (n = 102) % | Partners (n = 92) % |
|---|---|---|
| Protestant | 45.1 | 37.0 |
| Catholic | 21.6 | 20.7 |
| Jewish | 4.9 | 6.5 |
| Other Eastern | 2.0 | 1.1 |
| Mennonite | 2.0 | 3.3 |
| Agnostic | 3.9 | 4.3 |
| No preference | 14.7 | 23.9 |
| Other | 5.9 | 3.3 |

| Self-identified ethnicity (n = 84) | % |
|---|---|
| Canadian | 42.9 |
| Anglo/British | 23.8 |
| German | 3.6 |
| Jewish | 3.6 |
| Ukrainian | 7.1 |
| Other European | 3.6 |
| Asian | 4.8 |
| Other | 10.7 |

the direction of higher-status occupations. The partners of 20% of the sample were employed in professional occupations, and 35.8% of women's partners held positions in supervisory and managerial positions.

Participants were asked to estimate their household and personal incomes in the previous year. Response categories were in grouped intervals to provide a measure of privacy to the respondents; consequently, they are not continuous-interval variables. The median household income was $60 000 to $64 999, and the modal household income was in excess of $100 000 per annum (12.8% of the sample) (these figures are from the raw data, and are not shown in Table 3). About one-quarter of the sample households earned less than $40 000, and the proportion with household incomes under $20 000 was just over 5% of the sample. Women's personal incomes were markedly lower on average than their household incomes. Nearly one-third of the women reported their personal income to be under $20 000. The median personal income was $28 000 to $29 999, and the modal personal income was $45 000 to $49 999 (9.8% of the sample) (these figures are from the raw data, and are not shown in Table 3).

Two ethnocultural variables are of interest — religion and self-identified ethnicity. A substantial portion of the sample was Protestant (45.1%), while 21.6% were Catholic. The remainder of the sample came from other religious groups (18.7%), had no religious preference (14.7%), or were agnostic (3.9%). (Women's partners were also similarly distributed on this variable, with 37.0% Protestant, 20.7% Catholic, 23.9% with no religious preference, and 4.3% agnostic.) Twenty-five percent of the sample indicated that their religious beliefs are currently strong, and 23.1% said that their religious beliefs are somewhat strong. The remainder of the sample (51.9%) indicated that their religious beliefs are not strong. When asked if their religion was important to them, approximately one-quarter indicated that they strongly agreed with that statement as a description of their beliefs at present. Slightly more than one-third of the sample described their beliefs when growing up in this manner.

Most of the women (42.9%) identified themselves as "Canadian." The next largest group consisted of those who identified themselves as of Anglo or British extraction (23.8%). This variable reflects self-identification and cannot be assessed in terms of the way that the Canadian census categorizes ethnicity.

Comparisons of the interview-questionnaire sample and questionnaire-only sample were made on selected demographic variables (age, gravidity, parity, education level, household and personal incomes, and occupational classification). On none of these variables were there statistically significant differences between these two categories of respondents (Table 4). Accordingly, all findings reported here refer to the entire sample who completed questionnaires.

To summarize, the typical respondent was 36.5 years of age, married, in her second pregnancy, and with one child. She was highly educated, typically having at least some university training. She was employed outside the home on a full-time basis, in a high-status occupation. Her household income was relatively high. The typical respondent was of the Protestant faith and identified herself as Canadian.

### Table 4. Comparison of Interview/Questionnaire vs. Questionnaire-Only Subsamples on Selected Demographic Characteristics

| Variable | Interview/questionnaire sample means | Questionnaire-only sample means | f | p |
|---|---|---|---|---|
| Age | 36.49 | 36.50 | 1.09 | 0.771 |
| Gravidity | 2.28 | 2.60 | 1.49 | 0.179 |
| Parity | 0.85 | 1.16 | 1.56 | 0.136 |
| Education level | 10.39 | 10.59 | 1.00 | 1.000 |
| Household income | 22.47 | 22.22 | 1.30 | 0.413 |
| Personal income | 13.40 | 12.49 | 1.26 | 0.481 |
| Occupational classification | | | | |
| (a) Respondent | 6.22 | 5.44 | 1.26 | 0.467 |
| (b) Partner | 7.62 | 6.41 | 1.07 | 0.859 |

Before proceeding with other areas of the survey, a brief methodological note is in order. Liebetrau (1983) noted that measures of association based on the chi-squared statistic are convenient when summarizing two-way contingency tables, but some difficulty may occur when attempting to derive a meaningful, probabilistic interpretation on the basis of these measures. Since the primary objective in these analyses is to ascertain the types of relationships and not to presume causal direction, contingency measures such as phi and Cramer's V are fully appropriate statistics to report. Accordingly, both PRE (proportional reduction in error) statistics and those based on chi-squared are reported in the discussion that follows.[19]

## Women's Experiences of Genetic Counselling

The first segment of the questionnaire sought information from respondents regarding their counselling session in the Section of Clinical Genetics. Many of the questions used in this portion of the survey were derived from Sorenson et al.'s (1981) study and provide women's perspectives on the information they have received and an assessment of their level of satisfaction with the counselling session.

Table 5 provides information about women's experiences with genetic counselling. For most of the sample (56.0%), the counselling session was 20 to 39 minutes long; the range was from under 20 minutes (17.4%) to an hour or longer (5.5%). When asked whether the genetic counsellor mentioned the possibility of the woman having a child with a birth defect or genetic disorder, 13.9% said that the counsellor just mentioned this possibility, while 86.1% indicated that the counsellor discussed this in some depth.

**Table 5. Length of Genetic Counselling Sessions**

|  | % |
|---|---|
| 20 minutes or less | 17.4 |
| 20 - 39 minutes | 56.0 |
| 40 - 59 minutes | 21.1 |
| 60 minutes or more | 5.5 |
| (n = 109) | |

Women were asked to indicate their chances of having a child with a birth defect or genetic disorder (Table 6). The questions included on this topic were derived from the Sorenson et al. (1981) study. In that study, and the present one as well, women were asked to state their risk of bearing a child with a genetic disorder. The question was worded as "What are your chances of having a child with a birth defect or genetic disorder? I know the chances are ____. I think the chances are ____." Whether what they reported are the actual risks cannot be ascertained; instead, women's responses to these questions reflect their interpretation of the risks as they understood them from the counselling session. For instance, of those who responded to the question of "known" risks of bearing a child with a birth defect, 18 (or 23.7%) said that they knew the risks to be 3:1000 and 1 (or 1.3%) said she knew the risks to be 3:100. One might assume that the different patterning of responses here reflects the evaluation done by counsellors to construct an estimated risk for women clients.

Because the reports that these questions yielded do not necessarily indicate the nature of risk, except in numerical form, women were also asked to interpret their risk status. Quite simply, two women who are both told that the risk of bearing a child with a genetic disorder is 1:100 might define their risk status quite differently — one might consider herself at high risk, while the other might define this as a moderate risk. When asked to characterize the probability of bearing a child with a genetic disorder, 13.1% judged the risk to be high or very high, 31.8% judged the risk to be moderate, and 55.2% judged the risk to be low or very low.

Counsellors mentioned a number of tests that could be done as part of PND. Among them were amniocentesis, chorionic villus sampling, ultrasound, and blood serum tests (maternal serum AFP). Most of the women studied indicated that they either had already had some testing done[20] or intended to have testing performed after counselling (87.1%).

### Table 6. Estimates of Risk of Bearing a Child with a Genetic Disorder and Self-Assessed Risk of a Genetic Abnormality

**(a) Estimates of risk**

| Probability (ratio) | % who *know* their chances are (n = 76) | % who *think* their chances are (n = 31) |
|---|---|---|
| 1: 1000   | 0.0  | 13.2 |
| 3: 1000   | 23.7 | 22.6 |
| 4: 1000   | 13.2 | 12.9 |
| 5: 1000   | 13.2 | 19.4 |
| 6: 1000   | 3.9  | 9.7  |
| 7: 1000   | 10.5 | 0.0  |
| 8: 1000   | 5.3  | 12.9 |
| 1: 100    | 7.9  | 9.7  |
| 1.3: 100  | 10.5 | 3.2  |
| 1.5: 100  | 2.6  | 0.0  |
| 2: 100    | 3.9  | 3.2  |
| 2.5: 100  | 2.6  | 0.0  |
| 2.9: 100  | 1.3  | 0.0  |
| 3: 100    | 1.3  | 0.0  |
| 18: 100   | 0.0  | 3.2  |

**(b) Self-assessed risk of a genetic abnormality (n = 107)**

| | |
|---|---|
| Very high | 1.9 |
| High      | 11.2 |
| Moderate  | 31.8 |
| Low       | 34.6 |
| Very low  | 20.6 |

Amniocentesis was the most commonly used (or planned) procedure (34.8% had had and 54.1% planned to have amniocentesis performed). Chorionic villus sampling had been performed in one case and was anticipated by 21.6% of the sample (Table 7).

If women judge their risks to be high, will they make use of PND testing? When these two variables were cross-tabulated, there was no clear pattern, in a statistical sense. An examination of Table 8 shows that regardless of whether women judged their risks to be high, there was an overwhelming tendency to use (or plan to use) testing.

### Table 7. Women's Intended Use of, and Intended Use of Types of, Prenatal Testing

| | | % |
|---|---|---|
| Intended use | Have had testing | 16.5 |
| | Will have testing | 70.6 |
| | Will not have testing | 12.8 |
| | (n = 109) | |
| Intended use of types | Chorionic villus sampling | 21.6 |
| | Amniocentesis | 54.1 |
| | Other (includes various combinations of prenatal tests) | 24.3 |
| | (n = 109) | |

### Table 8. Cross-Tabulation of Chance of Risk by Intention to Use PND Tests

| | Risk | | | |
|---|---|---|---|---|
| | High | Medium | Low | |
| Had/will have tests | 13 (92.8%) | 30 (88.2%) | 50 (84.7%) | 93 (86.9%) |
| Will not have tests | 1 (7.2%) | 4 (11.8%) | 9 (15.3%) | 14 (13.1%) |
| Total | 14 (13.1%) | 34 (31.8%) | 59 (55.1%) | 107 |

$\chi^2 = 0.69$ (n.s.).

When asked to indicate why they had had or planned to have testing performed as part of their ante-natal care, the most commonly cited reason was concern over the possibility of bearing and needing to care for a child with a genetic abnormality (58.1% of those responding) (Table 9). Statements such as the following were not uncommon:

> Both my husband and I do not want to bring a severely physically disabled child into the world, and deal with that child dying at birth or in infancy. Nor do we feel we can deal with a severely mentally disabled child [in terms of the] quality of life of our existing child, responsibilities to careers and [the] financial need to work, and [we] do not want to have to institutionalize a child. (#109)

### Table 9. Reasons for Using or Not Using PND

| | | % |
|---|---|---|
| Why women will use PND | Concern about age | 12.9 |
| | Concern about disability | 58.1 |
| | Recommendation of physician | 2.2 |
| | Concerns about age and disability | 17.2 |
| | Concerns about age and/or disability and/or recommendation of physician | 7.5 |
| | Other | 2.2 |
| | (n = 93) | |
| Why women will not use PND | Not willing to have an abortion | 8.3 |
| | Fear of miscarriage | 16.7 |
| | Perceived low risk | 16.7 |
| | Not willing to have an abortion and/or fear of miscarriage and/or perceived low risk | 58.3 |
| | (n = 12) | |

Another stated:

> We have two healthy children that are very active. At times I haven't the patience with them. To me it takes a very special, patient person to be able to deal with a child that has a genetic disorder or Down syndrome, and I don't think I could handle it. (#123)

One woman commented:

> I want to know to the best extent possible whether my baby is free of any serious abnormalities — mental or physical. As a single parent I do not feel capable of raising a child with significant extra needs to those of a normally healthy child. (#340)

Other reasons cited included reference solely to age (12.9%) or because the woman's doctor had recommended testing (2.2%). Many women gave reasons from two or more categories — age and concern about disability (17.2%) or age and/or disability and/or a recommendation from their doctors (7.5%). Many of the women spoke of wanting to put their minds at ease or to have some reassurance regarding the health of the fetus. Some women spoke of wanting the testing so that they could "enjoy" their pregnancies.[21] Many indicated that the testing was being used to prepare them — either for the remainder of their pregnancy or for a pregnancy termination.

Of those having had or planning to have testing, 14.7% specifically mentioned the intention to abort the pregnancy if positive results were reported from testing. Two women specifically mentioned the desire to know the sex of the fetus, although neither said that this information was wanted in connection with selective abortion.

Some women talked about the testing as just another part of routine ante-natal care for someone their age — in other words, something that they had come to expect or that was automatically done for older mothers. Sometimes, though, the technology created its own burdens or ambivalence for the women. For example, one woman commented:

> Although at first I thought that the risk was sufficiently low that I would not have an "invasive test" that carries an almost comparable risk to the baby, I found that after the barrage of appointment dates, letter, etc., and my obstetrician's very blunt advice, I needed the reassurance of a test. (#332)

Another noted:

> I have read of increased risk of having a child with Down syndrome or other genetic abnormality (sic) as age increases; both parents 38 years old. Also, every doctor I have seen thus far has suggested it. (#110)

Speaking about the options for testing, one woman commented:

> [I] have decided not to have chorionic villus sampling because the extra risk thought to be involved is too scary for me. A miscarriage due to a test would cause me a lifetime of guilt and pain. (#122)

Many women indicated in their comments that they understood the limitations of the testing — that the tests could identify some, but not all, genetic abnormalities and that testing was not foolproof. This understanding is important since there are limitations to the testing. PND does not necessarily reduce the incidence of genetic abnormalities in the population (Asch 1989; Asch and Fine 1988; Boss 1990; Hook 1988; Jackson 1990; Mikkelsen 1988; Oliver 1990; Saxton 1987a, 1987b, 1989; Stratford and Steele 1985). Some women spoke of PND helping to eliminate certain risks, the most commonly cited being Down syndrome and spina bifida. Women rarely mentioned the possibility of teratogenic factors such as environmental exposures that might cause an abnormality. When age was mentioned, only maternal age was cited. Both of these findings may provide some evidence that the discourse in routine ante-natal care continues to emphasize maternal factors, and maternal age in particular, as likely contributors to increased risk of genetic abnormalities. This reflects scientific knowledge at this time. (These findings corroborate the qualitative data reported in Chapter 4.)

Of those women who intended not to have testing done (n = 12), the most commonly cited reasons related to an unwillingness to terminate a pregnancy, fear of miscarriage from the testing, a perception that the risk of abnormal findings was low, or some combination of these three factors (58.3%) (see Table 9). Some women believed that since the tests cannot guarantee that something else is not present, it was not worthwhile to have them, and they would add to their risk rather than alleviate it. A few women mentioned that they were "positive" that theirs was a normal pregnancy, that the baby was healthy, and thus it seemed pointless to undergo testing. One woman mentioned this in connection with her belief in God. The following comments of one respondent capture the essence of many women's thoughts on testing:

> I am currently scheduled for amniocentesis but plan to cancel. The additional risk of miscarriage is comparable to the risk of a birth defect. Even if a defect was found, I do not believe I could terminate the pregnancy. The benefits of knowing the state of the baby's health are not sufficient to take the risk of miscarriage. I don't like the idea of medical procedures that are invasive unless there are definite benefits. (#142)

Another woman wrote:

> If there was something wrong with the baby, I don't believe in abortion. If there was something wrong with the baby, I would probably sit and worry and be upset for the remainder of the pregnancy. There are some risks involved in having amniocentesis done — possibility of miscarriage. I'm 42 and this might be my only chance to have a baby. My husband and I will deal with any abnormality at birth. (#103)

One woman commented:

> I see no point in the test. I have a positive attitude on the health of the baby. My husband and I do not believe in abortion. I do not believe you should violate the baby's space. (#157)

Another said:

> My husband and I discussed it and decided that if the tests show an abnormal child, we would not terminate the pregnancy anyway so why put ourselves through extra months of knowing and worrying. We feel that a child is a gift, even if it is "abnormal." (#163)

Turning to the information that women received in the counselling session, most (63.9%) said that they got all of the medical information they wanted from the counsellor (Table 10). Of those who said that they got most (32.4%) or some (3.7%) of the medical facts they wanted, most thought that what they wanted was simply not known by medical science at this time (67.6%). Some women said that the counsellor needed to gather more information (10.8%) or would not discuss some facts that were asked about (2.7%). For 16.2% of the sample, the women did not want to know certain facts and therefore did not ask for information.

When asked whether the counselling session helped them with the types of personal concerns they had, over half said that it had helped with all (52.3%), most (32.7%), or some (12.1%) concerns (Table 10). A few women (2.8%) said that counselling had not helped to alleviate any of their concerns. Those who did not believe counselling had helped to alleviate their concerns most often said that medicine cannot deal with the things

### Table 10. Women's Perceptions Regarding the Information Received in Counselling

| | | % |
|---|---|---|
| Counselling gave: | All the facts I wanted | 63.9 |
| | Most of the facts I wanted | 32.4 |
| | Some of the facts I wanted | 3.7 |
| | None of the facts I wanted | 0.0 |
| | (n = 108) | |
| Facts not provided because: | Facts are not known by medical science | 67.6 |
| | Counsellor needed to get more information | 10.8 |
| | Counsellor did not want to discuss some facts | 2.7 |
| | I did not ask about some facts I wanted to know | 16.2 |
| | Other (includes combinations of above categories) | 2.7 |
| | (n = 37) | |
| Counselling helped with: | All the concerns I had | 52.3 |
| | Most of the concerns I had | 32.7 |
| | Some of the concerns I had | 12.1 |
| | None of the concerns I had | 2.8 |
| | (n = 107) | |
| Perceived reasons for concerns/ not being satisfied: | Concerns can't be dealt with medically | 73.5 |
| | Counsellor needed to get more information | 2.0 |
| | Counsellor did not want to discuss concerns | 2.0 |
| | I did not ask counsellor about my concerns | 14.3 |
| | Other (includes combinations of above categories) | 8.1 |
| | (n = 49) | |

that are of concern (73.5%). Some women did not ask about the concerns brought to counselling (14.3%). Very few thought that the counsellor needed more information to help with their concerns (2.0%). A few women (8.1%) cited more than one of these reasons why their concerns had not been alleviated.

When asked whether the counselling session had raised new concerns, 75.9% said "no." Of those for whom new concerns were raised (n = 26), many indicated that the counselling had given them a clear, sometimes "graphic" understanding of what the testing involved. Several women were concerned about the risks of miscarriage associated with testing (26.9%), and the risks and limitations of the procedures themselves (15.3%) — for example, infection, the fear of false-positive results, the inability to get clear results when there is a multiple pregnancy. Nearly one-third of those responding to this question said that they had new concerns about genetic defects and testing. From their written comments, it would seem that some women found the counselling session had revealed risks other than age that might be relevant (e.g., Tay-Sachs disease, fragile X syndrome).

A few women's comments about new concerns deserve note because they highlight the ambivalence and apprehension toward the technology that has been reported in Chapter 4 and in the literature. One woman wrote:

> Before the session I was only slightly concerned about birth defects, but I find that I am very much worried now. (#110)

Another said:

> It made the whole question of genetic defects seem more omnipresent. I also was confirmed in my concern re: the risk from prenatal testing to the baby (albeit low risk) — one that was not so far removed from the risk of a genetic problem. Also, I was not happy to find that the length of time it took for results was indeed as long as I had thought (it is very stressful, waiting). (#332)

Finally, one woman noted:

> [I] feel there is too much emphasis on the "average." With no history of Down's in the family, [I] don't feel comfortable lumped in the middle with those who perhaps do. (#146)

In connection with these comments, most women found the counselling session very informative (85.7%) and very helpful (75.2%) (Table 11). Most thought that counselling was not very stressful (68.6%), although 15.2% found the experience very stressful. About as many women found the counselling session very reassuring (43.2%) as those who thought of it in more neutral terms (44.1%). Some women (12.7%) did not find counselling to be at all reassuring.

The correlations between the satisfaction variables and selected demographic characteristics are shown in Table 12. Only marital status was significantly related to women's perceptions that their concerns had been satisfied in counselling (gamma = 0.24, Cramer's V = 0.35, $p < 0.0112$). Statistically significant associations were found between whether women found counselling to be informative and marital status (gamma = 0.63, phi = 0.50, $p < 0.0000$) and household income (gamma = -0.22, Cramer's V = 0.57, $p < 0.0000$). Women who had had other children tended to consider counselling as less helpful (gamma = -0.36, Cramer's V = 0.25, $p < 0.0381$). Women with higher household incomes also tended to view counselling as less helpful, but the relationship is extremely small, albeit statistically significant (gamma = –0.01, Cramer's V = 0.42 p < 0.0487). Women who had experienced more pregnancies found counselling to be less stressful (gamma = –0.26, Cramer's V = 0.23, p < 0.0270). Those with higher levels of education found counselling to be more reassuring (gamma = 0.36, Cramer's V = 0.30, p < 0.0275). Age was not significantly associated with any of the satisfaction variables, nor were occupational status and personal income.

**Table 11. Women's Assessments of the Genetic Counselling Session**

|  |  | % |
|---|---|---|
| Counselling informative | 1 (not very) | 0.0 |
|  | 2 | 1.9 |
|  | 3 | 12.4 |
|  | 4 | 39.0 |
|  | 5 (very) | 46.7 |
|  | (n = 105) |  |
| Counselling helpful | 1 (not very) | 0.0 |
|  | 2 | 5.7 |
|  | 3 | 19.0 |
|  | 4 | 37.1 |
|  | 5 (very) | 38.1 |
|  | (n = 105) |  |
| Counselling stressful | 1 (not very) | 44.8 |
|  | 2 | 23.8 |
|  | 3 | 16.2 |
|  | 4 | 6.7 |
|  | 5 (very) | 8.6 |
|  | (n = 105) |  |
| Counselling reassuring | 1 (not very) | 3.9 |
|  | 2 | 8.8 |
|  | 3 | 44.1 |
|  | 4 | 21.6 |
|  | 5 (very) | 21.6 |
|  | (n = 102) |  |

At the end of the section of the survey dealing with the counselling session, women were invited to add additional comments; 37 did so. Many (43.2%) provided positive comments on the nature and quality of the

Table 12. Satisfaction with Counselling by Selected Demographic Characteristics

| | Age | | Marital status | | Gravidity | | Parity | |
|---|---|---|---|---|---|---|---|---|
| | Cramer's V | Gamma | Cramer's V | Gamma | Cramer's V | Gamma | Cramer's V | Gamma |
| Satisfied concerns | 0.29 | 0.15 | 0.35* | 0.24 | -0.16 | -0.15 | 0.19 | -0.30 |
| Counselling informative | 0.35 | 0.11 | 0.50* (phi) | 0.63 | -0.20 | -0.43 | 0.24 | -0.56 |
| Counselling helpful | 0.25 | -0.05 | 0.20 (phi) | 0.11 | -0.19 | -0.34 | 0.25* | -0.36 |
| Counselling stressful | 0.26 | -0.01 | 0.13 (phi) | -0.19 | -0.23* | -0.26 | 0.14 | -0.15 |
| Counselling reassuring | 0.28 | -0.00 | 0.13 (phi) | 0.35 | 0.05 | 0.04 | 0.09 | -0.02 |

| | Occupational status | | Educational level | | Household income | | Personal income | |
|---|---|---|---|---|---|---|---|---|
| | Cramer's V | Gamma | Cramer's V | Gamma | Cramer's V | Gamma | Cramer's V | Gamma |
| Satisfied concerns | 0.34 | 0.03 | 0.18 | 0.21 | 0.34 | -0.03 | 0.25 | 0.04 |
| Counselling informative | 0.20 | -0.17 | 0.17 | -0.13 | 0.57** | -0.22 | 0.37 | 0.01 |
| Counselling helpful | 0.22 | -0.26 | 0.18 | 0.09 | 0.42 | -0.01 | 0.35 | 0.07 |
| Counselling stressful | 0.33 | 0.02 | 0.22 | -0.18 | 0.27 | 0.01 | 0.32 | -0.03 |
| Counselling reassuring | 0.33 | -0.25 | 0.30* | 0.36 | 0.40 | -0.06 | 0.29 | -0.02 |

\* $p < 0.05$.
\*\* $p > 0.01$.

encounter (reiterating their satisfaction with the counsellor and the information provided). Counsellors were described as "informed," "helpful," "personable," "professional," "thorough," "understanding," "reassuring," "approachable," "knowledgeable," "accommodating," "non-intimidating," and "non-judgmental."

At the same time, some women reported that the session was redundant — that, for example, they already had the facts, in written form (21.6%), or that some aspects of the counselling were not sufficiently explained (e.g., the pedigree) or attended to (most notably, women's or couples' feelings). A few women eloquently commented that the counselling had emphasized medical and technical facts to the exclusion of feelings. This was also reflected in the frustration of one woman that the counselling session was conducted in a medical examining room. Another woman said:

> We would have liked a bit more "counselling" in the sense of dealing with issues and feelings confronting us in this situation. For example, a question we posed was "what is advisable for people in our situation?" (more or less the question). We got *information* (good, solid medical information) but not a lot of discussion about feelings, etc. (respondent's emphasis) (#160)

Another wrote:

> I know they are trying to be neutral but if a patient wants to talk about the ethical dimensions of a medical situation it would be nice if doctors could engage in such a discussion. (#340)

Another woman commented:

> I would like to hear from the women who lost their babies due to having the tests. I wonder what they would choose next time. (#122)

And finally, these comments from one woman:

> The book of genetic information displayed pictures of Down syndrome children — (1) only (no other disorders) and (2) on several occasions the page was turned back to the page with the photos and left open almost to the point of displaying the pictures — very powerful subliminal message. (My mind unconsciously brings forward the memory of the pictures.) (#136)

Two women commented that they felt pressure to sign consent forms for testing. (It is customary in the Section of Clinical Genetics to try to obtain a woman's consent to testing, even if she should later decline the testing. Also, women are asked to sign a consent form to have pregnancy outcome information released back to the Section of Clinical Genetics for record keeping.) One woman wrote:

> [They] asked you right after you have all these facts thrown at you if you want tests. There is no time to think about it. [I] felt pressured to say yes. (#146)

Another woman said:

Even though I felt my mind was made up to take the test before counselling (my husband was undecided), I felt some pressure to sign the consent form. This may have only been my feelings, but it really bothered me at the time. (#315)

To summarize, women's perceptions of genetic counselling span a diverse spectrum (as has been reported elsewhere in the literature). Generally, this sample of women reported a relatively high level of satisfaction with regard to the quality and process of care received at the Section of Clinical Genetics, although several said that they found the experience difficult. Many of the themes presented in the open-ended comments of women highlight the concerns about the counselling experience, the testing process, and the consequences of testing (i.e., the implications of having a child with a genetic abnormality). Several of these themes have been elaborated earlier in Chapter 4, which dealt with the qualitative interview data.

## Psychosocial Correlates of the PND Experience

In the development of the survey instrument, three major psychosocial variables were incorporated as potentially important predictors of women's experiences with PND. These measures were general well-being (GWB), health-specific locus of control (HLOC), and access to and satisfaction with social support both in general and related specifically to reproductive decision making. As noted in Chapter 3, standardized measures of each of these concepts were used.

### *General Well-Being*

The measure of GWB was a modification of an 18-item instrument designed by Dupuy (1978) for the U.S. National Health and Nutrition Examination Survey. GWB measures psychological well-being in terms of six major dimensions: anxiety, depression, general health, positive well-being, self-control, and vitality. This measure is not a measure of psychological morbidity, nor is it a screening device.

Using the standard scoring recommended by Dupuy, we found no variation on this measure; that is, the entire sample was categorized as having positive well-being. However, looking at individual items reveals some variability (Table 13). Of particular note is the observation that nearly three-quarters of the sample was feeling at least a little worried or anxious. However, the women in the sample were relatively positive and in good spirits, untroubled by their health or life. Several respondents made marginal comments in connection with some questions in the measure of GWB to the effect of "but I'm pregnant!" (A factor analysis was performed on these variables but did not yield interpretable factors. Accordingly, the decision was made to treat items individually, and not as part of a larger scale.)

Table 14 shows the association between the various indicators of GWB and selected demographic variables (age, marital status, gravidity, parity, occupational status, educational level, household and personal incomes). A perusal of this table shows that most relationships are in the moderately weak to moderate range. There was no common (nor intuitively explicable) pattern among the variables, in terms of statistically significant associations. For example, age was in a statistically significant association with waking fresh (gamma = 0.08, Cramer's V = 0.34, $p < 0.0173$), feeling depressed (gamma = 0.00, Cramer's V = 0.34, $p < 0.0214$), and feeling emotionally stable (gamma = 0.27, Cramer's V = 0.35, $p < 0.0083$). Marital status was significantly related to feeling in control of one's behaviour (gamma = 0.52, Cramer's V = 0.29, $p < 0.0491$), feeling satisfied with one's personal life (gamma = 0.67, Cramer's V = 0.29, $p < 0.0210$), feeling down-hearted and blue (gamma = −0.63, Cramer's V = 0.29, $p < 0.0213$), feeling that anything in life is worthwhile (gamma = 0.67, Cramer's V = 0.51, $p < 0.0000$), and feeling anxious (gamma = −0.81, Cramer's V = 0.36, $p < 0.0014$). Gravidity was in a significant relationship to feeling that one is losing control of one's behaviour (gamma = −0.50, Cramer's V = 0.33, $p < 0.0129$); parity was significantly related to feeling emotionally stable (gamma = −0.07, Cramer's V = 0.31, $p < 0.0112$).

Several of the socioeconomic variables were significantly associated with indicators of GWB. Education level was significantly related to feeling stable (gamma = 0.07, Cramer's V = 0.53, $p < 0.0000$). Occupational status was in a significant relationship with each of the following: wake fresh (gamma = −0.07, Cramer's V = 0.40, $p < 0.0452$), concerned about health (gamma = −0.05, Cramer's V = 0.38, $p < 0.0505$), and energy level (gamma = 0.02, Cramer's V = 0.39, $p < 0.0271$). Although the respondent's personal income was found to be significantly associated only with how one is feeling generally (gamma = −0.20, Cramer's V = 0.40, $p < 0.0146$), household income was significantly associated with how one is feeling generally (gamma = −0.17, Cramer's V = 0.38, $p < 0.0443$), feeling anxious (gamma = 0.23, Cramer's V = 0.39, $p < 0.0182$), wake fresh (gamma = −0.03, Cramer's V = 0.39, $p < 0.0269$), feeling that anything in life is worthwhile (gamma = 0.27, Cramer's V = 0.40, $p < 0.0142$), and feeling down-hearted and blue (gamma = 0.22, Cramer's V = 0.42, $p < 0.0059$).

### Table 13. Distribution of Respondents on Selected Indicators of General Well-Being

|  |  | % |
|---|---|---|
| General feelings | Excellent | 11.0 |
|  | Very good | 20.2 |
|  | Good | 38.5 |
|  | Up and down | 24.8 |
|  | Low | 4.6 |
|  | Very low | 0.9 |
|  | (n = 109) |  |
| Feeling nervous | Very nervous | 7.3 |
|  | Quite nervous | 6.4 |
|  | Bothered some | 17.4 |
|  | Bothered a bit | 35.8 |
|  | Not bothered at all | 33.0 |
|  | (n = 109) |  |
| Feeling stress or pressure | Too much stress | 1.9 |
|  | Quite stressful | 13.9 |
|  | More stress than usual | 20.4 |
|  | As much stress as usual | 24.1 |
|  | A little stress | 22.2 |
|  | No stress at all | 17.6 |
|  | (n = 10) |  |
| Feeling anxious or worried | Extremely anxious/worried | 2.8 |
|  | Very anxious/worried | 2.8 |
|  | Quite anxious/worried | 8.3 |
|  | Worried some | 13.9 |
|  | A little bit anxious/worried | 40.7 |
|  | Not anxious/worried | 31.5 |
|  | (n = 108) |  |
| Satisfied with personal life | Extremely satisfied | 14.8 |
|  | Very satisfied | 34.3 |
|  | Fairly satisfied | 33.3 |
|  | Satisfied | 8.3 |
|  | Somewhat dissatisfied | 9.3 |
|  | (n = 108) |  |

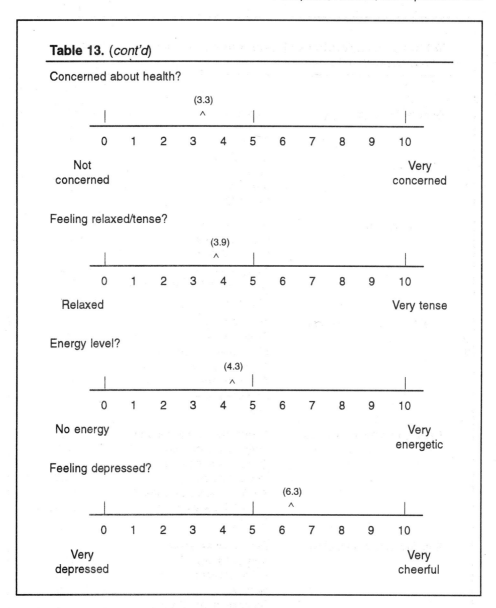

Table 13. (cont'd)

## Health Locus of Control

Locus of control is defined as "the degree to which individuals perceive events in their lives as being a consequence of their own actions, and thereby controllable (internal control), or as being unrelated to their own behaviour, and therefore beyond personal control (external control)" (Lau and Ware 1981, 1147). A measure of HLOC considers specifically the ways in which individuals perceive that their health is the product of internal, external, or chance factors. Of the original scale developed by Lau and

Ware, 15 items were included in this survey (with 5 items for each of the dimensions of HLOC). Table 15 reports the mean scores (on a scale of 1 to 5) on each of the HLOC items.

Reliability analysis involving all of the HLOC variables produced a Cronbach's alpha of 0.58. Factor analysis, with varimax rotation, was conducted with all of the HLOC variables, but no interpretable factors emerged in this exercise. The factors that did emerge do not fit, in any way, the preconceived categories of "chance," "provider control," and "self-control." The differences between this sample and the samples reported in previous research using the HLOC measure may be sufficiently great to expect that the patterns of response would not necessarily be replicated. At this point, one can only speculate why the hypothesized factors did not emerge. As a result of the factor analyses, a decision was made to treat the items individually.

## *Social Supports*

The concept of social support has become a major area of research interest in health sociology and health psychology. The reasons for the surge of research interest stem from the fact that there has been a growing recognition of the importance of affiliation with others in influencing individuals' health and well-being. House (1981) has identified the following major classes of supportive behaviours or acts: (1) emotional support (that which makes us feel we are loved and cared for by others); (2) instrumental support (the kind of help that is given when needed and that is often contrasted with emotional support; this type of support takes the form of doing things for others, taking care of them, giving them money or help, and so on); (3) informational support (information that helps people cope with daily life; this type of support "helps the person help himself or herself"); and (4) appraisal support (which, without the affect associated with emotional support, fosters self-evaluation or social comparison on behalf of the recipient).

In the present study, social support was measured using an abbreviated version of Sarason's Social Support Questionnaire (SSQ), which quantifies the availability of, and satisfaction with, social support (Sarason 1983). The seven circumstances that were considered in the measurement of social support were (1) who women can count on to listen to them when they need to talk; (2) who women can count on to help out in a crisis situation; (3) who women can count on to distract them from their worries when feeling stressed; (4) who women can count on to be dependable when in need of help; (5) who women felt would help if a close family member died; (6) who women felt truly loved them deeply; and (7) who women can count on to console them when upset. Considering each of these items, we see that they measure primarily either the emotional (affective) or instrumental nature of social support that has been described above.

Table 14. Correlations Between Measures of General Well-Being and Selected Demographic Characteristics

| General well-being | Age Cramer's V | Age Gamma | Marital status Cramer's V | Marital status Gamma | Gravidity Cramer's V | Gravidity Gamma | Parity Cramer's V | Parity Gamma |
|---|---|---|---|---|---|---|---|---|
| (a) general feeling | 0.26 | 0.15 | 0.10 | 0.21 | 0.21 | 0.19 | 0.18 | 0.12 |
| (b) bothered by nerves | 0.25 | -0.15 | 0.17 | 0.04 | 0.12 | 0.00 | 0.16 | 0.02 |
| (c) control behaviour | 0.27 | 0.07 | 0.29 | 0.52* | 0.25 | -0.19 | 0.25 | -0.15 |
| (d) feeling anything is worthwhile | 0.27 | -0.16 | 0.51 | 0.67** | 0.21 | 0.11 | 0.18 | 0.06 |
| (e) feeling strain or stress | 0.31 | -0.19 | 0.28 | -0.76 | 0.19 | 0.03 | 0.19 | 0.07 |
| (f) feeling satisfied | 0.30 | 0.11 | 0.29 | 0.67* | 0.26 | 0.02 | 0.23 | 0.06 |
| (g) feeling losing mind | 0.31 | 0.10 | 0.23 | -0.07 | 0.33 | -0.50* | 0.22 | -0.52 |
| (h) feeling anxious | 0.28 | -0.24 | 0.36 | -0.81** | 0.18 | -0.07 | 0.19 | -0.09 |
| (i) wake fresh | 0.34 | 0.08* | 0.16 | -0.05 | 0.24 | -0.16 | 0.26 | -0.15 |
| (j) bothered by illness | 0.28 | -0.06 | 0.14 | 0.01 | 0.19 | 0.04 | 0.18 | 0.05 |
| (k) life interesting | 0.29 | -0.08 | 0.22 | 0.26 | 0.16 | -0.10 | 0.16 | -0.08 |
| (l) feeling down-hearted | 0.30 | -0.15 | 0.29 | -0.63* | 0.23 | -0.10 | 0.22 | -0.09 |
| (m) emotionally stable | 0.35 | 0.27** | 0.27 | 0.76 | 0.20 | -0.08 | 0.31 | -0.07* |
| (n) feeling tired | 0.27 | -0.08 | 0.18 | 0.16 | 0.23 | 0.11 | 0.18 | 0.11 |
| (o) concerned about health | 0.25 | -0.05 | 0.24 | 0.11 | 0.32 | -0.10 | 0.34 | -0.18 |
| (p) feeling tense/relaxed | 0.25 | 0.07 | 0.24 | 0.40 | 0.26 | -0.02 | 0.31 | -0.11 |
| (q) energy level | 0.33 | 0.04 | 0.18 | -0.21 | 0.27 | 0.10 | 0.27 | 0.20 |
| (r) feeling depressed | 0.34 | 0.00** | 0.33 | 0.44 | 0.29 | 0.00 | 0.22 | -0.03 |

\* p < 0.05.
\*\* p < 0.01.

Table 14. (cont'd)

| General well-being | Occupational status | | Educational level | | Household income | | Personal income | |
|---|---|---|---|---|---|---|---|---|
| | Cramer's V | Gamma | Cramer's V | Gamma | Cramer's V | Gamma | Cramer's V | Gamma |
| (a) general feeling | 0.36 | 0.02 | 0.24 | 0.09 | 0.38 | -0.17* | 0.40 | -0.20* |
| (b) bothered by nerves | 0.33 | 0.01 | 0.18 | 0.04 | 0.36 | 0.15 | 0.36 | 0.06 |
| (c) control behaviour | 0.34 | -0.02 | 0.21 | 0.18 | 0.33 | -0.13 | 0.32 | 0.02 |
| (d) feeling anything is worthwhile | 0.32 | -0.03 | 0.14 | -0.17 | 0.40 | 0.27* | 0.33 | 0.12 |
| (e) feeling strain or stress | 0.35 | 0.04 | 0.23 | -0.10 | 0.35 | 0.12 | 0.34 | -0.06 |
| (f) feeling satisfied | 0.33 | -0.04 | 0.19 | 0.09 | 0.30 | -0.26 | 0.29 | -0.08 |
| (g) feeling losing mind | 0.33 | 0.10 | 0.19 | 0.06 | 0.36 | -0.05 | 0.31 | -0.05 |
| (h) feeling anxious | 0.31 | 0.07 | 0.15 | -0.02 | 0.39 | 0.23* | 0.35 | 0.09 |
| (i) wake fresh | 0.40 | -0.07* | 0.19 | 0.07 | 0.39 | -0.03* | 0.28 | 0.11 |
| (j) bothered by illness | 0.31 | -0.05 | 0.21 | -0.05 | 0.35 | 0.22 | 0.30 | 0.23 |
| (k) life interesting | 0.32 | 0.14 | 0.20 | -0.00 | 0.34 | -0.28 | 0.33 | -0.17 |
| (l) feeling down-hearted | 0.29 | 0.01 | 0.18 | -0.03 | 0.42 | 0.22* | 0.35 | 0.12 |
| (m) emotionally stable | 0.34 | 0.02 | 0.53 | 0.07* | 0.36 | -0.19 | 0.34 | -0.12 |
| (n) feeling tired | 0.37 | 0.02 | 0.17 | -0.05 | 0.26 | 0.09 | 0.31 | 0.02 |
| (o) concerned about health | 0.38 | -0.05* | 0.31 | 0.07 | 0.31 | -0.17 | 0.29 | -0.03 |
| (p) feeling tense/relaxed | 0.37 | -0.21 | 0.31 | 0.25 | 0.31 | -0.05 | 0.33 | 0.09 |
| (q) energy level | 0.39 | 0.02* | 0.27 | -0.15 | 0.33 | 0.09 | 0.29 | -0.01 |
| (r) feeling depressed | 0.33 | 0.06 | 0.32 | -0.14 | 0.36 | 0.20 | 0.35 | 0.10 |

\* $p < 0.05$.
\*\* $p < 0.01$.

### Table 15. Mean Scores on Measures of Health Locus of Control

| | | | Mean score |
|---|---|---|---|
| Provider control factors (external) | 1. | Seeing a doctor for regular check-ups is a key factor in staying healthy. | 3.9 |
| | 2. | Doctors relieve or cure only a few of the medical problems their patients have.* | 3.2 |
| | 3. | Doctors can almost always help their patients feel better. | 3.2 |
| | 4. | Recovery from illness requires good medical care more than anything else. | 3.0 |
| | 5. | Doctors can do very little to prevent illness.* | 3.6 |
| Self-control factors (internal) | 1. | People's ill health results from their own carelessness. | 2.7 |
| | 2. | There is little one can do to prevent illness.* | 4.0 |
| | 3. | I have a lot of confidence in my ability to cure myself once I get sick. | 3.3 |
| | 4. | In the long run, people who take very good care of themselves stay healthy and get well quick. | 4.0 |
| | 5. | Health-wise, there isn't much you can do for yourself when you get sick.* | 4.1 |
| Chance factors | 1. | Staying well has little or nothing to do with chance. | 3.4 |
| | 2. | Whether or not people get well is often a matter of chance.* | 4.0 |
| | 3. | People who never get sick are just plain lucky.* | 3.6 |
| | 4. | Recovery from illness has nothing to do with luck. | 3.4 |
| | 5. | Good health is largely a matter of fortune.* | 3.7 |

Coding of responses was as follows: strongly agree = 5, agree = 4, undecided = 3, disagree = 2, strongly disagree = 1. Items marked with an asterisk (*) have reverse coding.

Looking at this sample, it seems that women are well supported in the areas that the survey measured; very few women said that they had no support whatsoever on any of these items. The mean number of supporters on each of the dimensions of social support is shown in Table 16. Many women reported that their spouse or partner was key in their support. Other family members commonly listed as providing support included mothers, fathers, in-laws, siblings, friends, and co-workers.

Respondents were not asked to rank order the supporters in terms of their importance; nevertheless, the listing of supporters seems to reflect the primacy of support provided by each of the individuals listed. The first supporter listed was usually the woman's spouse or partner. The second supporter listed was typically a woman's friend or her mother. Physicians were listed by some women as strategic support on the various dimensions listed. Members of the clergy were also listed by some women. The range of support listed by women was quite extensive. Due to limitations in the time for extensive analysis of the social support variables, attention was focussed more on the amount of support and women's satisfaction with support, and less on who the supporters were.

Most women seem to be at least fairly satisfied with the support they have available. For instance, 88.7% were either fairly or very satisfied with the support they have when they need someone to talk to; 93.5% were either fairly or very satisfied with the support they have when in a crisis situation; 82.2% were either fairly or very satisfied with the support they have when needing distraction from their worries; 93.4% were either fairly or very satisfied with the support they have when in need of help; 92.3% were either fairly or very satisfied with the support they have in the death of a close family member; 92.4% were either fairly or very satisfied that they are truly loved deeply; and 86.9% were either fairly or very satisfied with the support they have when upset. In short, these measures yielded little variation with respect to women's satisfaction with social support. Because some researchers have found little variation on the measurement of satisfaction with social support, there is a tendency to focus more on the amount and quality of support (House 1981).

Table 17 shows the correlation between the amount of support available to a woman and her level of satisfaction with that support. This table shows significant associations ($p < 0.05$) on each of these associations. When the measures of social support were correlated with demographic variables, moderate associations were usually found, although only one such association was statistically significant (the correlation between age and the number of supports available to help with the death of a loved one) (see Table 18).

### Table 16. Women's Access to, and Satisfaction with, Social Support

| | Mean number of supporters | Satisfaction with support | % |
|---|---|---|---|
| Those one can count on to listen when you need to talk? | 4.6 | Very dissatisfied | 3.8 |
| | | Fairly dissatisfied | 0.9 |
| | | A little dissatisfied | 1.9 |
| | | A little satisfied | 4.7 |
| | | Fairly satisfied | 43.4 |
| | | Very satisfied | 45.3 |
| | | (n = 106) | |
| Those one can count on to help in a crisis situation? | 4.9 | Very dissatisfied | 1.9 |
| | | Fairly dissatisfied | 0.9 |
| | | A little dissatisfied | 0.9 |
| | | A little satisfied | 2.8 |
| | | Fairly satisfied | 40.2 |
| | | Very satisfied | 53.3 |
| | | (n = 107) | |
| Those one can count on to distract worries when stressed? | 3.0 | Very dissatisfied | 4.7 |
| | | Fairly dissatisfied | 0.9 |
| | | A little dissatisfied | 3.7 |
| | | A little satisfied | 8.4 |
| | | Fairly satisfied | 38.3 |
| | | Very satisfied | 43.9 |
| | | (n = 107) | |
| Those one can count on to be dependable when help is needed? | 4.1 | Very dissatisfied | 2.8 |
| | | Fairly dissatisfied | 0.9 |
| | | A little dissatisfied | 0.0 |
| | | A little satisfied | 2.8 |
| | | Fairly satisfied | 43.4 |
| | | Very satisfied | 50.0 |
| | | (n = 106) | |
| Those who would help if a close family member died? | 4.3 | Very dissatisfied | 1.9 |
| | | Fairly dissatisfied | 0.0 |
| | | A little dissatisfied | 2.9 |
| | | A little satisfied | 2.9 |
| | | Fairly satisfied | 47.1 |
| | | Very satisfied | 45.2 |
| | | (n = 104) | |

### Table 16. (cont'd)

| | Mean number of supporters | Satisfaction with support | % |
|---|---|---|---|
| Those who love you deeply? | 4.5 | Very dissatisfied | 3.8 |
| | | Fairly dissatisfied | 0.9 |
| | | A little dissatisfied | 0.9 |
| | | A little satisfied | 1.9 |
| | | Fairly satisfied | 35.8 |
| | | Very satisfied | 56.6 |
| | | (n = 106) | |
| Those one can count on to console? | 3.1 | Very dissatisfied | 3.7 |
| | | Fairly dissatisfied | 0.9 |
| | | A little dissatisfied | 0.0 |
| | | A little satisfied | 8.4 |
| | | Fairly satisfied | 41.1 |
| | | Very satisfied | 45.8 |
| | | (n = 107) | |

### Table 17. Correlations Between Social Support Available and Satisfaction with Social Support

| | Cramer's V | r |
|---|---|---|
| When you need to talk | 0.37 | 0.47* |
| Help in a crisis | 0.42 | 0.45* |
| Distract one from worries | 0.32 | 0.38* |
| Depend on for help | 0.45 | 0.34* |
| Help with the death of a loved one | 0.27 | 0.46* |
| Loves respondent | 0.34 | 0.39* |
| Consoles respondent | 0.45 | 0.47* |

\* $p < 0.05$.

## Social Support in Reproductive Decision Making

The measures of general social support indicate that women are well supported and generally satisfied with that support. We were interested to discover the type of support women receive in making key reproductive decisions. The measures of support in reproductive decision making included in the survey provide an insight into whether women make these decisions autonomously or in consultation with others, and whether they are effectively removed from the decision-making process. Four questions were asked: who makes decisions with respect to (1) when to have children; (2) how many children to have; (3) whether to use PND; and (4) how to use the information from PND. For each question, the women indicated who made the decision (self or self and others), what the relationship was of the others participating in the decision-making process, who the most important person was participating in the decision-making process, and the level of satisfaction with respect to the decision-making process.[22]

As shown in Table 19, women generally make decisions about reproduction in conjunction with others. In most cases, the other key person participating in decision making was the woman's spouse or partner. A few women listed other family members (parents and siblings), friends, or their personal physician as being the most important person participating in the decision-making process. Most of the decisions about when and how many children to have and whether and how to use PND are made by women and their partners. Some women make these decisions alone (nearly one-quarter of the sample on the decision to use PND), and in some cases others make these decisions for them, but the proportion is quite small.

Women are generally pleased with the decision-making process. As shown in Table 19, the mean scores on the measure of satisfaction with the decision-making process indicate that most women are relatively or very satisfied with this process.[23]

When the decision-making variables were cross-tabulated with the corresponding satisfaction variables, significant associations were found on the variables pertaining to when to have children (gamma = 0.21, Cramer's V = 0.39, $p < 0.0000$) and how many children to have (gamma = $-0.23$, Cramer's V = 0.37, $p < 0.0004$). Although a moderately weak association was found on the variables pertaining to whether to use PND, this was not significant (gamma = 0.17, Cramer's V = 0.12, $p < 0.8457$). A moderate association was found on the variables dealing with how to use PND information, but this was not significant (gamma = 0.38, Cramer's V = 0.25, $p < 0.1561$). No significant associations were found when the decision-making variable dealing with the use of PND information was cross-tabulated with women's intended use of testing.

The inclusion of the decision-making variables was considered to be important in this survey, but upon completing the analyses, these variables did not reveal as much as had been hoped; the reasons are not entirely clear.

**Table 18. Correlations Between Social Support Measures (Quantity of Support and Satisfaction) and Selected Demographic Characteristics**

| | Age | | Marital status | | Gravidity | | Parity | |
|---|---|---|---|---|---|---|---|---|
| | Cramer's V | r | Cramer's V | Gamma | Cramer's V | r | Cramer's V | r |
| **Social supports** | | | | | | | | |
| When need to talk | 0.36 | −0.11 | 0.41 | 0.08 | 0.19 | −0.15 | 0.18 | −0.13 |
| Help in crisis | 0.34 | −0.13 | 0.32 | −0.19 | 0.17 | −0.06 | 0.21 | −0.13 |
| Distract worries | 0.30 | 0.03 | 0.29 | 0.04 | 0.19 | 0.19 | 0.23 | 0.15 |
| Depend on | 0.28 | 0.13 | 0.37 | −0.12 | 0.17 | 0.00 | 0.18 | −0.06 |
| Help re: death | 0.34 | 0.26* | 0.19 | −0.30 | 0.14 | 0.12 | 0.13 | 0.12 |
| Loves respondent | 0.31 | −0.07 | 0.51 | 0.11 | 0.21 | 0.05 | 0.21 | 0.00 |
| Consoles respondent | 0.32 | −0.04 | 0.47 | −0.36 | 0.18 | 0.05 | 0.14 | −0.02 |
| **Satisfaction** | | | | | | | | |
| When need to talk | 0.37 | −0.09 | 0.53 | −0.32 | 0.27 | 0.29 | 0.22 | 0.14 |
| Help in crisis | 0.34 | −0.17 | 0.57 | −0.43 | 0.23 | 0.31 | 0.23 | 0.08 |
| Distract worries | 0.35 | −0.08 | 0.42 | −0.44 | 0.21 | 0.25 | 0.15 | 0.11 |
| Depend on | 0.47 | −0.08 | 0.36 | −0.41 | 0.27 | 0.35 | 0.18 | 0.08 |
| Help re: death | 0.37 | 0.05 | 0.35 | −0.10 | 0.30 | 0.41 | 0.18 | 0.27 |
| Loves respondent | 0.44 | −0.08 | 0.51 | −0.54 | 0.24 | 0.26 | 0.17 | 0.12 |
| Consoles respondent | 0.37 | −0.10 | 0.51 | −0.45 | 0.28 | 0.42 | 0.21 | 0.31 |

Table 18. (cont'd)

| | Occupation | | Education | | | Household income | | | Personal income | | |
|---|---|---|---|---|---|---|---|---|---|---|---|
| | Cramer's V | Gamma | Cramer's V | Gamma | | Cramer's V | r | | Cramer's V | r | |
| **Social supports** | | | | | | | | | | | |
| When need to talk | 0.36 | −0.14 | 0.21 | −0.03 | | 0.38 | 0.13 | | 0.26 | 0.16 | |
| Help in crisis | 0.42 | −0.20 | 0.15 | 0.06 | | 0.40 | 0.15 | | 0.36 | 0.04 | |
| Distract worries | 0.37 | −0.05 | 0.19 | −0.06 | | 0.37 | −0.13 | | 0.31 | −0.12 | |
| Depend on | 0.39 | −0.15 | 0.17 | 0.06 | | 0.38 | 0.13 | | 0.32 | −0.00 | |
| Help re: death | 0.35 | −0.03 | 0.13 | −0.01 | | 0.35 | 0.01 | | 0.38 | −0.08 | |
| Loves respondent | 0.31 | 0.03 | 0.18 | −0.32 | | 0.38 | 0.10 | | 0.31 | 0.09 | |
| Consoles respondent | 0.35 | −0.04 | 0.15 | −0.08 | | 0.30 | 0.00 | | 0.28 | 0.03 | |
| **Satisfaction** | | | | | | | | | | Gamma | |
| When need to talk | 0.25 | −0.10 | 0.32 | −0.19 | | 0.33 | 0.27 | | 0.30 | 0.24 | |
| Help in crisis | 0.30 | −0.16 | 0.19 | −0.13 | | 0.37 | 0.39 | | 0.26 | 0.29 | |
| Distract worries | 0.32 | −0.06 | 0.26 | −0.20 | | 0.32 | 0.29 | | 0.35 | 0.21 | |
| Depend on | 0.38 | −0.05 | 0.17 | −0.31 | | 0.41 | 0.28 | | 0.26 | 0.12 | |
| Help re: death | 0.29 | −0.01 | 0.22 | −0.28 | | 0.44 | 0.17 | | 0.27 | −0.02 | |
| Loves respondent | 0.33 | −0.15 | 0.20 | −0.13 | | 0.38 | 0.33 | | 0.24 | 0.09 | |
| Consoles respondent | 0.30 | −0.10 | 0.15 | −0.17 | | 0.40 | 0.24 | | 0.28 | 0.01 | |

\* $p < 0.05$.

## Predictors of Women's Satisfaction with Genetic Counselling

One of the objectives of this research was to examine women's satisfaction with genetic counselling (objective 3). In an earlier section of this chapter, the distribution of the sample on the various components of women's satisfaction with genetic counselling was presented (i.e., whether their concerns were met in counselling; whether they found counselling to be informative, reassuring, helpful, and stressful). To explore this area further, cross-tabular analyses were conducted, considering the importance of selected aspects of the counselling experience and session and the sociodemographic variables measured in this study.

**Table 19. Women's Support in Reproductive Decision Making**

| Who decides | | % |
|---|---|---|
| a) When to have children? | Decision made by woman alone | 15.0 |
| | Decision made with others | 83.2 |
| | Decision made by others | 1.9 |
| | (n = 107) | |

**Satisfaction with decision making (mean scores)**

```
                              (4.3)
   |       |       |       | ^     |
   1       2       3       4       5
(Very dissatisfied)                (Very satisfied)
```

| | | |
|---|---|---|
| b) How many children to have? | Decision made by woman alone | 5.7 |
| | Decision made with others | 93.4 |
| | Decision made by others | 0.9 |
| | (n = 106) | |

**Satisfaction with decision making (mean scores)**

```
                              (4.4)
   |       |       |       | ^     |
   1       2       3       4       5
(Very dissatisfied)                (Very satisfied)
```

| Table 19. (cont'd) | | |
|---|---|---|
| **Who decides** | | **%** |
| c) Whether to access PND? | Decision made by woman alone | 23.1 |
| | Decision made with others | 75.9 |
| | Decision made by others | 0.9 |
| | (n = 108) | |

**Satisfaction with decision making (mean scores)**

```
                         (4.5)
  |     |     |     |  ^  |
  1     2     3     4     5
(Very dissatisfied)    (Very satisfied)
```

| | | |
|---|---|---|
| d) How to use information from PND? | Decision made by woman alone | 13.0 |
| | Decision made with others | 87.0 |
| | Decision made by others | 0.0 |
| | (n = 108) | |

**Satisfaction with decision making (mean scores)**

```
                         (4.6)
  |     |     |     |  ^  |
  1     2     3     4     5
(Very dissatisfied)    (Very satisfied)
```

Some research has indicated that the gender of the counsellor is an important predictor of women's satisfaction with genetic counselling (Zare et al. 1984). In this study, most counselling sessions were conducted by men (87 with men, 21 with women). A weak, non-significant association was found between the gender of the counsellor and women's satisfaction that their concerns had been met in the session (Cramer's $V = 0.13$, $p < 0.5891$). A moderate inverse association was found between the gender of the counsellor and women's perceptions that they had received all of the facts they needed in the session, although this was not statistically significant (gamma = $-0.36$, Cramer's $V = 0.14$, $p < 0.3366$). In other words, women were more likely to be satisfied that they had received all of the facts when counselled by a woman.

When the gender of the counsellor was cross-tabulated with the other aspects of women's satisfaction, a similar pattern was repeated; that is, women were more likely to see counselling as informative (gamma = $-0.60$, Cramer's $V = 0.14$, $p < 0.3663$) and helpful (gamma = $-0.40$,

Cramer's V = 0.14, p < 0.3336) when the counsellor was female. A very weak, non-significant association was found when the gender of the counsellor was cross-tabulated with the women's experience of counselling as stressful (gamma = –0.11, Cramer's V = 0.06, p < 0.8044). No discernible association was found between the counsellor's gender and the women's view of counselling as reassuring (gamma = 0.02, Cramer's V = 0.06, p < 0.8192).

Moderately strong and statistically significant associations were found between the length of the counselling session and women's perceptions of it as informative (gamma = –0.58, Cramer's V = 0.22, p < 0.0386) and helpful (gamma = –0.45, Cramer's V = 0.23, p < 0.0255); those who had longer sessions were more satisfied about the session on these two dimensions. Weaker, non-significant associations were found when the length of the session was correlated with women's views of counselling as stressful (gamma = –0.11, Cramer's V = 0.16, p < 0.2823) and as reassuring (gamma = –0.06, Cramer's V = 0.12, p < 0.5378).

When we look at the data in terms of the gender of the counsellor, it seems that those counselled by women were somewhat more likely to assess the session favourably on whether it was informative and helpful. The picture is somewhat less clear when we look at the counsellor's gender and the other aspects of the women's assessments of genetic counselling. It is difficult to know for certain what accounts for women's assessments of same- versus other-gender counsellors (i.e., is it the counsellor's gender that explains client satisfaction or is satisfaction due to the qualitative aspects of the encounter?). This is an area of some importance and merits further attention.

Satisfaction variables were also correlated with women's demographic characteristics (previously shown in Table 12). Age was not significantly associated with any of the satisfaction variables. Marital status was significantly associated with women's assessment that counselling had satisfied their concerns (gamma = 0.24, Cramer's V = 0.35, p < 0.0112) and with the view of counselling as informative (gamma = 0.63, phi = 0.50, p < 0.0000). Women who had had more pregnancies were significantly more likely to judge counselling to be stressful (gamma = –0.26, Cramer's V = 0.23, p < 0.0270). A significant association was found between parity and the perception of counselling as helpful (gamma = –0.36, Cramer's V = 0.25, p < 0.0381); women who had given birth to more children were more likely to consider counselling to have been helpful. No significant associations were found between occupational status and any of the satisfaction variables. Education level was significantly associated with women's perceptions of counselling as reassuring (gamma = 0.36, Cramer's V = 0.30, p < 0.0097); those with less education were more likely to be reassured from counselling. Although personal income was not significantly associated with any of the satisfaction measures, household income was significantly associated with the perception of counselling as informative (gamma = –0.22, Cramer's V = 0.57, p < 0.0000) and helpful (gamma = –0.01, Cramer's V = 0.42, $p < 0.0487$); women from more affluent households were more likely to rate the counselling as informative and as helpful, although the relationship is admittedly negligible for the latter of these two dimensions.

To summarize the bivariate associations between the demographic variables and the measures of women's satisfaction, there is no clear pattern of association in that some variables are always in a particular correlation with women's satisfaction with counselling. Given the less than compelling findings at the bivariate level in predicting women's satisfaction with counselling, it would have been justified to end the analyses at this point. Clearly, the size of the sample and perhaps, too, aspects of measurement were confounding efforts to explain women's satisfaction with genetic counselling. However, it was decided that regression analyses would be undertaken, even if doing so would provide only a rough approximation of the predictors of women's satisfaction with counselling.

From a methodological standpoint, this poses some difficulty. First, because the sample size is comparatively small, it is possible that the hypothesized relationships are theoretically correct, but the small sample size renders them statistically incorrect. As will be discussed in the closing chapter, a much larger sample would be required and some modifications to the instrument would be needed to carry out the analyses that would be most appropriate. In addition, the form of multivariate analyses chosen (stepwise regression) presupposes that variables are measured at the interval level (Kleinbaum and Kupper 1978). Some researchers violate this assumption, treating ordinal variables as if they are interval variables. To do so means that an examination of beta coefficients requires some caution — the direction of the association may be meaningful but the strength of the association is not. This is because the underlying premise in regression analysis is that you can show how change in one variable is associated with change in another, using standard units of measure. With ordinal variables, the difference between categories cannot be assumed to be equidistant and therefore the proportional change is meaningless.

Alternative methods of multivariate analyses were considered (e.g., loglinear analysis), but the issue of sample size again made the use of these other analytic approaches problematic. In the end, multiple regression was conducted. The following results are tentative and caution is exercised in their interpretation.

Multiple regression allows for the inclusion of several variables simultaneously, to determine which variables are related to a specific dependent variable while controlling for the effects of all others in the model. In stepwise regression, which was used in this study, independent variables are added sequentially to the regression equation based upon their additional contribution in predicting the dependent variable. The order in which variables are entered into the regression equations is a function of the explanatory power of each variable. The results reported here show only the significant predictors of the dependent variables.

Regression analyses were run for each of the dependent variables measuring women's satisfaction with genetic counselling. Where variables were operationalized at the nominal (categorical) level, dummy variables were created. Separate regressions were run, with only demographic variables entered as independent variables, and with psychosocial variables (HLOC, selected items within the GWB measure, and amount of support in general). These separate regression analyses did not yield useful information.

A second set of regression analyses was run, with the demographic and psychosocial variables entered as possible predictors of women's satisfaction with genetic counselling. Also included in these analyses was the gender of the genetic counsellor. It is the latter group of analyses that is reported here. Table 20 provides a complete list of the independent variables entered into the regression models.

### Women's Perceptions That Counselling Satisfied Their Concerns (Table 21)

The first regression examined the predictors of women's perception that their concerns had been satisfied in the genetic counselling session. Being married was the most salient predictor, accounting for 20% of the variance, although some caution is necessary here since a significant majority of the sample was married. Two items in the GWB measures were significant predictors of women's satisfaction that their concerns had been met. Women who were anxious were more likely to have thought that their concerns were satisfied in counselling; this variable accounted for 7% of the variance. In contrast, women who did not feel under stress or pressure were more likely to be satisfied that their concerns had been met in counselling (accounting for 3% of the total variance). Both of these items in the measure of GWB are aspects of the "anxiety" subscale, so this contradictory pattern is somewhat puzzling.

Women who perceived their risk to be low believed that their concerns were met in counselling. Self-assessed risk explained 9% of the total variance. Women who identified themselves as having a Canadian ethnic background considered that their concerns had been satisfied in counselling (this variable accounted for 4% of the variance in the regression equation). Finally, 3% of the variance was accounted for by the woman's personal income. The women with more income considered that their concerns had been met more fully in the counselling session.

### Table 20. Independent Variables Entered into Regression Equations

*Demographic independent variables*
1. Age of respondent
2. Gravidity
3. Parity
4. Married vs. other (dummy variable created from living arrangement variable)
5. Respondent's educational level
6. Employed vs. other (dummy variable created from employment status variable)
7. Skilled worker vs. other (dummy variable created from respondent's Pineo-Porter McRoberts Occupational Classification variable)
8. Respondent's personal income
9. Protestant vs. other (dummy variable created from religious preference variable)
10. Catholic vs. other (dummy variable created from religious preference variable)
11. Strength of religious beliefs
12. Canadian ethnicity vs. other (dummy variable created from self-identified ethnicity variable)
13. English/Anglo ethnicity vs. other (dummy variable created from self-identified ethnicity variable)

*Psychosocial independent variables*
1. How one is feeling generally (from GWB)
2. Feeling anxious or worried (from GWB)
3. Feeling stress or pressure (from GWB)
4. Feeling nervous (from GWB)
5. Number of supporters when one needs to talk (from SSQ)
6. Number of supporters who help in a crisis (from SSQ)
7. Number of supporters who distract one from worries (from SSQ)
8. Number of supporters one can depend on for help (from SSQ)
9. Number of supporters who help with the death of a loved one (from SSQ)
10. Number of supporters who love respondent (from SSQ)
11. Number of supporters who console respondent (from SSQ)
12. "Chance" factors (from HLOC)
13. "Provider control" factor (from HLOC)
14. "Self-control" factors (from HLOC)

*Other independent variables*
1. Self-assessed risk of bearing a child with a genetic abnormality
2. Gender of genetic counsellor

### Table 21. Women's Perceptions That Genetic Counselling Satisfied Their Concerns

| Independent variables | b | beta | $r^2$ | f | p |
|---|---|---|---|---|---|
| Married | −1.38 | −0.48 | 0.20 | 29.04 | 0.0000 |
| Feeling anxious or worried | 0.33 | 0.48 | 0.07 | 15.63 | 0.0002 |
| Self-assessed risk | −0.32 | −0.34 | 0.09 | 14.43 | 0.0003 |
| Canadian ethnicity | 0.37 | 0.22 | 0.04 | 6.16 | 0.0154 |
| Respondent's income | −0.02 | −0.22 | 0.03 | 5.44 | 0.0226 |
| Feeling stress or pressure | −0.15 | −0.23 | 0.03 | 3.74 | 0.0572 |
| Constant | 3.29 | | | 46.07 | 0.0000 |

$r^2 = 0.46$; df = 6 and 71; f = 9.91; p < 0.0000.

Of the remaining independent variables entered into the regression model, none reached statistical significance. In total, six independent variables accounted for 46% of the variance. The proportion of variance explained here is inflated by the contribution of marital status, which was not highly variable in this sample.

### Women's Perceptions of Counselling as Informative (Table 22)

The second regression model examined which set of predictors best explained women's perceptions of counselling as informative. Only three variables emerged as significant predictors of this dependent variable. Women who were multiparous were more likely to judge counselling as informative. This variable accounted for the largest proportion of the total variance in this regression model, 15% of 22%. Women employed outside the home also tended to see the counselling as informative; this variable explained an additional 4% of the total variance. Women who had more support available when they lost a loved one found counselling to be more informative (3% of the variance explained).

### Table 22. Women's Perceptions of Genetic Counselling as Informative

| Independent variables | b | beta | $r^2$ | f | p |
|---|---|---|---|---|---|
| Number of children born | 0.45 | 0.49 | 0.15 | 18.34 | 0.0001 |
| Employed outside home | 0.58 | 0.25 | 0.04 | 4.66 | 0.0341 |
| Supporters at the death of a loved one | 0.01 | 0.00 | 0.03 | 3.16 | 0.0796 |
| Constant | 3.24 | | | 111.20 | 0.0000 |

$r^2 = 0.22$; df = 3 and 74; f = 7.12; p < 0.0003.

### Women's Perceptions of Counselling as Helpful (Table 23)

The third regression model examined which set of predictors best explained women's perceptions of counselling as helpful. Only three variables emerged as significant predictors of this dependent variable, and the pattern was identical to the previous regression model; that is, women who were multiparous were more likely to judge counselling as helpful. This variable accounted for the largest proportion of the total variance in this regression model, 10% of 20%. Women employed outside the home also tended to see the counselling as helpful. This variable explained an additional 6% of the total variance. Women who had more support available to them at the death of a loved one found counselling to be more informative (4% of the variance explained).

Table 23. Women's Perceptions of Genetic Counselling as Helpful

| Independent variables | b | beta | $r^2$ | f | p |
|---|---|---|---|---|---|
| Number of children born | 0.47 | 0.44 | 0.10 | 14.50 | 0.0003 |
| Employed outside home | 0.79 | 0.29 | 0.06 | 6.32 | 0.0141 |
| Supporters at the death of a loved one | 0.01 | 0.20 | 0.04 | 3.78 | 0.0558 |
| Constant | 2.78 | | | 60.23 | 0.0000 |

$r^2 = 0.20$; df = 3 and 74; f = 6.25; $p < 0.0008$.

### Women's Perceptions of Counselling as Stressful (Table 24)

The fourth regression model examined which predictors explained women's perceptions of genetic counselling as stressful. Of all of the demographic and psychosocial variables entered into the equation, only two variables emerged as significant predictors: the number of children a woman had had (accounting for 5% of the variance explained) and if a woman was married (accounting for an additional 4% of the variance explained). Women with fewer children tended to see the counselling session as more stressful. Married women, more than their counterparts, found counselling to be more stressful.

Table 24. Women's Perceptions of Genetic Counselling as Stressful

| Independent variables | b | beta | $r^2$ | f | p |
|---|---|---|---|---|---|
| Number of children born | −0.23 | −0.22 | 0.05 | 4.02 | 0.0486 |
| Married | 0.74 | 0.19 | 0.04 | 3.07 | 0.0838 |
| Constant | 3.94 | | | 68.16 | 0.0000 |

$r^2 = 0.09$; df = 2 and 75; f = 3.55; $p < 0.0337$.

## Women's Perceptions of Counselling as Reassuring (Table 25)

The final regression equation considered which factors best explained women's perceptions of counselling as reassuring. In total, four variables accounted for 23% of the variance in this dependent variable. Women who had more support available to them at the death of a loved one were more likely to be reassured by counselling. This variable accounted for 8% of the total variance. Also accounting for 8% of the variance was Canadian ethnicity; women identifying themselves as such were less likely to be reassured by counselling. Both marital status and self-assessed risk of bearing a child with a genetic disorder accounted for 3% of the variance in the dependent variable. Women who were married were more likely to experience reassurance in the counselling session. Those rating their risk as high were less likely to be reassured by counselling.

Table 25. Women's Perceptions of Genetic Counselling as Reassuring

| Independent variables | b | beta | $r^2$ | f | p |
|---|---|---|---|---|---|
| Supporters at the death of a loved one | 0.02 | 0.30 | 0.08 | 8.28 | 0.0053 |
| Canadian ethnicity | −0.60 | −0.29 | 0.08 | 8.12 | 0.0057 |
| Married | 0.68 | 0.19 | 0.03 | 3.54 | 0.0638 |
| Self-assessed risk | 0.20 | 0.18 | 0.03 | 2.97 | 0.0892 |
| Constant | 2.21 | | | 14.30 | 0.0003 |

$r^2 = 0.23$; df = 4 and 73; f = 5.38; p < 0.0007.

## Conclusions

Stepwise regression was used in this study instead of hierarchical regression. It is a technique that permits one to enter variables into the equation based on theoretical or logical criteria, thus indicating the distinct contribution of any particular independent variable or variables in predicting the dependent variable. This study was primarily interested in identifying the set of factors that best helped to account for variation in the dependent variables measuring women's satisfaction with genetic counselling. In this regard, the present research was not intended to test models as much as it was intended to identify predictive factors. Since stepwise regression is commonly criticized for capitalizing on chance, it is recommended that findings be cross-validated with a second sample. The findings here are exploratory at best; additional research on women's satisfaction with genetic counselling is indicated.

Although the regression analyses do not necessarily provide us with a clear understanding of the predictors of women's satisfaction (much of the variance remains unexplained here), we do have some evidence that the women referred to this program are essentially pleased with the services they received. Yet, it is equally pressing that issues of concern raised by some women in this study be given attention in future research. In particular, it is important to get an understanding of women's attitudes toward counselling and PND, and not just whether they are satisfied with what is already there. This presupposes asking questions such as "should we have these services?" (a question that was not explored in this study), and not simply "since we have these services, how do you feel about them?" (the focus of this study). Given the time constraints of this study, such a broad scope of empirical questions could not be explored fully.

Another point deserves comment: the identification of who uses genetic counselling (and presumably PND) at the Section of Clinical Genetics. We have seen in this chapter that the AMA women obtaining this service are mostly women of high social standing (i.e., high education, occupational, and economic status), and comparatively few are drawn from the lower social classes. This finding compares with research done at other centres and in other countries, which shows that these services are not used equally within the population. What cannot be known from this study is whether, for example, there is a systematic under-representation of women from the lower social classes. To know this with any certainty would require population-based demographic profiles of childbearing women and profiles of women using and declining genetic counselling. There is no basis in these data to conclude that certain segments of the population are excluded from this process. However, it is notable that the women who do use genetic counselling seem to derive from the middle and upper classes. If women in the middle and upper classes are using PND while those in the lower classes are not, might PND actually serve to reinforce inequalities in the population (owing to the unequal distribution of genetic abnormalities where screening has not occurred) (Lippman 1986, 1991)? There are profound social and health policy implications associated with the use of PND that deserve further attention by the providers of genetic counselling and prenatal screening services.

## Chapter 6. Discussion

What should be a public policy, disease prevention stance towards genetic disorders that are not life-threatening, but which make for lifetime dependency, or which are simply unaesthetic? The power of the technological advances is such that there is now a possible new attitude waiting to be adopted — that "the defective fetus" can be eliminated. The elimination or prevention of the "defective fetus" is the most likely consequence and ultimate meaning of a genetic screen. In a heterogeneous mix, the public forum for this debate needs to be vigorous and informed, not just by modest levels of technical knowledge about genetic or molecular biological developments, but about the role of power and the relative social locations of key actors in the determination of the knowledge, and its application ... There are ... "hidden arguments" underneath the surface language of neutrality of disease prevention and treatment. These need to be examined and addressed. I do not mean merely a discussion among elites about how these technologies can and should be deployed. *Those who will be consumers of the technology need to be part of the discussion. Out of this, an informed public policy could be generated and shaped.* (emphasis added)

(Duster 1990, 128-29)

## Introduction

This study was designed to explore the experience of a sample of AMA women with genetic counselling and PND. To that end, the research was guided by the premise that women's experiences with prenatal testing could best be understood by speaking directly to women themselves. It is not that women have been totally absent from discussions about the impact of PND on their pregnancies and their lives more generally; rather, much of the previous research conducted on women's experiences of genetic counselling and prenatal testing tells us only part of the story. Many studies have documented women's recall of counselling information, women's level of knowledge about PND, women's preferences for one form of testing over another, women's attitudes toward abortion in relation to PND, and women's acceptance or rejection of PND. Also, there have been studies on how women cope with the uncertainty associated with prenatal screening, and how their attitudes toward the disabled might influence their own personal behaviour in relation to testing. Each of these types of research provides a view of women's experiences of PND. But that view is partial.

Of course, the research discussed in this report is also incomplete, but it is incomplete in a somewhat different way than many of the studies done previously. Although the sample for this research is relatively small, and although data collection was of short duration, this research has given us an indication of perceptions and experience relevant to the debate about PND. It also has given a sample of AMA women an opportunity to describe in some detail how they experience this technology and the genetic counselling that accompanies PND. Relating the process that they experience, from referral to genetic counselling, we are able to see revealed some of the complexities — indeed, paradoxes — of this technological innovation through the prism of women's experiences.

In this closing chapter, we examine what has been learned during this study and what remains to be learned in future research. Organizationally, this discussion will first focus on the continuities of this study with existing research. Then we look critically at the strengths and limitations of the study, with a view to directions for future research. Finally, a set of recommendations to the Commission is proposed on the basis of this research experience.

## Prenatal Diagnosis: A Study of Women's Attitudes, Perceptions, and Experiences

In many ways, this study followed two streams — first, to document women's perceptions and experiences of PND and, second, to determine the level of satisfaction with the services they were receiving from the Section of Clinical Genetics. As has already been discussed, the second of these two dimensions of the research has limitations and, although we can say that women in this study were satisfied, many questions about why remain unanswered.

If we consider the qualitative data from this study, we get a sense of women's experiences with PND because their narratives provide an account for us. Based on the findings of this study, we can see the paradoxical nature of this technology as it is experienced by women. In many ways, PND is both a boon and bane to those who use it. PND gives women the technological potential to have information about the genetic state of the fetus they are carrying. With this information in hand, women can exercise control over whether to carry a pregnancy to term; with this information in hand, women for whom abortion is not an option can prepare themselves for the birth of a child with a genetic abnormality. Women in this study described the ways in which PND afforded them this knowledge and how empowered they were by the prospect of learning about their fetus.

However, women repeatedly commented that PND carries with it the weight of deciding that abortion would be preferable to bearing and raising a child with a genetic abnormality. Such a decision was, for many women in this study, a choice of no real choice, because of the perception that this society does not provide adequately for those who are disabled, in terms of social, economic, or other resources. This decision did as much to disempower women as the technological knowledge had done to empower them. For many women, the personal and social costs of having a child with a disability were simply too great to pass up the option of testing and abortion of an affected fetus.

As difficult as many women in this study found the genetic screening process to be, it seemed to be the path of least resistance. Although not all women were prepared to abort a fetus on finding an abnormality, many simply believed that — for many reasons — they could not proceed with their pregnancy without the information that PND would afford them. And along the way, some were prepared to treat their pregnancies as "tentative" (Rothman 1987; Tymstra et al. 1991).

The women in this study, even without someone coercing them into using this technology, felt pressure to use PND. The women in this study, as in Rothman's (1987) study and Farrant's (1985) study, were expected to take, and did take, responsibility for the prevention of fetal abnormality. Not all women in the study were content with the ideology underlying this technology — an ideology that "poses solutions to disability in terms of medical science and maternal responsibility, rather than social and political change" (Farrant 1985, 117). Yet, for most women here, the choice was between what is bad (anticipating an abortion in the face of a positive finding) and what is worse (having a child with a genetic abnormality) (Rothman 1987).

The women in this study realized that there really is no neutral ground when one looks at the field of genetic screening. As satisfied as they were with the services they had received, many also wanted an acknowledgment of what genetic screening means — for them, for their offspring, and for society. Not enough of a dialogue on these difficult issues has occurred. Clearly, there is a need for such a dialogue. This research is only a beginning to uncovering the complexities of prenatal screening. Much remains to be done in this area.

## The Strengths and Limitations of This Study

This research was conducted, from start to finish, in less than one year, which is not a long time to develop a project from the ground up, and to collect all of the data and assemble them into a coherent whole. Even with its methodological limitations, this study helps to provide an understanding of what the participating women think, and some suggestions as to how we should be considering the use of PND technologies and services in the future.

As has been noted earlier in this report, relatively little sociological research has been done into women's experiences with PND (Farrant 1985; Kolker and Burke 1987; Rothman 1987). There have been many more studies guided by psychological and health services research perspectives. Although the scope of this study was limited, it does provide data that illustrate the social basis of women's experiences of PND. In this regard, the present study, although exploratory, is important. However, several aspects of the methodology are subject to criticism and, for that reason, aspects of the sample and study design, interview, and questionnaire are considered below.

### *The Sample*

Whether the sample in this study is considered to be small or large depends on whether one refers to the qualitative or the quantitative components of the research. As noted in Chapter 5, a sample consisting of 122 AMA women was likely too small to detect differences between these women on some of the quantitative measures in this research (some measurement issues may have confounded aspects of the quantitative analysis as well). Although it has not been possible to discern whether the women in this study are significantly different from the AMA women normally seen at the Section of Clinical Genetics or if they differ in tangible ways from women declining the services offered at the clinic, this sample likely provides a reasonable approximation of the population of AMA women referred to and accepting genetic counselling at this central clinic in Manitoba.

In terms of the qualitative data, the sample size of 70 AMA women was noteworthy. Granted, more detailed accounts from the women who were interviewed would have been preferable. Regardless, we do have the narratives of these 70 women, thereby giving a great many women who use this service an opportunity to be heard by the Commission.

This sample is representative in a theoretical, rather than statistical, sense (Glaser and Strauss 1967). At the same time, with the high level of response to the study (90.9% overall), and no differences revealed on key demographic measures between women who were interviewed and women who participated only in the questionnaire component of the study, there is reason to believe that the women studied here probably do represent their peers served at the Section of Clinical Genetics. Having had exclusive access to this client population was not only efficient from the standpoint of the logistics of this study, but also ideal, as there was uniformity in at least some aspects of the likely experiences of the women involved.

### *Exclusions from the Study*

The second issue that merits comment concerns the exclusions from the study. On the basis of previous research, the women participating in this study were probably different from those who declined referral to genetic counselling and PND. Logistically, it was not possible to investigate those who declined PND, and thus the narrow focus on the users of this service was built into the design. Clearly, the differences between users and refusers of PND needs to be clearly established. No doubt these two groups of AMA women have important differences in their attitudes toward PND. Women declining PND should be heard in the debates about PND. Having such comparative data would have been desirable here, because it would have shed important light not only on why some women accept and others reject PND but also on the factors that lead women to make such decisions. This is a vital area that requires further investigation.

This research focussed primarily on the experiences of AMA women and not those of men, because it was not possible to study the men's experiences systematically, given limitations of time and resources. Another justification for the focus on women is that PND and other new reproductive technologies affect women's bodies (and lives) more intimately than they do men's. It is not suggested that men are unaffected by PND or that they are absent in decision making about PND; on the contrary, this study has shown that most women customarily make decisions about reproduction and about PND with their male partners. In interviews, women detailed how they believed that their own lives and those of their partners had been and would be affected by the testing process and the possibility of bearing a child with a genetic abnormality. In addition, when men were present during the pre-counselling interviews, they were not actively discouraged from participating, but most did defer to their wives or partners on the understanding that this was a study of women's attitudes, perceptions, and experiences, and all literature received about this study had stated quite clearly that this was a woman-centred study. Future research should study men's experiences of PND as well. Future studies might explore the nature and extent of men's involvement in this process and the effects of PND on men and their marital relationships, as perceived by the men. Studies could be done to establish what the differences are in the experience of PND between women and men. Ideally, such research would interview women and their partners separately, together, or both, to uncover how individuals and couples experience PND.

### *Time and Timing of the Interviews*

The time and the timing of the interviews have been an issue in this research. We decided for reasons of practicality that interviews in this study would be conducted before genetic counselling only. This allowed us to interview women to find out about their expectations about genetic counselling and their concerns about both counselling and prenatal testing. We assumed that women had received some minimal information about genetic counselling (i.e., all were to have received a brochure from the Section of Clinical Genetics). The interviews were brief; this was because our intent was to reach as many women as possible without disrupting the flow of clients through the Section of Clinical Genetics. From the logs kept by the interviewer and from a review of the transcripts, it seemed clear that the women had as much of an opportunity as possible to talk about their experiences — within the boundaries set by the interview guide and the clinic schedule. Obviously, the range of questions was limited and many areas could not be pursued in depth.

To do justice to the question of women's attitudes toward and experiences with PND, it would have been necessary to probe deeply into matters such as women's attitudes toward disability; women's experiences with uncertainty; women's attitudes toward abortion; and the psychosocial, emotional, socioeconomic, and other implications of PND for women, their partners, and their immediate (and extended) families, to name a few. Such detailed delving would necessitate at least 60 to 90 minutes per interview; this was beyond what could be accomplished in this study. However, the interviews that were conducted did tell us something about how women saw the counselling experience or, more accurately, what they expected from counselling, and what process they had already been through as they anticipated counselling, PND, or both.

It is also relevant that conducting interviews only at one point presents a limited view of women's experiences with PND. It would have been most desirable to speak to women at several other points during their pregnancies — for example, directly after counselling or before testing, after testing and receipt of results, and at the end of the pregnancy, whether terminated or carried to term.[24] It is well appreciated that the effects of PND are experienced not only at the time women are receiving genetic counselling, but throughout a pregnancy and well beyond. Future research could address this.

### *Measurement*

The range of information gathered in the interviews was relatively limited. To be clear, the interviews were intended to fulfil the first two objectives of this research — (1) to determine patterns of utilization of, and referral to, PND, and (2) to determine women's perceptions, attitudes, and knowledge of PND. Consequently, the interviews did not primarily gather attitudinal data because they were intended to gather experiential data. An attitudinal study would have included a broader range of questions on the use of PND, women's perceptions of the appropriateness of PND, and so on. However, as documented in Chapter 4, some women did express their attitudes toward this technology in pregnancy and about issues such as disability in relation to PND. When a woman did delve into these areas, she was encouraged to express her views.

The experiential data presented here do provide something that no amount of attitudinal data can ever offer. It is widely recognized that there is often a huge gulf between what people say and what people do (Babbie 1986). Documenting experience is about what people do; studying attitudes is about what people say they do, not necessarily what they actually do. A study of attitudes would have meant researching women's experiences of PND along the various dimensions noted previously and was not the focus of this exploratory study. The small sample, studied at one point for a short duration, was intentional. Although much more might have been done to unravel this complex experience, what we received is a glimpse of women's experiences. These experiences have allowed this group of AMA women an opportunity to be heard by the Commission. As the opening quotation in this chapter noted, this is far from inconsequential, as it has given AMA women in this sample a chance to contribute to the debate about such technologies.

Other measurement issues arise when we consider the second methodology used in this study — the post-counselling mail-questionnaire. This instrument was designed to measure the more easily quantifiable aspects of women's experiences with genetic counselling and, specifically, to provide them with an opportunity to comment on their satisfaction with the counselling they received (the latter being the third objective of this study). The questions dealing with satisfaction drew extensively on the work of Sorenson et al. (1981); however, because the samples used in these two studies are so different (i.e., this study was restricted to AMA women, while the Sorenson et al. study included women with family or genetic histories predisposing them to risk), the findings are not comparable.

As shown in Chapter 5, the findings from the survey provide interesting descriptive information about the users of genetic counselling, particularly when identifying the profile of such AMA users at the Section of Clinical Genetics.

In terms of the other substantive components of the questionnaire, some difficulties were encountered in the measurement of psychosocial variables. As noted in Chapter 5, the measure of general well-being was not particularly informative. Although there is considerable heterogeneity among pregnant women, this measure was unable to identify sources of difference in women's well-being. Perhaps another psychological measure like Bradburn's Affect Balance Scale, Macmillan's Health Opinion Survey, or the CES-Depression Scale would have proved more discriminating (McDowell and Newell 1987).

The measurement of health-specific locus of control raised other problems, which may be related either to the sample or to the fact that significant modifications were made to the instrument to reduce the length of the survey (i.e., several items were removed). Why this variable, which one would expect intuitively to have an impact on women's experiences, did not emerge as an important predictor of their attitudes toward counselling is unknown. Similarly, the measurement of social support did not provide important clues to women's attitudes toward counselling.

A careful examination of the questionnaire shows that, aside from providing descriptive information on the users of genetic counselling, the only aspects of the study that could be subject to scrutiny were the measures of satisfaction. The issue is, are the psychosocial variables measured likely to be critical in explaining women's satisfaction? Or are these variables more relevant in terms of explaining women's decisions about accessing PND and the whole range of experiences related to that decision? The latter is likely the case. In this study, no quantitative data were included to allow such an analysis. Where attitudinal information was obtained (in the interviews), it could not be analyzed statistically to disentangle the demographic and psychosocial correlates of women's attitudes toward PND. Future research clearly needs to be undertaken in this area.

These measurement issues, and the relatively small sample size in the quantitative component of the research, have meant that the research reported is still exploratory. As has been noted previously, there was a high variable-to-sample-size ratio and, consequently, any type of multivariate analysis was difficult to do. This (or a revised) methodology, used on a much larger sample, could have resulted in different (possibly clearer) findings at the multivariate level.

The study findings reported here provide an important piece of a complex puzzle. Notwithstanding the limitations of the study methodology, it has an important message to convey. The subjective experiences of women documented in the interview component tell us much more than might be possible by having women complete a structured questionnaire, in which they were asked to fit their experience into preconceived categories that, at best, approximate the "typical" response and, more often than not, appeal to the lowest common denominator. Although the process of interviewing is laborious, there really is no better way to understand subjective experiences. Recalling the words of John Stuart Mill, we must ask the women themselves if we want to understand their experience.

## Recommendations to the Royal Commission on New Reproductive Technologies

The mandate of the Royal Commission on New Reproductive Technologies specifies that it shall conduct an inquiry into, and make recommendations regarding, the new reproductive technologies "in terms of their social, legal, ethical, economic, research and health implications for women, men and children and for society as a whole." Integral to such an inquiry are data that illuminate the experiences of Canadians who are exposed to these technologies; this research is part of the overall research process.

Because the qualitative data provide a clearer picture of this sample's experiences with genetic services, this segment of the study has been used to compile the following recommendations. These recommendations reflect the content of the interviews and the comments women made in the open-ended questions of the survey.

### *Recommendation #1:*

Consumers of PND need and want to be able to make informed decisions about the care they receive from clinical geneticists and genetic counsellors. This requires disclosure of sufficient information to allow women to feel that they are able to exercise whatever choices are available.

### *Recommendation #2:*

Some reconsideration of the nature of genetic counselling — the values guiding it and the direction it takes — is indicated and necessary. Genetic counsellors should be encouraged to assess, for example, the meaning for their clients of whether they take a directive or non-directive approach (assuming that the latter is possible). Also, further consideration should be given to the content of genetic counselling. The finding in this study that some women thought their concerns could not be addressed by medical science, and their comments that they wished the counsellor had provided them with counselling about and an outlet for their feelings about PND and related matters (e.g., attitudes toward disability, attitudes toward selective abortion), suggest that women do not consider the current format involving the presentation of medical facts alone to be sufficient. Although most women in this study were satisfied with the counselling sessions overall, the fact that this issue was mentioned by some women suggests that there are sources of dissatisfaction for some.

### *Recommendation #3:*

Related to Recommendation #2, open and frank dialogue needs to take place on the relation between attitudes toward disability and the use of PND. This is essential to prevent what some researchers in the area of disability fear — that is, an increasing intolerance of disability in our society because PND is used to screen out particular forms of disability.

## A Final Word

In closing this report, it is fitting to quote the words of one of the women in this study. These comments, written on the back of her questionnaire, draw on many of the issues that have been discussed in this report.

> While at first I was reluctant to be "studied" by any group I came to see that this was an important opportunity to have input into a very important, personal, and yet societal concern. I think I understand the rationale behind offering prenatal testing to various "high risk" patients. Women over 35 seem to have been tagged as such. I understand the statistical curve increases in risk at this point; however, the risk is still less than 1%, for Down's for example. The risk from the various tests has been quoted as from 0.5% to 3%. Why is the first percentage of risk "high risk," but the second seems a risk factor that is "acceptable"? The whole process starting with my obstetrician on through the genetic counselling [to] testing felt de-humanized. No sense of happy potential joy, so often associated with pregnancy. Indeed, my other pregnancies had a much less clinical and more joyful sense attached to them vis-à-vis my interface with the medical world. My obstetrician was quite blunt and really assumed I would want/need amnio. I felt that he thought the only reasons that I could possibly have for not having it would be a lack of knowledge (not the case). The medical staff were not so upsetting but still the process by definition is not a positive experience. An acquaintance who had genetic counselling said she felt it was "scare tactics." I understand what she meant. The information is not incorrect but the overall impression one gets is not one of "there is a 98% chance of an okay pregnancy" but rather "oh-oh! this is a potential problem." At times, one feels that there is an element of the eugenics orientation to the whole business. Allowing personal choice is important but so is offering a positive environment in which to make said choice. I know that this is a difficult issue and often the nuances are dependent upon a given doctor's manner, etc., but at a stressful and vulnerable time, people need more than statistical tables. Do we have a clear perspective on where this is going? (#332)

Do we have a clear picture? Probably not. This research has, one hopes, identified areas of concern, as expressed by some of the women using PND. Public policy makers would do well to listen to what these consumers — the women — have to say. Ultimately, not only will women's health and well-being be affected by the decisions reached by policy makers in this area, but the health and well-being of all Canadians will be touched in some way by policies and practice in this branch of reproductive medicine.

# Appendix 1. Information Sheets and Consent Forms

(INTERVIEW)
**A Study of Women's Perceptions and Attitudes Toward Prenatal Diagnosis**

The use of prenatal diagnostic services by pregnant women aged 35 years and older has steadily increased over the past few years. In order to ensure that we are meeting the needs of women using prenatal diagnosis, we are conducting a study of women's concerns, perceptions and attitudes regarding prenatal diagnosis. Since you have been referred for prenatal diagnosis at the Section of Clinical Genetics, Health Sciences Centre, we would like to invite you to participate in this study.

In conducting this research, we will be studying a sample of women referred to the Section of Clinical Genetics. You have been selected to be interviewed prior to receiving genetic counselling, and to complete a questionnaire following genetic counselling. The interview and questionnaire will both contain questions concerning women's attitudes and perceptions regarding prenatal diagnosis. As well, we will be asking for some personal information such as age, marital status, educational level, and the like, in order that we can understand how different women perceive prenatal diagnostic services.

All information gathered through the pre-counselling (in-person) interview and post-counselling (mail) questionnaire will be kept completely confidential. The pre-counselling interview will be audiotaped for later transcription, so that we can analyze these data more completely. None of the information you disclose to the research team will be communicated to the genetic counsellors at the Section of Clinical Genetics at the Health Sciences Centre. Furthermore, none of the information you provide us with will be included in any hospital records. You are free to refuse to answer any of the questions you are asked in this research. You are also free to withdraw from the study at any time. Your decision on whether to participate in this study will in no way affect the care you receive through the Section of Clinical Genetics. In order to protect your identity, all information will be aggregated and analyzed with identification numbers only.

This research has been requested by the Royal Commission on New Reproductive Technologies. While there may be no direct benefit to you as a study participant, the findings will be incorporated into the final report of the Royal Commission to the federal government, and will influence the policy recommendations that the Royal Commission makes regarding prenatal services in Canada. In other words, we are certain that this study will help us in meeting women's needs in the area of prenatal diagnosis, in the long term.

## A Study of Women's Perceptions and Attitudes Toward Prenatal Diagnosis

I, _____, agree to participate in the study about women's attitudes regarding prenatal diagnostic services.

I have read the attached information sheet on this study. I understand that if I agree to participate in the study, my pre-counselling interview will be audiotaped. Any information provided by me in the interview and the questionnaire will be kept in strict confidence. I am free to refuse to answer any questions I consider too personal or objectionable. I understand that my identity will not be revealed at any time or to anyone. None of the information I provide will be given to the genetic counsellors at the Section of Clinical Genetics or to my physician. None of this information will be placed on my medical records.

I understand that my participation in this study is entirely voluntary. I also understand that I may withdraw my participation at any time, without my care at the Health Sciences Centre being affected in any way.

_____  
(Date)

_____  
(Signature in ink)

_____  
(Date)

_____  
(Witness)

## (QUESTIONNAIRE ONLY)
## A Study of Women's Perceptions and Attitudes Toward Prenatal Diagnosis

The use of prenatal diagnostic services by pregnant women aged 35 years and older has steadily increased over the past few years. In order to ensure that we are meeting the needs of women using prenatal diagnosis, we are conducting a study of women's concerns, perceptions and attitudes regarding prenatal diagnosis. Since you have been referred for prenatal diagnosis at the Section of Clinical Genetics, Health Sciences Centre, we would like to invite you to participate in this study.

In conducting this research, we will be studying a sample of women referred to the Section of Clinical Genetics. You have been selected to complete a questionnaire following genetic counselling. The questionnaire will contain questions concerning women's attitudes and perceptions regarding prenatal diagnosis. As well, we will be asking for some personal information such as age, marital status, educational level, and the like, in order that we can understand how different women perceive prenatal diagnostic services.

All information gathered through the post-counselling (mail) questionnaire will be kept completely confidential. None of the information you disclose to the research team will be communicated to the genetic counsellors at the Section of Clinical Genetics at the Health Sciences Centre. Furthermore, none of the information you provide us with will be included in any hospital records. You are free to refuse to answer any of the questions you are asked in this research. You are also free to withdraw from the study at any time. Your decision on whether to participate in this study will in no way affect the care you receive through the Section of Clinical Genetics. In order to protect your identity, all information will be aggregated and analyzed with identification numbers only.

This research has been requested by the Royal Commission on New Reproductive Technologies. While there may be no direct benefit to you as a study participant, the findings will be incorporated into the final report of the Royal Commission to the federal government, and will influence the policy recommendations that the Royal Commission makes regarding prenatal services in Canada. In other words, we are certain that this study will help us in meeting women's needs in the area of prenatal diagnosis, in the long term.

## A Study of Women's Perceptions and Attitudes Toward Prenatal Diagnosis

I, _____, agree to participate in the study about women's attitudes regarding prenatal diagnostic services.

I have read the attached information sheet on this study. I understand that if I agree to participate in the study, any information provided by me in the questionnaire will be kept in strict confidence. I am free to refuse to answer any questions I consider too personal or objectionable. I understand that my identity will not be revealed at any time or to anyone. None of the information I provide will be given to the genetic counsellors at the Section of Clinical Genetics or to my physician. None of this information will be placed on my medical records.

I understand that my participation in this study is entirely voluntary. I also understand that I may withdraw my participation at any time, without my care at the Health Sciences Centre being affected in any way.

_____          _____
(Date)                                                   (Signature in ink)


_____          _____
(Date)                                                              (Witness)

## Appendix 2. Interview Guide

Interview
Number _____ (1-3)

**A Study of Women's Perceptions and Attitudes
Toward Prenatal Diagnosis
*Pre-Counselling Interview***

Thank you for agreeing to participate in this study. Before you go in to consult with the counsellor, I would like to ask you some questions about why you are here today. This interview should take no more than 30 minutes to complete. I want to remind you that you are free not to answer any questions you consider too personal or objectionable. However, I assure you that all your answers will be kept completely confidential. Furthermore, your involvement in this study will in no way affect the care you receive through the Section of Clinical Genetics.

1.  Date of interview  _____ (4-9)
    (year/month/day)

2.  Start time of interview: _____ (10-13)
    (2400 clock)

3.  Finish time of interview: _____ (14-17)
    (2400 clock)

4.  Total length of interview: _____ (18-19)
    (minutes)

5.  Clinic:

    Children's Hospital Clinic ................. 1
    Women's Hospital Clinic ................. 2 (20)

6.  Interview subject(s):

    woman client only ....................... 1
    woman client with other ................. 2 (21)

    (a) <u>Gender of other</u> in attendance for interview:
    male ................................. 1
    female ............................... 2 (22)

(b) <u>Relationship of other</u> to interview subject:
spouse/partner ............................ 1
friend ..................................... 2
child(ren) ................................. 3
relative ................................... 4
other, please specify ...................... 5

not volunteered ........................... 6    (23)

**FIRST OF ALL, I'D LIKE TO GET SOME INFORMATION ABOUT YOU.**

7. What is your age?   _____    (24-25)
   (years)

8. a. What is your current living arrangement? (READ RESPONSES, CODE LOWEST NUMBER)

   now married and living with spouse ... 1 (ASK b)
   common-law relationship or live-in
     partner ............................ 2 (ASK b)
   single — never married ............... 3 (Skip to Q. 9)
   divorced ............................. 4 (Skip to Q. 9)
   separated ............................ 5 (Skip to Q. 9)
   widowed .............................. 6 (Skip to Q. 9)
   NR ................................... 9 (Skip to Q. 9)    (26)

   b. What was your marital status before your present relationship? Were you:

   divorced ............................. 1
   separated ............................ 2
   widowed .............................. 3
   single — never married ............... 4
   NA ................................... 7
   NR ................................... 9    (27)

**NOW, I'D LIKE TO ASK YOU SOME QUESTIONS ABOUT YOUR VISIT TO THE CLINIC TODAY.**

9. Could you tell me, in your own words, how you happened to be referred to the Section of Clinical Genetics?

    - What did the doctor tell you?
    - Did you request PND or did your doctor tell you to come?

10. What is your understanding of the purpose of the counselling session that will follow this interview?

11. What type(s) of information do you hope to receive in your counselling session today?

12. Do you have any particular concerns that you want addressed by the counsellor? What is the nature of these concerns? Why are they of concern to you? (Please be as specific as possible.)

    Probe for specific issues:

    - the pregnancy
    - the counselling session
    - the testing procedures and consequences

13. Have you thought about how you will use the information you get in the counselling session today? If so, please elaborate on how you expect that the counselling session or information will influence your reproductive decision-making.

14. Are there any other issues of interest or concern regarding prenatal diagnosis that you would care to comment on?

---

**Thank interview subject(s), and direct her/them back into the waiting area to await genetic counselling session.**

---

*Interview Process Form*

15. Quality of interview:

    high quality . . . . . . . . . . . . . . . . . . . . . . . . . . . . . 1
    adequate . . . . . . . . . . . . . . . . . . . . . . . . . . . . . . 2
    questionable . . . . . . . . . . . . . . . . . . . . . . . . . . . . 3     (28)

16. Respondent's cooperation:

    cooperative ............................. 1
    indifferent ............................. 2
    uncooperative ........................... 3          (29)

17. (If relevant) Did **the woman** ask spouse/partner or others for privacy?

    yes ..................................... 1
    no ...................................... 2
    NA ...................................... 7          (30)

18. Sources of interview interference, if any?

    |  | Yes | No |  |
    |---|---|---|---|
    | language | 1 | 2 | (31) |
    | noise | 1 | 2 | (32) |
    | presence of spouse | 1 | 2 | (33) |
    | presence of children | 1 | 2 | (34) |
    | presence of others | 1 | 2 | (35) |
    | other | 1 | 2 | (36) |

19. How would you rate the interview subject on the following:

    a) the pregnancy

        1    2    3    4    5

    very excited          very blasé          (37)

    b) the counselling session

        1    2    3    4    5

    very concerned      not at all concerned          (38)

    c) the testing process

        1    2    3    4    5

    very concerned      not at all concerned          (39)

20. (If relevant) How would you rate the interview subject's partner on the following:

   a) the pregnancy

         1    2    3    4    5

   very excited                 very blasé     (40)

   b) the counselling session

         1    2    3    4    5

   very concerned            not at all concerned     (41)

   c) the testing process

         1    2    3    4    5

   very concerned            not at all concerned     (42)

21. If the interview was terminated, what reasons were given? (To be recorded **on tape**.)

22. Did the woman indicate that she wished to continue her discussion of genetic counselling? Please elaborate with details. (To be recorded **on tape**.)

23. **THUMBNAIL SKETCH**: Anything about the respondent, the interview situation, the dynamics between the client and her partner (if relevant), etc., that seems important? (To be recorded **on tape**.)

*****************

I declare that this interview was conducted in accordance with the interviewing instructions given by the researchers. I agree that the content of all the respondent's responses will be kept confidential.

                                                                    (43)

_____
(Interviewer's signature)

## Appendix 3. Questionnaire

### A Study of Women's Perceptions and Attitudes Toward Prenatal Diagnosis

Thank you for agreeing to participate in this study. As you know, we are interested in finding out what **women** think about prenatal diagnosis. This questionnaire contains several questions about the counselling session you have completed. As well, there are some general questions about your health, about your relationships with others, and about you personally.

Completing this questionnaire should take about 20 minutes. We would ask that you complete this questionnaire as soon as possible after your visit today. This section of the study is for you to complete **on your own**.

Please be assured that the information you provide on this questionnaire will be kept **in strict confidence**. You are free to refuse to answer any questions you find too personal or objectionable. No one — including the genetic counsellor, your doctor, or the hospital — will learn of your answers to this survey. Furthermore, your identity will be protected.

We would ask that you **complete all of the questions on the survey**. There are no right or wrong answers to any of the questions contained in this survey. What we are interested in are your thoughts, feelings and attitudes. Please circle the answer that best describes your feelings. If you have any additional thoughts that you wish to record at the end of the survey, please do so on the back page of the questionnaire.

**If you are having any difficulties with any of the questions contained in this survey, please don't hesitate to contact the Research Office for some clarification and/or assistance. The phone number of the Research Office is 474-8298. Dr. Grant, the Principal Investigator of the study, can also be contacted if you have questions or concerns. She can be reached at 474-9831.**

When you have completed the questionnaire, please place it in the self-addressed, stamped envelope you were given. Seal the envelope, and drop it in the mail to:

Karen R. Grant, Ph.D.
Prenatal Diagnosis Study
Department of Sociology
University of Manitoba
Winnipeg, Manitoba
R3T 2N2

Once again, thank you for participating in this study.

* * * * * * * * * * * * * * * * * *

Questionnaire
Number _____ (1-3)

**TO BEGIN, WE WOULD LIKE TO KNOW A LITTLE ABOUT YOUR RECENT GENETIC COUNSELLING SESSION.**

1. On what day did you see the genetic counsellor?

   _____ (4-9)
   year/month/day

2. About how much time did you spend with the genetic counsellor?

   under 20 minutes ..................... 1
   20-39 minutes ........................ 2
   40-59 minutes ........................ 3
   an hour or more ...................... 4      (10)

3. Did the counsellor talk to you about your chances of having a child with a birth defect or genetic disorder?

   not discussed ........................ 1
   just mentioned ....................... 2
   discussed in some depth .............. 3
   not sure/can't remember ...... 8 (skip to Q. 5)   (11)

4. What are your chances of having a child with a birth defect or genetic disorder? (Give numbers or a percent.)

   I know the chances are _____.   (12-14)

   I think the chances are _____.   (15-17)

   The counsellor told me,
   but I don't remember what
   the chances are ....... ( ) (check if applicable)   (18)

5. Even though you may not know what the specific chances are, what kind of chance do you think there is of your having a child with a birth defect or genetic disorder?

   very high ............................ 1
   high ................................. 2
   moderate ............................. 3

> low ............................. 4
> very low ........................ 5                        (19)

6. Did the counsellor talk to you about tests that can be performed that can tell if the chromosomes of an unborn baby will be affected by genetic problems?

   > yes ............................. 1
   > no ...................... 2 (skip to Q. 8)
   > not sure/can't remember ...... 8 (skip to Q. 8)          (20)

7. What test(s) did the counsellor talk to you about?

   _____

   _____          (21)

8. a. Did you have any tests performed following your counselling session?

   > yes, I had tests performed .... 1 (answer part b)
   > no, but I am scheduled to have
   > tests performed ........... 2 (answer part b)
   > no and I will not have
   > any tests done ............ 3 (skip to Q. 10)            (22)

   b. What test(s) were (or will be) performed?

      Tests already performed:

      _____

      _____       (23)

      Tests to be performed:

      _____

      _____       (24)

9. Why did you or why will you have the prenatal diagnostic test(s)? Please be specific.

   _____

   _____

   _____

   _____          (25-26)

10. If you have decided not to have any prenatal tests, please indicate why. Please be specific.

   _____

   _____

   _____

   _____ (27-28)

11. Did the counselling session give you the medical (genetic) facts you wanted? It gave me:

    all the facts I wanted ........ 1 (skip to Q. 13)
    most of the facts I wanted ................. 2
    some of the facts I wanted ................ 3
    none of the facts I wanted ................ 4         (29)

12. If you did not get all the facts you wanted, was it because (circle as many as apply):

    some of the facts are not known by medical
    science ................................. 1
    the counsellor has to gather more facts ....... 2
    the counsellor did not want to discuss
    some facts I asked about ................ 3
    I did not ask about certain facts I wanted
    to know ............................... 4         (30-31)

13. Did the counselling session help you with the types of personal concerns that you had? It helped me with:

    all the concerns I had ........ 1 (skip to Q. 15)
    most of the concerns I had ................ 2
    some of the concerns I had ................ 3
    none of the concerns I had ............... 4         (32)

14. If counselling did not help you with all the personal concerns you had, was it because (circle as many as apply):

    some of the things I am concerned about
    can't be dealt with medically ............... 1
    the counsellor has to get more information .... 2
    the counsellor did not want to discuss
    the concerns I have .................... 3

I did not ask about some of the concerns
I have ............................... 4          (33-34)

15. Did the counselling session raise any new concerns for you?

    yes ................................. 1
    no ...................... 2 (skip to Q. 17)    (35)

16. If yes, what are these new concerns? Please be specific.

    _____

    _____

    _____  (36-37)

**FOR THE NEXT QUESTION, PLEASE CIRCLE THE NUMBER ON THE 1-5 SCALE THAT BEST DESCRIBES YOUR OPINION REGARDING THE GENETIC COUNSELLING SESSION.**

17. Thinking about the genetic counselling session as a whole, would you describe it as:

    (a)     5      4      3      2      1
         very                        not very
       informative                  informative         (38)

    (b)     5      4      3      2      1
        very helpful                  not very
                                      helpful          (39)

    (c)     5      4      3      2      1
       very stressful                 not very
                                      stressful        (40)

    (d)     5      4      3      2      1
         very                       not at all
       reassuring                   reassuring         (41)

18. Is there anything else you would like to comment on regarding your genetic counselling session?

   _____

   _____

   _____ (42-43)

**THIS NEXT SECTION OF THE SURVEY CONTAINS QUESTIONS ABOUT HOW YOU FEEL AND HOW THINGS HAVE BEEN GOING WITH YOU. FOR EACH QUESTION, CIRCLE THE NUMBER BESIDE THE ANSWER THAT BEST APPLIES TO YOU.**

19. How have you been feeling in general (during the past month)?

    in excellent spirits .................... 1
    in very good spirits .................... 2
    in good spirits mostly .................. 3
    I have been up and down in spirits a lot ...... 4
    in low spirits mostly ................... 5
    in very low spirits ..................... 6          (44)

20. Have you been bothered by nervousness or your "nerves" (during the past month)?

    extremely so — to the point where I could
    not work or take care of things ........... 1
    very much so ........................... 2
    quite a bit ............................ 3
    some — enough to bother me ............. 4
    a little bit ........................... 5
    not at all ............................. 6          (45)

21. Have you been in firm control of your behaviour, thoughts, emotions or feelings (during the past month)?

    yes, definitely so ...................... 1
    yes, for the most part .................. 2
    generally so ........................... 3
    not too well ........................... 4
    no, and I am somewhat disturbed .......... 5
    no, and I am very disturbed .............. 6         (46)

22. Have you felt so sad, discouraged, hopeless or had so many problems that you wondered if anything was worthwhile (during the past month)?

>   extremely so — to the point that I have
>   just about given up ...................... 1
>   very much so ........................... 2
>   quite a bit ............................. 3
>   some — enough to bother me ............. 4
>   a little bit ............................. 5
>   not at all ............................. 6         (47)

23. Have you been under or felt you were under any strain, stress, or pressure (during the past month)?

>   yes, almost more than I could bear
>   or stand ............................... 1
>   yes, quite a bit of pressure ............... 2
>   yes, some — more than usual ............. 3
>   yes, some — but about usual ............. 4
>   yes, a little ........................... 5
>   not at all ............................. 6         (48)

24. How happy, satisfied, or pleased have you been with your personal life (during the past month)?

>   extremely happy — could not have been
>   more satisfied or pleased ................ 1
>   very happy ............................ 2
>   fairly happy ........................... 3
>   satisfied — pleased ..................... 4
>   somewhat dissatisfied ................... 5
>   very dissatisfied ....................... 6         (49)

25. Have you had any reason to wonder if you were losing your mind, or losing control over the way you act, talk, think, feel or of your memory (during the past month)?

>   not at all ............................. 1
>   only a little ........................... 2
>   some — but not enough to be concerned
>   or worried about ...................... 3
>   some and I have been a little concerned ...... 4
>   some and I am quite concerned ............ 5
>   yes, very much so and I am very concerned ... 6     (50)

26. Have you been anxious, worried or upset (during the past month)?

    extremely so — to the point of being sick
    or almost sick .......................... 1
    very much so ........................... 2
    quite a bit ............................. 3
    some — enough to bother me ............ 4
    a little bit ............................. 5
    not at all .............................. 6     (51)

27. Have you been waking up fresh and rested (during the past month)?

    every day .............................. 1
    most every day ......................... 2
    fairly often ............................ 3
    less than half the time .................. 4
    rarely ................................. 5
    none of the time ....................... 6     (52)

28. Have you been bothered by any illness, bodily disorder, pains or fears about your health (during the past month)?

    all the time ............................ 1
    most of the time ....................... 2
    a good bit of the time .................. 3
    some of the time ....................... 4
    a little of the time ..................... 5
    none of the time ....................... 6     (53)

29. Has your daily life been full of things that were interesting to you (during the past month)?

    all the time ............................ 1
    most of the time ....................... 2
    a good bit of the time .................. 3
    some of the time ....................... 4
    a little of the time ..................... 5
    none of the time ....................... 6     (54)

30. Have you felt down-hearted and blue (during the past month)?

    all the time ............................ 1
    most of the time ....................... 2
    a good bit of the time .................. 3
    some of the time ....................... 4

```
    a little of the time .................. 5
    none of the time ..................... 6         (55)
```

31. Have you been feeling emotionally stable and sure of yourself (during the past month)?

```
    all the time ......................... 1
    most of the time ..................... 2
    a good bit of the time ............... 3
    some of the time ..................... 4
    a little of the time ................. 5
    none of the time ..................... 6         (56)
```

32. Have you felt tired, worn out, used-up, or exhausted (during the past month)?

```
    all the time ......................... 1
    most of the time ..................... 2
    a good bit of the time ............... 3
    some of the time ..................... 4
    a little of the time ................. 5
    none of the time ..................... 6         (57)
```

**FOR EACH OF THE FOLLOWING FOUR SCALES, NOTE THAT THE WORDS AT EACH END OF THE 0-10 SCALE DESCRIBE OPPOSITE FEELINGS. CIRCLE THE NUMBER ALONG THE SCALE WHICH SEEMS CLOSEST TO HOW YOU HAVE GENERALLY FELT DURING THE PAST MONTH.**

33. How concerned or worried about your health have you been (during the past month)?

    0  1  2  3  4  5  6  7  8  9  10

    not                                very
    concerned                          concerned
    at all
                                                     (58)

34. How relaxed or tense have you been (during the past month)?

    0  1  2  3  4  5  6  7  8  9  10

    very                               very tense
    relaxed
                                                     (59)

35. How much energy, pep, vitality have you felt (during the past month)?

       0   1   2   3   4   5   6   7   8   9   10

no energy at all, listless                          very energetic, dynamic

(60)

36. How depressed or cheerful have you been (during the past month)?

       0   1   2   3   4   5   6   7   8   9   10

very depressed                        very cheerful

(61)

**NOW, WE WOULD LIKE TO KNOW A LITTLE BIT ABOUT YOUR HEALTH.**

37. The following statements are designed to help us learn about your opinions regarding health and illness in general. Please indicate whether you agree or disagree with each statement.

| | strongly agree | agree | undecided | disagree | strongly disagree | |
|---|---|---|---|---|---|---|
| a. Staying well has little or nothing to do with chance. | 5 | 4 | 3 | 2 | 1 | (62) |
| b. Seeing a doctor for regular check-ups is a key factor in staying healthy. | 5 | 4 | 3 | 2 | 1 | (63) |

|   |   | strongly agree | agree | undecided | disagree | strongly disagree |   |
|---|---|---|---|---|---|---|---|
| c. | People's ill health results from their own carelessness. | 5 | 4 | 3 | 2 | 1 | (64) |
| d. | Doctors relieve or cure only a few of the medical problems their patients have. | 5 | 4 | 3 | 2 | 1 | (65) |
| e. | There is little one can do to prevent illness. | 5 | 4 | 3 | 2 | 1 | (66) |
| f. | Whether or not people get well is often a matter of chance. | 5 | 4 | 3 | 2 | 1 | (67) |
| g. | I have a lot of confidence in my ability to cure myself once I get sick. | 5 | 4 | 3 | 2 | 1 | (68) |

|   |   | strongly agree | agree | undecided | disagree | strongly disagree |   |
|---|---|---|---|---|---|---|---|
| h. | People who never get sick are just plain lucky. | 5 | 4 | 3 | 2 | 1 | (69) |
| i. | Doctors can almost always help their patients feel better. | 5 | 4 | 3 | 2 | 1 | (70) |
| j. | In the long run, people who take very good care of themselves stay healthy and get well quick. | 5 | 4 | 3 | 2 | 1 | (71) |
| k. | Recovery from illness requires good medical care more than anything else. | 5 | 4 | 3 | 2 | 1 | (72) |
| l. | Health-wise, there isn't much you can do for yourself when you get sick. | 5 | 4 | 3 | 2 | 1 | (73) |

|   | strongly agree | agree | undecided | disagree | strongly disagree |   |
|---|---|---|---|---|---|---|
| m. Doctors can do very little to prevent illness. | 5 | 4 | 3 | 2 | 1 | (74) |
| n. Recovery from illness has nothing to do with luck. | 5 | 4 | 3 | 2 | 1 | (75) |
| o. Good health is largely a matter of fortune. | 5 | 4 | 3 | 2 | 1 | (76) |

**IN THIS NEXT SECTION, WE WOULD LIKE TO FIND OUT A LITTLE INFORMATION ABOUT YOUR RELATIONSHIPS WITH OTHER PEOPLE.** (77-80 BL)

(1-3 ID)

38. a. What is your current living arrangement?

      now married and living with
      spouse .................... 1 (answer part b)
      common-law relationship or
      live-in partner ............. 2 (answer part b)
      single — never married ....... 3 (Skip to Q. 39)
      divorced .................. 4 (Skip to Q. 39)
      separated ................. 5 (Skip to Q. 39)
      widowed .................. 6 (Skip to Q. 39)          (4)

   b. What was your marital status before your present relationship? Were you:

      divorced ............................... 1
      separated .............................. 2

widowed . . . . . . . . . . . . . . . . . . . . . . . . . . . . . 3
single — never married . . . . . . . . . . . . . . . . . . . 4    (5)

THE FOLLOWING QUESTIONS ASK ABOUT PEOPLE IN YOUR ENVIRONMENT WHO PROVIDE YOU WITH HELP OR SUPPORT. EACH QUESTION HAS TWO PARTS. **FOR THE FIRST PART**, LIST ALL THE PEOPLE YOU KNOW, EXCLUDING YOURSELF, WHOM YOU CAN COUNT ON FOR HELP OR SUPPORT IN THE MANNER DESCRIBED. GIVE THE PERSONS' INITIALS, AND THEIR RELATIONSHIP TO YOU (SEE EXAMPLE). DO NOT LIST MORE THAN ONE PERSON NEXT TO EACH OF THE LETTERS BENEATH THE QUESTION. **FOR THE SECOND PART**, CIRCLE ONE ANSWER FOR HOW SATISFIED YOU ARE WITH THE OVERALL SUPPORT YOU HAVE. IF YOU HAVE NO SUPPORT FOR A QUESTION, CIRCLE THE WORDS "NO ONE", BUT STILL RATE YOUR LEVEL OF SATISFACTION. DO NOT LIST MORE THAN NINE PERSONS PER QUESTION. PLEASE ANSWER ALL QUESTIONS AS BEST YOU CAN.

\* \* \* \* \* \* \* \* **EXAMPLE** \* \* \* \* \* \* \* \*

(a) Who do you know whom you can trust with information that could get you into trouble?

no one    1) T.N. (brother)    4) T.N. (father)    7) _____

            2) L.M. (friend)    5) L.N. (boss)    8) _____

            3) R.S. (friend)    6) _____    9) _____

(b) **Circle one answer** for how satisfied you are with the overall support you have:

| ⑥ | 5 | 4 | 3 | 2 | 1 |
|---|---|---|---|---|---|
| very satisfied | fairly satisfied | a little satisfied | a little dissatisfied | fairly dissatisfied | very dissatisfied |

\* \* \* \* \* \* \* \* \* \* \* \* \* \* \* \* \* \* \* \* \* \* \* \*

39. (a) Whom can you really count on to listen to you when you need to talk? (6)
(7-24)

no one  1) _____  4) _____  7) _____

2) _____  5) _____  8) _____

3) _____  6) _____  9) _____

(b) **Circle one answer** for how satisfied you are with the overall support you have:

| 6 | 5 | 4 | 3 | 2 | 1 |
|---|---|---|---|---|---|
| very satisfied | fairly satisfied | a little satisfied | a little dissatisfied | fairly dis-satisfied | very dissatisfied |

(25)

40. (a) Whom could you really count on to help you out in a crisis situation, even though they would have to go out of their way to do so? (26)
(27-44)

no one  1) _____  4) _____  7) _____

2) _____  5) _____  8) _____

3) _____  6) _____  9) _____

(b) **Circle one answer** for how satisfied you are with the overall support you have:

| 6 | 5 | 4 | 3 | 2 | 1 |
|---|---|---|---|---|---|
| very satisfied | fairly satisfied | a little satisfied | a little dissatisfied | fairly dis-satisfied | very dissatisfied |

(45)

41. (a) Whom can you really count on to distract you from your worries when you feel under stress? (46)
(47-64)

no one  1) _____     4) _____     7) _____

        2) _____     5) _____     8) _____

        3) _____     6) _____     9) _____

(b) **Circle one answer** for how satisfied you are with the overall support you have:

| 6 | 5 | 4 | 3 | 2 | 1 |
|---|---|---|---|---|---|
| very satisfied | fairly satisfied | a little satisfied | a little dissatisfied | fairly dis-satisfied | very dissatisfied |

(65)
(66-80 BL)
(1-3 ID)

42. (a) Whom can you really count on to be dependable when you need help? (4)
(5-22)

no one  1) _____     4) _____     7) _____

        2) _____     5) _____     8) _____

        3) _____     6) _____     9) _____

(b) **Circle one answer** for how satisfied you are with the overall support you have:

| 6 | 5 | 4 | 3 | 2 | 1 |
|---|---|---|---|---|---|
| very satisfied | fairly satisfied | a little satisfied | a little dissatisfied | fairly dis-satisfied | very dissatisfied |

(23)

43. (a) Whom do you feel would help if a family member very close to you died? (24)
    (25-42)

   no one  1) _____   4) _____   7) _____
           2) _____   5) _____   8) _____
           3) _____   6) _____   9) _____

   (b) **Circle one answer** for how satisfied you are with the overall support you have:

   | 6 | 5 | 4 | 3 | 2 | 1 |
   |---|---|---|---|---|---|
   | very satisfied | fairly satisfied | a little satisfied | a little dissatisfied | fairly dis-satisfied | very dissatisfied |

   (43)

44. (a) Whom do you feel truly loves you deeply? (44)
    (45-62)

   no one  1) _____   4) _____   7) _____
           2) _____   5) _____   8) _____
           3) _____   6) _____   9) _____

   (b) **Circle one answer** for how satisfied you are with the overall support you have:

   | 6 | 5 | 4 | 3 | 2 | 1 |
   |---|---|---|---|---|---|
   | very satisfied | fairly satisfied | a little satisfied | a little dissatisfied | fairly dis-satisfied | very dissatisfied |

   (63)
   (64-80 BL)
   (1-3 ID)

45. (a) Whom can you count on to console you when you are very
    upset? (4)
    (5-22)

no one  1) _____  4) _____  7) _____

        2) _____  5) _____  8) _____

        3) _____  6) _____  9) _____

  (b) **Circle one answer** for how satisfied you are with the overall
      support you have:

  6          5          4          3          2          1
                                            fairly
  very      fairly    a little   a little    dis-      very
  satisfied satisfied satisfied  dissatisfied satisfied dissatisfied
                                                                    (23)

**NOW, WE WOULD LIKE TO ASK YOU A FEW MORE SPECIFIC
QUESTIONS ON THE SUPPORT YOU HAVE IN RELATION TO
REPRODUCTIVE DECISION-MAKING.**

46. (a) When it comes to deciding **when to have children**, who
        makes these decisions?

        me alone .................................. 1
        me, in consultation with others ........... 2
        others .................................... 3          (24)

  (b) How satisfied are you with this decision-making process?

                    5        4        3        2        1

              very                                     very
           satisfied                                 dissatisfied
                                                                    (25)

> **IF THIS DECISION IS MADE BY YOU ALONE, SKIP TO Q. 47. ALL OTHERS SHOULD ANSWER PARTS (c) AND (d) BEFORE ANSWERING Q. 47.**

(c) Who are the individuals participating in decision-making regarding when to have children? Please circle all of the numbers that apply.

```
spouse/partner ........................ 1
mother ................................ 2
father ................................ 3
mother-in-law ......................... 4
father-in-law ......................... 5
sister(s)/sister(s)-in-law ............ 6
brother(s)/brother(s)-in-law .......... 7
friend(s) ............................. 8
member of the clergy .................. 9
physician ............................ 10
others (please specify) .............. 11
```

_____

_____ (26-27)

(d) Of the individuals noted in part (c), who would you say was/is the single most important person involved in the decision-making process? **Please indicate only one number, corresponding to the individual listed above.**

_____
(number of person)                                         (28-29)

47. (a) When it comes to deciding **how many children to have**, who makes these decisions?

    ```
    me alone ............................... 1
    me, in consultation with others ........ 2
    others ................................. 3         (30)
    ```

    (b) How satisfied are you with this decision-making process?

             5      4      3      2      1

    very                          very
    satisfied              dissatisfied

                                      (31)

> **IF THIS DECISION IS MADE BY YOU ALONE, SKIP TO Q. 48. ALL OTHERS SHOULD ANSWER PARTS (c) AND (d) BEFORE ANSWERING Q. 48.**

(c) Who are the individuals participating in decision-making regarding how many children to have? Please circle all of the numbers that apply.

```
spouse/partner ........................ 1
mother ................................ 2
father ................................ 3
mother-in-law ......................... 4
father-in-law ......................... 5
sister(s)/sister(s)-in-law ............ 6
brother(s)/brother(s)-in-law .......... 7
friend(s) ............................. 8
member of the clergy .................. 9
physician ............................. 10
others (please specify) ............... 11
```

_____

_____ (32-33)

(d) Of the individuals noted in part (c), who would you say was/is the single most important person involved in the decision-making process? **Please indicate only one number, corresponding to the individual listed above.**

_____
(number of person)                                          (34-35)

48. (a) When it comes to deciding **whether to undergo prenatal diagnosis**, who makes these decisions?

    ```
    me alone ............................ 1
    me, in consultation with others ..... 2
    others .............................. 3      (36)
    ```

    (b) How satisfied are you with this decision-making process?

    |   | 5 | 4 | 3 | 2 | 1 |   |
    |---|---|---|---|---|---|---|
    |   | very satisfied |   |   |   | very dissatisfied |   |

                                                               (37)

> **IF THIS DECISION IS MADE BY YOU ALONE, SKIP TO Q. 49. ALL OTHERS SHOULD ANSWER PARTS (c) AND (d) BEFORE ANSWERING Q. 49.**

(c) Who are the individuals participating in decision-making regarding whether to undergo prenatal diagnosis? Please circle all of the numbers that apply.

```
spouse/partner ........................ 1
mother ................................ 2
father ................................ 3
mother-in-law ......................... 4
father-in-law ......................... 5
sister(s)/sister(s)-in-law ............ 6
brother(s)/brother(s)-in-law .......... 7
friend(s) ............................. 8
member of the clergy .................. 9
physician ............................. 10
others (please specify) ............... 11
```

_____

_____ (38-39)

(d) Of the individuals noted in part (c), who would you say was/is the single most important person involved in the decision-making process? **Please indicate only one number, corresponding to the individual listed above.**

_____
(number of person)                                                (40-41)

49. (a) When it comes to deciding **how to use the information obtained in prenatal diagnosis**, who makes these decisions?

```
me alone ................................ 1
me, in consultation with others ......... 2
others .................................. 3
```
(42)

(b) How satisfied are you with this decision-making process?

              5      4      3      2      1

    very                            very
satisfied                    dissatisfied

(43)

> **IF THIS DECISION IS MADE BY YOU ALONE, SKIP TO Q. 50. ALL OTHERS SHOULD ANSWER PARTS (c) AND (d) BEFORE ANSWERING Q. 50.**

(c) Who are the individuals participating in decision-making regarding how to use the information obtained in prenatal diagnosis? Please circle all of the numbers that apply.

```
spouse/partner ........................ 1
mother ................................ 2
father ................................ 3
mother-in-law ......................... 4
father-in-law ......................... 5
sister(s)/sister(s)-in-law ............ 6
brother(s)/brother(s)-in-law .......... 7
friend(s) ............................. 8
member of the clergy .................. 9
physician ............................. 10
others (please specify) ............... 11
```

_____

_____ (44-45)

(d) Of the individuals noted in part (c), who would you say was/is the single most important person involved in the decision-making process? **Please indicate only one number, corresponding to the individual listed above.**

_____ (46-47)
(number of person)

**FINALLY, WE WOULD LIKE TO KNOW A LITTLE BIT ABOUT YOU PERSONALLY.**

50. How old are you at the present time?

    _____ years (48-49)

51. How many pregnancies have you had in total (including this one)?

    _____ pregnancies (50-51)

52. How many children have you given birth to?

    _____ children born (52)

53. Currently, are you employed outside the home?

    employed full-time ........................ 1
    employed part-time ....................... 2
    employed both full-time and part-time ....... 3
    not employed outside
    the home ................. 4 (skip to Q. 57)         (53)

54. What kind of work do/did you normally do? That is, what is/was your job title?

    _____

55. What does/did that job involve? (Please describe your job.)

    _____
    _____
    _____

56. What kind of place do/did you work for?

    _____ (54-57)

> **IF YOU HAVE NO SPOUSE/PARTNER, SKIP TO Q. 61.**

**NOW, SOME QUESTIONS ABOUT YOUR SPOUSE/PARTNER.**

57. What is your spouse/partner's current employment or work situation?

    employed full-time ........................ 1
    employed part-time ....................... 2
    employed both full-time and part-time ....... 3
    not employed outside
    the home ................. 4 (skip to Q. 61)         (58)

58. What kind of work does/did your spouse/partner normally do? That is, what is/was your spouse/partner's job title?

    _____

59. What does/did that job involve?   (Please describe your spouse/partner's job.)

    _____

    _____

    _____

60. What kind of place does/did your spouse/partner work for?

    _____ (59-62)

**NEXT, WE WOULD LIKE TO GET SOME INFORMATION ABOUT EDUCATION.**

61. What is the highest level of education that you and your spouse/partner have completed?

|  | **Respondent** | **Spouse/Partner** |
|---|---|---|
| No Schooling | 01 | 01 |
| <u>Elementary School</u> | | |
| incomplete | 02 | 02 |
| complete | 03 | 03 |
| <u>Junior High School</u> | | |
| incomplete | 04 | 04 |
| complete | 05 | 05 |
| <u>High School</u> | | |
| incomplete | 06 | 06 |
| complete (GED) | 07 | 07 |
| <u>Non-University (Voc/Tech, Nursing Schools)</u> | | |
| incomplete | 08 | 08 |
| complete | 09 | 09 |
| <u>University</u> | | |
| incomplete | 10 | 10 |
| diploma/certificate (hygienists) | 11 | 11 |
| Bachelor's degree | 12 | 12 |
| medical degree (vets, drs., dentists) | 13 | 13 |
| Master's degree | 14 | 14 |
| Doctorate | 15 | 15 (63-64) |

No spouse/partner .............. 97   (65-66)

**NEXT ARE A FEW QUESTIONS ABOUT PERSONAL FINANCES. ALL INFORMATION WILL BE KEPT CONFIDENTIAL AND YOU ARE FREE, OF COURSE, TO NOT ANSWER ANY QUESTIONS YOU FIND OBJECTIONABLE.**

62. Which number comes closest to the total income for this past year, before tax and deductions, of **all members living in your household**? (CIRCLE NUMBER)

| | | | |
|---|---|---|---|
| No income | 00 | $36,000 - 37,999 | 17 |
| Under $6,000 | 01 | $38,000 - 39,999 | 18 |
| $6,000 - 7,999 | 02 | $40,000 - 44,999 | 19 |
| $8,000 - 9,999 | 03 | $45,000 - 49,999 | 20 |
| $10,000 - 11,999 | 04 | $50,000 - 54,999 | 21 |
| $12,000 - 13,999 | 05 | $55,000 - 59,999 | 22 |
| $14,000 - 15,999 | 06 | $60,000 - 64,999 | 23 |
| $16,000 - 17,999 | 07 | $65,000 - 69,999 | 24 |
| $18,000 - 19,999 | 08 | $70,000 - 74,999 | 25 |
| $20,000 - 21,999 | 09 | $75,000 - 79,999 | 26 |
| $22,000 - 23,999 | 10 | $80,000 - 84,999 | 27 |
| $24,000 - 25,999 | 11 | $85,000 - 89,999 | 28 |
| $26,000 - 27,999 | 12 | $90,000 - 94,999 | 29 |
| $28,000 - 29,999 | 13 | $95,000 - 99,999 | 30 |
| $30,000 - 31,999 | 14 | $100,000+ | 31 |
| $32,000 - 33,999 | 15 | Don't know | 98 |
| $34,000 - 35,999 | 16 | | |

(67-68)

63. Which number comes closest to your **total individual** income for this past year? (CIRCLE NUMBER)

| | | | |
|---|---|---|---|
| No income | 00 | $36,000 - 37,999 | 17 |
| Under $6,000 | 01 | $38,000 - 39,999 | 18 |
| $6,000 - 7,999 | 02 | $40,000 - 44,999 | 19 |
| $8,000 - 9,999 | 03 | $45,000 - 49,999 | 20 |
| $10,000 - 11,999 | 04 | $50,000 - 54,999 | 21 |
| $12,000 - 13,999 | 05 | $55,000 - 59,999 | 22 |
| $14,000 - 15,999 | 06 | $60,000 - 64,999 | 23 |
| $16,000 - 17,999 | 07 | $65,000 - 69,999 | 24 |
| $18,000 - 19,999 | 08 | $70,000 - 74,999 | 25 |
| $20,000 - 21,999 | 09 | $75,000 - 79,999 | 26 |
| $22,000 - 23,999 | 10 | $80,000 - 84,999 | 27 |
| $24,000 - 25,999 | 11 | $85,000 - 89,999 | 28 |
| $26,000 - 27,999 | 12 | $90,000 - 94,999 | 29 |
| $28,000 - 29,999 | 13 | $95,000 - 99,999 | 30 |

$30,000 - 31,999 ... 14    $100,000+ ....... 31
$32,000 - 33,999 ... 15    Don't know ....... 98
$34,000 - 35,999 ... 16                                (69-70)

**NOW A FEW QUESTIONS ABOUT YOUR RELIGION.**

64. How much do you agree or disagree with this statement?

    My religion is important to me now.

    | strongly disagree | | | | | | strongly agree | don't know |
    |---|---|---|---|---|---|---|---|
    | 1 | 2 | 3 | 4 | 5 | 6 | 7 | 8 |

    (71)

65. Religion was important to me when I was growing up.

    | strongly disagree | | | | | | strongly agree | don't know |
    |---|---|---|---|---|---|---|---|
    | 1 | 2 | 3 | 4 | 5 | 6 | 7 | 8 |

    (72)

66. What is your religious preference, if any?  Your spouse/partner?

    |  | **Respondent** | **Spouse/Partner** |
    |---|---|---|
    | Protestant | 01 | 01 |
    | Catholic | 02 | 02 |
    | Jewish | 03 | 03 |
    | Moslem | 04 | 04 |
    | other Eastern religions | 05 | 05 |
    | Mennonite | 06 | 06 |
    | atheist | 07 | 07 |
    | agnostic | 08 | 08 |
    | no preference/affiliation | 09 | 09 |
    | other, please specify | 10 | 10 |

    _____  (73-74)
    No spouse/partner ............. 97              (75-76)

67. Would you say that your religious beliefs are strong or not very strong?

    strong .......................... 1
    not very strong ................... 2
    somewhat strong ................. 3          (77)

68. How would you describe your ethnic identity?

    _____ (78-79)

---

**Thank you for completing this survey. If you have any comments on the survey as a whole, or any questions in particular, please write them on the back of the survey.**

---

## Notes

1. The use of "mother" instead of "parent" is intentional.

2. Related to this, the development of fetal medicine is very much a product of the technological innovations in PND. Increasingly, it appears that these technologies will be used on women's bodies, for the sake of the embryo or fetus, who is seen increasingly as a "bona fide patient" (Reece et al. 1991).

3. Second-trimester amniocentesis is currently the standard of care in Canada. However, many centres worldwide offer early amniocentesis, done around the 10th week of pregnancy.

4. Kessler (1979) noted, as well, that previously the mandate of genetic counselling practice was defined as the prevention of birth defects. To that end, the only method of prevention would entail directing clients to abort an affected fetus, since no medical treatment options exist that will cure conditions such as trisomies. The shift away from prevention to communication of risks in a non-directive fashion in the mid-1970s reflected the realization of this limitation of medicine, no doubt coupled with a trend toward affording patients greater autonomy in (reproductive) decision making.

5. Although data collection was only three weeks shorter in duration, in reality clinics in which data collection could be done totalled only 16 weeks. Clinics were cancelled during the study period because of long weekends and holidays, and one was cancelled because all of the counsellors were attending a genetics conference outside Winnipeg.

6. Women routinely had an appointment made for testing (either amniocentesis or chorionic villus sampling) at the time that their counselling appointment was arranged. Customarily, the women coming into Winnipeg from rural areas had appointments for counselling and testing booked for the same day. This was done to minimize the need for multiple trips into Winnipeg, and ensured that women had

been counselled before testing. It is important to note that while appointments for testing are pre-arranged, some women ultimately opt not to undergo the testing; this is a personal decision.

7. All identifiers have been deleted.

8. Although 70 interviews were conducted, the summary of the interviewing process reports on a sample of 68 cases because two interview subjects did not complete questionnaires. The entry of data from the interview process was based on completion of the questionnaire. The quantitative element of the interviews also contained a select number of demographic questions. However, in terms of the thematic content analysis, all 70 interviews are considered.

9. Some difficulty was encountered in making assessments of women's concern about testing. When this occurred, there might have been concern about one form of testing (e.g., chorionic villus sampling vs. amniocentesis), or about some but not all aspects of testing (e.g., the pain of the procedure vs. worry about results). Consequently, some caution should be used in drawing inferences on these criteria.

10. The brochure from the Section of Clinical Genetics provides details on the testing procedures (amniocentesis and chorionic villus sampling), including how each is performed, what risks are associated with testing, and so on. This pamphlet also provides information on the risks of bearing a child with genetic abnormalities and of bearing a child with Down syndrome at different ages. In some instances, women's responses to questions of what they thought the purpose of counselling was echoed quite closely the substantive content of the brochure. The brochure seems to be an important source of information and education for women regarding PND.

11. This may be an area that the Section of Clinical Genetics should consider carefully in enhancing its service to AMA women.

12. Many women mentioned other women's experiences of pregnancy (mothers, sisters, sisters-in-law, friends), although they were not specifically related to testing. This highlights the extent to which women rely on other women's experiences as an important reservoir of information about reproduction.

13. The reference was to a woman who understood from testing that she was likely to bear a child with spina bifida. Despite this information, she opted not to terminate the pregnancy. When the child was born, there were no signs of spina bifida or any other genetic defect. The reaction of the woman interviewed was "well, what if they make a mistake?" Clearly, the realization that false-positives can occur in testing was cause for some concern in this woman (and others). At the time of her interview, this woman was not certain that she would have testing.

14. Only two women mentioned the desire to have information on the sex of the fetus. In neither instance was this information wanted for reasons related to selective abortion. One woman was simply curious; the other wanted to know the sex of the fetus so that she could plan for the birth (she would arrange for friends to keep children's clothing). Three women specifically mentioned that they did not want to know the sex of the fetus.

15. Rothman (1987, 99) noted that some women would rather pretend to have gained weight than admit to a pregnancy. There is a certain amount of what social psychologists call "impression management" occurring. Presumably, some women interpret the potential stigma of a late abortion as greater than the stigma of

obesity. This is an interesting, if somewhat paradoxical, observation in a society so concerned with appearance.

16. Almost all women in the study mentioned concerns over miscarriage. To some degree, it would seem that women recognize this is an integral aspect to the testing process. The 38 women cited as concerned about miscarriage typically expressed their concern more emphatically.

17. J. Halliday, personal communication, 1992; J. Lumley, personal communication, 1992.

18. Two of the women in the questionnaire-only sample returned questionnaires that were not completed. One woman withdrew her participation over concerns that her name had been given to the research team by the Health Sciences Centre. The other woman miscarried and no longer thought that it was appropriate or relevant for her to complete the questionnaire. Although these two cases are "returns," they are not included in the analysis. If these two cases are considered incomplete returns, then the response rate for the questionnaire-only sample is reduced to 78.8%, and for the entire sample the response rate reduces to 89.3%.

19. Gamma is a PRE (proportional reduction in error) measure commonly used in sociological research. This measure can take on a value between 0 and 1, where gamma = 0 indicates no association and gamma = 1 indicates a perfect correlation between the variables. Phi and Cramer's V are statistics based on $\chi^2$. Phi is used with contingency tables 2 × 2 in size, while Cramer's V is used with tables larger than 2 × 2. Both of these statistics vary between 0 and 1. The stronger the association, the larger the values of these measures. There is no set agreement on what is a weak, moderate, or strong relationship, only when no relationship or a perfect relationship exists. Accordingly, in the present study, the following descriptions will be applied to various sizes of measures of association reported: 0.00 to 0.15 — weak association; 0.16 to 0.30 — moderately weak association; 0.31 to 0.45 — moderate association; 0.46 to 0.60 — moderately strong association; 0.61 or greater — strong association.

20. Since the protocol at the Section of Clinical Genetics is that a woman is first counselled and then tested, the women indicating they had already had testing might have been referring to a previous pregnancy.

21. Recall the discussion in Chapter 4 on the "tentative pregnancy."

22. Mid-way through the data collection, a typographical error was discovered in the survey instrument (this error occurs in part (c) of questions 46 through 49, inclusive). When the mistake was discovered, a series of statistical analyses were undertaken to see if women were answering the question as written, rather than as intended. From an examination of the data mid-way through and at the end of the data collection, it can be concluded that women seemed to identify the structure of the question series, and responded in kind. Different patterns of response are noted for each of the four questions in this section of the survey. However, some might argue that caution should be used in the interpretation of this segment of the data.

23. This finding supports information obtained during the interviews. Women generally said that they discussed their options with respect to PND with their spouse or partner. Although not all women said that they agreed with their spouse or partner on everything (e.g., whether to continue a pregnancy given a positive finding or attitudes regarding disability), there was a strong tendency for women to

seek some kind of consensus with their partner on various aspects of reproductive decision making. Some women indicated that their partners left decision making up to the woman.

24. A follow-up study of the AMA women in this research was conducted during the fall and winter of 1992-93, with funding from the Manitoba Health Research Council. More than 75% of the original interview sample was recontacted, and in-depth interviews were carried out on a wide array of issues, some of which have been listed previously. Analysis of the findings is under way. Data from the pre-counselling and post-testing/post-delivery interviews will be linked, in order to show the range of experiences of the women in this research.

## Bibliography

Abramsky, L., and C.H. Rodeck. 1991. "Women's Choices for Fetal Chromosome Analysis." *Prenatal Diagnosis* 11: 23-28.

Ajjimakorn, S., C. Thanuntaseth, and P. Sugkraroek. 1988. "Knowledge, Attitudes and Acceptances of Pregnant Women Toward Prenatal Diagnosis." *Journal of the Medical Association of Thailand* 71 (Suppl. 1): 9-12.

Ales, K.L., M.K. Druzin, and D.L. Santini. 1990. "Impact of Advanced Maternal Age on the Outcome of Pregnancy." *Surgery, Gynecology and Obstetrics* 171: 209-16.

al-Jader, L.N., et al. 1990. "Attitudes of Parents of Cystic Fibrosis Children Towards Neonatal Screening and Antenatal Diagnosis." *Clinical Genetics* 38: 460-65.

Anderson, K., and D.C. Jack. 1991. "Learning to Listen: Interview Techniques and Analyses." In *Women's Words: The Feminist Practice of Oral History*, ed. S.B. Gluck and D. Patai. New York: Routledge.

Antley, R.M. 1979. "The Genetic Counselor as Facilitator of the Counselee's Decision Process." In *Genetic Counseling: Facts, Values, and Norms*, ed. A.M. Capron et al. New York: Alan R. Liss.

Arditti, R., R.D. Klein, and S. Minden, eds. 1989. *Test-Tube Women: What Future for Motherhood?* London: Pandora Press.

Asch, A. 1989. "Reproductive Technology and Disability." In *Reproductive Laws for the 1990s*, ed. S. Cohen and N. Taub. Clifton: Humana Press.

Asch, A., and M. Fine. 1988. "Shared Dreams: A Left Perspective on Disability Rights." In *Women with Disabilities: Essays in Psychology, Culture and Politics*, ed. M. Fine and A. Asch. Philadelphia: Temple University Press.

Babbie, E.R. 1986. *The Practice of Social Research*. 4th ed. Belmont: Wadsworth.

Baird, P.A., and A.D. Sadovnick. 1988. "Maternal Age-Specific Rates for Down Syndrome: Changes over Time." *American Journal of Medical Genetics* 29: 917-27.

Baird, P.A., A.D. Sadovnick, and B.C. McGillivray. 1985. "Temporal Changes in the Utilization of Amniocentesis for Prenatal Diagnosis by Women of Advanced Maternal Age, 1976-1983." *Prenatal Diagnosis* 5: 191-98.

Beck, M.N. 1990. "Eugenic Abortion: An Ethical Critique." *Canadian Medical Association Journal* 143: 181-86.

Beckwith, J. 1991. "Foreword: The Human Genome Initiative: Genetics' Lightning Rod." *American Journal of Law & Medicine* 17: 1-13.

Bell, J., et al. 1986. "The Impact of Prenatal Diagnosis on the Occurrence of Chromosome Abnormalities." *Prenatal Diagnosis* 6: 1-11.

Berkman, L.F., and S.L. Syme. 1979. "Social Networks, Host Resistance, and Mortality: A Nine-Year Follow-Up Study of Alameda County Residents." *American Journal of Epidemiology* 109: 186-204.

Black, R.B. 1989. "A 1 and 6 Month Follow-Up of Prenatal Diagnosis Patients Who Lost Pregnancies." *Prenatal Diagnosis* 9: 795-804.

Black, R.B., and R. Furlong. 1984. "Impact of Prenatal Diagnosis in Families." *Social Work in Health Care* 9 (Spring): 37-50.

Blank, R.H. 1982. "Public Policy Implications of Human Genetic Technology: Genetic Screening." *Journal of Medicine and Philosophy* 7: 355-74.

Blumberg, B. 1984. "The Emotional Implications of Prenatal Diagnosis." In *Psychological Aspects of Genetic Counselling*, ed. A.E.H. Emery and I. Pullen. London: Academic Press.

Blumberg, B.D., M.S. Golbus, and K.H. Hanson. 1975. "The Psychological Sequelae of Abortion Performed for a Genetic Indication." *American Journal of Obstetrics and Gynecology* 122: 799-808.

Bortner, M.A. 1990. "The Necessity and Inadequacy of the Reproductive Rights Discourse." *Social Justice* 17 (Fall): 99-110.

Boss, J.A. 1990. "How Voluntary Prenatal Diagnosis and Selective Abortion Increase the Abnormal Human Gene Pool." *Birth* 17: 75-79.

Bradish, P. 1987. "From Genetic Counselling and Genetic Analysis, to Genetic Ideal and Genetic Fate?" In *Made to Order: The Myth of Reproductive and Genetic Progress*, ed. P. Spallone and D.L. Steinberg. Oxford: Pergamon Press.

Brandenburg, H., et al. 1991. "Prenatal Diagnosis in Advanced Maternal Age. Amniocentesis or CVS, A Patient's Choice or Lack of Information?" *Prenatal Diagnosis* 11: 685-90.

Brown, J. 1989. "The Choice." *JAMA* 262: 2735.

Bryce, R.L., M.T. Bradley, and S.M. McCormick. 1989. "To What Extent Would Women Prefer Chorionic Villus Sampling to Amniocentesis for Prenatal Diagnosis?" *Paediatric and Perinatal Epidemiology* 3 (2)(April): 137-45.

Bundey, S., and E. Broughton. 1989. "Are Abortions More or Less Frequent Once Prenatal Diagnosis Is Available?" *Journal of Medical Genetics* 26: 794-96.

Bunker, J. 1985. "When Doctors Disagree." *New York Review of Books* 32 (25 April): 7-12.

Campbell, S., et al. 1982. "Ultrasound Scanning in Pregnancy: The Short-Term Psychological Effects of Early Real-Time Scans." *Journal of Psychosomatic Obstetrics and Gynaecology* 1: 57-61.

Canadian Collaborative CVS-Amniocentesis Clinical Trial Group. 1989. "Multicentre Randomised Clinical Trial of Chorion Villus Sampling and Amniocentesis." *Lancet* (7 January): 1-6.

Capron, A.M., et al., eds. 1979. *Genetic Counseling: Facts, Values, and Norms.* New York: Alan R. Liss.

Chadwick, R.F. 1987. "The Perfect Baby: Introduction." In *Ethics, Reproduction and Genetic Control,* ed. R.F. Chadwick. New York: Routledge.

Chodirker, B.N. 1991. "Prenatal Diagnosis of Down Syndrome." *Manitoba Medicine* 61 (2): 57-59.

Clark, S.L., and G.R. DeVore. 1989. "Prenatal Diagnosis for Couples Who Would Not Consider Abortion." *Obstetrics and Gynecology* 73: 1035-37.

Clarke, A. 1990. "Genetics, Ethics, and Audit." *Lancet* (12 May): 1145-47.

—. 1991. "Is Non-Directive Genetic Counselling Possible?" *Lancet* (19 October): 998-1001.

Clarke, A.E. 1990. "Controversy and the Development of Reproductive Sciences." *Social Problems* 37 (February): 18-37.

Cohen, L., and H. Rothschild. 1979. "The Bandwagons of Medicine." *Perspectives in Biology and Medicine* 22: 531-38.

Corea, G. 1985. *The Mother Machine: Reproductive Technologies from Artificial Insemination to Artificial Wombs.* New York: Harper and Row.

—. 1991. "How the New Reproductive Technologies Will Affect All Women." In *Reconstructing Babylon: Essays on Women and Technology,* ed. H.P. Hynes. Bloomington: Indiana University Press.

Crandall, B.F., T.B. Lebherz, and K. Tabsh. 1986. "Maternal Age and Amniocentesis: Should This Be Lowered to 30 Years?" *Prenatal Diagnosis* 6: 237-42.

Currie, D. 1988. "Re-Thinking What We Do and How We Do It: A Study of Reproductive Decisions." *Canadian Review of Sociology and Anthropology* 25: 231-53.

Daker, M., and M. Bobrow. 1989. "Screening for Genetic Disease and Fetal Anomaly During Pregnancy." In *Effective Care in Pregnancy and Childbirth,* Vol. 1, ed. I. Chalmers, M. Enkin, and M.J.N.C. Keirse. Toronto: Oxford University Press.

Dickens, B.M. 1986. "Prenatal Diagnosis and Female Abortion: A Case Study in Medical Law and Ethics." *Journal of Medical Ethics* 12: 143-44, 150.

Dillman, D.A. 1978. *Mail and Telephone Surveys: The Total Design Method.* Toronto: Wiley.

Dupuy, H.J. 1978. "Self-Representation of General Psychological Well-Being in American Adults." In *The Official Program and Abstracts. 106th Annual Meeting of the American Public Health Association and Related Organizations,* held in Los Angeles, October. Washington, DC: American Public Health Association.

Duster, T. 1990. *Backdoor to Eugenics.* New York: Routledge.

d'Ydewalle, G., and G. Evers-Kiebooms. 1987. "Experiments on Genetic Risk Perception and Decision Making: Explorative Studies." *Birth Defects: Original Article Series* 23: 209-25.

Earley, K.J., et al. 1991. "Patient Attitudes Toward Testing for Maternal Serum Alpha-Fetoprotein Values When Results Are False-Positive or True-Negative." *Southern Medical Journal* 84: 439-42.

Ekwo, E.E., J.O. Kim, and C.A. Gosselink. 1987. "Parental Perceptions of the Burden of Genetic Disease." *American Journal of Medical Genetics* 28: 955-63.

Elder, S.H., and K.M. Laurence. 1991. "The Impact of Supportive Intervention After Second Trimester Termination of Pregnancy for Fetal Abnormality." *Prenatal Diagnosis* 11: 47-54.

Elias, S., and G.J. Annas. 1987. *Reproductive Genetics and the Law*. Chicago: Year Book Medical Publishers.

Elkins, T.E., et al. 1986. "Attitudes of Mothers of Children with Down Syndrome Concerning Amniocentesis, Abortion, and Prenatal Genetic Counseling Techniques." *Obstetrics and Gynecology* 68: 181-84.

Evans, M.I., et al. 1988. "Determinants of Altered Anxiety After Abnormal Maternal Serum Alpha-Fetoprotein Screening." *American Journal of Obstetrics and Gynecology* 159: 1501-1504.

—. 1990. "Parental Perceptions of Genetic Risk: Correlation with Choice of Prenatal Diagnostic Procedures." *International Journal of Gynaecology and Obstetrics* 31: 25-28.

Evers-Kiebooms, G., et al., eds. 1987. *Genetic Risk, Risk Perception, and Decision Making*. Proceedings of a conference held July 28-29, 1986, Leuven, Belgium. New York: Alan R. Liss.

Faden, R.R., et al. 1985. "What Participants Understand About a Maternal Serum Alpha-Fetoprotein Screening Program." *American Journal of Public Health* 75: 1381-84.

—. 1987. "Prenatal Screening and Pregnant Women's Attitudes Toward the Abortion of Defective Fetuses." *American Journal of Public Health* 77: 288-90.

Fahy, M.J., and A. Lippman. 1988. "Prenatal Diagnosis and the Canadian Collaborative Randomized Trial of Chorionic Villi Sampling: The Physician's View." *American Journal of Medical Genetics* 31: 953-61.

Farrant, W. 1985. "Who's for Amniocentesis? The Politics of Prenatal Screening." In *The Sexual Politics of Reproduction*, ed. H. Homans. London: Gower.

Finger, A. 1989. "Claiming *All* of Our Bodies: Reproductive Rights and Disability." In *Test-Tube Women: What Future for Motherhood?* ed. R. Arditti, R.D. Klein, and S. Minden. London: Pandora Press.

Fletcher, J.C. 1980. "Ethics and Amniocentesis for Fetal Sex Identification." *Hastings Center Report* 10 (February): 15-17.

—. 1984. "The Prenatal State: Screening and Treating Neural Tube Defects." In *The Machine at the Bedside: Strategies for Using Technology in Patient Care*, ed. S.J. Reiser and M. Anbar. New York: Cambridge University Press.

Fletcher, J.C., et al. 1980. "Ethical, Legal and Societal Considerations of Prenatal Diagnosis." *Prenatal Diagnosis* 1 (Special Issue): 43-51.

Fost, N. 1989. "Guiding Principles for Prenatal Diagnosis." *Prenatal Diagnosis* 9: 335-37.

Fraser, F.C. 1974. "Genetic Counseling." *American Journal of Human Genetics* 26: 636-59.

—. 1988. "Genetic Counseling: Using the Information Wisely." *Hospital Practice* 23 (15 June): 245-62, 266.

Fresco, N., and D. Silvestre. 1982. "The Medical Child — Comments on Prenatal Diagnosis." *Journal of Psychosomatic Obstetrics and Gynaecology* 1: 3-8.

Frets, P.G., et al. 1990a. "Factors Influencing the Reproductive Decision After Genetic Counseling." *American Journal of Medical Genetics* 35: 496-502.

—. 1990b. "Model Identifying the Reproductive Decision After Genetic Counseling." *American Journal of Medical Genetics* 35: 503-509.

Fuchs, V.R. 1968. "The Growing Demand for Medical Care." *New England Journal of Medicine* 279: 190-95.

Furhmann, W. 1989. "Impact, Logistics and Prospects of Traditional Prenatal Diagnosis." *Clinical Genetics* 36: 378-85.

Garcia, J. 1982. "Women's Views of Antenatal Care." In *Effectiveness and Satisfaction in Antenatal Care*, ed. M. Enkin and I. Chalmers. London: William Heinemann Medical Books.

Gill, M., V. Murday, and J. Slack. 1987. "An Economic Appraisal of Screening for Down's Syndrome in Pregnancy Using Maternal Age and Serum Alpha Fetoprotein Concentration." *Social Science and Medicine* 24: 725-31.

Gillot-de Vries, F. 1988. "Social and Psychological Research Methods in the Evaluation of Prenatal Screening Procedures." *European Journal of Obstetrics, Gynecology and Reproductive Biology* 28 (Suppl.): 93-103.

Glaser, B.G., and A.L. Strauss. 1967. *The Discovery of Grounded Theory: Strategies for Qualitative Research*. Chicago: Aldine.

Gluck, S.B., and D. Patai, eds. 1991. *Women's Words: The Feminist Practice of Oral History*. New York: Routledge.

Golbus, M.S., et al. 1979. "Prenatal Genetic Diagnosis in 3000 Amniocenteses." *New England Journal of Medicine* 300: 157-63.

Goodwin, B.A., and C.A. Huether. 1987. "Revised Estimates and Projections of Down Syndrome Births in the United States, and the Effects of Prenatal Diagnosis Utilization, 1970-2002." *Prenatal Diagnosis* 7: 261-71.

Grant, A., and P. Mohide. 1982. "Screening and Diagnostic Tests in Antenatal Care." In *Effectiveness and Satisfaction in Antenatal Care*, ed. M. Enkin and I. Chalmers. London: William Heinemann Medical Books.

Grant, K.R. 1981. "Social Control in Medicine: On the Medicalization of Pregnancy and Childbirth." Master's thesis, Department of Sociology, University of Manitoba.

Green, D., and J. Malin. 1988. "Prenatal Diagnosis: When Reality Shatters Parents' Dreams." *Nursing* 18 (February): 61-64.

Green, J.M. 1990. "Prenatal Screening and Diagnosis: Some Psychological and Social Issues." *British Journal of Obstetrics and Gynaecology* 97: 1074-76.

Greenberg, F. 1988. "The Impact of MSAFP Screening on Genetic Services, 1984-1986." *American Journal of Medical Genetics* 31: 223-30.

Gruenberg, E.M. 1982. "The Failures of Success." In *Technology and the Future of Health Care*, ed. J.B. McKinlay. Cambridge: MIT Press.

Heidrich, S.M., and M.S. Cranley. 1989. "Effect of Fetal Movement, Ultrasound Scans, and Amniocentesis on Maternal-Fetal Attachment." *Nursing Research* 38 (March-April): 81-84.

Henifen, M.S., R. Hubbard, and J. Norsigian. 1988. "Prenatal Screening." In *Reproductive Laws for the 1990s*, ed. S. Cohen and N. Taub. Clifton: Humana Press.

Holloway, S., and D.J.H. Brock. 1988. "Changes in Maternal Age Distribution and Their Possible Impact on Demand for Prenatal Diagnostic Services." *British Medical Journal* (Clinical Research Edition) (2 April): 978-81.

Holmes-Siedle, M., M. Ryynanen, and R.H. Lindenbaum. 1987. "Parental Decisions Regarding Termination of Pregnancy Following Prenatal Detection of Sex Chromosome Abnormality." *Prenatal Diagnosis* 7: 239-44.

Hook, E.B. 1988. "Variability in Predicted Rates of Down Syndrome Associated with Elevated Maternal Serum Alpha-Fetoprotein Levels in Older Women." *American Journal of Human Genetics* 43: 160-64.

———. 1991. "Economics of Prenatal Diagnosis." *Lancet* (27 April): 1042.

House, J.S. 1981. *Work Stress and Social Support*. Reading: Addison-Wesley.

Hubbard, R. 1986. "Eugenics and Prenatal Testing." *International Journal of Health Services* 16: 227-42.

———. 1989. "Personal Courage Is Not Enough: Some Hazards of Childbearing in the 1980s." In *Test-Tube Women: What Future for Motherhood?* ed. R. Arditti, R.D. Klein, and S. Minden. London: Pandora Press.

———. 1990. *The Politics of Women's Biology*. New Brunswick: Rutgers University Press.

Humphreys, P., and D. Berkeley. 1987. "Representing Risk: Supporting Genetic Counseling." In *Genetic Risk, Risk Perception, and Decision Making*. Proceedings of a conference held July 28-29, 1986, Leuven, Belgium, ed. G. Evers-Kiebooms et al. New York: Alan R. Liss.

Hunter, M.S., et al. 1987. "Ultrasound Scanning in Women with Raised Serum Alpha Fetoprotein: Long Term Psychological Effects." *Journal of Psychosomatic Obstetrics and Gynaecology* 6: 25-31.

Hyde, B. 1986. "An Interview Study of Pregnant Women's Attitudes to Ultrasound Scanning." *Social Science and Medicine* 22: 587-92.

Illich, I. 1977. *Medical Nemesis: The Expropriation of Health*. New York: Bantam Books.

Jackson, L.G. 1990. "Commentary: Prenatal Diagnosis: The Magnitude of Dysgenic Effects Is Small, the Human Benefits, Great." *Birth* 17 (2): 80.

Jahoda, M.G.J., et al. 1987. "Role of Maternal Age in Assessment of Risk of Abortion After Prenatal Diagnosis During First Trimester." *British Medical Journal* (Clinical Research Edition) (14 November): 1237.

Johnson, J.M., and N. Caccia. 1991. "Prenatal Diagnosis: Patient Attitudes and Acceptance." *Journal of the Society of Obstetricians and Gynaecologists of Canada* 13 (June-July): 43-48.

Jones, D. 1991. "Use of Amniocentesis Dependent on Doctors' Referrals, Attitudes." *Family Practice* (3 August).

Keenan, K.L., et al. 1991. "Low Level of Maternal Serum Alpha-Fetoprotein: Its Associated Anxiety and the Effects of Genetic Counseling." *American Journal of Obstetrics and Gynecology* 164: 54-56.

Kessler, S., ed. 1979. *Genetic Counseling: Psychological Dimensions.* New York: Academic Press.

Kessler, S. 1989. "Psychological Aspects of Genetic Counseling: VI. A Critical Review of the Literature Dealing with Education and Reproduction." *American Journal of Medical Genetics* 34: 340-53.

Kessler, S., and E.K. Levine. 1987. "Psychological Aspects of Genetic Counseling: IV. The Subjective Assessment of Probability." *American Journal of Medical Genetics* 28: 361-70.

Klein, R. 1991. "Women as Body Parts in the Era of Reproductive and Genetic Engineering." *Health Care for Women International* 12: 393-405.

Kleinbaum, D.G., and L.L. Kupper. 1978. *Applied Regression Analysis and Other Multivariable Methods.* North Scituate: Duxbury Press.

Knott, P.D., R.J.A. Penketh, and M.K. Lucas. 1986. "Uptake of Amniocentesis in Women Aged 38 or More by the Time of the Expected Date of Delivery: A Two-Year Retrospective Study." *British Journal of Obstetrics and Gynaecology* 93: 1246-50.

Koch, L., and J. Morgall. 1987. "Towards a Feminist Assessment of Reproductive Technology." *Acta Sociologica* 30: 173-91.

Kolata, G. 1983. "Beyond Amniocentesis: New Techniques in Fetal Testing." *Ms.* (December): 91-94.

Kolker, A., and B.M. Burke. 1987. "Amniocentesis and the Social Construction of Pregnancy." *Marriage and Family Review* 11 (3-4): 95-116.

Kromberg, J.G.R., et al. 1989. "A Decade of Mid-Trimester Amniocentesis in Johannesburg: Prenatal Diagnosis, Problems, and Counselling." *South African Medical Journal* 76: 344-49.

Kyle, D., C. Cummins, and S. Evans. 1988. "Factors Affecting the Uptake of Screening for Neural Tube Defect." *British Journal of Obstetrics and Gynaecology* 95: 560-64.

Laborie, F. 1987. "Looking for Mothers You Only Find Fetuses." In *Made to Order: The Myth of Reproductive and Genetic Progress*, ed. P. Spallone and D.L. Steinberg. Oxford: Pergamon Press.

Landenburger, G., and K.J. Delp. 1987. "An Approach for Supportive Care Before, During and After Selective Abortion." *Birth Defects: Original Article Series* 23 (6): 84-88.

Lappe, M. 1984. "The Predictive Power of the New Genetics." *Hastings Center Report* 14 (October): 18-21.

Lau, R.R., and J.F. Ware, Jr. 1981. "Refinements in the Measurement of Health-Specific Locus-of-Control Beliefs." *Medical Care* 19: 1147-58.

Laurence, K.M., and J. Morris. 1981. "The Effect of the Introduction of Prenatal Diagnosis on the Reproductive History of Women at Increased Risk from Neural Tube Defects." *Prenatal Diagnosis* 1: 51-60.

Leff, P.T. 1987. "Here I Am, Ma: The Emotional Impact of Pregnancy Loss on Parents and Health-Care Professionals." *Family Systems Medicine* 5 (1): 105-14.

Leschot, N.J., M. Verjaal, and P.E. Treffers. 1982. "Therapeutic Abortion on Genetic Indications — A Detailed Follow-Up Study of 20 Patients." *Journal of Psychosomatic Obstetrics and Gynaecology* 1: 47-56.

Liebetrau, A.M. 1983. *Measures of Association*. Beverly Hills: Sage Publications.

Lippman, A. 1986. "Access to Prenatal Screening Services: Who Decides?" *Canadian Journal of Women and the Law* 1: 434-45.

—. 1991. "Prenatal Genetic Testing and Screening: Constructing Needs and Reinforcing Inequities." *American Journal of Law & Medicine* 17: 15-50.

Lippman, A., et al. 1992. "Canadian Multicentre Randomized Clinical Trial of Chorion Villus Sampling and Amniocentesis. Final Report." *Prenatal Diagnosis* 12: 385-476.

Lippman-Hand, A., and F.C. Fraser. 1979. "Genetic Counseling — The Post-Counseling Period: I. Parents' Perceptions of Uncertainty." *American Journal of Medical Genetics* 4: 51-71.

Lippman-Hand, A., and M. Piper. 1981. "Prenatal Diagnosis for the Detection of Down Syndrome: Why Are So Few Eligible Women Tested?" *Prenatal Diagnosis* 1: 249-57.

Loader, S., et al. 1991. "Prenatal Screening for Hemoglobinopathies. II. Evaluation of Counseling." *American Journal of Human Genetics* 48: 447-51.

Lofland, J. 1984. *Analyzing Social Settings: A Guide to Qualitative Observation and Analysis*. 2d ed. Belmont: Wadsworth.

McCance, D. 1984. "Limits of Burden: Toward an Ethical Framework for Prenatal Diagnosis." Ph.D. dissertation, University of Manitoba.

MacDiarmid, W.D. 1991. "Ethics and Birth Defects." *Manitoba Medicine* 61 (2): 74-75.

McDonnell, K. 1988. "Saying No to Amnio." *Healthsharing* 9 (Fall): 23-24.

McDowell, I., and C. Newell. 1987. *Measuring Health: A Guide to Rating Scales and Questionnaires*. New York: Oxford University Press.

McGovern, M.M., J.D. Goldberg, and R.J. Desnick. 1986. "Acceptability of Chorionic Villi Sampling for Prenatal Diagnosis." *American Journal of Obstetrics and Gynecology* 155: 25-29.

McKinlay, J.B. 1982. "From 'Promising Report' to 'Standard Procedure': Seven Stages in the Career of a Medical Innovation." In *Technology and the Future of Health Care*, ed. J.B. McKinlay. Cambridge: MIT Press.

Macklin, R. 1977. "Moral Issues in Human Genetics: Counseling or Control." *Dialogue* 16: 375-96.

Macri, J.N. 1986. "Critical Issues in Prenatal Maternal Serum Alpha-Fetoprotein Screening for Genetic Anomalies." *American Journal of Obstetrics and Gynecology* 155: 240-46.

Magyari, P.A., et al. 1987. "A Supportive Intervention Protocol for Couples Terminating a Pregnancy for Genetic Reasons." *Birth Defects: Original Article Series* 23 (6): 75-83.

Maier, K.E. 1989. "Pregnant Women: Fetal Containers or People with Rights?" *Affilia* 4 (2): 8-20.

Marks, J.H., et al. 1989. "The Ambiguous Amnio." *Birth Defects: Original Article Series* 25 (5): 65-78.

Marteau, T.M. 1989. "Psychological Costs of Screening May Sometimes Be Bad Enough to Undermine the Benefits of Screening." *British Medical Journal* (26 August): 527.

Marteau, T.M., et al. 1988a. "Development of a Self-Administered Questionnaire to Measure Women's Knowledge of Prenatal Screening and Diagnostic Tests." *Journal of Psychosomatic Research* 32: 403-408.

—. 1988b. "Screening for Down's Syndrome." *British Medical Journal* (3 December): 1469.

—. 1989a. "Factors Influencing the Uptake of Screening for Open Neural-Tube Defects and Amniocentesis to Test for Down's Syndrome." *British Journal of Obstetrics and Gynaecology* 96: 739-41.

—. 1989b. "The Impact of Prenatal Screening and Diagnostic Testing upon the Cognitions, Emotions and Behaviour of Pregnant Women." *Journal of Psychosomatic Research* 33: 7-16.

Mikkelsen, M. 1988. "The Incidence of Down's Syndrome and Progress Towards Its Reduction." *Philosophical Transactions of the Royal Society of London (Biology)* 319: 315-24.

Milunsky, A. 1975. *The Prevention of Genetic Disease and Mental Retardation.* Philadelphia: W.B. Saunders.

Minister, K. 1991. "A Feminist Frame for the Oral History Interview." In *Women's Words: The Feminist Practice of Oral History*, ed. S.B. Gluck and D. Patai. New York: Routledge.

Minogue, J.P., and N.J. Reedy. 1988. "Companioning Parents in Perinatal Decision Making." *Journal of Perinatal and Neonatal Nursing* 1 (January): 25-35.

Moatti, J.P., et al. 1990. "Socio-Cultural Inequities in Access to Prenatal Diagnosis: The Role of Insurance Coverage and Regulatory Policies." *Prenatal Diagnosis* 10: 313-25.

Mohide, P., and A. Grant. 1989. "Evaluating Diagnosis and Screening During Pregnancy and Childbirth." In *Effective Care in Pregnancy and Childbirth*, Vol. 2, ed. I. Chalmers, M. Enkin, and M.J.N.C. Keirse. Toronto: Oxford University Press.

Motulsky, A.G. 1989. "Societal Problems in Human and Medical Genetics." *Genome* 31: 870-75.

Naylor, E.W. 1975. "Genetic Screening and Genetic Counseling: Knowledge, Attitudes, and Practices in Two Groups of Family Planning Professionals." *Social Biology* 22: 304-14.

Nuckolls, K.B., J. Cassel, and B.H. Kaplan. 1972. "Psychosocial Assets, Life Crisis and the Prognosis of Pregnancy." *American Journal of Epidemiology* 95: 431-41.

Oakley, A. 1981. "Interviewing Women: A Contradiction in Terms." In *Doing Feminist Research*, ed. H. Roberts. London: Routledge and Kegan Paul.

Oliver, M. 1990. *The Politics of Disablement*. London: Macmillan.

Overall, C. 1987. *Ethics and Human Reproduction: A Feminist Analysis*. Boston: Unwin Hyman.

—, ed. 1989. *The Future of Human Reproduction*. Toronto: Women's Press.

Paez-Victor, M.E. 1988. "Risks and Values: A Study of the Social Context of Prenatal Diagnosis and Counselling." Ph.D. dissertation, York University.

Papp, Z. 1989. "Genetic Counseling and Termination of Pregnancy in Hungary." *Journal of Medicine and Philosophy* 14: 323-33.

Parikh, M. 1990. "Sex-Selective Abortions in India: Parental Choice or Sexist Discrimination?" *Feminist Issues* 10 (Fall): 19-32.

Pauker, S.G., and S.P. Pauker. 1987a. "Prescriptive Models to Support Decision Making in Genetics." *Birth Defects: Original Article Series* 23 (2): 279-96.

Pauker, S.P., and S.G. Pauker. 1987b. "The Amniocentesis Decision: Ten Years of Decision Analytic Experience." *Birth Defects: Original Article Series* 23 (2): 151-69.

Pelosi, A.J., and A.S. David. 1989. "Ethical Implications of the New Genetics for Psychiatry." *International Review of Psychiatry* 1: 315-20.

Phipps, S., and A.B. Zinn. 1986a. "Psychological Response to Amniocentesis: I. Mood State and Adaptation to Pregnancy." *American Journal of Medical Genetics* 25: 131-42.

—. 1986b. "Psychological Response to Amniocentesis: II. Effects of Coping Style." *American Journal of Medical Genetics* 25: 143-48.

Pineo, P.C. 1985. *Revisions of the Pineo-Porter-McRoberts Socioeconomic Classification of Occupations for the 1981 Census*. Research report 125. Hamilton: McMaster University, Program for Quantitative Studies in Economics and Population.

Pitz, G.F. 1987. "Evaluating Decision Aiding Technologies for Genetic Counseling." *Birth Defects: Original Article Series* 23 (2): 251-78.

Rapp, R. 1984. "The Ethics of Choice: After My Amniocentesis, Mike and I Faced the Toughest Decision of Our Lives." *Ms.* (April): 97-100.

—. 1987. "Moral Pioneers: Women, Men and Fetuses on a Frontier of Reproductive Technology." *Women and Health* 13 (1-2): 101-16.

—. 1989. "XYLO: A True Story." In *Test-Tube Women: What Future for Motherhood?* ed. R. Arditti, R.D. Klein, and S. Minden. London: Pandora Press.

Ratcliff, K.S., et al., eds. 1989. *Healing Technology: Feminist Perspectives.* Ann Arbor: University of Michigan Press.

Raymond, J.G. 1987. "Fetalists and Feminists: They Are Not the Same." In *Made to Order: The Myth of Reproductive and Genetic Progress,* ed. P. Spallone and D.L. Steinberg. Oxford: Pergamon Press.

Reading, A.E., and D.N. Cox. 1982. "The Effects of Ultrasound Examination on Maternal Anxiety Levels." *Journal of Behavioral Medicine* 5: 237-47.

Reading, A.E., D.N. Cox, and S. Campbell. 1988. "A Controlled, Prospective Evaluation of the Acceptability of Ultrasound in Prenatal Care." *Journal of Psychosomatic Obstetrics and Gynaecology* 8: 191-98.

Redman, S., et al. 1988. "Assessing Women's Health Needs." *Medical Journal of Australia* (1 February): 123-27.

Reece, E.A., et al. 1991. "A Viewpoint of Future Prenatal Diagnosis." *Prenatal Diagnosis* 11: 125-28.

Reid, M. 1988. "Consumer-Oriented Studies in Relation to Prenatal Screening Tests." *European Journal of Obstetrics, Gynecology and Reproductive Biology* 28 (Suppl.): 79-92.

Reid, M., and J. Garcia. 1989. "Women's Views of Care During Pregnancy and Childbirth." In *Effective Care in Pregnancy and Childbirth,* Vol. 1, ed. I. Chalmers, M. Enkin, and M.J.N.C. Keirse. Toronto: Oxford University Press.

Rice, N., and R. Doherty. 1982. "Reflections on Prenatal Diagnosis: The Consumers' Views." *Social Work in Health Care* 8 (Fall): 47-57.

Richards, M.P.M. 1989. "Social and Ethical Problems of Fetal Diagnosis and Screening." *Journal of Reproductive and Infant Psychology* 7: 171-85.

Riessman, C.K. 1983. "Women and Medicalization: A New Perspective." *Social Policy* 14 (Summer): 3-18.

Robinson, G.E., et al. 1988. "Anxiety Reduction After Chorionic Villus Sampling and Genetic Amniocentesis." *American Journal of Obstetrics and Gynecology* 159: 953-56.

—. 1991. "Psychological Reactions to Pregnancy Loss After Prenatal Diagnostic Testing: Preliminary Results." *Journal of Psychosomatic Obstetrics and Gynaecology* 12: 181-92.

Robinson, J.O., B.M. Hibbard, and K.M. Laurence. 1984. "Anxiety During a Crisis: Emotional Effects of Screening for Neural Tube Defects." *Journal of Psychosomatic Research* 28: 163-69.

Rose, H. 1987. "Victorian Values in the Test-Tube: The Politics of Reproductive Science and Technology." In *Reproductive Technologies: Gender, Motherhood and Medicine*, ed. M. Stanworth. Minneapolis: University of Minnesota Press.

Rothman, B.K. 1986. "Reflections: On Hard Work." *Qualitative Sociology* 9 (Spring): 48-53.

—. 1987. *The Tentative Pregnancy: Prenatal Diagnosis and the Future of Motherhood.* New York: Penguin.

—. 1990. "Commentary: Women Feel Social and Economic Pressures to Abort Abnormal Fetuses." *Birth* 17 (2): 81.

Rowland, R. 1987. "Of Women Born, But for How Long? The Relationship of Women to the New Reproductive Technologies and the Issue of Choice." In *Made to Order: The Myth of Reproductive and Genetic Progress*, ed. P. Spallone and D.L. Steinberg. Oxford: Pergamon Press.

Rowley, P.T., et al. 1991a. "Prenatal Screening for Hemoglobinopathies. I. A Prospective Regional Trial." *American Journal of Human Genetics* 48: 439-46.

—. 1991b. "Prenatal Screening for Hemoglobinopathies. III. Applicability of the Health Belief Model." *American Journal of Human Genetics* 48: 452-59.

Roy, D.J. 1986. "First-Trimester Fetal Diagnosis: Prudential Ethics." *Canadian Medical Association Journal* 135: 737-39.

Ruse, M. 1980. "Genetics and the Quality of Life." *Social Indicators Research* 7: 419-41.

St. Peter, C. 1989. "Feminist Discourse, Infertility, and Reproductive Technologies." *National Women's Studies Association Journal* 1: 353-67.

Sandelowski, M., B.G. Harris, and D. Holditch-Davis. 1991. "Amniocentesis in the Context of Infertility." *Health Care of Women International* 12: 167-78.

Sanden, M.L., and P. Bjurulf. 1988a. "Pregnant Women's Attitudes and Knowledge in Relation to Access to Serum-Alpha-Fetoprotein Test." *Scandinavian Journal of Social Medicine* 16: 197-204.

—. 1988b. "Pregnant Women's Attitudes for Accepting or Declining a Serum-Alpha-Fetoprotein Test." *Scandinavian Journal of Social Medicine* 16: 265-71.

Sarason, I.G. 1983. "Assessing Social Support: The Social Support Questionnaire." *Journal of Personality and Social Psychology* 44: 127-39.

Sawicki, J. 1991. "Disciplining Mothers: Feminism and the New Reproductive Technologies." In *Disciplining Foucault: Feminism, Power and the Body*. New York: Routledge.

Saxton, M. 1987a. "The Politics of Empowerment: Enabling the Disabled." *Update: Newsletter of the Evangelical Women's Caucus* 11: 1-2, 14.

—. 1987b. "Prenatal Screening and Discriminatory Attitudes About Disability." *Women and Health* 13 (1-2): 217-24.

—. 1989. "Born and Unborn: The Implications of Reproductive Technologies for People with Disabilities." In *Test-Tube Women: What Future for Motherhood?* ed. R. Arditti, R.D. Klein, and S. Minden. London: Pandora Press.

Scutt, J.A. 1988. "Women's Bodies, Patriarchal Principles: Genetic and Reproductive Engineering and the Law." In *The Baby Machine: Commercialisation of Motherhood*, ed. J.A. Scutt. Carlton (Victoria, Australia): McCulloch Publishing.

Seals, B.F., et al. 1985. "Moral and Religious Influences on the Amniocentesis Decision." *Social Biology* 32: 13-30.

Sell, R.R., K.J. Roghmann, and R.A. Doherty. 1978. "Attitudes Toward Abortion and Prenatal Diagnosis of Fetal Abnormalities: Implications for Educational Programs." *Social Biology* 25: 288-301.

Shiloh, S., and L. Saxe. 1989. "Perception of Risk in Genetic Counseling." *Psychology and Health* 3: 45-61.

Sissine, F.J., et al. 1981. "Statistical Analysis of Genetic Counseling Impacts: A Multi-Method Approach to Retrospective Data." *Evaluation Review* 5: 745-57.

Sjögren, B. 1992. "Future Use and Development of Prenatal Diagnosis. Consumers' Attitudes." *Prenatal Diagnosis* 12: 1-8.

Sjögren, B., and N. Uddenberg. 1987. "Attitudes Towards Disabled Persons and the Possible Effects of Prenatal Diagnosis: An Interview Study Among 53 Women Participating in Prenatal Diagnosis and 20 of Their Husbands." *Journal of Psychosomatic Obstetrics and Gynaecology* 6: 187-96.

—. 1988a. "Decision Making During the Prenatal Diagnostic Procedure. A Questionnaire and Interview Study of 211 Women Participating in Prenatal Diagnosis." *Prenatal Diagnosis* 8: 263-73.

—. 1988b. "Prenatal Diagnosis and Maternal Attachment to the Child-to-Be: A Prospective Study of 211 Women Undergoing Prenatal Diagnosis with Amniocentesis or Chorionic Villi Biopsy." *Journal of Psychosomatic Obstetrics and Gynaecology* 9: 73-87.

—. 1990. "Prenatal Diagnosis for Psychological Reasons: Comparison with Other Indications, Advanced Maternal Age and Known Genetic Risk." *Prenatal Diagnosis* 10: 111-20.

Somer, M., H. Mustonen, and R. Norio. 1988. "Evaluation of Genetic Counselling: Recall of Information, Post-Counselling Reproduction, and Attitude of the Counsellees." *Clinical Genetics* 34 (6)(December): 352-65.

Sorenson, J.R., and D.C. Wertz. 1986. "Couple Agreement Before and After Genetic Counseling." *American Journal of Medical Genetics* 25: 549-55.

Sorenson, J.R., J.P. Swazey, and N.A. Scotch. 1981. *Reproductive Pasts, Reproductive Futures: Genetic Counseling and Its Effectiveness*. New York: Alan R. Liss.

Sorenson, J.R., et al. 1987. "Reproductive Plans of Genetic Counseling Clients Not Eligible for Prenatal Diagnosis." *American Journal of Medical Genetics* 28: 345-52.

Spallone, P. 1989. *Beyond Conception: The New Politics of Reproduction*. Houndmills: Macmillan Education.

Sparling, J.W., J.W. Seeds, and D.C. Farran. 1988. "The Relationship of Obstetric Ultrasound to Parent and Infant Behavior." *Obstetrics and Gynecology* 72: 902-907.

Stanworth, M. 1987. "Reproductive Technologies and the Deconstruction of Motherhood." In *Reproductive Technologies: Gender, Motherhood and Medicine*, ed. M. Stanworth. Minneapolis: University of Minnesota Press.

Stein, E.J., and C.W.G. Redman. 1990. "Maternal-Fetal Conflict: A Definition." *Medico-Legal Journal* 58: 230-35.

Stewart, N. 1986. "Women's Views of Ultrasonography in Obstetrics." *Birth* 13 (1): 39-43.

Stoeber, W., C.R. Greenberg, and A.E. Chudley. 1991. "The Essentials of Genetic Counselling." *Manitoba Medicine* 61 (2): 71-73.

Stratford, B., and J. Steele. 1985. "Incidence and Prevalence of Down's Syndrome — A Discussion and Report." *Journal of Mental Deficiency Research* 29: 95-107.

Swerts, A. 1987. "Impact of Genetic Counseling and Prenatal Diagnosis for Down Syndrome and Neural Tube Defects." In *Genetic Risk, Risk Perception, and Decision Making*. Proceedings of a conference held July 28-29, 1986, Leuven, Belgium, ed. G. Evers-Kiebooms et al. New York: Alan R. Liss.

Swint, J.M., and F. Greenberg. 1988. "Maternal Serum Alpha-Fetoprotein Screening for Down Syndrome: Economic Considerations." *American Journal of Medical Genetics* 31: 231-45.

Tait, J.J. 1986. "Reproductive Technology and the Rights of Disabled Persons." *Canadian Journal of Women and the Law* 1: 446-55.

Tedgärd, U., et al. 1989. "How Do Carriers of Hemophilia Experience Prenatal Diagnosis (PND)? Carriers' Immediate and Later Reactions to Amniocentesis and Fetal Blood Sampling." *Acta Paediatrica Scandinavica* 78: 692-700.

Thomas, L. 1979. "On the Science and Technology of Medicine." In *Health, Illness and Medicine: A Reader in Medical Sociology*, ed. G.L. Albrecht and P.C. Higgins. Chicago: Rand McNally.

Thomassen-Brepols, L.J. 1987. "Psychological Implications of Fetal Diagnosis and Therapy." *Fetal Therapy* 2: 169-74.

Tsoi, M.M., et al. 1987. "Ultrasound Scanning in Women with Raised Serum Alpha Fetoprotein: Short Term Psychological Effect." *Journal of Psychosomatic Research* 31 (1): 35-39.

Tunis, S.L., et al. 1990a. "Normative Scores and Factor Structure of the Profile of Mood States for Women Seeking Prenatal Diagnosis for Advanced Maternal Age." *Educational and Psychological Measurement* 50: 309-24.

—. 1990b. "Patterns of Mood States in Pregnant Women Undergoing Chorionic Villus Sampling or Amniocentesis." *American Journal of Medical Genetics* 37: 191-99.

Tyler, A. 1987. "Genetic Counseling in Huntington's Chorea." In *Genetic Risk, Risk Perception, and Decision Making*. Proceedings of a conference held July 28-29, 1986, Leuven, Belgium, ed. G. Evers-Kiebooms et al. New York: Alan R. Liss.

Tymstra, T. 1991. "Prenatal Diagnosis, Prenatal Screening, and the Rise of the Tentative Pregnancy." *International Journal of Technology Assessment in Health Care* 7: 509-16.

Tymstra, T.J., et al. 1991. "Women's Opinions on the Offer and Use of Prenatal Diagnosis." *Prenatal Diagnosis* 11: 893-98.

Varekamp, I., et al. 1990. "Carrier Testing and Prenatal Diagnosis for Hemophilia: Experiences and Attitudes of 549 Potential and Obligate Carriers." *American Journal of Medical Genetics* 37: 147-54.

Verjaal, M., N.J. Leschot, and P.E. Treffers. 1982. "Women's Experiences with Second Trimester Prenatal Diagnosis." *Prenatal Diagnosis* 2: 195-209.

Verp, M.S., et al. 1988. "Parental Decision Following Prenatal Diagnosis of Fetal Chromosome Abnormality." *American Journal of Medical Genetics* 29: 613-22.

Villeneuve, C., et al. 1988. "Psychological Aspects of Ultrasound Imaging During Pregnancy." *Canadian Journal of Psychiatry* 33: 530-36.

Vlek, C. 1987. "Risk Assessment, Risk Perception and Decision Making About Courses of Action Involving Genetic Risk: An Overview of Concepts and Methods." *Birth Defects: Original Article Series* 23 (2): 171-207.

Wajcman, J. 1990. "Reproductive Technology: Delivered into Men's Hands." In *Feminism Confronts Technology*. University Park: Pennsylvania State University Press.

Waltz, J.R., and C.R. Thigpen. 1973. "Genetic Screening and Counseling: Legal and Ethical Issues." *Northwestern University Law Review* 68: 696-768.

Welch, J.P., et al. 1991. "Eugenic Abortion: An Ethical Critique." *Canadian Medical Association Journal* 144: 8-13.

Welshimer, K.J., and J.A.L. Earp. 1989. "Genetic Counseling Within the Context of Existing Attitudes and Beliefs." *Patient Education and Counseling* 13: 237-55.

Wertz, D.C., and J.C. Fletcher. 1988. "Attitudes of Genetic Counselors: A Multinational Survey." *American Journal of Human Genetics* 42: 592-600.

—. 1989. "Ethical Problems in Prenatal Diagnosis: A Cross-Cultural Survey of Medical Geneticists in 18 Nations." *Prenatal Diagnosis* 9: 145-57.

Wertz, D.C., J.C. Fletcher, and J.J. Mulvihill. 1990. "Medical Geneticists Confront Ethical Dilemmas: Cross-Cultural Comparisons Among 18 Nations." *American Journal of Human Genetics* 46: 1200-1213.

Wertz, D.C., J.R. Sorenson, and T.C. Heeren. 1984. "Genetic Counseling and Reproductive Uncertainty." *American Journal of Medical Genetics* 18: 79-88.

—. 1986. "Clients' Interpretation of Risks Provided in Genetic Counseling." *American Journal of Human Genetics* 39: 253-64.

Wertz, D.C., et al. 1991. "Attitudes Toward Abortion Among Parents of Children with Cystic Fibrosis." *American Journal of Public Health* 81: 992-96.

Winestine, M.C. 1989. "To Know or Not to Know: Some Observations on Women's Reactions to the Availability of Prenatal Knowledge of Their Babies' Sex." *Journal of the American Psychoanalytic Association* 37: 1015-30.

Woliver, L.R. 1989. "The Deflective Power of Reproductive Technologies: The Impact on Women." *Women and Politics* 9 (3): 17-47.

—. 1991. "The Influence of Technology on the Politics of Motherhood: An Overview of the United States." *Women's Studies International Forum* 14: 479-90.

Wright, B.D. 1989. "Reproductive Technologies: Economic and Social Implications: Introduction." In *Healing Technology: Feminist Perspectives*, ed. K.S. Ratcliff et al. Ann Arbor: University of Michigan Press.

Yarborough, M., J.A. Scott, and L.K. Dixon. 1989. "The Role of Beneficence in Clinical Genetics: Non-Directive Counseling Reconsidered." *Theoretical Medicine* 10: 139-49.

Youings, S., N. Gregson, and P. Jacobs. 1991. "The Efficacy of Maternal Age Screening for Down's Syndrome in Wessex." *Prenatal Diagnosis* 11: 419-25.

Young, G., and C. Robinson. 1984. "Attitudes Toward Genetic Engineering: The Dilemma of the Genetically Abnormal Child." *Journal of Applied Behavioral Science* 20: 155-66.

Yoxen, E. 1982. "Constructing Genetic Diseases." In *The Problem of Medical Knowledge: Examining the Social Construction of Medicine*, ed. P. Wright and A. Treacher. Edinburgh: Edinburgh University Press.

Zare, N., J.R. Sorenson, and T. Heeren. 1984. "Sex of Provider as a Variable in Effective Genetic Counseling." *Social Science and Medicine* 19: 671-75.

Zeitune, M., et al. 1991. "Screening for Down's Syndrome in Older Women Based on Maternal Serum Alpha-Fetoprotein Levels and Age: Preliminary Results." *Prenatal Diagnosis* 11: 393-98.

Zimmerman, J. 1981. "Technology and the Future of Women: Haven't We Met Somewhere Before?" *Women's Studies International Quarterly* 4: 355-67.

Zola, I.K. 1983. *Socio-Medical Inquiries: Recollections, Reflections, and Reconsiderations*. Philadelphia: Temple University Press.

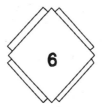

# Manitoba Voices: A Qualitative Study of Women's Experiences with Technology in Pregnancy

## Sari Tudiver

**Executive Summary**

This qualitative research study explores how 37 Manitoba women perceive their experiences with prenatal tests and technologies. The focus of the study was on women's experiences with ultrasound and fetal assessments, maternal serum alpha-fetoprotein (MSAFP) screening, and amniocentesis. These tests are either routinely used in prenatal care (ultrasound) or frequently suggested for use in certain categories of women. The sample also included women who refused testing. The research explored the women's perceptions, cultural beliefs, and attitudes pertaining to uses of technologies during pregnancy and birthing; how the women perceived their needs for information during pregnancy; how the women (and their partners) made decisions, at times in stressful situations; the women's beliefs and attitudes toward disability and abortion; and what the women believed was necessary for good care during pregnancy, specifically in relation to prenatal testing.

Thirty-seven women from diverse backgrounds were each interviewed for approximately two hours. The project was housed at a community health centre and took a participatory feminist approach, recruiting women ranging in age from 16 to 42. The majority of the women had a low income, and English was not the first language of 15.

---

This paper was completed for the Royal Commission on New Reproductive Technologies in July 1992. The research was carried out by the author on behalf of the Women's Health Clinic, Winnipeg.

They varied in education from primary level to post-graduate and were ethnically diverse. They included 10 immigrant and refugee women, three women with disabilities, five teenagers, and three deaf women. The women raised a broad range of issues and concerns pertaining to prenatal testing and prenatal care in general. Despite the considerable social and cultural diversity of the women, a number of common themes emerged.

The study analyzes the women's narratives in terms of both medium and messages. The narratives demonstrate the richness and complexities of the women's perceptions and knowledge of pregnancy and prenatal technologies, some of the ways they integrate and give meaning to these experiences, and how the women express a unique sense of self. The study suggests that health professionals must learn to hear and understand some of these meanings in order to provide better quality care.

Eight major themes are identified from the women's narratives. The women describe "competing constructs of pregnancy" — their subjective, quasi-scientific constructs that reveal pregnancy as a complex physiological, cultural, social, and psychological life event; and a medicalized, disease-oriented construct presented or assumed in most medical encounters, including testing. The women provide detailed examples and insights into the fragmentation of prenatal care and how prenatal testing further reinforces such fragmentation. They identify the contexts and settings within which tests occur and suggest that the meaning of a test cannot be understood apart from the context of how tests are explained and carried out. The women also call attention to the fact that tests occur in a microsetting to which a woman brings her individual history, fears, hopes, stored memories of abuse, and other past experiences, and that these experiences may be triggered in test settings and shape the nature of a woman's anxieties. The medical ideology of testing tends to deny that the context of the tests is important to the patient's health and well-being.

The women identify questioning or refusing tests or procedures as fraught with difficulty and ambivalence. Their stories reveal the delicate balance in medical encounters and in making decisions between trusting the health care provider, receiving sound and appropriate information about the meaning of risks, and having established procedures to ensure informed choices and informed consent. Women also require the self-esteem and assertiveness to ask questions and seek needed supports. A major theme focusses on the women's struggle for respect and empowerment.

The study reveals a continuum of complex attitudes held by these women concerning disability and abortion, which are rooted in personal experiences, culture, and an evaluation of what is possible in a woman's (or family's) circumstances. The women address the promises and contradictions of prenatal testing, providing examples of the desire for reassurance and feelings of alienation. The narratives reveal how the women grappled with and tried to reconcile the contradictions and tensions inherent in testing. They processed complex technical medical/scientific information and risk scores in relation to subjective feelings of wellness; balanced the desire to know as much as possible and control the outcome of the pregnancy with feelings of acceptance; and experienced the discomforts and sometimes the pain of tests and the anguish of waiting for results, while trying to enjoy the wonder of a pregnancy and positive emotions. The study indicates that as prenatal technologies become increasingly routine, testing becomes a kind of metaphor for how women describe the progression of their pregnancies. Pregnancies are socially constructed in new ways.

The women in this study describe a medical system that is fragmented and uncoordinated, and that isolates clients. Whatever a woman's background and circumstances, she perceives a need for support and advocacy to deal with the system. The study suggests that medical care pertaining to pregnancy and childbirth requires serious reforms in institutions and procedures, and profound transformations in philosophy and approach. Social policy decisions pertaining to the introduction and application of prenatal technologies must be evaluated in new ways, paying prime attention to psychological and societal impacts.

The research study provided an opportunity for the women to make recommendations about how prenatal care might be improved and to address specific suggestions pertaining to tests and technologies. Their responses provide profound insights and a vision of a more humane system of prenatal care. Their recommendations have been grouped by area of focus: (1) needed supports and services during pregnancy, birthing, and the post-partum period; (2) improved communication between health professionals and clients; (3) prenatal screening and diagnostic tests, including informed consent, the setting of tests, and philosophical and social policy issues; (4) genetic and fetal research; (5) alternative models of prenatal care and birthing; and (6) general social transformations.

The women express a strong desire to have the options of prenatal screening and testing, but stress the need for informed choices and informed consent pertaining to such tests. They do not support mass screening programs, but an opt-in process with supportive services and resources appropriate to the diversity and needs of all Manitoba women. Alongside a desire for reproductive information and reproductive choices, they have deep concerns about the social, eugenic[1] implications of screening and about negative attitudes toward persons with disabilities in Canadian society. The women hope to live in a society that positively values differences. The conclusions and recommendations of the research study provide some guideposts for balancing these humane goals.

> If none listen, nevertheless the tale is told aloud, to oneself, to prove that there is existence, to tame the chaos of the world, to give meaning. The tale certifies the act of being and gives sense at the same time. Perhaps these are the same, because people everywhere have always needed to narrate their lives and worlds, as surely as they have needed food, love, sex, and safety.
>
> Barbara Myerhoff, *Number Our Days*, 271

## Background, Goals, and Rationale

### Evolution of the Project

The idea for this study was conceived by the members of the Manitoba Working Group on New Reproductive Technologies. The Working Group was formed in 1988 by individuals and representatives of a number of Manitoba community health centres, agencies, and women's organizations in anticipation of a Royal Commission on New Reproductive Technologies being established. The goals were to educate group members and local organizations and to initiate public discussion about reproductive technologies in order to provide optimal input to the Commission's consultation process.

The suggestion for a research study was predicated on the Working Group's goal to ensure the Commission would hear from women from a wide range of backgrounds, reflecting the client base of the community health centres and agencies represented in the Working Group and in Manitoba generally.

There was a particular interest in understanding how women perceive their experiences with diagnostic tests and reproductive technologies that are increasing in use. Working Group members suggested a study to explore how women perceive the increasingly "routine" prenatal testing and procedures and the decisions they and their partners may have to make about these procedures. There was a sense that there was not enough documentation of these experiences from women's perspectives. The Working Group was concerned that issues around making technologies routine might not be given the same prominence by the Commission as high-technology approaches to infertility or prenatal diagnosis.

In the spring of 1991, after the Commission had held public hearings and other meetings in Winnipeg and after the research program of the Commission was under way, the Women's Health Clinic, with the involvement of other interested community health centres and agencies, submitted a proposal for a qualitative research project to interview a sample of women about their experiences with tests and technologies during pregnancy. One goal was to reach women who would not come forward to the Commission in any other way due to social or other barriers.

Specifics of the study evolved as the proposal was developed, reworked, and negotiated with the Commission. The rationale, ethics, and methodology were refined and decisions made about the key emphases.

It was seen as important to permit a woman to explore the overall experiences of a pregnancy and post-partum period in order to understand the context within which tests were perceived and experienced. Therefore, the primary emphasis of the study would be on tests related to prenatal diagnosis, but would also include other tests and technological interventions (including those related to birth) if the woman wished to discuss these tests and saw them as relevant. In the course of the interviews, women also spoke about interventions related to miscarriage and abortion.

It was also seen as essential that the questions address the women's attitudes toward disability and abortion — sensitive issues that affect decisions about prenatal tests. Other areas given priority were communication between clients and health care providers, informed choice, and informed consent.

From the start, the project was consciously community-based. It was located at a community health centre and cultivated a broad base of community support. These features were seen as essential to the integrity and success of the project. Thus, while addressing research questions relevant to the mandate of the Commission, the project was designed to generate information about women's experiences with tests and technology during pregnancy that would be useful to the community from which the information emerged. It was hoped that the study would provide insights into how health care for women during pregnancy might be improved. The Women's Health Clinic provided these rationales to the Commission. The project was approved in October 1991 for completion by the end of April 1992.

I was hired as research coordinator, that is, as principal investigator and project manager. I acted as a liaison between agencies, including the Commission and a variety of resource persons, coordinated recruitment of the women interviewed, conducted all the interviews, analyzed the data, and wrote the final report. A research assistant transcribed the taped interviews and helped code and organize descriptive data.

An Advisory Committee of representatives from interested community health centres and agencies was formed and provided expertise on a wide range of issues, including the design of appropriate questions for immigrant and refugee women, women with disabilities, teenagers, and Aboriginal women — groups with whom these agencies worked directly.[2] The members of the committee vetted criteria and ideas and helped recruit women to the study, they reviewed major issues and recommendations included in the final report, and they will help with follow-up initiatives to ensure that information and conclusions from the research are directed to appropriate Manitoba agencies.

## Goals and Objectives of the Study

The study was designed to provide the Commission with an account of the experiences of some Winnipeg women with medical technologies during pregnancy. Participants in the study were women who had experiences with prenatal screening and testing, but were not likely to come forward and speak to the Commission for various reasons: for example, they experienced barriers of socioeconomic status, cultural differences, or disability; they were not part of an organization that took an interest in these issues; they lacked knowledge about developments in the new reproductive technologies and about the Commission.

The project had three specific objectives:

1. Provide individual women from a variety of backgrounds with the opportunity to tell in their own words their experiences with technologies used during pregnancy, and through this to explore

    (a) their perceptions, cultural beliefs, and attitudes pertaining to uses of technologies during pregnancy and birth;

    (b) how the women perceive their needs for information during pregnancy;

    (c) the ways the women make decisions, at times in stressful situations;

    (d) their beliefs and attitudes toward disability and toward the possibility of having a child with a disability, including how these attitudes may differ among women from different cultural backgrounds, socioeconomic positions, and abilities; and

    (e) what they believe is necessary for good care during pregnancy and birthing.

2. Synthesize and analyze the information provided and present it in a written report to the Royal Commission on New Reproductive Technologies.

3. Provide feedback and other relevant information about the results of the study to the individual participants and to the participating institutions.

It is hoped that from this qualitative research, the Commission, the participants, and the participating institutions will gain additional insights into issues of policy and practice — for example, the following:

- the types of support services that may be needed when particular technologies are used;
- ways to avoid gaps or miscommunication between health care providers and clients concerning the uses of reproductive technologies;

- issues of informed consent and refusal of tests or treatment; and
- how, when, and why technologies are made routine.

As we will see, the conclusions and recommendations address and go beyond some of these anticipated issues.

## Rationale for the Research

The rationale for this research is rooted in a number of complex and conflicting trends in prenatal medical care in Canada. On the one hand, Canada has made significant improvements over the past century in perinatal mortality rates for most sectors of the population — gains due to improved public health measures, better nutrition, birth spacing, and falling birth rates, as well as to prenatal care.[3] As well, over this period pregnancy has become highly medicalized; the dominant disease paradigm is one that promotes the management of women, preferably by specialists, through the course of a potentially dangerous period.[4] There is considerable debate and increasing evidence to demonstrate that increased medicalization of pregnancy has not improved outcomes.[5]

Since the 1960s, strong consumer-driven movements have emerged in North America to de-medicalize pregnancy and childbirth.[6] These movements have stimulated a crucial re-examination of the practice of medicine in pregnancy and childbirth, including the cultural and ideological roots of Western medicine in the oppression and control of women. They have encouraged many consumers to be highly informed and educated about pregnancy and birthing and to explore and press for a range of options, including birthing rooms in hospitals and legalized midwifery in some jurisdictions. They have had some impact on changing the practices and protocols of doctors and institutions to acknowledge the desires of the mother and her partner and to eliminate unnecessary or repressive practices.[7]

There has also been a large increase in the use of diagnostic machinery in prenatal care and birthing over the past 20 years. The use of ultrasound is routine in most pregnancies in Manitoba.[8] Fetal monitoring is widely used during birth, although there seems to be a reconsideration of its benefits.[9] This technology-driven model of care profits product manufacturers, researchers, and technicians. Often technologies are introduced and clear guidelines for appropriate uses are developed only after millions of woman-hours of experience.[10]

In addition, since the early 1980s, research has flourished in biotechnology and human genetics with increased capabilities for various types of genetic screening through fetal and maternal blood serum samples. Through deoxyribonucleic acid (DNA) probes, screening for genes or gene sequences that cause particular disabilities has become possible. The Human Genome Project will extend the capabilities for such screening to include susceptibilities for particular diseases. Currently, the capabilities of screening and diagnosis far outstrip the potential for treatment or cures.[11]

The system of prenatal care is increasingly constructed around testing and diagnosis. Decisions about funding and implementing new technologies and screening programs are made by policy makers, physicians, researchers, and manufacturers of biotechnology processes, products, and equipment used in medical research and diagnostics. Such decision making is largely invisible to the individual client presenting herself for prenatal care and is usually outside an arena of public debate. Increasing numbers of pregnant women find themselves at the intersection of complex trends of scientific advances in genetic screening, increasing medicalization, and routine uses of technology in pregnancy, with the promises tests offer of more information about the health of a fetus. While the results of some tests can provide reassurance about how a pregnancy is progressing, the process of testing can also create anxieties and have an impact on a woman's overall well-being. Women and their partners often must make difficult decisions; they must grapple with possible scenarios of how their family would be changed by the birth of a child with a particular disability, and they must deal with their attitudes toward abortion. At the same time, women are strongly drawn by the ideology that pregnancy is not a disease, but a life experience.

The study focusses on women's experiences when confronted with particular prenatal tests and technologies. How do these experiences shape a woman's perceptions and experiences of her pregnancy as a whole? The study contributes to a deeper understanding of how prenatal technologies have the potential to transform a woman's understanding and consciousness of her pregnancy and her self.

There are recognized gaps in the research literature on how women perceive screening and diagnostic tests during pregnancy.[12] Despite the fact that particular forms of prenatal screening and diagnosis have become routine, women clients (and their partners) are often unclear about the nature and reasons for such testing. Unless they know of a particular hereditary disease or condition in their family, it is difficult to relate to risk factors in particular populations or age groups. Health care providers vary considerably in what types of information they provide about tests. Most have little time and are not trained or financially compensated to explore how well their clients understand the meaning of testing and the further decisions that must sometimes be made due to test results.

In addition, there are few studies about the meanings tests have for pregnant women from different ethnic, class, and social backgrounds, and for pregnant women who have particular disabilities.[13] Yet in Manitoba, the client base of many of the community health centres, urban hospitals, individual practices (of family physicians, obstetricians, and gynaecologists), and agencies providing prenatal education reflects considerable cultural and social diversity. Meeting the physical and emotional needs of a diverse client base is a difficult challenge, especially when most doctors have different social backgrounds and life experiences from many of their clients. As well, male doctors are especially challenged to empathize with the experiences of pregnant women.

In medical encounters, listening carefully and being able to "decode" a woman's narrative are crucial skills for health professionals. For example, women and health care providers may have very different concepts of science and knowledge about pregnancy; they may interpret symptoms and perceive testing in different ways. Profound gaps in communication between health professionals and clients can undermine good care.

## Methodology and Ethics

In this study, the research methods were suited to the specific research problem. Ethical principles were applied throughout the conduct of the inquiry.

### Taking a Feminist, Participatory Approach

Care was taken to articulate and clarify a participatory, feminist approach to research.[14] This approach included six factors:

1. researching a problem identified by and relevant to the local community and the women interviewed;
2. seeking community involvement in the design and evolution of the project;
3. ensuring that the women could participate in the study in ways that were comfortable to them and maximized their input (women were asked not only about their experiences but about what specific changes, if any, they might have wanted in their own prenatal care; they were encouraged to provide recommendations for inclusion in this report);
4. ensuring that feedback from the study would be provided to local agencies and the wider community;
5. ensuring feedback to the women in ways appropriate to them and to be discussed with them; and
6. commitment to encouraging empowerment and self-esteem, especially among women who are marginalized by the health care system. (The study attempted to hear from women who did not have opportunities to speak out about their situations, perspectives, and needs. On this basis, the participating agencies might be in a position to advocate for necessary changes in policies and practices in the health care system.)

## The Value of Qualitative Research to the Study

Research methods that primarily generate qualitative data have always been recognized as appropriate to many of the questions posed by cultural and social anthropologists. Ethnographies, detailed interviews, and life histories have been widely used by medical anthropologists. There is increasing recognition among the health professions of the place and value of qualitative research in understanding complex issues and processes in primary health care. Qualitative research is also being used in the design and evaluation of health programs.[15]

In this study, an approach involving in-depth, semi-structured interviews with 37 individual women, and a detailed analysis by the author of their recorded stories (narratives) to identify the range of issues and common themes, was determined to be the most appropriate. Such interviews have a number of strengths:

1. Flexible, semi-structured interviews provide the scope for listening in depth to a woman's version of her experiences. They allow a woman to express her understanding of what happened to her, in retrospect, and why. The interviews permit a deeper level of detail, including the time to go back and clarify issues, to remember.

2. The interviews provide an easier mode of communication for women who are not literate in English or who may present other barriers in research studies that require more formal protocols (e.g., difficulty with writing because of a disability, or English being their second language).

3. Qualitative research helps us understand the woman's frame of reference; her explanatory model of pregnancy (nature, cause, onset, symptoms); the physiological and emotional aspects of pregnancy; how a woman perceives the state of pregnancy in general and her pregnancy in particular; how the woman thinks her pregnancy should be treated, including her view of appropriate medical interventions.

4. Qualitative research permits a more sensitive exploration of how a woman sees her relationship to her changing body; how in touch she feels with the fetus; how she expresses the process of bonding — or the absence of bonding; her fears, anxieties, and happiness. Women are more apt to express their feelings in detailed interviews.

5. Qualitative research brings insight into how a woman perceives her experience of illness, abortion, or crisis. The depth of the interviews permits exploration of attitudes concerning disability.

6. Qualitative research can explore alternative options about past experiences and future visions — how situations and circumstan-

ces might be different. It gave these women the rare opportunity to analyze, review, and test alternative models of care in a supportive atmosphere.

On the other hand, interviews with the women provide only the women's perspective. There is no direct access to medical files or to information from the health care provider about the rationales for individual treatment. The analysis must be clearly focussed on the women's perceptions and construction of the situations as presented to a third party. The researcher must be aware of and take into account many "silent participants."

## Confidentiality, Consent, and Other Ethical Issues

A number of ethical issues were addressed in the study's design.

- The confidentiality of each woman was assured by removing all identifiers from transcripts; by having secure procedures for storing tapes and notes; and by taking particular care that individual women could not be identified through the report.[16] Individuals' names have been changed, as have specific circumstances that might have resulted in the identification of any of the women. The researcher worked only with trained individuals who were approved or requested by the women themselves and who adhered to protocols of confidentiality.

- A consent form was developed and reviewed. Every woman interviewed signed the form (see Appendix 1).

- As the researcher, I had to be trusted. I went into women's homes and recorded, with permission, some of their deepest feelings and experiences. I attempted to conduct myself appropriately in different cultural settings.

- The women interviewed were each paid an honorarium of $25. This was based on the rationale that the women were being asked to provide considerable time for the study and might incur expenses such as babysitting or transportation. It was a small way to show that we valued their time and effort. As one agency director noted, many researchers draw information from immigrant and other communities with only a letter of thanks in English in return. The money did not appear to be an incentive, per se, to the women, but it was certainly appreciated and made the researcher feel much more comfortable with the time commitment involved.

- Follow-up referral for counselling was available for the participants, if necessary.

## The Sample of Women

### Selection of the Sample

The research proposal for the study indicated several criteria for the sample:

- A minimum of 35 women currently living in Winnipeg would be interviewed.
- The women would have had some experiences with prenatal diagnostic tests or screening during pregnancy. These might include ultrasound and fetal assessment, maternal serum alpha-fetoprotein (MSAFP) screening, amniocentesis, or other forms of prenatal diagnosis or therapy. Experiences might include refusing tests.
- The women would reflect considerable diversity in age, economic backgrounds, levels of formal education, ethnic backgrounds, and abilities.
- Minimum numbers of women in particular social categories would be sought: Aboriginal women (5); immigrant and refugee women (10); women with chronic illness or disabilities (5); adolescents; and others with relevant experiences.
- Participants would not otherwise be screened for whether their experiences with technologies were positive or negative.

Further criteria were elaborated once the project was approved:

- Participants would be limited to women who had been pregnant within the past three years. This was thought to be a reasonable time within which women would be apt to remember explicit details of a pregnancy.
- Women whose pregnancy did not result in a live birth, including women who decided to terminate a pregnancy because of a particular prenatal diagnosis, were to be interviewed, if they came forward.
- After considerable discussion by the Advisory Committee (and consultation with the Commission) it was decided to include but minimize the numbers of women currently pregnant in order to be able to explore the overall experience of a pregnancy. In addition, it might be sensitive or produce anxiety for some women to talk about issues of potential disability and abortion during a current pregnancy, especially if they were waiting for test results. The interview might be blurred with counselling.[17]
- Some women currently pregnant would be interviewed, since women who have two or more pregnancies within a three-year period might otherwise have been excluded from the study.

Women having frequent pregnancies form a significant subset of the client base of some of the community health centres in Winnipeg.

- At the suggestion of the Advisory Committee, the study actively sought women from the deaf community in Winnipeg in order to reach women who rarely have the opportunity to address these issues. It became clear that interviewing one deaf woman would be perceived as a kind of tokenism. I was given the names of three women and interviewed all three, broadening the range of issues facing deaf women in prenatal care.

## Reaching the Women

The potential population from which the sample for this study could be drawn was any woman who had a pregnancy in the past three years currently living in Winnipeg. Since ultrasound, fetal assessments, and maternal serum AFP are widely used in Manitoba during prenatal care, almost any woman who had prenatal care had experiences relevant to this study. Women who actively refused tests or went out of their way to avoid them in a particular pregnancy also had crucial perspectives to share on why they refused.

As specified in the proposal, recruitment took place primarily through a variety of community health centres and other community organizations in Winnipeg. I contacted directors of organizations by phone to discuss the study. When they expressed interest in participating, they were sent a formal letter of request for help in recruiting women and a written description of the goals, methods, ethical principles, and sample questions. In most cases, this information was taken to their boards of directors or appropriate staff, and decisions were made about the nature of the organization's participation.[18] No agency contacted directly refused to participate. Notices about the study were also circulated to other community health centres and selected agencies.

Thirty-seven women were recruited as follows:

- Fourteen women were referred by the health centre or agency staff; these women were asked whether they wished to participate and agreed before having their names passed on to me.

- Ten immigrant and refugee women were recruited through the Immigrant and Refugee Program of Planned Parenthood Manitoba and through a consultant on immigrant and refugee issues at Mount Carmel Clinic. The women were contacted by the staff of these agencies, who explained the study and then obtained their agreement. For the eight women who required interpretation, the staff made the appointments. For the two women not requiring interpretation, once they had agreed to have their names released, I arranged to meet them.

- Seven women who had seen the notice at the community health centres or other agencies called directly to offer to be interviewed.
- Three deaf women were identified and contacted by an outreach worker in their community, who had been informed about the study by me using a deaf access line. When they agreed to participate, I set up the appointments using the deaf access line at the Women's Health Clinic.
- Two women were referred by other participants.
- One woman was referred by another woman who knew about the study.

## A Brief Profile of the Women Interviewed

At the time of the interview, the 37 women ranged in age from 16 to 42, with an average age of 30.4 (Table 1). All the women interviewed had been pregnant at least once during the previous three years. All but one of the women had at least one live birth during that period as well (Table 2). Of the six pregnant women included in the study, all had experienced at least one previous pregnancy.

**Table 1. Ages of Participants**

|  | Range | Average |
| --- | --- | --- |
| Age at time of interview | 16-42 | 30.43 |
| Age at first pregnancy | 14-40 | 25.60 |
| Age at last pregnancy | 16-40 | 29.40 |

**Source:** Transcribed interviews.

### Social Profile

The social profile of the women follows closely the outline in the original proposal:

- Five women were interviewed who had experienced pregnancies between the ages of 14 and 18.
- Ten immigrant and refugee women were interviewed. Their countries or regions of origin were China, Southeast Asia, Africa, and Central America.
- Three women were interviewed who had particular physical disabilities: two had cerebral palsy and one woman had been blind since the age of 18 as a result of retinitis pigmentosa. As

noted above, three deaf women were also interviewed. Since two of the women explicitly made the point that they did not perceive themselves to be disabled or handicapped but part of a deaf culture, the report lists these six as "women with disabilities and deaf women."[19]

- Four rather than five women of Aboriginal descent were interviewed. This was a matter of time and circumstance. One young woman was unable to meet her appointments because of difficulties in her life. She reflected many of the problems facing some teenage mothers. Other Aboriginal women were identified after the study time limit was past.

**Table 2. Pregnancy Outcomes**

| Description | Number of pregnancies | Number of children | Number of women |
|---|---|---|---|
| Live births | 68 | 71[a] | 36[b] |
| Pregnancies not resulting in live birth | 19 | | 11[c] |
| Miscarriages | 12 | | 8 |
| Abortions | 4 | | 4 |
| Ectopic pregnancies | 2 | | 1 |
| Fetal death in third trimester | 1 | | 1 |
| Newborn death | 1 | | 1 |
| Adoptions | | 2 | 1 |
| Currently pregnant | 6 | 7[d] | 6 |
| Total current and expected | 94 | 80 | 37[e] |

a. Three of the pregnancies resulted in twin births.
b. Of the sample of 37 women, one is currently pregnant and has had no live births.
c. Some women experienced more than one pregnancy not resulting in a live birth.
d. One of the women is pregnant with twins.
e. Subtotals in this column do not add up because some women are counted in more than one category.

**Source:** Transcribed interviews.

- Other ethnic backgrounds of the women included Ukrainian, German-Mennonite, English, French, Scottish, and Irish.
- The women's religious backgrounds included Catholic, Protestant, and Buddhist. Some of the women said they had strong religious beliefs; others did not.

### *Education, Work Backgrounds, and Income*

The women's educational experiences were varied. Six women had completed primary school. Sixteen had completed high school and another three were in the process of finishing high school. Twelve women had some university training or had graduated from university. Of these, three had post-graduate degrees or training. Of the women who had completed primary and high school, most had taken some type of training course or program.

Most of the women were currently working or had worked at a variety of industrial, clerical, and professional jobs. These jobs included that of secretary, hairdresser, maintenance worker or cleaner, waitress, meat-packing plant worker, garment factory worker, vegetable cleaner in a factory, sheltered workshop employee, outreach or community worker, part-time student, store manager, self-employed business person, teacher (in home country), education consultant, nurse, midwife, medical assistant, and full-time homemaker. Many women indicated that they had aspirations to return to school or to seek training once their children were a bit older. In particular, some of the teenagers who had difficult early years hoped to go into such fields as social work and corrections.

As Table 3 notes, approximately 65 percent of the women in this sample were classified as low income on the basis of direct information they provided — in some cases supplemented by the researcher's assessment of the woman's situation through visiting her home. About 25 percent of the sample (nine women) were single mothers. This included four of the five teenagers and five other women, all of whom were low income.

### *Medical Profiles*

As Table 4 summarizes, the women reported a number of pre-existing medical conditions, conditions that developed during or as a result of their pregnancies, and several fetal conditions. This information provided a basis from which to interpret the kinds of testing and interventions described and the woman's overall discussion of her pregnancy. Where a condition or procedure was not clearly explained, I sought some professional medical advice, including such issues as why a woman might have had two amniocenteses, and the implications of active herpes for vaginal delivery. All the information provided is self-reported and thus gives insight into the ways the women perceived, interpreted, understood, and labelled their medical conditions and symptoms. Similarly, all the information reported in Tables 5 to 8 is based on self-reports and forms the outlines for understanding how the women perceived the rationales for prenatal screening and diagnostic tests and how they came to make the decisions they did.

## Table 3. Social Information

| Category | Number |
|---|---|
| General | |
|     Teenagers[a] | 5 |
|     Women of Aboriginal descent | 4 |
|     Women with disabilities and deaf women | 6 |
|     Women who were immigrants or refugees | 10 |
|     Mothers of children with disabilities or genetic anomalies | 3[b] |
|     Single mothers | 9 |
| Income | |
|     Low income[c] | 24 |
|     Middle income | 13 |
| Education range | primary to master's |
| Language | |
|     First language is English | 22 |
|     First language is other than English[d] | 15 |
|     Number of interviews using interpretation | 11[e] |

a. The teenagers in this study had pregnancies between the ages of 14 and 19.
b. One of these children was adopted.
c. These rough categories indicate that a majority of women interviewed experienced barriers of poverty. Criteria for low income are direct information provided by the woman about social assistance or limited income; the researcher's assessment of the woman's resources through visiting her home; indications of financial precariousness — e.g., her husband is laid off; she is a single mother in school. A woman who indicated she worked in a secure job or was on maternity leave, or whose resources appeared to support a reasonable standard of living, was categorized as middle income.
d. Includes American sign language.
e. Includes three using American sign language.

**Source:** Transcribed interviews.

**Table 4. Medical Conditions Identified by the Women**

| Pre-existing medical conditions | Conditions associated with pregnancy or post-partum period | Fetal medical conditions |
|---|---|---|
| cerebral palsy | gestational diabetes | hereditary webbing of fingers and extra fingers |
| retinitis pigmentosa | hyperemesis | thoracic dystrophy |
| congenital hip problem | severe and mild post-partum stress | intrauterine death at 35 weeks |
| hereditary, congenital, and childhood deafness | infections | fetal hernia |
| hand deformity | pneumonia | |
| intestinal bypass surgery | severe back pain | |
| herpes | adhesions from previous Caesarian section | |
| narrow pelvis | high blood pressure | |
| obesity | headaches | |
| migraines | migraines | |
| anaemia | numbness | |
| depression | cardiac arrhythmias | |
| infertility (causes unknown) | abnormal Pap results — early-stage uterine cancer | |

Source: Transcribed interviews.

## Table 5. Prenatal Tests and Birth Situations

| Prenatal tests | N |
|---|---|
| Women who actively refused tests | 9 |
| Women who had at least one ultrasound | 33 |
| Women who had one fetal assessment | 1 |
| Women who had more than one fetal assessment | 14[a] |
| Women who knew they had a maternal serum AFP test in one or more pregnancies | 14 |
| Women who thought they might have had a maternal serum AFP test | 2 |
| Women with positive maternal serum AFP test results | 10 |
| Women who had amniocentesis | 7 |
| Women who had other prenatal diagnostic tests[b] | 2 |
| Birth situations | |
| Women who had at least one Caesarian section | 13 |
| Women who had two Caesarian sections | 2 |
| Women who had three Caesarian sections | 2 |
| Women who had breech births | 3 |
| Women who had home births | 2[c] |
| Women who had or were currently pregnant with twins | 4 |

a. The number ranged from two to seven.
b. Scraping of the fetal sac and cordocentesis.
c. One in Manitoba and one in Cambodia.

**Source:** Transcribed interviews.

### Table 6. Women Having Amniocentesis or Related Procedures

| Number | Age at pregnancy | Procedure | Time (woman's estimate) | Reason for procedure | Outcome |
|---|---|---|---|---|---|
| 4 | 31 | amniocentesis attempted; scraping of fetal sac | not stated | positive alpha-fetoprotein (AFP); risk of Down syndrome; scraping done since amniocentesis attempt failed | negative |
| 11 | 35 | amniocentesis | "early in pregnancy" | maternal age | negative |
|  |  | amniocentesis | 35 weeks | gestational diabetes | diagnostic |
| 12 | 35 | amniocentesis | 6 months | maternal age; risk of handicap; requested by mother | negative |
| 13 | 32 | amniocentesis and cordocentesis | not stated | requested by mother; artery missing in umbilical cord | negative |
| 16 | 35 | amniocentesis | not stated | AFP count high | negative |
| 19 | 37 | amniocentesis | not stated | maternal age; fear of Down syndrome; requested by mother | negative |
| 28 | 16 | amniocentesis | 18 weeks | high AFP and fetal hernia | results unknown at interview |

**Source:** Transcribed interviews.

Table 7. Women Refusing Prenatal Screening or Diagnostic Tests

| Number | Age at pregnancy | Test refused | Indication for test | Reasons for refusal |
|---|---|---|---|---|
| 5 | 34 | amniocentesis | AFP levels high | fear of miscarriage; risk of miscarriage equivalent to risk of fetal abnormality |
| 10 | 34 | amniocentesis | AFP levels high | couldn't live with herself if she miscarried due to amniocentesis; fear of miscarriage; experience with persons with disabilities |
| 15 | 29 | AFP | "routine screening" | mother saw no point in taking it; would never consider abortion |
| 16 | 37 | amniocentesis | high AFP; maternal age | twins and higher risk of miscarriage |
| 21 | 40 | AFP and amniocentesis | maternal age | doesn't feel she could terminate; mother is aware of false positives; felt healthy; did not want amniocentesis; experience with children with disabilities |
| 27 | 39 | amniocentesis | AFP levels high; maternal age | wouldn't consider abortion |
| 29 | 37 | amniocentesis | AFP levels high; maternal age | would abort if baby had Down syndrome or severely handicapped; did not feel risk was high; past experience fine; "has not sinned" |

### Table 7. (cont'd)

| Number | Age at pregnancy | Test refused | Indication for test | Reasons for refusal |
|---|---|---|---|---|
| 30 | 30 | amniocentesis | suggested by doctor for better information | wouldn't terminate pregnancy if disability found; felt she would miscarry; personal experience with cerebral palsy and with children with disabilities |
| 32 | 24 and 26 | ultrasound | to check dates | non-interventionist philosophy; had concerns about possible effects of ultrasound on fetus |

Source: Transcribed interviews.

### Table 8. Women with Positive Maternal Serum AFP Results

| Number | Age at pregnancy | Time of AFP (according to mother) | Results ("high," "low," "positive") | Follow-up (e.g., repeat AFP; genetic counselling; ultrasound; fetal assessments) | Outcome (healthy baby; twins) |
|---|---|---|---|---|---|
| 1 | 16 | 3 months 4 months | positive high level at 3 months; negative at 4 months | repeat AFP; genetic counselling; fetal assessments | healthy baby |
| 4 | 31 | not stated | positive levels high | repeat AFP; attempted amniocentesis; fetal sac scraping | healthy baby |
| 5 | 34 | not stated | positive levels high | genetic counselling; refused amniocentesis | healthy baby |

Table 8. (cont'd)

| Number | Age at pregnancy | Time of AFP (according to mother) | Results ("high," "low," "positive") | Follow-up (e.g., repeat AFP; genetic counselling; ultrasound; fetal assessments) | Outcome (healthy baby; twins) |
|---|---|---|---|---|---|
| 6 | 32 | not stated | positive levels low | counselling; went for amniocentesis; determined her dates wrong, so MSAFP normal | healthy baby |
| 7 | 28 | not stated | positive levels high | ultrasound | twins |
| 10 | 34 | 3 months | positive levels high | ultrasound; fetal assessments; refused amniocentesis; repeat AFPs through pregnancy | healthy baby |
| 16 | 35 | 4 months | positive levels | repeat AFP; genetic counselling; amniocentesis | healthy baby |
|    | 37 | 4 months | positive levels | ultrasound; refused amniocentesis | twins |
| 27 | 39 | not stated | positive | counselling; refused amniocentesis | healthy baby |
| 28 | 16 | not stated | positive | ultrasound; amniocentesis | fetal hernia; currently pregnant |
| 29 | 37 | not stated | positive levels high | counselling; refused amniocentesis | breech delivery; healthy baby |

Source: Transcribed interviews.

## Strengths and Limitations of the Sample

The sample of 37 women is reasonably large by the standards of many qualitative research projects and relative to the time frame.[20] The study provided considerable depth and diversity in the issues put forward. A number of common themes emerged through analysis of the data. The variety of medical conditions, ages, and social backgrounds of the women permitted insight into a significant range of experiences during pregnancy.

No generalizations based on percentages from this group of women can be made to the wider population of Manitoba women of those same ages or backgrounds.[21] However, the experiences of these women have many elements in common with others receiving prenatal care in Manitoba. Many of the situations and conditions of these women are readily recognized within the obstetrical practices of Manitoba doctors and genetic counsellors and in prenatal clinics.[22]

A limited group of immigrant and refugee women was interviewed, reached through agencies advisory to the research study. The women interviewed were likely more knowledgeable about tests and technologies and prenatal care in Canada because of their contacts with programs specifically providing health education and health advocacy services to immigrant and refugee women. Additional issues and concerns might have been raised by women who had no contacts with such programs. Women from India, Eastern European countries, and other backgrounds might have identified additional issues as well.

The study drew a proportionately large number of women with positive maternal serum AFP results (10 women out of 37, or 27 percent). In contrast, approximately 8 percent of Manitoba women who received the maternal serum AFP test in 1990 had positive results.[23] Women with positive results might have come forward or been referred to the study because they felt they had something to say about testing or because health care providers thought they would be interesting subjects. Given the goals of the study, they proved to be an important subset of women because they were able to share the diverse and common ways in which anxiety is experienced. They described a range of experiences with doctors and technicians.

The study drew a relatively large number of women who had experienced at least one Caesarian section (13 women out of 37). Reasons for Caesarian sections included cerebral palsy, herpes, breech births, narrow pelvis, and numerous complications surrounding the birth of twins. The women's experiences thus captured some of the diversity surrounding the reasons for Caesarian sections in major teaching hospitals in Winnipeg.[24] The sample also included three women who had had twins and one who was currently pregnant with twins. Again, the women came forward because they or their practitioners believed they would have something to say about technological interventions.

The data provided on this non-probability, purposive-convenience sample of women are descriptive. No attempts were made to manipulate variables — for example, using non-parametric statistics for small samples.

## The Interview Process

### Sites of the Interviews

The women were given a choice of where they would prefer to have the interview conducted. They were also offered transportation to and from the interview. Sixteen interviews were conducted at the Women's Health Clinic in a private counselling room. Four were conducted in private rooms in other agencies involved in the study. Four women brought nursing infants with them. Seventeen interviews were conducted in the women's homes, while children slept, played, were held, or were at day-care. In one interview, the husband stayed throughout the interview and participated actively through the interpreter.

### Use of Interpreters

In seeking women from diverse backgrounds, I was assisted by the skills of seven women who provided interpretation in 11 interviews. Eight of the interviews involved the professional assistance of four health educators working in Planned Parenthood Manitoba's Immigrant and Refugee Health Program.

The health educators provided services to the study beyond language interpretation. They, along with another immigrant woman consultant, advised on design of the interview questions and the consent form to ensure they were culturally appropriate and clear to the women from their communities. They identified potential participants, contacted the women to discuss the study, and secured their approval. They served as a point of entry into these communities. They provided crucial information since they had, in many cases, also attended the medical appointments with the women interviewed. During the interview, they clarified questions and comments where necessary and eased the situation through humour and talking with children and husbands. They debriefed with me about how they felt during the interviews and were able to explain cultural beliefs and medical issues.

Three of the 11 interviews were conducted with deaf women and used the skills of professional interpreters working in American sign language (ASL) for the Independent Interpreter Referral Service in Winnipeg. At the request of the woman, one of these interviews involved the use of two interpreters, one deaf ASL "relay" interpreter and one hearing ASL interpreter.[25]

### Format of the Interviews

The interviews began with my discussing the reasons for the study and a brief background of the Commission (six of the women had heard of it); I also stated that the report presented to the Commission would try to reflect the concerns and issues raised by the women. There would also be feedback to the local agencies and to them, if they wished.

I summarized the key points in the consent form. Most of the women then read it themselves. I read the form to the visually impaired woman; two of the deaf women asked that it be read aloud and signed to them. The health educators translated the form orally and presented it to the women; in all cases, the women signed the English version.

I asked if they had any questions or concerns and reiterated that they were free to ask anything during the course of the interview. For those who permitted a tape recorder, I turned it on and began the interview. If they refused, I wrote detailed notes of their answers.[26] I did not refer to a list of questions, although they remained in a file folder, accessible if needed.

The interviews generally followed a generic set of questions (see Appendix 2). Questions were adapted to the specific situation of each woman, as well as to the broader circumstances of her life (e.g., whether she was an immigrant, teenager, etc.). Depending on the flow of the discussion, we covered the issues in different sequences, sometimes coming back to clarify and explore issues raised earlier.

The women were asked to set aside approximately two hours for the interview. This generally proved appropriate to the task. Individual interviews ranged between 1.5 and 4.5 hours.

## Assessing the Reliability of the Interviews

### The Women's Voices

The interviews provide a narrative (transcribed or summary version) of what the women chose to tell me about their experiences with tests during pregnancy and about their pregnancies in general. Except where interpreters had something to add, there are no other sources available concerning what happened during the particular medical encounters.

As qualitative social documents, the narratives can be evaluated systematically for their consistency and reliability.[27] These can be assessed by consciously examining the internal consistencies within each interview, the consistencies across interviews, the role of the interviewer, and the nature of the interaction between interviewer and participant. A number of elements were examined in these narratives. They suggest that the narratives satisfy criteria of reliability and that a similar sample of women interviewed about the same issues would come forward with a highly similar set of issues and concerns.

#### *Consistency Within the Narrative*

If there are specific inconsistencies (e.g., dates of tests and other references), one must ask why. Was the woman nervous during the interview or under stress? Is English her second language? Were there problems understanding my question or the interpretation? Did her confusion reflect the difficulty of absorbing information provided to her by others? Did she wish to avoid talking about a certain topic? Was the information not particularly important to her? If so, why? Was I confused about her response? Overall, there were few inconsistencies that could not be clarified during the interview or with interpreters, or puzzled out once the transcript was read several times.

### The Woman's Attempts to Clarify and Provide Explanations

The woman's efforts to go back and correct a version when she thought she made errors or misinterpretations suggest her own criteria for accuracy.

### The Woman's Analysis and Balance of Viewpoints

How she presents her own situation and whether she tries to take into account alternative points of view can indicate reliability. Many women attempted to look at a situation from the point of view of the health care provider, even when describing a personally difficult situation. Others noted that given their own experiences, the situations of women who had multiple barriers (e.g., poverty, single parenthood, etc.) would be even more difficult.

### The Woman's Involvement in the Process of the Interview, Including Whether It Changed After the Recorder Was Turned Off

Assessing involvement is sometimes difficult, especially when there are different cultural styles and differentials of power between interviewer and participant. The interview was a delicate process of building trust and assessing some shared meanings. Two hours usually provided enough time to build a basic sense of trust and for me to gauge the woman's involvement in the interview.

The intangibles of interviewing — the comfort levels between interviewer and participant — are key here and differed with each woman. With some there was quick rapport; with others it built more slowly. Overall, I experienced very good communication; no one looked at her watch or sought to terminate the interview early.

In the interviews with interpreters, rapport between interpreters and the women appeared excellent. The interpreters were known to the women beforehand. Laughter, warm interactions, and a sense of comfort transmitted across the language barrier.

### The Nature of Disclosure

Pregnancy was recognized as a personal experience. No woman questioned the need to talk a bit about her background and, in many cases, to share some very personal feelings and experiences, because she considered them relevant to the discussion. For example, most of the women offered personal information about relationships with partners and family; some discussed sexuality and sexual relations (questions about these were not asked); some shared information about depression.

Sometimes a woman indicated that something was confidential, but that she believed it was important for me to know so that I could better understand her other experiences.

This confidence suggests that most women did feel comfortable with the interview process, agreed with the goals of the study, and saw that it was appropriate to make these things known. There was less disclosure of very personal issues with the immigrant, refugee, and deaf women, given the presence of interpreters and cultural differences, such as differences in what constitute polite questions. However, when women felt close to the health educators, they often provided deep insights and details about their personal feelings throughout the pregnancy. There were only a few instances where I sensed that a woman did not wish to talk about an issue, and I never probed beyond that.

### Sensitive Questions and How They Were Handled

Sometimes a seemingly straightforward question raised difficult issues early in the interview, before a higher degree of trust was established. For example, when I asked "How many pregnancies have you had?" one woman paused slightly and answered, "Two — I will tell you about the second one later on." As it turned out, she had very recently had an abortion and had told no one except her husband, one friend, and me. Certainly her desire to tell her story as completely as possible and provide reliable information overrode her reticence. The setting also gave her an opportunity to explore her feelings in a structured and secure way.

### Listening for the Voices That Are Not There — The Physician, the Technician, the Nurse

As the interviewer, I tried to ask myself what a woman might have said in a particular setting. Is the woman's version stressing one of many things said by herself or by the health care provider? How do I explore this in order to better understand why she is telling me certain things and not others?

### Completeness or Closure

In most of the interviews, we seemed toward the end to circle around to themes identified earlier. I gave the women an opportunity to add some last points before closing. I asked, "Do you feel you had your say? Are there other things you want to raise?" Often, the woman added something.

### Consistency Across the Interviews

Despite the differences in social background, age, and experience among the women, the interviews raised a number of common themes and issues. To validate these, I had several discussions with health care providers — a nurse-midwife working in fetal assessment, an obstetrician-gynaecologist, a geneticist, and the health professionals involved in the project Advisory Committee. They confirmed that many of these issues were very relevant and current in their settings of client care.

## The Role and Reactions of the Interviewer

The interviewer is an integral part of the interview process and as such my role must be scrutinized for its impact on the setting and the information secured.

For me, interviewing is a delicate balance of encouraging the woman to feel comfortable to talk in her own way; listening very carefully; being genuinely engaged and supportive while at the same time watchful for nuances that might lead to other questions; clarifying what I don't understand; intervening when appropriate about views or issues a woman might want to reflect on; and recognizing, yet trying to step beyond, barriers of class, education, culture, and race by acknowledging them. In some cases, the woman may have held back from saying certain things because I was white, educated, and more obviously identified with the health professionals she was being asked to discuss than with herself.

I had to trust my intuition. For example, when I thought someone was describing negative attitudes toward Aboriginal people but did not name it as racism, I tried to give the woman scope to identify it as a social issue. I waited, and if she did not name the issue, I proposed it, saying, "I have talked with others who think that Aboriginal women receive poorer treatment from some health professionals just because they are Aboriginal. Do you feel this was true for you in this case? I'm not trying to put words in your mouth. I really want to understand what it meant to you."

With each interview, I attempted to assess my comfort level. Did I interject too often? appropriately or not? How did I react to particular disclosures? Sometimes I was ignorant — as, for example, concerning the strength of positive attitudes toward deafness in the deaf community. For example, one woman would like there to be a prenatal test for deafness; she *wants* her children to be deaf. "English is my second language. Being deaf is a culture." I attempted to explore these issues with deaf women in subsequent interviews and through reading.[28]

This interview process cannot be romanticized. It was not "friendship" or "two women sharing equally." I had an explicit agenda, and in some cases the women came with their own agenda: to tell about experiences during pregnancy that mattered to them very much. There was no expectation that I would be their friend, just that I would facilitate the telling of their stories. With a few women I felt very deep rapport; with the others, I was engaged, often fascinated, and entirely drawn into the process. They did not choose to ask or know anything about me specifically in the course of the interview — they saw the Women's Health Clinic and the Commission as legitimate institutions and me as their representative. Often it is easier to tell one's story to an empathetic stranger.

My own reactions to the process of the interviews were complex. The interviews took considerable emotional energy. They raised memories both sad and joyful about my own pregnancy and stories my late mother told me about hers. At the same time, to hear and watch what the women said and the strength with which they said it was energizing and hopeful. It pushed me to see beyond my normal daily boundaries, to visit parts of Winnipeg I had never seen and sit in homes I could not have entered any other way. Working with interpreters taught me to watch facial expressions and body language, and to feel connections to women in new ways. The interviews with women with disabilities challenged me the most — it took me a while to understand that their pregnancies were not much different from those of any of the other women; it was the social attitudes of others against their daring to become mothers that created the really important differences. The stories of all the women and the strong emotions with which they were told are now part of my knowledge base. This is very privileged information and I feel a tremendous responsibility to transmit their experiences and recommendations with integrity.

## The Women's Narratives

The raw data of the study are narrative documents, transcriptions of the taped interviews, and detailed summaries of what the women said. The narratives are documents rich in descriptive detail, imagery, dialogue, and nuance.[29] They provide the content from which the major themes are drawn in the following sections.

What the women said is also embedded in how they said it, how they wove themes, issues, stories, and answers to particular questions into a narrative whole. In this study, it became increasingly clear that the medium was a crucial part of the message.

This section of the report examines some of the narrative styles and diversity of the women's knowledge as reflected in the interviews. This attempt to decode the narratives seeks to show (1) the richness and complexities of the women's perceptions and understandings about pregnancy and prenatal technologies; (2) some of the ways the women process, integrate, and give meaning to these experiences; and (3) how the women express a unique sense of self.

Throughout the interviews, women noted how their attempts to tell their stories in depth are excluded from most medical encounters. There is limited value placed on useful exchanges between client and health care provider in the health care system. In contrast to these non-linear narratives, communication with health care providers emphasizes a linear sequence of symptoms and physiological changes and rarely the meanings people assign to these. Almost all of the women interviewed expressed some degree of dissatisfaction with their medical encounters. While some women provided examples of caring health professionals, the many negative comments highlight the need for much more sensitive ways of listening and decoding information by health care providers and for basic transformations in how medical encounters are structured. Focussing on the narrative styles, kinds of knowledge, and how the women came to have some of the knowledge they do alerts us to the fact that what women say and how they say it, including their silences, are important clues to the meaning their stories hold. One implication of this study is that health professionals must be able to hear and understand some of these meanings to provide good care.

## Narrative Styles

The women were told that they had considerable control over the interview. Some women began more timidly and built toward a powerful crescendo. A few needed a steady flow of questions and encouragement. They provided details when we reached a particular issue or set of issues that they wanted to discuss in depth. Others had a story to tell and jumped in; I sometimes had to interrupt to clarify dates of tests and other details. These women used the opportunity to place prenatal tests in the context of their life story. In answer to specific questions, they told me they were getting to that or they needed to tell me something else first so I would understand.

Despite the common questions, each woman shaped the narrative to cover particular themes of importance to her. For example, Sue emphasized her lack of self-esteem when she was pregnant previously and placed her discussion of prenatal testing in that framework. She had felt dominated by her ex-husband and went along with anything suggested to her by doctors. At that time, she said, she had little interest in knowing about tests. Information was hard to secure because she is deaf. She wanted to have an ultrasound in her current pregnancy and saw it as a sign of her growing self-esteem and desire for knowledge about the pregnancy.

Ruth spoke movingly and in detail about her post-partum stress following the birth of her first child and linked it to her experiences during pregnancy and a traumatic breech birth. Despite numerous questions about prenatal testing, which she had experienced, it was the post-partum period that dominated her story. Her post-partum experiences influenced her fears and actions in subsequent pregnancies, including demanding more testing to ensure she would not have another breech. A study that asked only about prenatal tests might have missed these important links.

Kathy's narrative theme highlighted the need for pregnant women to be critical consumers of prenatal health care services. She documented her own evolution as a critical consumer through her three pregnancies, as she increasingly questioned whether ultrasounds and AFP screening were necessary to what she believed were normal, healthy pregnancies. She recently trained to be a childbirth educator.

Each story reflects choices made by the woman to share, withhold, or otherwise control information. Sometimes a woman decided to speak about certain personal experiences at the end of the interview, once we had built up enough trust and once other parts of the story had been told. A few women said they came forward because they believed it was important for the Commission to hear of such experiences. Some really wanted an opportunity to talk — they were personally involved in trying to understand what happened to them, or what to do in current or future pregnancies regarding tests and technologies. In the time between speaking with me and arranging the appointment, many of the women had thought about what they wanted to say and had made some decisions about what they might disclose. It appeared to be a therapeutic retelling and working through of issues. As Jean put it, "When I saw the notice about the study, I had been thinking a lot about the tests I had and what to do now that I'm pregnant again. I'm really confused." Sally had been waiting for an opportunity to talk: "It's incredible. Someone is allowing me to do this. How many weeks do you have?"

The women's narrative styles varied even within a single narrative. For example, many women spoke in dialogue to depict particular situations. The dialogue does not indicate accurate recall but suggests the importance of the interaction: how the woman was engaged, how she integrated the information, and how she perceived what others said.

Ina used dialogue to exaggerate and make her points much more dramatic. She is a highly articulate 25-year-old who must speak slowly and has trouble pronouncing certain letters clearly because of cerebral palsy. Early in the interview she described her struggle to have people listen to her, to accept her as the intelligent, humorous person that she is.

> Ina: I was kind of excited when I found out I was pregnant because all my life as I was growing up and I was a teenager I asked the doctor straight out in Ontario I asked him, "Can I ever conceive a child?" and he goes, "No, you're just a stupid cripple, you'll never conceive," and I'm like, "How can you say that when you haven't really seen me or seen what my body is like?"
>
> Interviewer: He actually said that?
>
> Ina: Not in so many words. But that's basically what he summed it up to. I said, "That's not fair, how do you know until I actually have conceived or have lost a few children?" But he goes, "Most people that are handicapped cannot have children." So when I actually found out that I was carrying my daughter I was quite happy but I was also very, very scared because I did not know how to handle the rest of my life. Because of the fact when I was growing up they said, "You'll never be able to conceive and you'll never be able to live alone and you'll never be able to do this and that."
>
> Interviewer: How old were you when you asked that doctor about whether you could have children?
>
> Ina: I think I was about 17 going on to 18. He goes, "No, you cannot and you never will conceive a child." I'm like, "Excuse me, this is me we're talking about, don't ever tell me that, I love kids, I want my own child one of these days." He turned around and he goes, "No, I want you

to go and have yourself tied." And he told my mother this too. "It's my life. What happens if I fall in love with somebody and I want to have their child, you cannot take that freedom away from me." He goes, "I want you to go have it tied," and I said, "Forget it."

Accuracy was not the point here. Ina wanted me to hear the meaning of her experiences and her perception of how one doctor tried to deny her sexuality and her hopes to have children some day. She went on to describe the real threat, once she became pregnant, that her child would be taken away by Child and Family Services because they did not think she could adequately care for her. The doctor who provided her prenatal care was very supportive and helped her mobilize financial and other resources for home care.

This background set the stage for my understanding Ina's satisfaction with her prenatal care and with her experiences with testing. She trusted her doctor and participated in decisions about her care. She had no genetic screening, went for regular check-ups and two ultrasounds, and had a planned Caesarian section. Ina's pregnancy was relatively unproblematic, quite normal despite her cerebral palsy and wheelchair mobility.

> The only extra precaution that he really took is that he had me come and see him more frequently than he would with anybody else, all through the pregnancy, I was going every two weeks ... My doctor was very concerned but also very understanding ... He just wanted to have an extra ultrasound to make sure the baby's lungs were developed and the odd X-ray to make sure my lungs and everything were intact. I wasn't having any problems ... I didn't need many tests. I was just lucky, I guess.

In the face of external threats, her doctor's attitudes were reassuring and kind. Unlike the first doctor, he did not judge her for wanting children, but supported her decision and helped it happen. Frequent ultrasounds or fetal assessments might have been justifiable to some doctors given her disability, but would have added to her stress and physical discomfort.

The style of Ina's narrative riveted my attention to her early negative experiences and allowed me to understand that the essence of her struggle as a woman with a disability was, to her, primarily social and systemic.

Other women's narratives described in gripping detail their anxieties about testing and provided a window into what they considered crucial to the experience.

In the first part of the narrative, Ruth talked about receiving positive maternal serum AFP results. To her, that meant the risk of Down syndrome.

> One problem we did have — it was Good Friday, the day before Good Friday. Two weeks before that I had gone in for my regular check-up — or a month before that, she took a blood test for the alpha-fetoprotein test. The test came back the Thursday before Good Friday and she phoned me and she said to come into the office, "I want to talk to you

about the results of this test." So I'm just ah ... I don't know what this alpha-fetoprotein test all does, but she wanted to talk to me about it. She said, "Don't worry, just come and talk." So I went, fine. So I went there, I'll never forget this, it's like it just happened yesterday, I sat down in her office and she looked at me and said, "The test came back saying either the fetus has died or your baby has Down syndrome," and I thought, "Oh, my God." I don't know what to say. She says, "I'm going to send you over to the hospital and you're going to have an emergency ultrasound just to see if the fetus is alive," because like this is Easter long weekend and I don't want to go through Easter and not knowing if this child is alive or not in me. So I went for the test, it's not a very clear one because I didn't have a chance to drink all the fluid, so here I am running to the store drinking all these drinks as fast as I can to get there, to get the test done, finally get in there, she says, "The fetus is alive," phew. "Of course we cannot tell if the child has Down syndrome or not. So you're going to have to go home and wait around and come back and we'll do an amniocentesis. Now we'll take you to the lab, we'll get another AFP test just to make sure, to see the results." So I go down for a blood test, they take my blood and I go home. Just bawling all the way home thinking, "I'm going to have a Down's child."

It was the most horrifying Easter I had. I went home crying, phoned my parents, not knowing what to do, how can I raise a Down syndrome child because my marriage is stable but it puts a big strain because it takes a lot to raise a Down syndrome child. So that Easter Monday, I go back to work and I talk to a lady at work, she has a Down syndrome grandson and she tells me how wonderful the child is and how loving and how caring and understanding but it takes a lot, a lot of work. So I'm going, "What am I going to do?" So I go back to see the doctor, she says, "The same test came back the same way. We're going to have to do an amniocentesis." Fine, okay. So by the time they book, by the time I get in to the hospital, I don't even know how much of this lapsed because I was just, I couldn't think about anything else, but thinking how am I going to raise the child like this. Going to have it done, during the ultrasound to insert the needle she goes into fetal distress, so they can't do it because they figure the fluid would not be able to be replaced because she was in distress and they figured that she might die if they take the fluid out. So here I go back home again waiting another week or so before they decide what they're going to do. They decided what they're going to do is do like a Pap smear but take a scraping of the sac and do the test with that because they can do the same amount of testing with the scraping of the sac. But there's a chance of the sac being nicked so you have to be very careful. I go back to the hospital, get this done, of course you have to wait, this is all DNA testing and all sorts of stuff, so you really have to take time to get the results back.

So we're waiting another two weeks or so. By this time, I'm at the border of having an abortion or not, I'm at the border within days. By that time she started to move, I remembered laying in bed and the baby started to move and I called my husband and he held me and we felt the baby move. I said, "I can't do it, I don't care if she has Down's or not, I can't

> do it, we'll have to raise a Down's child. I just can't abort it." I've always been against it anyways, in a way. If it's severely — I can see it, but with Down's I was going to try. So we decided, we got the results back saying there's a certain percent of chance that she'll come out totally normal. That they're not 100 percent these tests, there's still a chance for error. So I phoned my mother back, she says, "Well, what have you decided?" "I've decided to have it." She says, "Well, I'll come in and help you as much as I can." So going through the rest of my pregnancy, I kept busy by working and trying not to think about it. I was just preparing for it and I was just hoping it was going to be healthy, that's all I cared.

I later went back and asked her if the doctor explained that other conditions, not just Down syndrome, might have caused the positive test result. She acknowledged that the doctor posed several possibilities, but clearly the option of Down syndrome affected her most. Her focus on Down syndrome suggests an attempt to confront her deepest fears of what might happen.

> She did to a point explain what an alpha-fetoprotein test is but not to an extent of, because when she said Down's, I was just, I wasn't expecting that. Oh sure, she said my dates could have been screwed up, my dates couldn't be exact on, that could have really screwed up the protein tests ... Sure, it wasn't told before. She tried to inform me as much as she could, I guess ... I think she gave me a piece of paper about it, but it was like a lot of mumble jumble, like you couldn't understand half the words that were on the paper. There was no list of what could come about with these tests, there was no detailed list of all the things that they look for. Just they say "abnormalities," and that's basically what they said.

The narratives provide rich detail about how women processed the medical and technical information presented. Woven through the women's descriptions are emotions of fear, guilt, shame, vulnerability, rage, anger, insecurity, joy, and sadness. The passion in these narratives reinforces how significant these life events are. It is through the often passionate telling and retelling of such stories that women construct the sequences of what happened to them and ascribe meaning to these major life events.

## Kinds of Knowledge

The narratives also reflect the complex kinds of knowledge that the women have about their bodies, pregnancy in general, the health care system, and medical technologies. What women know is rarely articulated in clinical encounters.

Such knowledge includes the woman's knowledge about how her body works, its biology and physiology, and her technical-scientific or folk-scientific knowledge base about physiology and reproduction in general.[30] This knowledge may be drawn from Western or non-Western modes of science, as in Chinese medicine.

The technical-scientific knowledge base of the women interviewed differed. Four women were trained as either nurses or midwives, two in

Canada and two in other countries. The women with cerebral palsy reflected a very deep understanding of their bodies; in addition, their encounters with the medical system had left them knowledgeable about medical approaches to their conditions. The women from China and Southeast Asia discussed many cultural practices that would facilitate an easy labour and restore the body to a healthy balance in the post-partum period. They frequently combined Chinese and Western approaches in discussing their pregnancies. Most of the 37 women had attended some form of prenatal classes and knew the basic language of Western medicine in relation to pregnancy.[31]

The women described symptoms of pregnancy and how they knew or failed to recognize they were pregnant, physical and emotional changes during pregnancy, and particular medical conditions or pain they experienced. Each narrative provides a unique glimpse into a "personal-quasi-scientific model" of how a woman experienced and understood her pregnancy. The physiology is described in the context of when and how body changes were noticed and is interwoven with the meanings and emotions that these experiences had for the women.

Leora shared her deep shock and frustration over an unexpected pregnancy. "I couldn't believe I was pregnant. We had been so careful. My stupid ovaries."

Several women offered their theories of why they had particular conditions, such as high blood pressure and body spasms. Some vividly described miscarriages and discussed the frustration of not knowing the reasons.

All the women discussed labour and birthing in considerable, often breathless, detail, including the perceived sequence of events and descriptions of feelings at particular times. For all the women, these were critical life experiences. Many of these birth stories describe technological interventions or the use of drugs and reflect the woman's attempt to reconstruct knowledge about the birth of her child. For example, one woman described being given Demerol® during labour and regretted it because it made her foggy and less conscious of the birth. As she described it,

> They came in and said, "We're not going to get an anaesthetist for you till midnight to do an epidural," there were a lot of babies that night and I thought, "I can't deal with this till midnight." I was in agony, beyond anything I'd ever imagined. I was so worn down from the pain of the past three months ... So I said, "OK give me Demerol," and that's my one true regret. I talked to some people and they said they had the same experience as me, I talked to others who didn't have the same experience ... I was stoned out of my mind, to the point that I fell asleep at one time which must have relieved the pain, but for days afterwards and to this day there's stuff I don't remember ... I remember saying to my husband, "I need you to tell me what happened during the process" because all of a sudden I started wondering what the progression was because it was

like snatches, it was in a dream, I remember being here, I remember being there but I have no clue how I got from A to B ... He's had to describe that to me over and over because I wish I had been able to see more of that.

In contrast, the majority of the women interviewed did not have a detailed scientific or personal language to discuss human genetics and the risk of fetal anomalies. The women found risk factors and the results of tests difficult to comprehend or interpret. As will be seen below, women drew on other sources of knowledge to address the issues raised by the tests.

Another kind of knowledge is about the roles of patient and health care provider and the procedures and practices of medical institutions. The role of patient was deeply learned from childhood and experienced in the contexts of a woman's race and ethnic group, social class position, and past medical encounters. Appropriate behaviours were learned through the professional demeanour and aura of power projected by health care providers and perceived by the patient, consciously and not.

Many of the immigrant and refugee women had a wide range of experiences with health care providers in their home countries. Six of these women had borne other children before coming to Manitoba; the children had been born in conditions such as refugee camps, small or large urban hospitals, or with the help of a local woman at home. However, the mothers saw this knowledge base to have limited use when they were confronted with Western hospitals and medical procedures and prenatal technologies. The women were fearful of ultrasound equipment and medical encounters generally. For example, Thida described her fears of having an internal examination as part of her early prenatal care; she had had three children in her home country where this was not routine practice. Going with a health advocate to a sympathetic female doctor helped. Other women commented that they felt more at ease when technicians permitted health educators to be present during tests.

Other women, more familiar with these institutions, still believed they did not know about routine practices. Several women sent for fetal assessments by their doctors did not know that they would have to return for repeat assessments, and repeats caused them much anxiety. The nurses in the study believed that, as clients, they had to negotiate around protocols and stand up for what they wanted.

As we will see below, several women accepted the role of client passively; others struggled to question procedures and assert their autonomy in particular contexts. Many of the women's stories captured how difficult it was to do this, within the settings and structure of medical encounters and the perceived and real power differential between patient and health care provider.

Moral knowledge formed the basis for actions and may have posed conflicts between what a woman thought she ought to do and what she felt compelled to do in a situation. Jan, a teenager, had a very clear situational ethic concerning abortion. Jan believed that if a pregnancy occurred because of being stupid and not taking precautions, abortion could not be condoned; if pregnancy was the result of contraceptive failure, there was more justification for abortion.

> I never thought about abortion, people brought it up. You can't do this, you're too young ... I told my mother straight out, "I got myself into this mess, I'm not going to kill the baby because I did something stupid. It's my thing I have to deal with and I'm going to deal with it, not get rid of the problem, can't run away from problems." She was shocked ... After I had him I thought I was pregnant again and I was thinking about abortion because after carrying a baby for nine months I don't think I could give it up and I don't think I could handle two at such an early age ... It depends on the situation. I don't agree with abortions, but when I thought I was pregnant using condoms, I was using foam, I couldn't use the pill because I was breast-feeding. If I was to get pregnant it would have been an accident, it wasn't stupidity. If it's stupidity, I don't agree with abortion at all.

The women expressed their feelings of spirituality, faith, and sin as they discussed pregnancy and the dilemmas of making decisions based on prenatal diagnosis. They offered instances when they drew from spiritual sources of knowledge they had and sought out new sources to come to decisions. For example, Kim, a 40-year-old refugee from Southeast Asia, had positive results from her AFP test. She and her husband were very worried and went for genetic counselling. She reviewed her genetic tree, including the fact that she had had three previous normal pregnancies, and she strongly believed that abnormalities would be the result of sin in her life, which she did not think she had. She refused amniocentesis and said she was able to put the worry out of her mind for the duration of the pregnancy; she gave birth to a healthy baby girl.

Intuitive knowledge is another kind of knowledge that the women exhibited. A majority of the women offered examples of their intuitive knowledge pertaining to pregnancy. Several women said they just knew the baby would be the particular sex that it was; some women had dreams or strong intuitions prior to a miscarriage. Other women cited experiences that were based on past knowledge of their bodies, applied in current situations. They believed they were right despite what a doctor said. One immigrant woman said she knew she did not have an ectopic pregnancy, because a pregnancy 12 years earlier had felt similar. Several women clearly stated that intuitive knowledge played a very strong role in their lives and that they trusted such knowledge in making major decisions. For example, Sally described feeling torn between her desire to be awake during the birth of her child, which would mean taking the advice of her doctor who said an epidural was indicated for her Caesarian section, and knowing that her back could not tolerate the epidural because of her cerebral palsy.

> I desperately wanted to see the baby born. My intuition kept going off, "Your back, your back, beware of your back, you're going to be sorry,

don't do an epidural," and I kept going, "The doctor knows what he's talking about," saying the epidural was the best way to go and it was safe, that was the way they normally do it. Part of me was saying, "Can I have a general anaesthetic if I really want it?" and he said, "Yes, you can if you really want it." I went through a lot of struggles ... They stuck this needle in my back, it was like they put my finger in a hydro pole. My whole body was like this inside, it was just exploding and I froze ... I was in so much pain ... I thought I'd be paralysed ... I got out a few words, "Stop, no more. Please put me out ..." My body had already told me that I shouldn't be going through this and I didn't listen and I found out that it was right and I better stop them from doing it. So they did put me out.

As the above examples indicate, the women's narratives provide a source for understanding how the women integrated knowledge and meaning. For many women, being pregnant gave them new insights from the start:

> When we found out it was twins, we changed our expectations; we knew we couldn't have a non-intervention pregnancy. (Kim)

> The pregnancy was an accident; a good accident, but still an accident. (Peggy)

> I had healthy, happy pregnancies. It was nice being pregnant ... I remembered how callous I used to be. I had heard about a woman who lost her baby in the third trimester and I had said, "Well, it wasn't born yet." I recalled that attitude after I was pregnant and I thought to myself, "If I lost this baby now it would be tragic." Oftentimes you have to experience these things in order to understand. It would have been awful even though I can't describe a relationship as such, but I know it would have been tragic if anything had happened. (Jocelyn)

## Some Sources of the Women's Knowledge

The narratives also reveal a great deal about how the women come to know what they do about pregnancy, their changing bodies, and medical interventions, including prenatal testing. Understanding some of the sources of women's knowledge provides insights into how a woman may respond in particular medical encounters, whether she actively seeks needed information and support when confronted with a new situation or dilemma, such as prenatal testing.

How women come to knowledge is complex and varied. It depends a great deal on past experiences forged in family relationships, schools, and through contacts with other significant individuals and institutions, including health professionals and medical institutions. How women learn is embedded in the power relationships that characterize these settings. What is learned carries the emotional weight of past experiences absorbed in the setting in which something is learned. What individual women know about their bodies and pregnancy is unique to each woman and learned in diverse settings often characterized by ambivalent messages. For example, women who have experienced physical or sexual abuse and other forms of violence "store" these experiences in their bodies in complex ways.[32] These experiences are a form of knowledge that may be remembered under particular circumstances. The women in this sample provided examples of the many ways they come to knowledge, and many women noted how they had changed in seeking knowledge.

### *Received Knowledge*

A few women characterized themselves as having until quite recently been silent — their knowledge came from others. They saw themselves in the past as voiceless, subject to the whims of external authorities, and unable to protest because they did not know how or what to question.

Sue, who is deaf, described how her first husband and mother-in-law determined everything when her first two children were born. She saw the nurses collaborating with them against her own desires.

> I was trying to breast feed and it was the first time and at the same time it was visiting hours. My husband at that time was there, my mother-in-law, all these people were coming in. My mother-in-law was saying you shouldn't be breast feeding, you should be bottle feeding and I wanted to have that bonding with my daughter ... The nurses and my mother-in-law and sister-in-law were into a discussion and they made the decision and I asked my husband what was going on and he said, "Mom says that breast feeding is not right and it's better to do the bottle because that's what she's used to," so I followed what she said because there was so much conflict happening.

Eleanor, born deaf into a hearing family, had a deficit of any language until about age seven. She too described having almost no information when pregnant the first time, largely because prenatal classes were difficult to follow without a relay interpreter. She has since talked with other women and learned more about pregnancy. Slowly, she is learning what to ask.

Some women described feeling silenced by health professionals. They saw it of no use to tell a doctor how they really felt, to ask questions, or to demand accountability if they felt wronged. For example, Marie, a 37-year-old from an Aboriginal background, was infertile for many years. She described feeling devalued by her specialist throughout her pregnancy, birth, and post-natal period. In the past she had tried to ask him things and felt rebuffed. She acquiesced to every procedure the doctor ordered, including two amniocenteses, although she didn't always understand clearly why the particular procedures were being done. "I felt angry. I didn't want to talk to him. I didn't want to make a fuss about it, so I just continued going back because I wanted to get through the pregnancy." Her knowledge came from her sisters and very supportive prenatal nurses at a community clinic.

A few women described themselves as receiving knowledge from health care providers and other formal authorities whom they believed to be the experts. They did not see themselves as capable of engaging in discussion with health professionals beyond asking them to clarify instructions or basic information. Cheryl took the attitude that "the doctor's the expert." Monique thought, "They watched everything and took good care of me, explained everything." Karen, describing her behaviour toward the end of her pregnancy when she had high blood pressure, said, "They told me to lie around and count fetal movements. I did not ask why, just [asked] what I was supposed to do. I was too scared to know, I guess."

## Intuition

Intuition is described by the women as both a kind of knowledge and a source of knowledge. Almost all of the women relied in some ways on subjective sources of knowledge, known as true or reliable from their personal experiences or from what they felt or intuited. There were several women who saw themselves as "very intuitive" and "in touch with themselves." They described a process of coming to trust what they knew. Their pregnancies were key life experiences that helped them recognize the strength and intuitions they did have.

> I guess there was enough in me to say I believe our bodies know how to make babies and our bodies are going to birth babies. I think you learn to trust instincts a bit more. (Kathy)

> With the first pregnancy I knew I was pregnant, I could tell at the moment that it all happened. I just had this, well, feeling inside me that I was pregnant. Everybody will tell you, "No, it's impossible," but I knew every single time when I was pregnant. This doctor refuses to believe me, he keeps telling me that I was wrong and I was two weeks later than I thought I was ... I knew it was a girl. I knew she was going to have red hair. I used to sing to her and hold my tummy. (Sally)

## Research and Creative Fact-Finding

All of the women tried to learn more about pregnancy, prenatal care, and medical tests. Depending on their backgrounds, they sought out a variety of sources of information and tried to apply their knowledge to their situations. Usually this was done because they couldn't get the information they felt they needed from busy doctors, nurses, or technicians, or because they wanted external verification about what was being done to them. Some of the women looked for more mainstream medical information, others combined that with less conventional approaches — for example, using garlic to reduce high blood pressure, or researching the option of home birth. The women in this study sought information from a wide range of sources, including health professionals and health educators, counsellors, prenatal classes, books, encyclopaedias, and talking to friends and relatives.

Mai, for example, consulted with family members in the United States and Hong Kong about the safety and advisability of amniocentesis. She felt reassured and decided to proceed. She also wanted information about how to be healthy in Canada, as part of adapting to a new country. Shirley attended three sets of prenatal classes offered by different community service groups, since she had the time. She pointed out that they each provided different information and perspectives and she found them useful. Several of the teenaged mothers praised the residential program for teen mothers where they were able to continue school, take prenatal classes, and receive support during their pregnancies and post-partum periods. They stated that the information and support were crucial to their handling of difficulties during their pregnancies, including experiences with testing, keeping their babies, and feeling confident to cope at the present time.

A few women expressed deep frustration with not having access to knowledge they needed. Phuong had a Caesarian section while being held in a refugee camp. Because of language and other barriers, she was never told why. Sally has had trouble gaining access to her substantial medical files in Winnipeg. Two Aboriginal women were adopted and had recently found their birth families. They had wanted to know more about their family medical histories for themselves and their children.

## *Critical Analysis*

A majority of the women interviewed valued knowledge gained in a variety of ways. They tried to understand their own experiences during pregnancy in a broader social and political context and were critical consumers of health services. They read widely and talked with others about how the system of health delivery might be transformed. They offered analyses of such issues as screening and eugenics, attitudes toward teen pregnancies in Canadian society, and biases toward women and minorities within the health care system.

> I didn't know sometimes what questions to ask and I would get the feeling I need to know more about this, go to the library and take out a whole stack of books and read like crazy. You put together from various sources the information that makes most sense to your own life, draw it together and sort out the stuff that you don't agree with. (Mira)

> I feel strongly that public health and hospital classes aren't geared towards teaching women to be consumers. They teach them to be good patients because that's what they want them to be, but it's not optimal for the women ... Women have a lot of knowledge and take classes and read the books but they don't have a good self-image, good self-esteem. It's really important to look at how can we build women's self-esteem and give ourselves better status, feeling within ourselves that we can take the responsibility for the lives that we're carrying and making those decisions, instead of feeling like we're just the little patient and we should listen to the father figure. Prenatal classes should focus more on personal growth because from that you gain strength that we need to

make women stand up for what you believe and implement the information you have. (Kathy)

Young girls do get pregnant. I don't think it's finally clicked with society yet, young girls are getting pregnant and they are keeping their babies; they are raising healthy babies. They are trying their best. They do what they can. They just need a little bit of support from the society. Just because I'm young doesn't mean I can't do anything. (Roseanne)

The medium of the narratives suggests a number of messages. In telling their stories, most women provided the links between discrete experiences, showing how each experience was in fact part of a whole to them. During a pregnancy, of course, the women could not know how the discrete pieces would fit together. Sequence, integration, and meaning emerge as the women retell particular details of their experiences. For many women, this is an ongoing, complex, and active process of "remembering." The elements may change over time. The forms and styles of the narratives provide important clues to the unique ways each woman constructs memory, meaning, and her sense of self.

Numerous issues and themes are woven into a single narrative. Each narrative reflects some of the dynamics of the Canadian medical system and suggests questions for further research. To appreciate the stories more fully, it is helpful to deconstruct the elements of the narratives; but to understand their meanings, they must be worked with, listened to carefully, and ultimately perceived as a whole.

The kinds of knowledge that women have about their bodies, pregnancy, and the medical system and how they come to know what they know are rarely considered in medical encounters. Medical interactions usually emphasize a linear presentation of facts and sequences, presented as "rational," "objective," and "scientific." There is little recognition that such interactions are the product of particular cultural and historical circumstances and power relations. The female patient is expected to participate in structured ways, to respond to questions, and to be compliant. Other types of discourse are usually considered inappropriate.

There is a message in these narratives for the kinds of medical care during pregnancy that women want. Deconstructed symptoms of pregnancy or of any disease have limited relevance without attention being paid to the rich and diverse meanings women give to their experiences as a whole. The next section identifies the major themes brought forward by the women and explores these issues in greater detail.

## Major Themes

Eight major themes emerged from repeated review of the narratives. Each woman interviewed touched in some ways on almost all of these. Two themes address pregnancy and medical care in general; five relate to prenatal screening and testing; one addresses what the women identified as a struggle for respect.

## Competing Constructs of Pregnancy

The women's discussions reveal pregnancy to be a complex physiological, social, cultural, and psychological process. Women saw their pregnancies as unique, but essentially normal, processes, even if they experienced near-constant nausea, severe headaches, or back pain. At the same time, each woman conceptualized her pregnancy in unique ways, depending on symptoms experienced, her own levels of comfort with changes in her body image, and how others supported her, or failed to support her, in this process.

> I had a long pregnancy. I was vomiting and lost weight. It was a very sickly pregnancy. Other than that there was really no major complications at all in my pregnancy ... I didn't mind being pregnant at all other than the migraines and the headaches and feeling sick and that sort of thing. (Sarah)

> I was really thrilled to be pregnant and felt great. But my husband was appalled at how fat I got and that was hard on me ... He made remarks about how thin other women were, thin and attractive. It really didn't help the way I felt. Then my cousin didn't want me in her wedding party because I was pregnant. I was really hurt. (Joan)

The women generally used common medical terms when they described their pregnancies, some women more knowledgeable of terminology than others. But the women's understandings of their pregnancies went beyond clinical medical descriptions of stages, symptoms, and tests. Some women had explicit theories of fetal growth. For example, many of the Southeast Asian and Chinese women articulated the theory that pregnant women should "look at beautiful images and think happy thoughts." The mother's mental state and emotions are believed by many Asian women to have an impact on the fetus.

> In our culture, when you are pregnant, you are supposed to look at beautiful things, think happy thoughts, use your imagination in positive ways. (Phuong)

> There is a Chinese tradition of "fetal education." We have to pay a lot of attention and be very careful in what we do, because what you do has an effect on the baby. For example, you cannot sit on a bed to sew, can't use scissors, can't hammer a nail on the wall, or cement something. It might leave a mark or scar on the baby ... Also, certain foods can cause illness. I followed these taboos, because if anything went wrong, I'd worry it was from that. (Fong)

Similarly, many Canadian-born women believed in the value of massage and music during pregnancy to calm themselves and the fetus. Monique, who is blind, enjoyed massaging her stomach throughout her pregnancy. Two of the teenagers described "playing with the fetus" or "waking it up." Some women felt there were links between the stresses they had experienced during pregnancy and their child's temperament. As Ellen elaborated,

> I feel that the more stressed the woman is the more stressed the baby is going to be. Even though I was stressed I did my best to calm myself, to get other things out of my thoughts. I know they can't read my thoughts while I'm pregnant but they can feel my emotions ... I would talk to the baby. I had read that after six months that they can hear you and I was thinking that even before I had read that, that it's only a stomach wall that's separating us, so they must be able to hear, they're in water so it's muffled but just the tone of your voice. One prenatal class, this one woman she had four children and she said she sang to every one of her babies while she was pregnant. She said when they were colicky she would sing these songs and it reminded them, they heard these songs before so it helped calm them down again. I did that to him while I was pregnant and I always rubbed my stomach and I rocked him while I was pregnant and I still rock him all the time, it's just a habit now. But I would just calm myself and get rid of the thoughts and play music. When I was pregnant with my older son ... I sang to him all the time, he likes those songs now and I know that those songs soothe him.

The women's descriptions of their pregnancies stand in marked contrast to how they described the medicalized construct of pregnancy that they assumed to be the norm in most medical encounters. This medicalized model presents pregnancy as a state of disease or potential disease to be closely monitored and watched for abnormal signs. Appointments with a doctor were regular and brief and involved physiological measurements, such as blood pressure, weight, fetal measurements, and heartbeat. Almost all of the women in the sample were sent for at least one ultrasound during pregnancy. Some had genetic screening as well. If some irregularity was found, further monitoring or testing was recommended.

Women sought doctors for their clinical skills and expertise and for the backup they could provide if something went wrong. They also said they wanted more time to talk, ask questions, and feel comfortable sharing the less measurable experiences of pregnancy. Some women felt care was being provided to their bodies, to the fetus, but not to themselves. As Heather, one of the teenagers, put it:

> I don't know, I just had this whole feeling most of the time when I was pregnant that I didn't really count. I had to do this for the baby, I had to do that, I had to eat properly, I had to sleep properly, I had to do everything right, get exercise, but you know, what about for me? Everything is done for the baby, everybody is talking about the baby, but not to me. I'm just left out, unless there's a problem and then they tell you about it and you're sitting there waiting for two weeks for the results.

Most of the women described feeling caught between the medicalized model and their intuitive and experiential knowledge of their changing bodies. They told about struggles with doctors over dates of conception, due dates, and whether they had in fact experienced a miscarriage rather than a heavy period. Many women felt their doctor did not acknowledge their experiences as valid, despite the expressed interest in "symptoms."

Seven of the women noted that their doctors clearly expressed the view that pregnancy is not a disease. These women described greater ease communicating with their doctors who took "a bit more time" and answered "stupid questions." Despite this, many of these women still had difficult situations during pregnancy and birthing through encounters with other health care providers. Having a doctor who subscribed to a less medicalized model of pregnancy did not necessarily ensure that a woman's birthing experience was managed much differently from that of those who saw more traditional doctors, since they, too, were rarely on call for the delivery or came only at the last minute. These doctors, however, did provide important support and follow-up in particular situations.

Many of the women had to negotiate their way between their personal construct of pregnancy and a medicalized construct. Sometimes, they tried to reconcile the models and were rebuffed.

> I tried to talk to my doctor about some of these feelings and intuitions about my body. At first he seemed understanding. Then after a while, he seemed to be thinking I was making mountains out of molehills ... He knew the kinds of things I wanted but when I actually experienced the situation, everybody at the hospital questioned everything. I couldn't understand why that was happening. The breakdown in communication I thought must have had something to do with me because he had to make all these special concessions because I wanted it a certain way. I never resolved that with him. (Sally)

Sally felt there was a widening gap between her knowledge of her body and the schema her doctor presented for her care. For example, he continued to suggest she have amniocentesis for subsequent pregnancies, despite knowing of her terror of it and her lack of interest in genetic screening.

Most women learned to keep their personal selves separate from their prenatal care. This seemed particularly true for the deaf women who needed interpretation and for some of the immigrant and refugee women who held cultural beliefs and practices that were not seen as relevant to the practice of Western medicine. They also held doctors in great esteem and offered little information unless asked.

As later sections of this report explain, when women were confronted with decisions about prenatal genetic screening and diagnostic tests, they had to try to reconcile the knowledge of these contrasting constructs of pregnancy. In those situations, they had to assess how they "felt" the pregnancy was going in relation to risk factors and indicators determined through "scientific" tests and technologies.

## Fragmentation of Medical Care

The women commonly perceived their doctors as the overall coordinator of client care, the node for information and for any plans for treatment. What the women described in relation to their care is vastly different. As the narratives show, many people are involved in the prenatal care of a single client, only some of whom may know each other or be part of a health care team. Based on the women's stories, persons involved in a woman's prenatal care, labour, delivery, and post-partum care might include the following:

- five or six obstetrical specialists who work in a group practice, each of whom the woman may see at least once during her regular visits, the rationale being that one of them will be on call when she delivers (specialists might also be called in by family physicians or general practitioners as consultants on a case)
- family physician or general practitioner
- technicians (a woman might see a different technician each time she goes for ultrasound, fetal assessment, amniocentesis, or other procedures)
- genetic counsellor(s)
- nurses, nurse-practitioners, or nurse-midwives, encountered if a woman goes for any hospital procedures, if she is treated at a community health centre or in a residential facility, when she is in labour, when she gives birth, and when she receives post-partum care
- residents and interns, who may be the ones to deliver the baby
- anaesthesiologist
- medical and nursing students in teaching hospitals
- health educator or other prenatal instructor(s)
- interpreters
- social workers, mental health counsellors, or other social agency workers
- labour companion
- other specialists, such as neonatologists
- other professionals, such as ethicists or priests who may be asked for input in making decisions

The women told of particular individuals among these health care providers who helped them at key times, with expertise and compassion. They also identified individuals who were harried, curt, and less than professional. But it was the overall fragmentation of care that drew criticisms. The women experienced fragmentation of care in a number of ways:

1. They found it difficult to have an overview of medical opinions concerning their pregnancy, especially where treatment was indicated. Women cited situations where health professionals did not communicate among themselves about their care; where reports went astray; where technicians told them they did not know why the doctor had wanted a fetal assessment done; where they were unsure how they would receive test results.

2. Women experienced anxiety confronting new health care providers whose skills were critical to the outcome of their pregnancies. For example, women did not think they could question the person performing amniocentesis or other invasive tests about their background or expertise.

3. The women believed that most health care providers barely knew or remembered them, even when they had seen them several times. They were "just another patient, or chart processed through."

4. The women experienced fragmentation of care during labour and delivery when nursing shifts changed and they felt abandoned at a crucial point in labour and when key decisions had to be made and their doctor (or someone from the group practice) was not present.

In one scenario of fragmented care, Heather, 16 years old and pregnant with her first child, described her experience of parallel care. Following a high maternal serum AFP result, she saw a social worker and genetic counsellor. She was sent for repeat maternal serum AFP testing and then for four fetal assessments. She continued going to her doctor for prenatal check-ups. According to Heather, the doctor never commented on the fetal assessments or asked her if she felt stressed because of the situation.

> Around this time, I barely had anything to do with my obstetrician, my prenatal doctor, barely anything to do with her. I was at the hospital all the time ... She got the results but never talked to me about it. I went in there for my regular check-ups ... She never said anything, never any emotional stuff. You know, it was just like how are you feeling today, took my blood pressure and that was it, I was gone.

Even when a woman had a sympathetic family physician or general practitioner, the woman saw them as "pushed aside" once other consultants were called in, or when the client went for other procedures or counselling.

The women who were themselves health care professionals or worked in health-related fields were highly critical of the fragmentation of care.

They expressed the view that those with insider knowledge and connections had a better chance of having the system work to their advantage than the average person. Jocelyn, a nurse, discussed how she put together a package of prenatal care involving a general practitioner and nurse-midwife based at a community health centre:

> I guess I felt sort of lucky, I felt like if I hadn't known how to work the system in certain ways and hadn't had friends and contacts, this wouldn't have been an option for me. I felt lucky I had some of the background knowledge to sort of put together a package for myself instead of just doing the routine of what the system offered. I felt people made certain exceptions, did nice things for me because I was their friend ... I had a little bit of guilt associated with that, since it isn't something that everybody can do, using the contacts and networks that they had. It goes along with being middle-class and having the resources.

Another woman who worked in a hospital setting knew the ultrasound technician and describes a setting of collaborative care quite different from those described by other women in the study. Leora had been sent for the test because of suspected gallstones:

> I knew the technician from somewhere, which was really nice because she treated me with a lot of respect. I said, "Could it be an ectopic pregnancy because of the pain?" and she says, "There's only one way to find out — through a vaginal ultrasound," which they do internally. Because I was too early to tell from outside with ultrasound. So we went in and I saw these two little blips and what does it mean to me, so she said to me: "Do twins run in your family?" I said, "As a matter of fact they do."

Another nurse who knew in advance her child had a fatal genetic anomaly arranged guidelines for treatment before the birth of her infant:

> They knew I was a nurse and listened more to my orders for non-intervention when our daughter was born. I knew what they would want to do when she was born. It took a lot of strength to ensure our wishes were carried out.

As the nurses' experiences indicate, women perceived a gap in coordination of care. Health professionals who were also clients were able to serve as their own coordinators. Others with less expertise, self-esteem, and power were hardly able to do so. As Sandy, 16 years old and pregnant, noted,

> They have people to support you like nurses, doctors, counsellors, but nobody really talks to you, never tells you what's wrong, it always comes through a different person. You worry if that's what's really wrong ... Doctors don't have time for you or someone else is waiting for them and they have to go.

A few women described examples where care was well coordinated. These involved situations where health educators provided supportive, linking roles for immigrant and refugee women. They attended appointments with doctors, went with the women and their partners for genetic counselling, ensured they understood clearly the decisions to be made. They also provided direct information back to the doctor on behalf of the clients.

One woman experienced some fragmentation of care during her pregnancy, but thought it was mitigated by the continuity of care provided by midwives. During her pregnancy, Anne had moved from California and shifted care from a group practice of midwives to a team of midwives in Manitoba. She saw a family practitioner in Manitoba several times during her pregnancy who agreed to serve as a hospital backup for her planned home birth. At eight and a half months pregnant, Anne was hospitalized for several days because of high blood pressure and was seen by a number of specialists. The midwives provided support throughout her pregnancy, came to the hospital with nutritious foods, and discussed in depth what her options for treatment were. Despite the specialists' disapproval, she felt supported by the family practitioner and the midwives to attempt a home birth and she delivered a healthy daughter. She felt truly informed about her decision. "I had done a tremendous amount of reading and talking to others. All the time, throughout the pregnancy and the birthing, I was making the choices."

## The Contexts of Prenatal Screening and Testing

The women provided scores of examples of their experiences with ultrasound, fetal assessments, and amniocentesis. As well, they were asked whether they had maternal serum AFP or other forms of genetic screening and, if they did, what they knew about the results. In their descriptions of prenatal screening and testing, a major theme emerged: tests do not take place in a social vacuum, but are part of the social relations of hospitals and other medical environments where they occur. How tests are explained and carried out are crucial parts of a woman's experiences with tests and technologies during pregnancy. The meaning of a test cannot be understood apart from the context within which it occurs.

Some of the different elements of these contexts are identified below. These elements were drawn from the women's descriptions of what happened to them during particular tests, including their discussion of what information was not provided. The context of prenatal testing includes many variables:

- Who offers the test? In what manner is it first mentioned and described, if it is?
- Who explains the test or procedure, if anyone? Did anyone explain the risks and benefits of having the testing?

- How is it explained? What are the rationale and degree of detail? Is it presented as urgent, or is the woman or couple able to take time to think about it? Are there written or verbal explanations? Who answers questions if there are any?
- Who administers the test? Does the client know anything about this person's professional credentials? Are there any set protocols for the client to evaluate the person or to receive information about the person in advance?
- Where is the testing done?
- Are instructions for the procedures and preparations for administering the test offered in a range of languages?
- Who else is permitted to be present during the test, such as interpreters, advocates, or partner? Are some people denied permission to be present?
- Do the technicians or other health workers provide information during the test? Do they speak more than minimally to the client? Are they perceived as kind, friendly, helpful, hurried, unfriendly? Do they inform the client about what to expect during the test and about any possible after-effects?
- What is the waiting period for test results? How is it addressed? Is it ignored? How long do clients actually wait for results? Is information provided beforehand about waiting and about how results will be provided?
- Are any supports offered during the waiting period?
- Are there certain protocols for how and when positive test results are given? Are clients told serious results over the phone? Are they told just before a weekend? Is it suggested that women come in with a partner or friend?
- Is any information provided by a technician after a test?
- Is consent pertaining to tests informed and meaningful? Are clients informed of screening before testing or when results come back?
- Given the implications of genetic screening for abortion and attitudes toward disability, are these issues discussed with the client beforehand as part of the process of consent?
- How is follow-up explained, if it is, and by whom?
- What if the client refuses the test?

The women described, often in vivid detail, the interpersonal dynamics surrounding particular tests and technologies. In the worst scenarios, women felt patronized and humiliated; in others, they felt ignored or treated as if their bodies had little to do with their minds. In positive situations, women felt respected and included in knowing about the procedures and guidelines for what was going on. These medical encounters can induce anxieties or be reassuring apart from the test's measurements and results. Indeed, research is needed to explore how the woman's feelings may influence particular test results and overall outcomes.

Brenda described a demeaning encounter with a technician during ultrasound. It is one of the more infuriating experiences of her pregnancy, recalled three years later:

> I had my ultrasound and it was a terrible experience. I was so excited about it weeks before. I had this ultrasound. This guy was cold as ice. A male technician as cold as ice. He said he'd been doing it for 18 years and I thought, "18 years." I had to drink 64 ounces of water, I was laying on the table shivering, I was so cold and this guy wouldn't put more covers on me. He kept telling me to keep still, I said, "I'm shivering, I can't keep still" ... I said, "Can't you even tell me what body parts those are?" The first time you see an ultrasound, you have no idea what you're looking at unless you see something distinct. He's going, "Just a minute, if you're a good girl" — he was treating me like I was 10 years old — "if you're a good girl and you keep still and you let me get all the pictures I need, I will go through them with you when I'm finished." I was so mad, but I thought, OK, so I just laid there and I just shivered to death ... So when it was over, that was the only thing that kept me from getting up and leaving, I was anticipating when he was going to show me something and he goes, "OK, this is the head, the body, the bottom, that's your baby and you're all done" ... I didn't see nothing ... Right away I thought maybe something is wrong with it, that's why he won't tell me, so I go home and I cry and I mean he didn't show me the limbs, I didn't know if the baby had limbs or not.

Some immigrant and refugee women had difficult experiences because the technician refused to permit their husband or a health educator to be present with them during the test. The protocols are erratic, since at the same hospital some technicians permit a companion to be present. Rosa, for example, was sent for ultrasound about a week before her due date to check for twins. They confirmed there was one heartbeat. The technician did not allow her husband to come in, even though he speaks English. During the ultrasound, she was worried because they spent a lot of time doing it. She thought they did it twice. During the test, they did not tell her anything. She did not see the baby's image. People came and went. They asked her to move to another table. A doctor was called and they talked in front of her, but she could not understand anything. No one tried to talk to her. Then she was told she was done. She understood that the technician could not say anything and that the report would be sent to the doctor. When she left, her husband asked why it took so long. He wanted to talk to the technician, but the technician had disappeared. For the next six days until she went into labour she was worried; she received no results. They later found out that the report had been sent to the wrong doctor and was forwarded after the baby was born. There was some concern that the baby's head size was too small, but there was no problem. As her husband said, "Perhaps too small for Canada, but not for Central America."

A number of women described being bypassed in deliberations or used as a vehicle through which health professionals communicated. After Adele's fetal assessment, a resident barely talked to her, sealed a letter in an envelope, and asked her to give it to her doctor. She felt uncomfortable about how things were being handled and opened the letter in the cafeteria. They were recommending she be induced or have a Caesarian section. A 40-year-old medical assistant, she felt she should have been included in the discussion about her care.

Ellen highlighted how technicians interacted with the machine, not the patient:

> They just said how big the baby's head was, the machine was right there, they interacted with the machine more. And in fact one of them, this company was coming to sell them a new machine and kept saying how good this machine was going to be. They were talking about this machine and saying, "Oh, it's too bad that you can't see" because through my pregnancy, the thickness of my stomach was hard on the ultrasounds in getting a good picture, and they're saying, "It's too bad the first one that you're doing this testing on you can't see the picture." Well, they're forgetting that I'm just lying right there. If I was the type of person that doesn't understand what they were doing, what would this say to another person, how would this make them feel? They're forgetting the patient is there and the machinery is just interpreting what's going on with the patient and not thinking how the patient is feeling.

The women's anxieties were of course compounded when there were positive test results. Cindy was told on the phone, and before a long weekend, that her fetus was dead and she had to wait over a week for an induction. Heather was told her maternal serum AFP results were high, but she felt unprepared to deal with it. She received support from the staff at her residential school for young mothers, but went to most medical tests or genetic counselling alone. She had a healthy son after a worried pregnancy.

> They had a social worker type who came and talked to me. Like I'm asking, "What the hell is this all about? Why are you guys doing this to me?" and she said, "The protein level is too high and we want to do some more tests." So I said, "What happens if it's too high?" She said, "Well, there could be problems. I have to ask you about your family history, baby's father's family history and see if there is any medical complications and stuff like that." She asked about loss of arms, mongoloid, heart problems, just everything at once. I think it was spina bifida she said, but she was saying something about where the skin is not going over the spinal cord. I'm sitting there, like WHAT? Or else the skull is not forming properly and I'm just like ... okay ... She was telling me all these things that could be wrong, I'm just like, "Okay, fine" you

know. "So we'll take these tests and you're going to have to come back every two months or every six weeks for fetal assessment and blood tests." "So when am I going to know the results?" She said, "In about one week to nine days we'll give you a call" and I just said "That long?" I was freaking out, I'm holding my stomach, feeling if it's moving still and I'm just still totally freaking out like I felt, my God, this baby is my life; if he dies, I'll die. I was all freaked out.

Some women did not know they had had maternal serum AFP screening until the results came back. This was particularly confusing for some of the immigrant women who did not speak English. Others described the long waiting period for results from amniocentesis, with no suggestions from health care providers about how to deal with the anxiety.

There are examples of testing performed sensitively in which the woman is addressed with respect, included in discussions, and informed about procedures and how she will receive the results. In contrast to her experience with the "icy technician," Brenda had a reassuring and very personal experience with fetal assessment, in which she got to see her baby. She was concerned that this baby would be breech like her first:

> It was really a good experience, we came out of the fetal assessment as happy as ever ... it was just wonderful. We were so worried and everything. We were told, "Don't worry, you'll feel a lot better after you have a fetal assessment this afternoon." The woman was wonderful, she was wonderful, she was perfect. She told us everything and we got to see her — she didn't say "her." She was more personal, asked about this and that, said the baby is in a good position — that was about two weeks before she was born ... She asked, "What would you like this time?" and I said, "I really want a girl, we have a little boy," and I asked, "Do you know what it is?" and she said, "Well, I had a pretty good look." So I said, "We don't want to know" and she said, "Oh, I wouldn't tell you." It was wonderful, it was so informative and she was showing the kidneys, went over the whole baby, it was just great.

Whether women see themselves treated with respect or not throughout the often lengthy process of testing is very important to their emotional and overall well-being during pregnancy. The medical ideology of testing tends to deny that the context of the tests is important to the patient's health and well-being, although good practitioners and the clients themselves know otherwise. It is left to the individual technician to make a woman feel comfortable. The woman may leave unhappy, anxious, hysterical, or relieved — apart from any information resulting directly from the test that she received. The experiences of testing become part of the memory each woman constructs of a particular pregnancy, and as these narratives indicate, such memories and their meaning are not readily forgotten.

## **The Interior Contexts: What Women Bring to the Tests**

The women's descriptions of test settings highlight another related theme: tests occur in a microsetting to which a woman brings her individual history, including fears, stored memories of abuse, previous relations to doctors and other health care providers, and past experiences with other tests. All these may surface in the current test settings and shape the nature of a woman's anxiety. These dynamics were articulated by Sally, who said simply, "You can't understand what all the tests meant to me unless you know a great deal about my life starting in my childhood." She proceeded to narrate her experiences as a child with a long history of medical interventions for cerebral palsy; and her complex relations to many doctors, some of whom used her as the subject of formal lectures. She talked about family relationships and friendships, experiences of isolation, cruelty and abuse from others because of her disability, her intense struggle to gain control over her body, and her strong desire for children. In the course of having three children and several miscarriages, Sally had tests (e.g., AFP, ultrasound), had procedures (D&C, epidurals), and had to make decisions about further tests (amniocentesis). The meaning tests have for her has to be put into the context of past fears and anxieties. Sometimes her body reacts through internal spasms when she is touched, especially in a medical setting. She relies on the knowledge of her body and intuition to decide about testing and procedures, and describes a struggle with her doctor to secure greater control over how her pregnancies are "managed." What Sally brings to a test and medical setting is inseparable from these life experiences.

> He sent me for tests, that's when it started, it was just awful. He sent me to the hospital to get an ultrasound and I walked in on the third floor and it was just like somebody had taken me from the world I was in to when I was a child and I was going through the whole realm all over again ... The smell of the hospital and all of this. I never dreamed it was going to affect me. They did their ultrasound and I got through it. I ended up having to talk to my doctor for hours about this whole thing. So I thought maybe I should change hospitals ... I have all this stuff going on in my head, all these old tapes ... This whole thing comes from my childhood, it isn't just the medical people, it's the stuff I've endured.

Sally's experiences underscore what many other women suggested: women imbue prenatal tests with a wide range of meanings and emotional weight. Past experiences are layered over current situations. Everyone brought baggage to the setting, some handling it more easily than others.

For example, some immigrant women identified anxieties associated with past traumas, such as having a Caesarian section while under guard in a refugee camp. Letti requested amniocentesis because she had a fear of people with Down syndrome, due in part to having been assaulted by a young man with Down syndrome years earlier. Yet she felt she should be able to love a child with Down's: "I cannot forgive myself that I cannot accept a Down's child."

A few women discussed feelings of guilt and unresolved grief because of previous fetal death or miscarriages. They saw current prenatal tests as particularly difficult ordeals to endure because they reminded them of what had happened and what they might have done differently. Jean had a fetal death at 35 weeks; the cord was found to be very short. It had been a normal pregnancy, and she had not had any testing. For her second child, she was extremely anxious and she wanted tests. The doctor sent her for fetal stress tests.

> She sent me for the stress tests. Maybe I could have asked not to go to them. I think she would have complied if I would have said I didn't want to go. But at the time, I think I wanted it. Because I was so anxious ... They did it on the baby once a week and they put the heart things on your stomach and they have these little things of how often the baby moves and then they can tell how fast the heart rate is and if it's normal. I was supposed to count every day how often the baby was moving. That bothered me in a way because of the heartbeat. I just didn't realize that they could, I had heard no heartbeat before. Then when I would go there and I was anxious for this baby to survive. When I heard that heartbeat it was like, like it was really hard for me to go for that test, because of the heartbeat. To hear it and to hear all the rumblings, the gurglings. I was waiting for the next one, and it would miss, it was really hard.

> I found that the staff there just applied the test and left me alone and one time I said to the nurse, "You know, this is really hard for me. I really get tensed when I have to listen to that. Could you turn the volume down?" She said, "We have to hear it." The funny thing was that she just said to me, "That's something that you sort of have to go through alone," because it was my particular experience. I tried to tell her that this test really, I'm also mental to go through it. She said, "I know it's hard for you but that's something you have to cope with alone. The doctor wanted it done and it needed to be done." As far as thinking about how you feel about these tests and having to have them done and they tell you, you have to be quiet and cope with it. When I expressed something she told me "Can you just deal with it?"

These feelings are rarely expressed by the women in normal medical encounters and rarely explored, considered, or checked out beforehand by any of the health care providers, unless a woman specifically seeks out a counsellor or finds a particularly sympathetic doctor or nurse. Yet, these dynamics are the unspoken essence of medical encounters. They can be heightened by someone uncaring or calmed by a warm and compassionate health care provider.

The women's stories contain examples of positive support from health care providers when they expressed anxieties about testing, but mostly medical staff do not seem trained, nor do they have the time to address these concerns. The medical ideology ignores such feelings of clients and considers them separate from the procedures and processes of testing. For most of the women, these were feelings they took home with them to ponder, worry about, and sometimes cry over. They were part of the test experience as much as results revealed from the technical probes of amniocentesis, ultrasound, and DNA screening.

## Questioning or Refusing Tests

Almost all the women raised concerns about questioning or refusing prenatal tests or procedures during pregnancy, labour, and delivery. This seemed to be an area fraught with difficulty and ambivalence. Decisions about what tests were necessary, and when, were seen by many women as the prerogative of the doctor because of his or her expertise. The women did not always understand clearly the rationale for particular tests being done and did not feel comfortable asking for further explanation. They were reluctant to challenge the expertise of the health care provider and thought that the consequences might be uncomfortable. Some women said their doctors encouraged questions, but they still felt uncertain about voicing their misgivings or confusion about proceeding with a test. They thought that in contrast to a scientific-medical model, they lacked real reasons to question. As Joanne, pregnant with twins, explained,

> That's when the fetal assessments started getting really frequent, from the 26th week to the 32nd week it was every two weeks and after that it was every week and I tried to argue that. Because I didn't really know quite enough about the whole situation, it was a very strange feeling to override a doctor's concern. The minute where you say, no, we don't want this, you're taking so much responsibility for something that you really don't have the training or the background for ... It did make some sense, although I'm not convinced that the frequency was necessary because there was no indication that anything was going wrong.

The specifics of these medical encounters were shaped in part by the personal styles and personalities of the health care provider and the client; by their cultural norms and beliefs concerning doctor-client relationships, such as politeness and respect; and by differences of gender, social class and power, race, and age. Whether an interpreter was present might also determine how readily a woman would speak her mind. For example, several immigrant and refugee women from Southeast Asia noted that they would not question a doctor if he or she ordered a test; in their culture, a doctor is like God. Some of these women did have to make decisions about amniocentesis following high maternal serum AFP results. They were able to do so because health advocates went with them to genetic counselling and clarified that in Canada they had a right to refuse.

The women discussed a wide range of examples of how they felt swept along by decisions made for them. Carla, 18 when pregnant, had a congenital hand deformity that she considered minor to her life:

> The doctor did ultrasounds to make sure everything was going fine. I had told him this wasn't hereditary, nobody else in my family has it, it was just a freak thing, but he wanted to make sure that nothing like this was going to show up on the baby. He wanted to keep an eye on it, just to be safe ... The hand is no big deal. I've been with it all my life and I do everything everybody else does. I can type better than girls in my

class who have all of their hand ... but he wanted to do it so I said fine, I'm not going to argue with him.

Another teenager felt swept up in the decision to go ahead with amniocentesis. A high maternal serum AFP result and ultrasound had determined a hernia in the fetus. As she described it, she was told she needed amniocentesis to "grow chromosomes to determine whether the baby was normal." Sandy was handed a consent form to read as she was being prepared for the test. Whatever the actual medical concerns, the young woman did not feel she gave consent. No family member or advocate was with her at this time:

> They told me I could refuse if I wanted to. But they told me there was no real risk to do it because the chances were very high. She told me that I had to sign a consent form and she gave me this list of things I understood were happening. But while I was reading this list they were getting me ready to do it and I never signed that thing to do it. They just shoved the list [in front of me] and they did it ... That was kind of weird. They did it right away from the ultrasound. The consent form said that I understood that this was happening to me and that it would hurt a little. There was this one part that said that I understand like for some women complications start when they're doing the test and beside that one paragraph that woman wrote in 1 in 200 are the chances. After I read that I wasn't going to do it, but I felt I had to ... No, I didn't tell her it worried me. They were just doing it, while I was reading the form. I just handed the form back without signing it. I don't really feel I had a choice over the test, but actually if they would have asked me, I would have done it. They didn't really ask me.

Sandy's experiences and those of several other teenagers in the study raise serious questions about procedures for informed choice and informed consent of minors. She also received no support during the waiting period for test results.

Some women were vocal in questioning tests and procedures. They described negotiating with doctors and other health professionals about the numbers of ultrasounds or fetal assessments they thought were necessary and having the numbers reduced. One woman, after her first pregnancy, strongly asserted that she wanted no ultrasounds, as she had concerns about the lack of research data on long-term effects of ultrasound on child development. Her doctor went along with her request.

Several women actively challenged doctors regarding treatment and procedures. Laura challenged a specialist in Regina who thought she was having a miscarriage and wanted to do a D&C. She spoke up and the doctor became annoyed:

> I've had three miscarriages. In between the two boys I had one miscarriage, so when I was pregnant with my second son, my cervix does not close properly, of course I had started bleeding early in my pregnancy and the doctor in the town near the reserve had sent me to Regina. The Regina doctor had said, "You're miscarrying again, we'd like to do a

D&C," and I said, "Well no, I don't think so." I said, "I've had a couple of miscarriages and this is not quite the same." He was actually a bit annoyed with me for second-guessing him. He had an intern with him, so he had turned around to his intern — I'll never forget this — he said, "Sometimes you need to prove to these women that they have miscarriages because it's so painful that they don't want to believe it." I was really glad I spoke up, I'm not a person that usually second-guesses a doctor. I've been brought up to believe "doctors know best," right? But I had had a couple of miscarriages, that's why I didn't, it was different, and so they did an ultrasound and just before the ultrasound, he didn't turn on the set, "You have polyps, that's why you're bleeding." I guess polyps was like a little sore at the end of your cervix and they pop periodically. He says, "You're still pregnant." But he wasn't going to check, he was just going to go and give me a D&C without checking. When they gave me the ultrasound, here's my son jumping up and down on the screen. I was so happy that I spoke up, I was so happy. I fought with polyps throughout my pregnancy until I was about six months, then they seemed to heal themselves.

Two women in the study refused maternal serum AFP screening when given the option. They believed they had sufficient information to make an informed decision. In both cases, they felt well, were wary of false-positive results, and had decided that they would not terminate a pregnancy on the basis of information about Down syndrome or spina bifida. They felt supported by their doctors. As Joanne expressed it,

> We turned down at the fourth month, or just the beginning of the fifth month, I can't remember the right time now, where they asked about the test, spina bifida and so on was tested. When we said to the doctor, "What good does it do?" and she said, "If you wanted to do something about it." I'm assuming she meant if we wanted to abort the child or the children, if there was anything wrong. We said, "No, at this point, we're in for the duration." It wouldn't have made any difference at all if that test had come out positive. There was no point taking it ... At that point it was too late as far as we were concerned. We were on the road and that's where we were going. There's no guarantees that you get any of these, we don't know what might happen later on if they get sick. We were just going to deal with whatever was ahead.

Adele, pregnant at 40, did feel a "silent judgment" from fetal assessment staff that she had refused both maternal serum AFP and amniocentesis.

> It was sort of their attitude, like when they said, "Oh, you didn't have amnio; oh, you didn't have AFP." It was disapproved. They were trying not to but it was obvious, like "Why didn't you do these things or why didn't your doctor." I guess on the prenatal sheet it says "refused" and I sort of declined.

Five women refused amniocentesis after positive maternal serum AFP results. These women all went for genetic counselling, which they experienced as informative and "not pressuring in any direction." They were then to make a decision appropriate to themselves, a process described as highly stressful. They had to gauge whether the risk of miscarriage from the test was worth the knowledge and reassurance the test could provide them. As Ellen described this complex process, it was a slippery slope of percentages and doctors' opinions of what information was good enough:

> They told me that they would give me the ultrasounds and they would check the spine to see if there is any openings. They made an appointment, I saw the doctor, and they had said through the ultrasounds, I was right there, they were doing the ultrasounds and he was telling me that because the wall of my stomach is too thick that he couldn't quite see, it was fuzzy, it wasn't as clear as it usually is and he wasn't completely positive. He says he likes to be 100 percent sure with the ultrasound that there's no opening in the spine. He said he was only 98 percent sure and he would like me to come back and I think it was two weeks because I was thinking, if I wanted to think of abortion, if there was something wrong with the baby, they would have to watch the dates. Also he said they might give longer time because if they find out there's a lot of brain damage or something with the baby. I had to wait two weeks and they said if at the time they think there's something wrong they could give me an amniocentesis at the time and that would tell 100 percent sure if there was something wrong with the baby. They also told me that there's a 2 percent chance of having a miscarriage and you could miscarry a perfectly normal baby, so that was an added stress. All this information was added stress on my pregnancy. I just went through pure hell. At the time I was thinking if this baby is badly brain damaged, is this baby going to live further, I had to think whether I wanted to go, the amniocentesis right at that time and they would give me the results then if I wanted to have an abortion I had to think, in a couple of weeks of what I was going to do, I wanted to have everything planned. They did the other ultrasounds, and the other doctor had measured the size of the brain and he saw the shape of the brain, they had another doctor do the ultrasound, so there would be a second opinion, and he saw the top part of his spine. The baby was not in the right position at the time. They had talked to me and they said if I wanted the amnio done they would do it but they weren't recommending it because they were 98 percent sure. But this other doctor kept saying he wanted to be 100 percent sure. They said if I wanted the amnio I could, the other doctor said, he saw the shape of the brain, he's seen as much of the spine as he could, he hasn't seen any problems, and what they've seen is more than if I never had any of these testings, the baby is moving so that is one sign that the baby wouldn't be paralysed. So they weren't recommending it, it was up to me if I wanted it or not. I refused.

The women in the study who questioned doctors or other health care providers about procedures and tests, or who decided to refuse tests, tended to be assertive. They had knowledge about the particular tests, procedures, and conditions. They received support and information from health advocates or midwives or from sympathetic doctors or nurses, or they had been through a formal process of genetic counselling and explored the implications of refusing diagnostic testing. In a few cases, the women believed they had to challenge a doctor to protect their pregnancy. Those who felt swept along in this process, such as the teenagers, believed they had much more limited information and support. The young woman who felt pressured into the amniocentesis had wanted to know more about maternal serum AFP screening and had gone to the library to look it up. As she said, "It was more scary reading about it there."

The women's concerns about questioning health professionals reflect the delicate balances among trusting the health care provider, receiving sound information about the meaning of risks, and having established procedures to ensure informed choices and informed consent. It is essential to this process that women have the self-esteem and assertiveness to ask questions, explore issues, and seek needed supports. As we see in the following sections, the decisions pertaining to prenatal tests and technologies entail a wide range of moral and ethical issues and underscore the importance of women feeling empowered to speak on their own behalf.

## The Moral Dilemmas of Testing: Attitudes Toward Disability and Abortion

Many of the women's stories reflect the moral and ethical dilemmas confronting them with prenatal testing. Where doctors provided information and discussed the choice of maternal serum AFP screening, women (and partners) grappled with the implications of testing in relation to their attitudes toward disability and abortion. Some women went ahead with screening, thinking they would only terminate a pregnancy for the most severe of situations; others wanted to know if anything was wrong, in order to have a choice about whether to proceed with the pregnancy; others refused tests because they were not convinced of the accuracy of such tests, did not feel they would act on the results, and did not want the worry of the tests. For a number of women, positive test results (that is, that identify an abnormality or give a result out of the normal range) were the first knowledge they had of maternal serum AFP, since it was carried out routinely by their doctors.

Where test results were positive (that is, they identified an abnormality or gave a result outside the normal range), the test became the trigger for a whole set of new options and pathways for making decisions. It was frequently labelled as a crisis requiring immediate attention to ensure any abortions would be done well within the second trimester. Few women anticipated what would happen when a result was positive and how quickly decisions would need to be made.

Positive results present women and couples with profound moral and existential decisions. These decisions may be rooted in people's attitudes toward those with particular kinds of disabilities and toward the concept of having a child or a "perfect" child; in the cultural, religious, and personal backgrounds of the women and their families; in the meaning of life; and in attitudes toward abortion, including the specific situations under which a woman might consider abortion. Feelings of hope, despair, or sin may be woven into these decisions, depending upon a woman's situation and how she felt generally about the pregnancy.

The women discussed a continuum of complex attitudes toward fetal disorders and concerning the kinds of decisions they made or thought they might make in particular circumstances. Several women clearly stated that they would not intervene in a pregnancy; they would raise a child with any disabilities and would cope with the sadness even if the infant were to die soon after birth. As Sally explained,

> I discussed the AFP test with my doctor and I said, "I really don't care what the tests said, if they said the child was abnormal that's fine ..." I think because I've done a lot of work in that area myself and I feel very confident in that way, that if I did end up with a child that had a disability, I would not discard it, or do that with a child. I think the struggles I had give me a lot of strength that a lot of other people don't possess, because they didn't have to do the things that I felt I had to do to survive. In some ways it maybe isn't so positive, but there's a lot more positive than there is negative. I think that I would only enhance that child's life because of my own personal experiences. I don't know how you would handle it or somebody else would handle it, but I wasn't at all concerned about that kind of thing happening ... Even in the situation where the child is to die soon after birth, I think I could probably handle that the same as I did with the miscarriage because it's really nothing I can change and a lot of my life is, well, you're going to go with the way the cookie crumbles. I've experienced some very high grief levels in the loss of animals that were very close to me ... it would be the same as losing a baby or a very close friend. Like that friend that died in my arms, I've been through lots of those experiences, so it makes a difference the way you look at it. That's where I think a lot of my strength came as a foster parent. They would say, "I can't understand how you can do all that." Well, it's just I drew on those experiences.

Several women from Aboriginal, Buddhist, and Euro-Canadian traditions expressed other positions in varied ways:

> I believe life starts at conception and that every life is sacred. I guess sort of believing in a higher knowledge or power ... I think we can't rule out that there are reasons for these little lives, however long or short they may be. It's not for us to judge whether they're appropriate or good or useful. There's just too much we don't know. (Kathy)

> Knowing she had a disability wouldn't have mattered. So long as she was there and I knew I wouldn't give her up because she was a part of my body. I love her for who she is, not what she is. (Monique)

> It wouldn't have mattered. I would have had the baby even with Down syndrome, 'cause I had waited so long to have a baby. I wanted a baby so badly. (Marie)

> In Buddhism, there is a great respect for life. Even when my mother had a miscarriage at three months, they buried it in a grave. I would not have an abortion. (Thida)

> The baby is my own flesh and blood. It is a sin to have an abortion. Religion is not that strong for me. These are my own very strong beliefs. (Sokhom)

A majority of women in the study, however, said they would consider terminating a pregnancy if they knew the infant would be severely disabled and would have a very short, "tortured" life. Jocelyn and her husband decided not to proceed with amniocentesis after she had a high maternal serum AFP.

> If it was a question of a severe handicap or retardation, I would consider abortion. There is a difference to me between Down syndrome where people can live quite normal lives and anencephaly or extreme retardation with a terrible quality of life. I'd have less difficulty making decisions in that case. On the other hand, I wouldn't want to reject a child. I wouldn't abort a deaf child.

Marilyn, a nurse whose infant had died shortly after birth from a genetic anomaly, was clear that she would want genetic screening and would abort if she knew the fetus had a lethal anomaly. However, she would not terminate a pregnancy "for things that people can live with, like spina bifida or Down syndrome." Most of these women were in stable relationships and thought they would be able to seek out supports and resources in the community. However, they did not underestimate the difficulties of raising a child with disabilities. Some of the women had experiences working with disabled children. Adele had an older, adopted son with multiple disabilities. Her attitudes came from deeper values, a particular social analysis, and her strong feeling that the pregnancy was healthy:

> I guess I never underestimate the difficulty with a child with disabilities ... I have found a lot of strength in other parents and supports. If we did have a child that was disabled, it would be a real grieving process, difficult, but I also get upset with what others think and my feeling would be that society would think, well, you didn't need to bring that child into the world. That's one of the things with this screening thing, it worries me that it's going to be seen as cost-effective and why would anybody have a child like this. I guess my values are that that shouldn't be involved.

Eight women explicitly stated that they would terminate a pregnancy if the child had Down syndrome or spina bifida. Their reasons varied. Some believed it would be too hard a life for parents and child in a "cruel world." Some of the teenagers thought they would not be able to cope as single parents; they would probably opt for early termination or would give the child for adoption. Three women of Chinese background felt strongly that having a child with a disability "gives a lot of harm and is a burden to society," as well as to the mother and the child. They requested whatever prenatal screening and testing were available to rule out any disabilities. The women also mentioned emotional and financial strains that would lead them to such a decision.

Most of these women were in stable relationships, and two had worked with or fostered children with disabilities. One of Laura's children was born with a hereditary webbing of fingers and toes, easily corrected by surgery. She had served as a foster parent to a child with fetal alcohol syndrome and stressed the need to provide supports to people with disabilities and for couples to have reproductive choices. These views were rooted in strong spiritual beliefs.

> Having a child born with extra fingers and webbing, I know how much easier it is to have a deformed child or a child with spina bifida or Down syndrome. For a while it became very important that I'd need to know that this child is OK. My husband and I discussed it and if I did find that I was carrying a Down syndrome child or deformed child I would have terminated. We agree it's not a fair life, you don't get a fair chance in life when you are born with so many strikes against you. To us, we both agreed that we would be best to terminate. At least it would go up to heaven, it wouldn't have all these problems. It's a very strong feeling, but we have discussed it ... Yes, I'm a strong believer in God, in the spiritual world ... If you were born deformed, let's deal with it, let's work with you, but love you the way you are. If you know about it early enough, I still think it's not fair to be born, to be always looked at, constantly, not thinking that you have no feelings and being stepped on.

Women confronted with positive screening results had to decide whether to risk amniocentesis on the basis of limited information. Some women noted that exactly how severely affected the individual would be by Down syndrome or spina bifida is not determined by the testing. They worried about miscarrying a normal fetus as a result of the test. They described feeling bonded and close to the fetus from the start of the pregnancy. As Rosa, a recent immigrant from Central America, said about her experiences with positive test results during her first pregnancy at age 35, "I felt sad, but I loved the baby. I felt sad for the baby. It didn't really matter to me if she had Down's, but my husband didn't want to have a child with disability. It was very hard to decide to have the test. My husband and I couldn't sleep." When Rosa found out she was carrying twins during her next pregnancy two years later and that the risk of miscarriage during amniocentesis was higher, she decided not to have the test. Similarly, Ellen struggled with limited information and decided against amniocentesis:

> I just couldn't live with myself if I had the amnio and I had a miscarriage and it was a perfectly normal baby, I just couldn't live with that decision

and I thought if this baby, if there's going to be anything wrong with it, I'll live. I made that decision, if there is something wrong with him I'll just have to live with that. I've already brought up my boyfriend's children who are slightly mentally handicapped, and I know a little bit, they aren't that much of a problem but I know somewhat of what I would get into. I thought, well, he's here and I'm just going to leave it at that.

The women's attitudes toward abortion were also woven into their views about fetal disability and influenced their decisions about screening and further testing. In speaking about abortion, the women revealed the complexities of what it would mean to them to abort what were wanted, if sometimes unexpected, pregnancies. Thus, while some of the women in the study might abort (or had aborted in the past) an unwanted pregnancy, deciding to abort a wanted pregnancy because of disability raised further dilemmas and issues.

All the women in this study held the view that abortion was a woman's choice. A number of women would not themselves consider abortion for an unplanned pregnancy or, as noted earlier, if a fetus were severely disabled. The vast majority held a variety of ethical positions on when they believed abortion might be condoned (e.g., as a result of sexual assault) and when it was not (e.g., if a woman got pregnant as a result of "stupidity"). At the same time as a woman spoke in greater detail about her views, she described situations in which she would consider or did have abortions that pushed the boundaries of her earlier views to encompass the hard realities of daily life. For example, Anna, who came from a strong Christian background, observed,

> The religious and moral values from my upbringing instilled my sense of the value of life and that you don't have the option to opt out if the baby or child isn't perfect. But I'd like to clarify this because something happened in my life that I never thought would happen and I suspect I haven't dealt with it fully yet. I became pregnant quite recently and it was unplanned ... I always said to people, I am pro-choice, but I always said personally I don't think I could ever have an abortion unless it was some health reason, if my health were in jeopardy ... because of my background I truly believe children are a gift ... I started to feel sick and I realized there's no way I can take care of three very young kids ... By the morning I had resolved to terminate and I just couldn't believe it ... Out of love for my children I made the decision and I'm positive I haven't begun to deal with it yet.

Some of the women's decisions about abortion were closely tied to timing. They said they would not be able to have an abortion once they felt fetal movement.

The women's attitudes and beliefs concerning disability and abortion are deeply personal and affect their decisions about prenatal screening and testing. Women weigh these attitudes and subjective feelings against the risk factors and uncertainties offered through early testing and interpreted in genetic counselling. As Jocelyn expressed it, this process has "nothing to do with science":

> There was information on the technical nature, what's this for, what is it trying to detect. Written information is hard to help you sort out what it means to have a 1 in 200 chance. How do you deal with that? It has nothing to do with science, it has to do with what does it mean to have a 1 in 200 chance of dying tomorrow or of having this thing happen to you or of having something wonderful happen to you, like win a lottery. I don't know if anybody can really help a person sort that out. I did feel a lot better when we talked to the genetic counsellor, she was much clearer about the testing, about my results, what they meant, the risk stuff and all of that. She was much clearer than my doctor was. I think it must be really difficult for GPs to keep up on the whole range of what are all specialty areas. I really felt better after we talked to her. But would I personally have an abortion, despite my political and social views after 20 weeks pregnant? I don't think you ever know until you are there.

The women in the study describe very limited engagement with health professionals about the profound issues confronting them. Only a few physicians raised the question of screening at initial appointments and asked their client's views or provided some additional written information about the testing. Some women were given the provincial brochure on maternal serum AFP screening, but said that this really did not provide information about specific anomalies, nor mention the issue of abortion.[33] Such information "routinizes" the screening and masks the underlying implications. The link between maternal serum AFP screening and abortion did not become clear until positive results indicated a need for action — a time of crisis. Genetic counselling provided a useful and important context for exploring relevant issues and decoding the test results, but it could only provide some guidelines along an unknown road. As Marcia said, "This is a screening test; it's helpful to us. It's sort of like you don't want to reject something that might be useful. But you don't realize what you're embarking on."

The moral dilemmas raised by some of the women pertaining to fetal disability, abortion, and genetic screening were rooted in a broader view of social attitudes and public policies. Several women explicitly identified what they perceived as discriminatory or eugenic implications of screening. Sheila stated:

> If it's a matter of aborting a fetus that isn't perfect, I am really deeply opposed to that because I think it sets a really wrong precedent for that end of the spectrum of life which will later have implications for the other end of the spectrum of life. I think we have to be bigger people than that, whether it's testing for the sex of the child or for other things, Mother Nature works things out really well and if it's a boy or a girl, then that's just what it is, you can't start playing with it. In a larger picture ... who knows what ends up happening if you start sorting out the redheads, it's ludicrous ... What happens if later on we know which part

of which chromosome has such and such information on intelligence, if there is some way of engaging intelligence or temperament or something if it doesn't suit you. If it gets to that point, it's getting into really dangerous turf.

As Gail commented,

Yes, I know ultrasounds are good and some of the testings are good because of defects, but then sometimes I think why should we be having an abortion just because of a defect. It's kind of going back and trying to make a perfect society and then are we saying that the people that we have here that have some problems, they're not valued. I really do have a big issue, I can see if the child is severely damaged and there is no way that the child might not even make the whole nine months or shortly after. But not if there's a little bit. Even if the child has muscular dystrophy or cerebral palsy or whatever, I think they're there for a reason. Children who are like that can still be a delight to the parents. It's just the way our society looks at them. A lot of these things, there are good sides to them, but I think it's too much knowledge sometimes. Putting their hands in and we're sort of wanting a perfect world and we're never going to have a perfect world, so why are we doing all these testings? ... Are we trying to create a perfect society, are we going back to how Hitler, he was wanting to do: devaluing people that have problems?

Sue addressed the way society defines deafness as a disability and framed the discussion of testing in terms of the question "Who decides what and who is normal?"

I'm very proud to be a deaf woman, I have no shame in the matter. I want this baby to be deaf, I really do. I value the deafness that we have in our family. I'm married to a deaf gentleman and my daughters are deaf ... When I'm talking about deaf, I'm talking about writing it with a big D, as you would put English with a big E, because you're quite proud of it ... I use a capital D when I describe who I am ... When my children were born, I never got them tested to see if they were deaf or not. It wasn't until my oldest was a year and a half and the youngest was three months. Of course, at that time I was thinking of preschool for my oldest so that's why we had some testing done because I didn't know how much hearing loss they had. So when I took them there, they put wires on them, they said to me, "I'm sorry, your daughter is deaf." And I was like YES, they were Deaf. I was so incredibly happy, it's nothing to be sorry about, that's the best news you can tell me. Normal is what they're looking for when they do these tests. Like the baby isn't normal on an ultrasound, that's when they're sorry ... I don't label myself as being disabled or handicapped.

Prenatal testing opened the door to many ethical and moral issues for the women in this study. Tests also offered the promise of hope and reassurance that a pregnancy would go well or could be helped when there were problems. The women speak to this theme in the following section.

## The Promises and Contradictions of Prenatal Testing

Depending on their particular experiences, the women described prenatal tests in a number of contradictory ways. Tests were "intrusive," a "window" to fetal development, a "trigger" for decisions, "inevitable," "pure hell," or "reassuring." Despite this ambivalence, a majority of the women characterized prenatal tests and technologies as potentially helpful to a woman's pregnancy by providing reassurance about the progress of the pregnancy, by identifying problems and helping to prevent or "manage" later crises or trauma. Women who had stressful experiences with false-positive maternal serum AFP results in fact chose to have the test with a subsequent pregnancy.

The women in this study gave a number of reasons for wanting prenatal testing:

1. To allay specific fears associated with previous traumatic experiences during pregnancy. For example, Ruth demanded ultrasound and fetal assessments to ensure that her second child was not a breech. In her first pregnancy, the doctor had missed the breech presentation; she required an emergency Caesarian section under a general anaesthetic and had serious post-partum stress, largely due to the trauma of the birth. Similarly, Jean had experienced a fetal death *in utero* at 35 weeks. Her pregnancy had seemed normal and her doctor had not sent her for any ultrasound or invasive testing. She was very anxious with subsequent pregnancies and asked for the reassurance of tests.

2. To determine whether they were carriers of a particular genetic anomaly known to be present in their family and to identify whether the fetus was affected. This would allow the woman or couple to prevent and treat the condition, if possible, to abort, or to prepare for the birth situation. Two women in the study had experienced lethal genetic defects in their children or in immediate family members and stressed the importance of being prepared for tragic situations, and for intervention where possible.

3. To screen for and diagnose the presence of particular disabilities in a fetus at the request of a mother who wishes to abort if the disabilities are determined to be present. The mother or parents may feel unable to care for a child with those types of disabilities for a variety of reasons and circumstances, including emotional and financial hardship; they may have particular fears stemming from past experiences; or they may express a strong ethic that disability is a burden on society.

4. To screen and diagnose particular disabilities, where indicated, in order for the mother or parents to be prepared for the birth and care of the child. As Louise, one of the deaf women, noted,

> I would not consider abortion but I would like to know as much as possible about the potential for the baby to be challenged. Then at least I'm not in total shock when the baby is born. I may not need to know all the details of the handicap, but if the doctor was not telling me, I think my devastation would be huge upon the baby's birth. If I knew those things, I could go to some workshops for older mothers, or about spina bifida or whatever, and be prepared in a sense.

5. To provide as much information as possible from existing prenatal tests and technologies because the technology is available, and the parents feel they have a right to know as much as they can. Some women expressed a kind of "technological imperative," wanting to know as much as they could, even if their doctors thought there were no indications for particular tests. These views may press some doctors to use more screening and testing to avoid liability. Jocelyn and Ada summarized this position in these ways:

> I would have been really angry if something had happened and I found out later that it would have been possible to detect it and nobody offered that to me. Because then I would never have had the choice even though the choices were difficult. (Jocelyn)

> I want to know everything. I don't like being kept in the dark about anything; if there's a way to find out, let's see if we can find out ... It's a lot harder to be in between and not know and wonder. I'd rather know that there is no cure or no treatment, then fine, I'll deal with that when it happens, but right now we're dealing with this ... If something went wrong with the test, I would not blame the reasons for miscarrying on that. To me it would have been that the test didn't go off right. It's not their fault, the baby obviously is not strong enough to withstand something like that. That's how I would feel. (Ada)

As prenatal technologies become increasingly routine in prenatal care, testing becomes integral to how women describe the progression of their pregnancies. Throughout the interviews, women spoke in a way where feelings, experiences, and symptoms were woven into the sequences of testing: "After I had my ultrasound, I came home and cried"; "I went for fetal assessments every two weeks — it drove me crazy"; "It was a nightmare waiting for the results of the amniocentesis"; "I felt great once I heard everything was okay." Bonding to the developing fetus was given elaborate meanings through such tests. Carla, a teenager, captures her everyday wonder at the pregnancy and her deep emotions when she saw her baby on the screen:

> At first I felt bad, thought I looked like a fat cow, but I thought it was just great, there's this little life inside of me and I can feel it kicking. I used to sit and watch my stomach move. I thought it was wonderful, I was really proud to be carrying a baby. It was the most amazing thing to me, he'd kick at night and I'd sit up and let him do his thing ... I cried at the ultrasound — here he is sucking on his thumb and laying back and his legs crossed and he moves. Till this day he still sits like that. I did cry and then I went home and phoned my mom and cried again because I was so excited. He still sits like he did when he was in my womb with his legs crossed at the ankles.

Prenatal testing dramatically transformed some women's pregnancies by introducing previously unknown worries and then providing the opportunity for reassurance. Marie was a 36-year-old Aboriginal woman who had recently come to Winnipeg from a northern reserve. She had to deal with a number of health care providers at several facilities and a long series of tests, including two amniocenteses. During these tests, she was asked if she wanted to know the sex of her child. Thus, testing further defined her experiences of pregnancy. Her story provides keen insights into how she tried to integrate the technical, medical information about how her pregnancy should be managed with her subjective feelings.

> And then for my age like they had to give me that test for 35 and older, the amniocentesis. He said like some women maybe they have their Down's syndrome babies and that's why he wanted me to have one because I was too old. They wanted me to have one so I could be [pause] prepared if I have it, if something is wrong with the baby.

> No, it didn't really matter to me beforehand. Not until after they explained it to me. They suggested to have that test and that's when my mind began to wonder what if my baby becomes like that because I'm too old to have — I'm older — what if I have a baby like that and it came to my mind lots of times during my pregnancy. But after I took that test they told me everything was OK and I was really pleased with that.

> They gave me another amniothesia [sic] where they take out fluid at 35 weeks. They told me they wanted to know how the baby is reacting and when the baby will come out, to know if they would have to do something, a C-section, if there were complications, maybe they would change something for the labour. I took another one and the doctor said he was going to phone me about the results and he said I gave him the wrong number.

> The doctor that did the amniothesia [sic] the first time asked me if I wanted to know what sex the baby was and I said OK. Then he told me it was a boy, but already I had a feeling that it was going to be a boy. It's a feeling ... I don't know. I talked to my sisters but they didn't have those feelings like I did during their pregnancies. But me I had that

feeling after a few weeks and I felt so happy about it. This baby was special that I was carrying, it's been special ever since he was born. It didn't matter what sex as long as it was a baby. When I saw the baby on the screen, it was a happy feeling. I was connected to him. Every time I used to look at him, I used to feel he was special. I wanted to be a mother for a long time.

Many of the women in the study persevered with such testing because they hoped the outcome would provide a healthy child and because they saw no other options to the management of their care. Women who had previous traumatic pregnancies were particularly wary of not proceeding with tests and close monitoring of their pregnancies. At the same time, women expressed considerable ambivalence about the effects of the anxieties produced by the tests on a woman's sense of well-being. As Sokhom and Thida noted, while they wanted the choice of prenatal testing, the stress undermined their ability to "think happy thoughts." As Kathy said, "The stress alone is difficult on the baby and the mother; it's not just the test, whether you are going to miscarry because of the tests. It's the stress on the pregnancy that is an important factor in the development and progress overall."

Testing made the pregnancy tentative for some women until they received reassuring results. They did not tell family or friends about what was happening and felt isolated as a result. Others described a more protective reaction, "taking the baby's point of view."

As a matter of fact I think it put me closer to her. It didn't put me any further away from her. I started thinking of her more as a person, more of a living thing rather than just a pregnancy. I started taking her point of view into consideration that I wouldn't want my parents to throw me away because there was something wrong with me. I would hope that my parents would do what they could for me and my parents would. So I kept thinking I should do what I can, no matter how minimal it is, even if she just lives for a short while ... It put me a lot closer. That's the only way I can think about it and keep my sanity about it and not worry as much. Taking it one day at a time basically is all I can do. (Erica)

When results were reassuring, some women were able to lay worries aside; for others, the seeds of doubt were planted and they continued to worry throughout the pregnancy. As Shawna described, "Through my whole pregnancy, even though the doctors are saying nothing is wrong, there's still that thought in my mind, he did put that thought in my mind and I went through my whole pregnancy worrying that there could be that chance, there's something wrong with him."

Throughout the narratives, women expressed their ambivalence about how prenatal testing is perceived and used. They commented that tests can provide information about some genetic disabilities, but not about others. It is not possible to have total knowledge about the outcome of pregnancy and birthing. They stated that many disabilities can occur at birth or later in childhood. A few women were concerned that negative test results may give a woman whose lifestyle or diet is unhealthy a false sense of reassurance that everything is going well. Many women expressed the view that tests and technologies tend to be over-used or used inappropriately in place of, rather than to supplement, sensitive clinical skills. Some raised the issue that the rising costs of routine testing could have detrimental effects on funding for services for persons with disabilities.

> There are so many disabilities where there are no markers and it can be due to the birth process. Some women are fooling themselves with testing thinking everything is fine and not realizing that things can happen all the way along. (Laura)
>
> Something I feel very strongly about is sometimes you do too much testing, like I went through hell with the AFP and my daughter is fine. Sometimes they don't do enough testing — my sister had an ultrasound too early and they missed the fact the baby had trisomy 13. He died two days after birth with horrible deformities. Had they taken another ultrasound later, they would have determined it, she would have been prepared. I can see too much testing being done and putting people through hell for no reason at all and sometimes I can see not enough testing and then what you go through at the end of your pregnancy. It's hard. I think I prefer to have the testing done and to know. (Ruth)
>
> A lot of what is done to women in the whole process of having a child seems for most women to just not be necessary. There are difficult pregnancies and all kinds of problems, but I think there's still quite a lot of people who could manage without a lot of the technology that's been applied. Seems a lot of it is not just intrusive and unnerving but also, if you think about the costs of medical care and so on, some of the tests and procedures seem to be wasteful in the cases of people, low-risk people who don't require it. People who've had healthy normal births in the past. I'm glad at the health centre I go to, they don't routinely put people through a whole series of tests unless there is some kind of indication. (Roxanne)
>
> Routine tests like for spina bifida aren't accurate all the time. So that's another thing that needs to be considered. Is it really necessary for a test which isn't conclusive to a high percentage to actually be routine, or should that just be administered in cases where it's a risk? ... We're so fascinated in this age of technology, computers and getting information down in nitty gritty tiny little pieces of smaller and smaller portions so we can dissect everything, but we're losing something else. We're losing the bigger picture while we're working so hard on the small picture. We need to get back to some of that regular human, born and die, getting more normalized again. (Joanne)

The narratives revealed how the women grappled with the contradictions and tensions inherent in prenatal testing. They processed complex technical, medical-scientific information and risk scores in relation to subjective feelings of wellness; explored profound moral and ethical issues about disability and abortion at a vulnerable time; balanced the desire to know as much as possible and control the outcome of the pregnancy with feelings of acceptance; and experienced the discomforts and sometimes the pain of tests and technologies and the anguish of waiting for results, while trying to enjoy the wonder of a pregnancy and other positive emotions. They tried not to feel fragmented into body, mind, and fetus while probed with technologies that could literally see through the boundaries of their bodies. Many did this while they worked full time at home, in offices, in clinics, or in factories, and faced other stresses and demands in their lives.

One woman's story captured the ambivalences of prenatal testing and indicated how the promises technology holds for reassurance could also drive a woman to feel deeply alienated from herself and her child. Jean had experienced a fetal death at 35 weeks due to an undetected defect in the umbilical cord. She grieved the death and was angry at her doctor who had not seen a need to send her for ultrasound or other tests in an otherwise normal pregnancy. During her next pregnancy three years later, she was highly anxious. She regularly saw two doctors, a general practitioner and a specialist, and asked for tests. As described earlier, she was sent for fetal stress tests, which provided some reassurance but also caused her considerable anxiety since it recalled feelings of her first pregnancy. She gave birth to a healthy son, by Caesarian section because of an active case of herpes. In a third pregnancy, Jean again asked for many tests and went regularly for ultrasounds. Close to term, her doctor informed her that the baby was ready and she could choose a date for the Caesarian section. She asked if it could be done in November rather than the beginning of December, since it might make a difference to get her child tax credit for that year. He agreed. That birth became a turning point for her.

> I was just walking down the street and it just kind of hit me, "Are you really thinking about the baby, is the baby ready? You're going with his advice, you're leaning towards his advice because you wanted your child tax credit ... maybe the baby could stay there for a few days longer." But this is the way it went. I went in there and the first time I had an epidural it turned out, and this time the guy couldn't get the epidural to take and they put me to sleep and the baby was born and the nurses were busy and I said, "I want to see her, I think she needs to see me." I had to come out of the dope, but I was conscious for a long time, so I knew she waited all that time, lying in the crib somewhere and it was a busy morning at the hospital. I thought, there's this little baby, I didn't have anybody in there with me, I was alone. The nurse said, "You're going to have to wait until we can go and get her" and it was a long time. Finally they brought her. Everybody said she's healthy, she's beautiful and there's nothing wrong with her. But I just felt, what have I done ... All these tests and I felt what have I done, I wanted to get back to something, I just felt I wanted to get back to something, something that I've kind of been ignorant of, I felt badly for the baby and I felt like I was kind of getting too technical. Leaning on these things and well the baby is going to be healthy so you might as well do it so I can get my money. I went along with that, I started to feel that I would put, I wasn't getting

myself attuned to something. All of a sudden I got to the point where after she was born that I felt that I needed to get back to something. I just felt, this whole experience, she's alive and I'm alive but I don't feel alive. I hadn't really stayed with her life, in spite of everything, in spite of all the tests. Somehow, I hadn't really made the right efforts. Maybe I could have had somebody there, they could have stayed with her while I was getting better. I wasn't really attuned in spite of everything to what was supposed to be going on or what was going on. The doctor, I don't think he was, the nurses, I don't think they were. I felt sort of sorry for the anaesthesiologist because he just couldn't, he just kind of said, "I'm sorry but we're going to have to put you under."

When she became pregnant a fourth time, Jean delayed going to a doctor. "[I] just sort of wanted to keep something to myself, not always running to the doctor. Just to keep it secret for a while. I thought, 'After a while, I'll go.'" The pregnancy ended in miscarriage in her fourth month. Jean chastised herself, wondering if prenatal care and testing in the early months might have made a difference. Even though the doctor reassured her that she would have miscarried, she continued to wonder whether she was to blame.

Over an eight-year period, Jean swung repeatedly between embracing prenatal technologies and rejecting them when she felt alienated and isolated from her child and from pregnancy and birthing. At the time of the interview she was pregnant and seeking greater integration and balance in her life.

I had a lot of anxiety with my daughter that she wasn't going to be normal. She's super normal, she's really wonderful. I think to enjoy your pregnancy is to learn not to encourage all these anxieties. It's important to have a doctor who tries to be very appropriate when they do give a test, it's because it has a true meaning. If a baby is going to be lost at 18 weeks old, maybe it's better not to be anxious and anxious, until it finally happens anyways. I think to enjoy it and not to worry all the time, to accept it ...

The days and the nights, minute after minute, your mind can be filled with all kinds of untruths, all kinds of horrible ideas, all kinds of worries. You get to the point where you're debilitated with having to know, wanting to know, wanting to get your mind at peace, and they say "just do it to get your mind at peace." But there's got to be a point at which to ride it out, settling the issue through tests and through knowing, through faith, or through acceptance, through learning that's just the way that life is. You have to be very strong to do that. I'm not there yet but I'm getting to know where it is.

In confronting their ambivalences, the women in the study began to articulate a vision of a better system of prenatal care. Some of the elements of this system are compassionate health care providers who use technologies wisely to supplement clinical skills, the provision of options for prenatal screening with sensitive counselling and information about tests and their implications, and a respect for the self-knowledge of women. Central to this vision is women having self-esteem and self-trust.

## The Struggle for Empowerment and Respect

The most compelling common theme in the women's narratives is their struggle for empowerment and respect. Despite their diversity of backgrounds and personal styles, every woman interviewed revealed numerous situations in which she confronted health care providers or institutions and tried to secure some acknowledgment of herself as an individual deserving of respect. Sometimes these attempts were vocal, even strident. Heather, one of the teenagers, dismissed an inexperienced "do-gooder" as her labour companion and found a supportive nurse; Ina, the young woman with cerebral palsy, demanded that hospital staff allow her to hold her baby; Elise made it clear to hospital staff that she and her husband did not wish to have an interpreter present during her labour and delivery — it was too personal an event for them to share with a stranger and they felt in control despite being deaf. Other women were more passive in their resistance. Marie was silent during final appointments with a specialist who she felt treated her and other Aboriginal women with disdain; Sandy, the young teenager, did not go back to a doctor she did not feel comfortable with. These women used the opportunity of the interviews to discuss their underlying feelings of anger, fear, and discomfort.

Most of the women described specific examples of considerate and compassionate care that they received at some point during their pregnancies, labour, and birthing. After the death of her newborn infant, Sheila's obstetrician took off her shoes, put her feet up on the bed, and talked with Sheila about their mothers. Throughout the ordeal she had felt supported by the chief neonatologist, who provided clear information and held out a slim ray of hope that technologies were fallible. Cheryl had a nurse who spent a good deal of time talking with her after her miscarriage. Roseanne's doctor was gentle in his examination — he did not ask her if she was scared because of an irregular Pap smear; he told her he knew she was scared. Marie was pleased to see the prenatal nurse at the community health centre she attended because she always remembered her baby's name and called to check if she did not make her appointment. Manuela's doctor took time to explain why she needed another Caesarian section and reassured her about the outcome.

All the women were extremely grateful for such kindnesses, as if provided a glimpse of another system in which there was time to talk about what mattered to women and where women were equal participants in their health care. However, the overwhelming message of their narratives is that the "real" system had little time for valuable interactions and could be indifferent or even abusive. Women recounted experiences with technicians, doctors, and nurses who were harried and dismissive of their concerns. A thoughtless remark to a woman already anxious about a test or immediately post-partum was remembered and pondered over for months, even years afterwards.

Such thoughtless remarks mattered because, as many women made the point, pregnancy and birthing were not medical events but life experiences. As Mira said,

> Every woman is an expert on her own pregnancy ... It seems that in some ways reproductive technology is still in the Dark Ages when it comes to sensitivities of the issues. We've got all this wonderful science out there and there's a lot of doctors who are just, yeah, let's use this stuff. But I think that the scientific developments are to some extent leaving the human and personal and individual aspects of the experience behind. As far as I'm concerned having a baby is not a medical event, it's a life experience.

Others described the wonder of being pregnant and a passionate process of bonding to their developing fetus and new child. Ada commented,

> I knew a baby was in there, we'd talk to her and stuff, but just having her for about a week or two after she was born and her little personality is forming already and everything and I'm thinking I wish I had known that was you, I wish I had met you face to face and known your personality while you were in there and I would have been able to talk to you the way I do now. It's weird, it's just incredible.

The women struggled to sustain such feelings of wonder despite difficult situations waiting for test results, threatened pregnancies, or tragedies.

The birth experiences were particularly crucial life events in this struggle for respect and empowerment. The narratives are filled with detailed birthing stories in which women tried to have a positive experience despite the procedures and protocols of an institutional environment. Women demanded more comfortable birthing positions despite residents and nurses remaining preoccupied with fetal monitors that rarely worked properly. They tried to make decisions under stressful conditions concerning epidurals, Demerol®, emergency Caesarian sections, or induction. Their own doctors were almost never present while they made those decisions. Approximately half the women's doctors were not available for their deliveries; those that came arrived at the last moment, or for a scheduled Caesarian section. Women who managed to birth in a low-intervention way, in a birthing room and in an alternative position, felt lucky that they were able to "slip through the cracks" in the system. As the culmination of the pregnancy, the birthing was a key life event that women tried to remember with meaning and fondness. This task was difficult for many of the women in this sample who experienced fragmentation of care and loss of dignity.

Many of the women interviewed have been led by their experiences with pregnancy and birthing to evaluate the health care system and their own behaviours, and become more critical consumers. As discussed in earlier sections, some women have started to find their voices and a stronger sense of self.

> Having my children and going through all of this like the post-partum stress has made me such a stronger person. I feel more vocal. Because I used to just take it. I used to just say, "Whatever the doctor says, fine. Whatever the nurses said, fine." I let people walk all over me, I would be just a doormat for everybody. Not anymore. And I feel really strongly about health care. I think there should be some kind of a humanitarian course that nurses and doctors have to take, some bedside manner courses before they get their licences because some of them don't deserve to work with people that are in vulnerable situations. (Ruth)

> The deaf training program I took changed my life. We talked about a lot of different issues that are happening to us and to the world and I always thought I couldn't do things, I can't because I'm deaf, I can't because I can't improve my English. I can't meet hearing people and that CAN'T can turn into the biggest can't you can possibly believe in. That was the way it was when I had my first two kids. I feel I'm independent now. This is going to be our birth and we're going to decide how it goes. I'm excited to see what it looks like for myself to be in labour, the way I am today. (Sue)

Sally spoke for most of the women when she indicated that her quest for respect and empowerment was a lifelong process:

> I wanted to find my way through this whole path. The part I wanted so much with the kids was to have it as smoothly as I could and be able to understand what was happening and why and not have people expect me to terminate my ability to be pregnant because of all the difficulties that I go through. Like my values as to why I would put myself through it was because a child was so important ... It's like my whole life is part of this pregnancy thing. I'm sure if I didn't have the kind of background I had and the cerebral palsy, it maybe wouldn't have been as difficult, but I've talked to other women who had normal pregnancies that have had a lot of the same concerns that I have and mine just got multiplied. The frustration, the feeling of not being able to control the situation when I knew what was going to happen to me and the staff getting all upset and throwing their hands up. Why couldn't I be respected for the things I wanted to do? I'm still working through all that stuff. I think it's going to be a lifetime thing for me.

Empowerment requires personal self-esteem and a medical system that is structured to facilitate trust, mutual respect, and informed decision making between clients and health care providers. The health care system must address the deep-rooted problems inherent in the themes identified by the women: conflicting constructs and understandings of the meaning of pregnancy and birthing, fragmentation of care, ideologies that discount the settings within which procedures are carried out and that devalue the selves that women bring to such settings, and the profound ambivalences of prenatal screening and testing with their moral and ethical implications.

The women in this study not only offered a critique of the system but suggested specific alternatives for more humane care. These are elaborated in the following recommendations.

## Recommendations of the Women Interviewed

The women were asked to make specific recommendations about the use of tests and technologies, including prenatal screening, during pregnancy. In addition, they were free to address how they thought that prenatal care for women, particularly women such as themselves (i.e., teenagers, immigrant women, women with particular disabilities, etc.), might be improved. They were told that the recommendations would be compiled and summarized and would go forward to the Royal Commission on New Reproductive Technologies through this report. Feedback would also be provided to community health centres and agencies.

Thirty-five women chose to make recommendations. About 170 recommendations were made in total pertaining to prenatal testing and prenatal care in general. The recommendations have been grouped into six basic categories:

1. needed supports and services during pregnancy, birthing, and the post-partum period;
2. improved communication between health professionals and clients;
3. recommendations concerning prenatal testing and diagnostic technologies;
4. recommendations concerning genetic and fetal research;
5. alternative models of prenatal care and birthing; and
6. general social transformations.

## Needed Supports and Services During Pregnancy, Birthing, and the Post-Partum Period

About one-quarter of the recommendations addressed the need for specific supports and services for pregnant women or new mothers. Many of the women noted that it was through services such as the following that they received support when confronted with decisions on prenatal testing and diagnosis. The women recognized that many of these services operated on shoestring budgets or had only year-to-year funding. Others were more stable, but the women thought these needed to be extended to other parts of the city and the province.

1.  Since language and interpreter services are crucial to ensure access to prenatal care and to informed consent for immigrant, refugee, and deaf women, particularly pertaining to tests, medical interventions, and hospital routines, it is essential:
    (a) that written and verbal information pertaining to prenatal care and testing be provided in their first language;
    (b) that interpreters be permitted to accompany women into test settings, such as ultrasound and amniocentesis;
    (c) that sign interpreters be available for medical appointments, including tests, for deaf women; that medical professionals recognize that for some deaf women English is a second language; and that some women may require the use of a deaf "relay" interpreter to ensure a good level of comprehension;
    (d) that sign interpretation for medical purposes be covered under the Manitoba Health Services Commission;
    (e) that deaf access equipment be more widely available in Manitoba hospitals; and
    (f) that programs be funded to train labour companions from a broad range of cultural communities.
2.  There should be ongoing core funding for community-based programs like Planned Parenthood Manitoba's Immigrant and Refugee Health Educator Program. Women identified a critical need for trained health care workers from ethnic communities who can provide information about prenatal care and birthing, including testing and informed consent, in their own language, and who can serve as advocates and interpreters in relation to health professionals and hospital bureaucracies. The need for such workers to maintain trust and confidentiality within their communities was stressed.
3.  The above model of community-based delivery of information and prenatal education should be extended to the deaf community where there are huge gaps in access to such education. Women recommended the establishment of training for deaf health educators, and support groups and specialized prenatal classes for deaf pregnant women and their partners.
4.  There should be safe places for pregnant teenagers to go to talk about problems and options and to feel supported; these should include drop-in centres in small towns and suburbs where young women often experience hostile attitudes. There should be more female school counsellors, and there should be support for residential settings that provide prenatal classes, other schooling, emotional support, and an environment promoting life skills for pregnant teenagers and new mothers.

5. There should be continued and expanded financial support for community health centres and agencies that take a proactive role toward clients (e.g., calling if an appointment is missed; offering a ride) where staff generally provide some personalized care.

6. There should be support for counselling and public awareness about post-partum stress. Women indicated that this needed to be recognized as a serious issue in the training of doctors and nurses.

7. Hospitals should ensure they have the necessary equipment (e.g., low changing tables) for women with disabilities to care for newborns more easily.

8. There should be ongoing support for prenatal classes and for evaluation and review of content to ensure they meet the needs of participants. Many women said that prenatal classes are a crucial setting for women to become educated and thoughtful consumers of health services. As some women noted, classes usually begin after many women have had some screening or testing and are faced with decisions about their care and about technological interventions. Numerous recommendations addressed the following needs:

    (a) the need for prenatal classes to address issues of women's self-esteem — how to ask for information or express concerns, and to explore ways to trust one's knowledge and judgment (one woman suggested that private prenatal classes were more readily able to provide such a critical framework; classes offered through hospitals and public health departments tended to teach women how to be "good patients");

    (b) the need for prenatal classes to provide general information about health services in Canada and about adjustment to immigrants and refugees;

    (c) the need for classes to provide realistic preparation for circumstances that might be encountered, particularly during birth, and for dealing with situations of crisis and decision making;

    (d) the need for classes to address post-partum issues and practical ways to cope with stress, lack of sleep, and potential effects on relationships; and the need for advice on where to seek post-partum stress counselling;

    (e) the need for specific classes to meet the needs of women with disabilities (these could provide support and information pertaining to prenatal care, labour, and delivery, and preparation for what might be encountered in hospital settings, including difficulties of access);

(f) the need for individualized support and information about labour and delivery for women or couples who are expecting to have a stillbirth or an infant with disabilities (information about the infant's condition often overshadows the preparation for childbirth, especially if this is a first birth experience; decisions concerning possible interventions at the birth might also be addressed); and

(g) the need for prenatal classes to occur throughout the pregnancy to help women learn relaxation techniques, be more focussed, and feel, as one woman said, "less helpless and more special."

## Improved Communication Between Health Professionals and Clients

The vast majority of the women's recommendations related to the need for improved communication between health professionals and clients. Doctors, notably specialists, were mentioned most often, but women also noted the need for changes in relation to nurses and technicians. The women tended to be more satisfied with counsellors (including genetic counsellors) and with staff encountered in community health centres than in hospitals.

1. Doctors must be trained to listen and to interact in sensitive, humanitarian ways with clients, to create an environment in which women can speak comfortably. The women put forward a composite view of such a professional:

    - offers something about himself or herself as a person, for example, about his or her philosophy of care and views of pregnancy;
    - is able to express compassion in a professional manner;
    - is able to admit to mistakes or uncertainties, and to apologize when necessary;
    - is able to establish the knowledge base and understanding of the particular woman about her pregnancy and what she understands about a particular condition, laying the basis for further communication;
    - is aware that medical encounters are intimidating to many women, and does not exploit this, but attempts to overcome it (as one woman, a nurse, stated, "You shouldn't intimidate with care");
    - takes more time than usually allocated (as one teenager said, "An extra five minutes to find out the woman's general background — where you stand in the world"; another said, "How about a half hour instead of 15 minutes — to be sure the information is

clear"; sometimes extra patience is needed to hear what a woman with disabilities is saying, etc.);
- "treats you more like a person" (women appreciated being remembered by a health professional and felt upset when they were not);
- treats a woman with respect for the choices she has made or is making and tries to understand her rationale even when the doctor may not agree (e.g., with home birth, or refusing routine tests); treats her concerns seriously;
- "explains more; not staying just on the surface of things"; offers more than just measurements (blood pressure, heart rate, fundal height) during the appointment;
- coordinates and helps the woman to understand the medical/technical information, such as test results, that comes from others in relation to her overall situation; is aware of and tries to combat the fragmentation of care;
- takes the initiative in providing information and encouraging questions, especially when it is clear that women do not know what to ask or are intimidated;
- encourages women in their control over decisions;
- takes the time to explore culturally appropriate ways of caring for the client and providing information (e.g., the client may wish a family member, first, to know a tentative diagnosis of her condition); or explores major fears, past traumas, and mistrust, as with many refugees who were political prisoners (this can reduce stress and enhance client care);
- does not penalize the care of clients from particular ethnic or other backgrounds (women specifically mentioned racist attitudes they experienced when their doctors found out they were from Aboriginal backgrounds);
- does not stereotype women with disabilities or make judgments about their sexuality, desire for children, or competence (women recommended specific training programs for health professionals to understand the diversity of women and their needs in more sensitive ways);
- attends to the specific needs of deaf clients by recognizing that English may be their second language; booking an interpreter when the health care provider knows the client is deaf ("without communication there is no information; it is not possible to build trust and rapport");

- attends to the language needs of immigrant women for whom English is a second language by ensuring access to interpreters; and
- respects the decisions of deaf women or couples; some may not want interpreters present in particular personal situations (e.g., labour).

2. With regard to nurses, the women had two main recommendations:
   (a) Nurses should be trained to be more supportive of new mothers and not critical. Several women specifically mentioned the need for kind support in relation to breast feeding.
   (b) Nurses should learn some basic signing to be able to care for the deaf patient and not feel uncomfortable with her care. As one deaf woman said, "The nurses seemed uneasy having a deaf patient. Gesture, swallow your pride; don't leave me!" Public health nurses should book interpreters when visiting deaf clients.

3. A number of women addressed the need to improve crisis management skills in labour and delivery. In fact, some indicated that they thought staff had treated situations as crises unnecessarily and had escalated the woman's or couple's anxieties.
   (a) Staff should coordinate information being provided to patients.
   (b) When the patient is present, staff should not discuss the patient's care as if she were a third party, not relevant to the discussion.
   (c) Securing informed consent must be done in a context sensitive to a woman's situation (is she in severe pain? is she informed enough to decide about these particular options for her care?), and not just to avoid the liability of the staff.
   (d) Nurses should not leave patients in a crisis point in labour if a shift is ending, but should provide continuity of care.
   (e) Where infant death or severe disability is anticipated, staff should respect the rights of parents to make informed decisions about possible interventions and adhere to these; the need for trust between staff and parents was stressed.

## Prenatal Testing and Diagnostic Technologies

The women addressed their recommendations to issues of informed consent, specific ways the testing process might be improved, and the need for broader philosophical discussions about testing.

## Informed Consent

1. Women or couples need clearer explanations of what tests are for and the implications of positive and negative results before tests are administered.
2. Doctors should indicate to patients if they do automatic screening for genetic disabilities and provide the choice to opt out.
3. Doctors should inform patients about what tests they perform or order routinely.
4. Genetic screening for particular disabilities should be available but it should be clear it is the woman's choice to participate. Accurate, up-to-date information needs to be provided for a woman to make that choice, including possible risks from having the testing. She must have the right to refuse.
5. Instructions should not be confused with explanations of tests.
6. The process of informed consent should be sensitive to social and cultural factors, recognizing that teenagers, immigrant women, Aboriginal women, and others might hesitate to raise concerns or questions, and to refuse or request particular tests. Advocates are needed in this process.
7. Decisions about whether to proceed with further testing can be helped with disability counselling. There is a need for a "non-judgmental sounding board" to help women or couples sort out their feelings about the genetic information and risk factors. Part of this process could include talking with the parents of children with certain disabilities and with adults or teenagers who experience forms of the disability.
8. The process of genetic and disability counselling should be non-directive; it should facilitate discussion of the issues of major importance to the woman or couple. The statistical risks are only one part of this process. Counselling should empower women to trust their judgments and intuition in making decisions.

## The Setting

9. Explanations about medical equipment should be provided. Many women, particularly from non-Western countries, indicated fears of medical equipment.
10. At the request of the woman, interpreters or companions should be allowed into the test setting.
11. A woman should never be treated as if she were absent when health professionals are discussing her situation and care.

12. Overbooking appointments for ultrasound creates physical and emotional discomfort.
13. There is a need for improved coordination among health professionals pertaining to test results and consultation about treatment or case management. The fragmentation of care must be addressed through new models of client care.
14. Test results, when positive, should be provided in a highly sensitive manner, ensuring that ongoing support is provided to the woman or couple. Health care providers must recognize that clients may not absorb information when in crisis and require follow-up emotional support.
15. Technicians, nurses, and doctors involved in testing must be carefully trained to be sensitive to a woman's emotional state and the psychological meaning of tests. Hospitals and clinics need to design more supportive, woman-centred approaches to testing.

## *Philosophical and Social Policy Issues*

16. The escalation of costs in prenatal testing should be closely reviewed. Several women noted that Canadians should be wary of following the lead of the United States in unnecessary uses of technologies and high costs.
17. Testing should be used appropriately, ideally with risk factors discussed between health care provider and client. As noted in earlier sections, the women indicated a wide range of attitudes in assessing the meaning and relevance of risk factors.
18. Public education about screening programs should emphasize that tests may be wrong and that they do not provide information about the severity of a disability. Women or couples must be clearly informed that negative test results are not a guarantee that everything is fine.
19. There needs to be much more public discussion about the philosophy and attitudes underlying genetic screening, the history of eugenic practices and attitudes in Canadian society, and the use of tests in a discriminatory or coercive way. Testing raises philosophical and moral issues for individuals pertaining to attitudes toward abortion. Women or couples are also confronted with assessing their attitudes and fears and societal attitudes about having and raising a child with a particular disability. The medical system does not easily find time or space to address these deeper issues. As some women noted, pregnancy is not the best time to examine these attitudes.
20. Public education and policies should strive to counter the negative social attitudes that de-value persons with disabilities and particularly women with disabilities in Canadian society.

## Genetic and Fetal Research

Several women made recommendations pertaining to research. One woman, whose infant died shortly after birth as a result of a chromosomal anomaly, and another whose sister's infant was born with multiple, fatal disabilities, spoke most eloquently on the need for research into such genetic anomalies. They hoped that research might lead to knowledge about prevention and possible treatment. They believed that if an anomaly could be determined with certainty early in a pregnancy, the woman could have the option to abort, or she and her family could be prepared and make prior decisions about intervention at birth. If a couple is found to be carriers, they can decide to risk pregnancy or not. Both women emphasized that it was crucial to address the social and philosophical implications of research and testing.

1. Funding for research into genetic anomalies should continue. This is crucial for lethal anomalies or where children born lead short lives with much suffering.

2. Genetic research is important for possible treatment and prevention of particular diseases and disabilities, and to provide women or couples with information to make informed choices about a particular pregnancy. Research should not be directed toward de-valuing persons with such disabilities, but toward enhancing their quality of life.

3. There should be funding for research on fetal tissue to determine the reasons for miscarriages. More emphasis should be placed on providing women with reasons to explain why miscarriages occur.

4. There should be ongoing research on the possible long-term effects of ultrasound used in prenatal diagnosis.

5. Research should focus on the effects on the newborn of the mother's well-being during pregnancy. Several women suggested research on how stress and anxiety during pregnancy (such as anxiety brought about through testing) may affect the labour and birthing and the infant's temperament. They also suggested such research look at impacts of a positive mental outlook, aided by relaxation techniques and music. They saw a need for research into the process of bonding and suggested that detailed stories of women's attitudes and behaviours during pregnancy and of their infants may provide some valuable information.

## Alternative Models of Prenatal Care and Birthing

As the above shows, the women interviewed recommended reforms to current practices of medical care during pregnancy. They called for major changes to rigid hospital procedures, and more flexibility and attention to the diverse needs of women such as immigrant women and women with disabilities. The overwhelming call for patient advocates suggests that current structures fall short in meeting most women's psychological and other needs.

A number of women identified alternative models and sites of care. They recommended the following.

1. The practice of midwifery should be legalized in Manitoba. Midwives should be trained, certified, and accepted as health professionals. Women identified many positive features of midwifery, including the continuity of care; better care; and the ability of the midwife to spend time providing health education, nutrition counselling, and emotional support. Midwives were seen as potentially of great benefit to women who felt particularly marginalized within the mainstream health care system, and who might need particular support for medical or other needs.

    Women wanted doctors for backup to midwives and referral if complications arose during pregnancy and labour. Some women noted that such services would probably be cost-effective in the long run since midwives tend to refer pregnant women less often for testing than specialists and rely on clinical skills. One woman, herself a midwife, cautioned that midwives would not be much different from doctors unless they were trained to understand "the psychology of women."

2. Birthing centres should be established where principles of care are woman-centred and where backup medical support is available, if needed.

3. There should be formal recognition by the medical profession in Manitoba of the option of home birth, with attending midwives or physicians and with available hospital backup. The one woman who had a home birth in Manitoba movingly identified the many benefits she felt from this experience, including the sense of personal power and control that she maintained throughout her labour and delivery, the deep trust she felt in herself and in the midwives, and the personal meaning of the experience for her and her daughter.

4. Support should be extended for community-based health care programs that pay attention to the broad needs of women during pregnancy and the post-partum period. As elaborated in the recommendations under "Needed Supports and Services During Pregnancy, Birthing, and the Post-Partum Period," creative programs that provide specialized services and supports (e.g., labour companions, health educators or advocates, interpreters, prenatal education, counselling, etc.) are perceived as "woman-friendly" contexts for health education, health promotion, and building self-esteem.

## General Social Transformations

Many of the women noted that improving their quality of health necessitated other changes in society. They frequently said, "I know this really isn't part of the study, but ..." They cited the need for better working conditions in factories, specifically for pregnant women; preventive health programs; and more economic and social supports, such as food co-ops, bursaries, and good day-care to allow women to finish high school or university or enter training courses.

The high proportion of low-income women in this study draws attention to the particular needs of women living in poverty or close to the poverty line. There is a direct and well-researched relationship between health and wealth. The circumstances of women's daily lives cannot be separated from their health and well-being nor from how they interact with the health care system. Low-income women tend to live in poor housing; they and their children experience higher rates of respiratory diseases; children may be exposed to hazards and have more accidents; and nutrition may be poor. Getting to medical appointments takes considerable effort and may be costly if a woman needs a babysitter and has no car. Many women called attention to the need for community and preventive health programs that attempt to address the broader context of a client's life.

Many women also identified a crucial need for changes in social attitudes. They told of experiencing hostility or discrimination because they were pregnant teenagers or young mothers; because they were of Aboriginal background, immigrants, or refugees; or because they had a particular condition such as cerebral palsy or deafness. They did not have specific recommendations for how the more subtle attitudes could be combatted except that people should try to be more open-minded and get to know individuals. Once people know each other personally, stereotypes are often hard to reconcile with individuals. As Ina told her fellow students, "Touch me. Did anything happen to you? Did you catch what I have?"

A few women were critical of fee-for-service reimbursement and thought that this means of payment contributed to fragmented care, to a lack of time for patient visits, and in some cases to placing greed above client interest. Doctors were not rewarded for spending caring time. The women envisioned a system in which they were treated as individuals in a holistic manner and in which their emotional, physical, and social well-being would be the focus of care.

The deaf women drew attention to what they believed was a medical, disease model of care for the deaf in general and one that disparaged and failed to recognize the value and validity of a deaf culture. They noted how everything is measured against the norm of a hearing world. As Sue said,

> This story might come as baffling for you. If a child has a hearing loss and they can have a cochlear implant, the Manitoba Health Services Commission will pay up to $70 000 for that implant for each child, if the

parents want to try it. But they won't pay $30 per hour for an interpreter. That's the medical perspective though. "The ear is broken, let's fix it. Oh no, they're deaf people, they just want to communicate and use their own language. Why pay $30 an hour?" They won't and it's really not fair and who suffers at the end is the deaf community.

The need for broad changes in social attitudes toward persons with disabilities and toward minorities was a strong theme among the recommendations.

## Conclusions[34]

### Principles of Care

All of the 37 women interviewed defined many of their medical encounters as arenas of struggle, not support. While the women described many health professionals as caring, attentive, and sometimes highly compassionate, they also described a medical system that was fragmented and uncoordinated, and that isolated clients. Whatever a woman's background and circumstances, she perceived a need for support and advocacy to deal with some aspects of the medical system. Many of the women believed they needed huge reserves of self-esteem, conviction, and courage to question what was happening to them and to ensure they were heard. The settings and nuances of care made them feel vulnerable. This was equally true of the nurses in the study who talked about needing considerable emotional resources to deal with the medical system as clients.

Despite the positive outcomes of healthy babies for the vast majority of the women, pregnancy and birthing held many disappointments because of medical encounters. As major life events, these experiences may have had undetermined effects on labour, birthing, and the post-partum period. The interviews suggest that medical care pertaining to pregnancy and childbirth requires serious reforms in institutions and profound transformations in philosophy and approach. The women's interviews provide some basic principles upon which reform should be predicated:

1. Prenatal care should be based on the assumption that pregnancy is not a disease, but a physiological, cultural, and social process engaged in by the majority of the world's women; pregnancy and birthing are major life experiences.

2. Prenatal care and birthing should be woman-centred; women should be supported to have the knowledge, skills, and confidence to birth in a secure and safe environment; protocols should not be geared to the convenience of doctors, staff, and bureaucratic procedures.

3. Health care providers must respect the subjective and objective knowledge that women bring to the medical encounter. This knowledge might be drawn from diverse cultural traditions; it might also be rooted in experiences of abuse and violence encountered by women and triggered in medical encounters. Good health care depends on the health care provider being sensitive to such issues and treating women and their bodies with respect.

4. Women should be full participants in their prenatal care and be treated as the social equals of the health care provider. There is no single model of ideal care, but it is in the interest of all for health care provider and client to explore their common ground and their differences and to develop good communication and rapport. Care should not be used to intimidate.

5. Health care providers must strive to overcome fragmentation by ensuring coordination of care and by finding new models for collegiality and for continuity of care.

6. Women should be involved in a process of informed choice and informed consent in relation to their care and to medical interventions such as screening and diagnostic testing. This involves access to accurate, balanced, and current information about options in care.

7. Technologies should be used appropriately and to enhance, not supplant, the development of excellent clinical skills in diagnosis.

Implementing these principles will require major changes in how doctors, nurses, and other health professionals are trained; alternative options of prenatal care such as legalizing midwifery; and alterations in how medical services are reimbursed. The various creative models suggested in the recommendations for delivery of prenatal care and birthing (e.g., birthing centres, health educators, and advocates) will need to be evaluated for their costs and benefits. As a few of the women suggested, pilot programs have been shown to be highly cost-effective in the delivery of certain types of health-promoting services and result in high levels of client satisfaction.

## Implications of Prenatal Testing for Woman-Centred Care

When a Manitoba woman becomes pregnant, she steps onto an escalator of decision making about prenatal diagnosis and testing. The woman becomes linked to a complex and confusing set of institutions and programs about which she most likely knew little or nothing before. It is also a system in flux. Maternal serum AFP screening in Manitoba over the past decade evolved from a pilot research project to a provincially funded program now screening 11 000 women per year. As data about outcomes were evaluated, guidelines for what are considered normal and abnormal results were adjusted. Recommended diagnostic testing has evolved and changed.[35] There has also been a large increase in the use of ultrasound and fetal assessment. Guidelines concerning the use of ultrasound and fetal assessments in pregnancy have also been changing, as outcomes and costs are weighed. Doctors and their associations concerned with providing up-to-date care and with liability, and manufacturers promoting technologies, are key factors sustaining the use of these tests and technologies. Once such technologies are available and promoted, consumer demand reinforces further use.

The women in this study were not aware of the history and economics of prenatal testing, nor of who made decisions that such programs should be offered in Manitoba. The tests are perceived to be part of the package of routine, modern prenatal care. For many of the women, ultrasound and maternal serum AFP provided assurance that their pregnancy was going well. They describe their pregnancy and fetal development in terms of when the tests occurred and what they revealed. As elaborated earlier, the tests became a metaphor for the progression of the pregnancy and a construct for how women experience pregnancy in new ways.

Confronted with decisions about whether to have a maternal serum AFP screening test or not, whether to pursue further diagnosis through amniocentesis if maternal serum AFP results are positive, and whether to agree to recommended ultrasounds or fetal assessments, each woman experiences a personal dilemma about her particular pregnancy. She may refuse to proceed, but it is nevertheless a choice and one that is perceived to involve the woman in a roulette of potential liability against herself. Either she must be sure enough of herself to confront the system and refuse tests or she must be prepared to take the consequences, if only in relation to herself and her doubts about whether she has done the "right" thing. As the interviews indicated, women can be ridden with tremendous conflicts and anxieties over what to do. Should they trust their gut feelings or the professional assessment that there is a risk, however small? Do they feel something is wrong? Should they proceed? What if they miscarry? Is it possible to reconcile the medical and the intuitive models and the tensions and contradiction inherent in prenatal testing?

The women describe a medical system that is not easily geared to decisions by pregnant clients and in which how and if informed consent is obtained in relation to prenatal testing are highly variable. For example, the study revealed considerable diversity in how women were informed by doctors about maternal serum AFP tests and about subsequent results. Some women attending community health centres were given detailed written information at least one week before the tests being done in addition to information provided by the provincial screening program; others had a brief oral explanation. Some women had no information at all beforehand and only knew they had received the test when results were positive and they were confronted with decisions about further testing.

Women with positive results were referred to other professionals and programs and sometimes experienced "parallel care," with little communication between their health care providers, as they saw it. Genetic counselling was generally described as helpful, but again was a specialized service apart from a woman's overall prenatal care. Some women, especially the teenagers, felt swept along by a process that did not involve informed choice or informed consent. Many women experienced weeks of anxious waiting for test results with no supportive word from a health care provider.

The stated goals of genetic screening programs are to avoid long-term pain and suffering for women, other family members, and the infants having particular, severe disabilities. Some proponents of testing advocate other reasons: those with severe disabilities who survive require the expenditures of tax dollars to be maintained and have a poor quality of life and are thus seen as a social burden.

Prenatal screening through maternal serum AFP can only identify a risk that something is wrong for a particular woman. It is not designed to make a definitive diagnosis, and it cannot specify the severity of a disability. Further diagnostic tests can be more accurate but, as in the case of amniocentesis, pose a risk of miscarriage. As the women in this study showed, women with positive screening results are confronted with hard decisions, weighing the risks of reassurance and uncertainty. The women in this study believed that women should be offered the opportunity of screening. In reference to infants with severe, lethal abnormalities, almost all the women stated that they would prefer to know in advance and would consider abortion if they had the opportunity.

The women differed among themselves regarding non-lethal, less severe disabilities. For example, eight of the 37 stated they would or might terminate a Down syndrome or spina bifida pregnancy and so risked amniocentesis; others decided they would not terminate either spina bifida or Down syndrome; they saw them as "things you can live with," and rejected amniocentesis. Almost all the women discussed the possibility of the child not being seriously disabled and being able to live a satisfying life.

In describing the difficult decisions or situations they were presented with, the women grappled with social and personal ethics rooted in their cultural backgrounds. Women from China expressed the view that persons with disabilities were a social burden. Some women, especially those who had experience with persons with disabilities, identified the eugenic implications of genetic screening. They saw screening leading to therapy as potentially valuable but were concerned that screening created an environment in which persons with disabilities were perceived as less valuable and unproductive members of society. They felt it important that persons with disabilities not be denied the opportunities and resources to access services and social institutions to lead fulfilling lives. Women can be made to feel guilty for continuing such pregnancies and for expecting society to respond with appropriate resources and services. They asked who decides what abilities are more valuable than others. They described a slippery slope and were concerned about where it led.

The women also expressed the view that all women should be able to make reproductive choices. This view was held whatever a woman's own personal beliefs and decisions concerning abortion. They said they wanted the option to know if there was a problem with a pregnancy and would decide what to do. Those critical of the trends toward routinization of testing felt that women had to be highly informed consumers in order to make choices in their own best interests. Since women are the primary caregivers in the family and the ones to bear the major responsibilities of caring for a child with disabilities, all 37 women thought they had to have the option to choose to continue a pregnancy or not.

The women's stories of their situations and the decisions they made reflect the struggle to balance the needs and resources of the fetus, other family members, society, and themselves. Women struggled to determine what was right in that situation, what they and their families could cope with, based on the knowledge they had. The women made those decisions by drawing on a variety of resources and knowledge — the opinions of doctors, counsellors, partners, and friends, and their intuition about what "felt right." They attempted to integrate the medical construct of pregnancy with their subjective construct and evaluate what risk factors really meant in the context of their values and the circumstances of their lives. In a stressful period, they were trying to put a fragmented system of prenatal care into a working whole.

There are no easy answers as to where prenatal screening and tests "fit" in the scenarios of holistic care suggested in the women's recommendations. Ideally, in a more woman-centred framework, women should have information about options for genetic screening, why screening is being carried out in Manitoba, and results of screening programs to date. How information about screening and testing is designed and packaged is very important. Information about genetic screening can be geared to reinforce the management and control of women[36] and can obscure the difficult decisions that results bring to the fore. If only simplistic information is provided, some professionals are making assumptions about the level of consent that is necessary or possible from Manitoba women.

Significantly, such information tends to obscure the fact that social policy decisions have been made to allocate resources for particular programs and for the introduction of technologies with limited or no public debate and with few guidelines about how and when the outcomes of such programs will be evaluated. The demand for such programs may then expand while resources remain the same. In the case of maternal serum AFP screening in Manitoba, more women are being screened, putting added pressure on limited services for counselling and follow-up.[37] Social policy decisions affect the ideologies, practices, and protocols of prenatal care and have profound personal impacts on how women experience their pregnancies.

There is no optimal consent process, nor is there a perfect way to provide information to women that links social policy decisions to the personal choices with which a woman is confronted. Information can be designed to take women through the steps of understanding what tests are able to do and what they cannot do at this point and, more importantly, what issues might confront women and their families through such screening. The latter reflects a more authentic process of informed consent. Such information could be designed with the help of women from diverse backgrounds who have experienced prenatal testing and the anxieties caused by positive results and with input from health advocates. Consultants should include women with disabilities who have a different understanding of the potential of persons with disabilities and the experiences of pregnant women. They can provide important insights into what information would have been useful to hear and in what formats.

In a more woman-centred system, how information is introduced and by whom can make a difference in how a woman approaches the decision to proceed or not with screening or with counselling for risk factors. A detailed family and medical history, including an assessment of how a woman copes with the various stressors in her life, and some of her views on disability and circumstances under which she might consider abortion, if any, can provide a basis for discussing the meaning of tests and how she might cope with future decisions. Talking about scenarios hypothetically is, of course, different from confronting the reality, but it helps to establish rapport and understanding between the woman and the health care provider — whether midwife, general practitioner, or specialist. It allows her time to consider her views, talk to others, and decide how she will exert control in this process. Broad public education should help to stimulate public discussion about the social and ideological issues underlying the introduction of particular technologies and the ways to evaluate their benefits and risks.

## Supplemental Recommendations of the Research Report

Drawing from the women's experiences and recommendations, the report calls attention to a number of key issues in relation to prenatal screening and testing and makes the following further recommendations, supplemental to those of the women.

1. Screening programs, such as maternal serum AFP, should be offered to clients only on an opt-in basis and if sufficient resources are allocated for counselling of clients, including follow-up counselling; for well-designed information that clarifies the potential and limitations of screening programs and are appropriate to the diversity of Manitoba

women, including immigrant women and deaf women; and for detailed education of physicians about such programs so they can evaluate outcomes. Technologies should not be introduced without attention being paid and adequate resources allocated to the psychological and societal implications of these technologies.

2. The above elements provide a basis from which to design appropriate, authentic procedures for informed choice and informed consent in relation to prenatal screening and testing. Such procedures should be implemented in Manitoba with particular attention paid to consent by minors and to women whose first language is not English.

3. Screening programs should be evaluated carefully in terms of the social and financial costs and benefits, taking into account the following factors:

    (a) the anxieties induced in women who have positive results but normal outcomes;

    (b) alternate methods (if any) for identifying cases of serious defects, such as ultrasound or more specific biochemical tests;

    (c) the long-term benefits of maternal serum AFP screening in terms of research, to allow more specific tests to be developed and information about other complications of pregnancy to be obtained;

    (d) how the concerns for liability of health providers and insurers relate to the use and expansion of screening programs;

    (e) whether the counselling program provides a balanced view of what it means to live with a particular disability;

    (f) if research is a major goal of current screening programs, the type of informed consent process that should be developed.

4. There is a need to understand much more profoundly how the routinization of prenatal testing affects a woman's attitudes toward her pregnancy and affects her bonding with the fetus. The impacts on fetal development, labour, and delivery and on the post-partum period need to be explored. More qualitative research is needed on these issues.

5. There is a need for more insight into and understanding of the social stigmas and isolation that persons with disabilities face and particularly into the issues facing women with disabilities. Health professionals and researchers need greater sensitivity in addressing reproductive health, sexuality, and prenatal care of women with disabilities. Social research and advocacy should be addressed to questions of valuing difference in society and transforming stereotypes. A wide range of issues pertaining to women with

disabilities and children with disabilities is raised in relation to the new reproductive technologies and deserves a separate inquiry.

6. Major transformations are needed in the training of health professionals to address fragmentation of care, particularly in prenatal care. The implications of a client's history as a victim of abuse and violence for medicalization and testing should be addressed in curricula and in continuing education of health professionals.

7. The creative models of health advocacy and delivery, such as those beginning in immigrant communities, should be expanded. These models can enhance culturally appropriate education about prenatal tests and technologies.

8. Health policy makers and administrators should look for ways to solicit client input and advice, specifically in relation to prenatal testing and reproductive technologies. As the study reveals, clients can be a crucial resource in design and evaluation of health services.

One of the strengths of this study has been the diversity of the women who participated in terms of age, class, abilities, ethnicity, and race. The study highlights how these women feel marginalized and fragmented by the medical system, particularly during a period in their lives that they felt ought to be life-affirming and enriching. Their stories reflect the passion with which children can be wanted and loved and the strong feelings women have toward exercising reproductive choices. The struggles of the minority women — women with disabilities, deaf women, Aboriginal women, immigrant and refugee women, and teenagers — are especially illuminating; they suggest how our society cannot deal with difference in an accepting way. The norm continues to be set from the perspective of the privileged, the able-bodied, and the male gender. Policies and practices largely alienate, isolate, and stigmatize those who are different from the norm or "make up for the difference" by "special arrangements" for marginal assistance. As this sample of women reflects, difference is a fact of life.

Reproductive technologies ought to be about making pregnancy, birthing, and mothering a healthy life experience. We are left with these social questions: How do we work with and support women of all circumstances in achieving these goals? How do we extricate our social policies and daily practices from the language and politics of "negative difference"? How do we integrate and value various kinds of knowledge from different sources and traditions to ensure quality prenatal care?[38]

This study indicates how profound understanding comes from the margins; these women offer eloquent insights into the potential of certain prenatal technologies to ease human suffering, but also into the pain and anguish that the technology-driven health care system can inflict. The study provided a forum for the women to recommend changes. The women speak with diverse voices and provide common visions of a humane and empowering system of care.

# Appendix 1. Consent Form for Participants

## "Women's Experiences with Technology in Pregnancy"

### Consent Form for Participants

I agree to participate in the study "Women's Experiences with Technology in Pregnancy" sponsored by the Women's Health Clinic.

I understand that I will be asked questions and talk about my experiences with prenatal tests and about my prenatal care in general. The main focus will be on experiences I have had with pregnancy in the last three years.

I understand that I will also be asked some questions about my background, work experiences and beliefs about pregnancy.

The interview will take approximately two hours. It will be held in the language of my choice with an interpreter, if necessary. This will be arranged beforehand.

At any time, I can choose not to answer particular questions. I can ask the researcher questions and raise any concerns.

At any time during the interview, I can decide not to continue. This will not in any way at all affect the care I receive from the agency that informed me about the study.

I understand that the information I give will be treated as confidential. My name and other ways to identify me will not be used. The information will be kept secure in a locked cabinet. If the interview is recorded, the tapes will be erased once the study is over.

I will have a chance to review a written version of what I say and make any corrections I wish.

If I choose, I will receive a summary of the conclusions of the study. I can choose to discuss the conclusions of the study in the language of my choice.

I will be paid $25.00 towards time and expenses for participating in the study.

I agree to participate in the study "Women's Experiences with Technology in Pregnancy."

Signed: _____

## Recording the Interview

I agree to have my interview tape recorded. I understand that this information will only be used so that what I say can be recorded accurately to prepare the summary for the report. The tape will be stored in a locked cabinet. It will not have my name on it. It will be erased after the study is completed.

Signed: _____

Date: _____

Witness: _____

## Honorarium

I have received $25.00 from the Women's Health Clinic for participating in the study "Women's Experiences with Technology in Pregnancy."

Signed: _____

Date: _____

Witness: _____

I would like to receive a summary of the conclusions of the final report.

Yes _____ No _____

# Appendix 2. Topic Areas and Questions

## Women's Health Clinic — Research Project
## "Women's Experiences with Technology in Pregnancy"
## Topic Areas and Questions (Final Draft)

Many of the questions are open-ended, to elicit each woman's narrative concerning her experiences with pregnancy and prenatal testing. While the range of topics covered will be the same for each woman, the specific questions will be suited to her particular situation. Questions will be in clear language. In some cases, the researcher will work with an interpreter.

Each interview is expected to take approximately two hours.

**BACKGROUND**

Birthdate

Number of pregnancies

Number of children — girls; boys?

When were the children born?

Where were the children born?

How old were you when you became pregnant the first time? How old were you each of the other times?

Where were you born? Where have you lived; when did you come to Canada/Manitoba (if relevant)?

(May be asked with some) What formal schooling, training or other education do you have? Did you have to quit school or training because of the pregnancy? Why? What happened? Do you have plans to return to school or training?

What work were you doing when you became pregnant?

Were there any hazards or stresses where you worked that you think may have affected your pregnancy? If so, what were these? How long did you keep working at your job(s) while you were pregnant? (if relevant) What type of work are you doing now?

Tell me about some of the other kinds of work you have done — for pay, volunteer, at home. Were there times when you wanted to work for wages but could not?

When you were pregnant, did someone help you with cleaning, cooking, other tasks? What help do/did you have from your partner, husband, extended family, friends, neighbours, etc.?

Who lives in your household? Who was living with you when you were pregnant or were you living by yourself?

What language(s) do you speak? What do you speak mostly at home? What other languages do you understand?

Is your ethnic background important to you? Your culture? In what ways?

Is religion important to you? How?

Given your background, are there certain things a woman is supposed to do when she is pregnant? What are some of these? If a woman has problems during her pregnancy, what might be some of the reasons? What could she do? How did you learn these? Were they important to you? Did you follow any of these practices?

What do you consider to be the ideal number of children? Do you have any preference or none for girls or for boys? Do you think your views about how many children to have or whether it's better to have boys or girls differ from those of your mother or grandmothers? In what ways?

## INFERTILITY

Did you have any problems getting pregnant? If yes, do you have any ideas about why this was/is so? What were your experiences?

## PREGNANCY

Please tell me about your pregnancy(ies). (Drawing from her descriptions, and focusing on a recent pregnancy, we will also ask):

Was the pregnancy planned or unplanned?

How did you know you were pregnant? What were your feelings about this? Who did you tell?

Did your experiences with previous pregnancy(ies) affect how you felt about this one? (if relevant) In what ways?

What was your health like before the pregnancy? Were you taking any drugs? Substance abuse?

When you found out you were pregnant, did you think about prenatal care? Why or why not? What kind of care did you want? How did you go about finding prenatal care?

Did you face any barriers such as language or physical access in trying to get prenatal care? Were you fearful, shy or anxious? Did you have access to interpreter services? Did these help? Were there other kinds of help that you needed (e.g., making contacts with Dept. of Immigration or Welfare)? Did you receive help? If not, how did you cope?

Did you go for prenatal care? Why or why not? Where did you go? How often did you go? Did anyone come to you? What was the care like?

## TESTS

What types of tests, medical technologies or treatments did you have during your pregnancy? Can you describe these?

Do you know the names of the tests, procedures or of any drugs you may have been given?

What is your understanding of why these were done? (We will ask specific questions about urine tests; blood tests — AFP, etc.; ultrasound; amniocentesis ... as relevant.)

Did your prenatal care include any forms of HIV testing? Any treatment for substance abuse?

Who suggested the tests or procedures? Did you (or your partner or anyone else in your family) ask for any particular tests? If so, what were these and why? What was the response?

Did anyone explain the tests/procedures to you? If yes, who? When did they do this? Were you alone at the time or with others? Was an interpreter present with you? If so, what training did they have?

Did you understand what was told to you? Did you raise any questions or concerns? If yes, do you feel these were heard and dealt with? If not, why not?

Did you receive counselling before the test?

Were you given anything to read about the tests? In what language? Did you have trouble reading it? Was it helpful? Did you have time to think about it and ask any questions?

How did you feel before the test (ultrasound, amnio, etc.)? Did you have any worries about pain or other worries?

How did you feel during the tests or procedures?

How did you feel after?

Did you experience any pain or discomfort? Were any of the tests, in your belief, risks to the pregnancy?

Do you feel having the test was your choice?

Was the interpreter present during the test? (if relevant) Did you want her to be there? Was she permitted to be there or denied admittance?

If no one explained the test, how did you feel? Did you ask for information? Did you feel you could raise questions and concerns? What did you want to know? Were there things that you preferred not to know but were told — about the tests, the pregnancy, etc.?

**RESULTS**

How long did you have to wait before getting results? What was this time like for you? Did you talk to anyone about how you were feeling? Counsellor? friends? relatives?

How were you told about the results? Who was with you, if anyone? What happened? Did you have any counselling at this time?

If the results were positive, tell me what happened then. (Questions will be shaped to specific tests — e.g., the results from amniocentesis or from tests for neural tube defects may have required more information and further decisions.)

If the results were negative, how did you feel?

Did you ever refuse any suggested tests or treatment? If so, why? What happened? If not, did you ever think of refusing? Did you know that you could refuse? Did you ever miss any appointments — e.g., for ultrasound? Why, and what happened?

Would you have liked your doctor to have used more tests? Why or why not?

During your pregnancy were you diagnosed as having any condition such as anemia? gestational diabetes? preeclampsia? (Women may not be familiar with the medical terms, so colloquial terms could be used — e.g., "sugar.") Other? If so, how did you feel?

What medical care and treatment did you have? Was it difficult for you? e.g., did you have to follow a diet, have other tests, or take particular drugs, etc.? Did you understand what you were expected to do? How did this affect your pregnancy?

**DISABILITY ISSUES**

Did you have any thoughts or concerns about having a child with disabilities when you became pregnant? During your pregnancy? What were these?

What are some of your own experiences with disability (e.g., as a woman with disability; in your family; friends; other)? What were you taught about disability as a child? How have these experiences affected your attitudes now? Could you explain how disability (or particular disabilities) might be seen in your culture, ethnic group? Is it different for a boy or a girl? For a man or woman?

If the results of the tests showed that the child would have Down syndrome, spina bifida, other ... what would you have done? or (where relevant): If you like, tell me about what happened when the test results indicated it was likely the baby would have a disability.

What kinds of information and counselling did you receive? Who gave you the information and counselling? What did they tell you about this type of disability? About how severe it might be? About the life a child or adult with such a disability would lead? Did they suggest anything? Was this helpful? How? If not, why not? (Questions about whether an interpreter was present will be asked, if relevant.)

Did you talk with someone who has that type of disability to know what their life is like? With parents of a child with that type of disability? If not, would you have liked to? Did you make contact with any resources such as support groups in the community? If so, what did you find out? If not, would you have liked to have these contacts?

What resources would have been available (are available) to you to care for, love and encourage a child with disability?

Would you (or did you) consider abortion, based on the test results? Why or why not?

Are you satisfied that you had enough knowledge about disability and were aware enough of your feelings at the time to make an informed choice?

## GENERAL IMPACTS OF TESTS

Did your experiences with tests during your pregnancy affect how you thought of the developing fetus? How did you think of it? Did you have a name for him/her? Did you see a fetal image during the tests? If you did, how did that affect you?

Did your experience with tests and procedures during your pregnancy have any impact on other parts of your life (e.g., on your relationships? on whether to have other children?)?

Did these experiences affect what you thought your birth would be like? In what ways?

## PREPARATION FOR THE BIRTH

How did you feel the pregnancy was going? What changes did you feel in yourself? Did you discuss these with anyone?

Did you feel prepared for the birth?

Did you do anything to prepare yourself (e.g., attend prenatal classes)? Did you seek out information or specific resources about what was happening during your pregnancy? What were some of these and how did you find them (e.g., TV, radio, magazines)?

Did you talk with your mother, mother-in-law, grandmother or other women about their pregnancies and birth experiences? If so, what were some of the things you learned? What were some of the main differences/similarities to your experiences? Were there any beliefs and rules about what to do during pregnancy that they wanted you to follow? Did you? Why or why not?

What did you find helpful in your prenatal care and what would you like to have changed or improved, if anything?

## BIRTH

What kind of birth did you want? What did you think it would be like?

Describe your birth experience (where appropriate). Did your experiences differ from your ideal? In what ways? What would you have liked to be different?

## MISCARRIAGE, STILLBIRTH OR THERAPEUTIC ABORTION

Where a woman experienced a miscarriage, stillbirth or a therapeutic abortion because of prenatal diagnosis, she may discuss the experience, if she chooses.

Did you receive counselling or other support immediately after this happened? Have you been involved in any longer term counselling, support groups, etc.? How did you get involved with these? If not, would you have liked to have had further support?

Did family and friends help you or did they not understand what you were going through?

What do you think would be the best type of help and advice for a woman who experienced what you did?

## GENERAL QUESTIONS

- Was there a "most difficult time" during the pregnancy? If so, what do you think the most difficult part of the pregnancy was? How did you cope with it? Did you have to make any hard decisions? If so, how were these made? Did you receive support and help from others? Would you change what you did? How might it have been an easier time?

- What was the best time in the pregnancy for you? Why? Do you think that has affected how you are now?

- Describe what the first few months after the birth were like for you (if relevant). Did you decide to breastfeed the baby? Why or why not?

- Tests during pregnancy can tell us many things about the developing fetus. What types of information would you like to have before the child is born, if any? Why would you like this information? Are there things you would prefer not to know? Why?

- Based on your experiences, do you have any specific recommendations for the Royal Commission on New Reproductive Technologies or for health professionals and institutions (e.g., clinics, hospitals) concerning prenatal testing or genetic screening, or about prenatal care in general? What are these?

- Is there anything else that you would like to say?

THANK YOU!
Sari Tudiver, Ph.D.
Research Coordinator — "Women's Experiences with Technology in Pregnancy"
Women's Health Clinic
3rd Floor — 419 Graham Ave.
Winnipeg, Manitoba R3C 0M3

November, 1991

## Acknowledgments

Without the 37 women interviewed, this study could not have taken place. I thank them for their honesty and wisdom, and hope that this report in some way does justice to their visions.

The project would have suffered without the help of Jackie Linklater, who served as research assistant. She efficiently transcribed all the taped interviews, coded and collated much of the data on the women's experiences with prenatal diagnosis, and provided support, insights, and encouragement in a number of ways, for which I am exceptionally grateful.

I deeply appreciate the time, insights, and specific expertise provided by the Advisory Committee to this project: Yvonne Peters, Canadian Disability Rights Council; Chris Ansons, Klinic Community Health Centre; Susan Marshall, Manitoba Association for Childbirth and Family Education; Laura Donatelli, Mount Carmel Clinic; Anna Ling, Planned Parenthood Manitoba; and Madeline Boscoe, Women's Health Clinic.

The Women's Health Clinic served as a wonderful anchor institution for this project. Thanks to all the staff and board members who provided much-needed administrative and emotional support, and to Jennifer Cooper, the past Executive Director, who nurtured the project in its early phases. Madeline Boscoe helped bring the project to fruition in many ways, and her enthusiasm, good humour, and incisive comments are particularly appreciated. Thanks to Linda DeRiviere for her accounting skills and to Gio Guzzi, Arlene Mak, Sheila Rainonen, Colleen Clark, Audrhea Lande, and Stephanie Van Nest for specific support and advice.

Thanks for considerable help and advice go to the Health Educators at Planned Parenthood Manitoba who provided interpretation services for some of the interviews. Anna Ling, Sonia Hernandez, Tuyet Nguyen, and San Nop spent many hours reviewing questions and consent forms to ensure they were "culturally appropriate," and with warmth, humour, and understanding took me into their communities.

Thanks as well to the interpreters working at the Independent Interpreter Referral Service who ably facilitated my discussions with the deaf women in the study.

Thanks to Linda Koskie at the Deaf Centre Manitoba; Laurie Shattuck at Villa Rosa; Rosa Mundaca at Mount Carmel Clinic; Sharon Spinks at Fort Garry Women's Resource Centre; and the staff at the Independent Living Resource Centre for specific help referring women to the study.

Over the course of the study, I consulted with a number of people in order to learn more about prenatal testing or for specific information and advice. Special thanks for considerable time to Barbara Lewthwaite, nurse-midwife at the Fetal Assessment Unit, St. Boniface Hospital, Winnipeg; Laurie Thompson and Sandra Gessler, Women's Health Branch, Government of Manitoba; Dr. Meera Sinha, obstetrician and gynaecologist; Dr. Jane Evans, Department of Human Genetics, University of Manitoba and Manitoba Maternal Serum AFP Screening Program; and Madeline Hall, Department of Sociology, University of Manitoba.

Several other people provided key input along the way. Dr. Karen Grant, Department of Sociology, University of Manitoba, served as advisor to the project and provided valuable help, especially in the early stages. Others from whose advice or past work I benefited were Dr. Patricia Kaufert, Laurel Garvie, Dr. Dale Berg, Miriam Baron, and Lea Smith.

Dolores Backman and Dr. F. Clarke Fraser from the Royal Commission on New Reproductive Technologies were understanding and a pleasure to deal with, as were Annie Hall and her library staff at the Commission.

I would particularly like to thank Neil Tudiver for his expertise and help getting the document to its final form. He and Simon Tudiver provided the many small things that make it all worthwhile.

## Notes

1. Eugenics is used in this study to refer to a range of attitudes, beliefs, and strategies to "improve" the human genetic make-up through selection of parents and/or genetic manipulation. Historically a response to declining birth rates among those of Anglo-Saxon ancestry and used to promote policies of racial purity, its proponents advocate that better-educated middle- and upper-class persons will transmit "desirable" traits and should be encouraged to reproduce, while the disabled, poor, and "socially marginal" should be discouraged from having children. In relation to the new reproductive technologies, eugenic attitudes are evident, for example, in sperm banks that limit their donors to men of high academic achievements; in negative attitudes on the part of some researchers and medical professionals toward the sexuality and desire for children of persons with disabilities; and in the potential for genetic manipulation of physical characteristics such as height through preimplantation diagnosis. See, for example, D. Suzuki and P. Knudtson, *Genethics: The Ethics of Engineering Life* (Toronto: Stoddart, 1988); J.E. Bishop and M. Waldholz, *Genome — The Story of the Most Astonishing Scientific Adventure of Our Time: The Attempt to Map All the Genes in the Human Body* (New York: Simon and Schuster, 1990); S. Trombley, *The Right to Reproduce: A History of Coercive Sterilization* (London: Weidenfeld and Nicolson, 1988); A. McLaren, *Our Own Master Race: Eugenics in Canada, 1885-1945* (Toronto: McClelland and Stewart, 1990).

2. The Advisory Committee to the project included representatives from the Women's Health Clinic, Klinic Community Health Centre, Mount Carmel Clinic, Manitoba Association for Childbirth and Family Education, Planned Parenthood Manitoba — Immigrant and Refugee Health Program, and the Canadian Disabilities Rights Council.

3. For a valuable summary of Canadian and international issues concerning prenatal health, see Ontario, Task Force on the Implementation of Midwifery in Ontario, *Report* (Toronto: The Task Force, 1987), and especially Appendix 1, 196-232 on the history of midwifery in Canada; and K. Arnup, A. Lévesque, and

R.R. Pierson, eds., *Delivering Motherhood: Maternal Ideologies and Practices in the 19th and 20th Centuries* (New York: Routledge, 1990).

4. For a superb analysis of medicalization and the social construction of pregnancy, see A. Lippman, "Prenatal Genetic Testing and Screening: Constructing Needs and Reinforcing Inequities," *American Journal of Law & Medicine* 17 (1991): 15-50. The work of Emily Martin is also important in deconstructing cultural meanings of pregnancy. See E. Martin, "Science and Women's Bodies: Forms of Anthropological Knowledge," in *Body/Politics: Women and the Discourses of Science*, ed. M. Jacobus, E.F. Keller, and S. Shuttleworth (New York: Routledge, 1990); E. Martin, *The Woman in the Body: A Cultural Analysis of Reproduction* (Boston: Beacon Press, 1987). See also A. Oakley, *The Captured Womb: A History of the Medical Care of Pregnant Women* (Oxford: Basil Blackwell, 1984); A. Oakley, *Women Confined: Towards a Sociology of Childbirth* (New York: Schocken Books, 1980); D.C. Wertz, "What Birth Has Done for Doctors: A Historical View," *Women and Health* 8 (1) (1983): 7-24; R.W. Wertz and D.C. Wertz, *Lying-In: A History of Childbirth in America* (New York: Free Press, 1977).

5. Medicalization is defined here as an ideology and a set of practices that introduce technological interventions before broad evaluation of their psychological and social impacts and their effectiveness.

6. See, for example, S.B. Rusek, *The Women's Health Movement: Feminist Alternatives to Medical Control* (New York: Praeger, 1979); and S. Romalis, ed., *Childbirth, Alternatives to Medical Control* (Austin: University of Texas Press, 1981).

7. While practices still vary considerably among hospitals, tying down a woman's arms while in labour is no longer practised; shaving, enemas, and routine episiotomies are on the way out. Many hospitals offer birthing rooms for low-risk deliveries.

8. Guidelines for the Society of Obstetricians and Gynaecologists of Canada recommend a minimum of two ultrasounds be carried out during a pregnancy where dates are uncertain or there are other indications. However, ultrasound is a routine procedure in Manitoba. For example, a 1990 report noted that an average of 3.95 obstetrical scans were conducted for each woman who gave birth in Manitoba in that year. See Manitoba, Provincial Ultrasound Advisory Committee, "Diagnostic Ultrasound in Manitoba: A Five Year Plan" (Winnipeg: Manitoba Health, 1990). For detailed references on ultrasound, see Lippman, "Prenatal Genetic Testing and Screening," 21.

9. Unpublished internal documents, Manitoba Working Group on Midwifery, 1991. For a critique of electronic fetal monitoring, see J.R. Kunisch, "Electronic Fetal Monitors: Marketing Forces and the Resulting Controversy," in *Healing Technology: Feminist Perspectives*, ed. K.S. Ratcliff et al. (Ann Arbor: University of Michigan Press, 1989).

10. For example, contraceptive technologies have followed this model. Oral contraceptives were first used in higher dosages for a very wide range of women. With clinical experience, dosages were lowered and contraindications were expanded. Women served unknowingly as a research population.

11. See, for example, E. Yoxen and B. Hyde, *The Social Impact of Biotechnology* (Dublin: European Foundation for the Improvement of Living and Working Conditions, 1987); U.S. Congress, Office of Technology Assessment, *Mapping Our*

*Genes: Genome Projects — How Big, How Fast?* (Washington, DC: Government Printing Office, 1988). For critical reviews and the social implications of such initiatives, see Council for Responsible Genetics, "Position Paper on Genetic Discrimination," and "Position Paper on Human Genome Initiative," *Issues in Reproductive and Genetic Engineering* 3 (1990): 287-95.

12. A good summary of limitations of current research and issues pertaining to the social costs of testing, including anxieties in testing, can be found in M. Reid, "Consumer-Oriented Studies in Relation to Prenatal Screening Tests," *European Journal of Obstetrics, Gynaecology and Reproductive Biology* 28 (Suppl.)(1988): 79-92. See also R.R. Faden et al., "What Participants Understand About a Maternal Serum Alpha-Fetoprotein Screening Program," *American Journal of Public Health* 75 (1985): 1381-84; J.O. Robinson, B.M. Hibbard, and K.M. Laurence, "Anxiety During a Crisis: Emotional Effects of Screening for Neural Tube Defects," *Journal of Psychosomatic Research* 28 (1984): 163-69; D.M. Zuskar, "The Psychological Impact of Prenatal Diagnosis of Fetal Abnormality: Strategies for Investigation and Intervention," *Women & Health* 12 (1)(1987): 91-103; and B.K. Rothman, *The Tentative Pregnancy: Prenatal Diagnosis and the Future of Motherhood* (New York: Viking, 1986).

13. Major work in this area is being done by Rayna Rapp. See R. Rapp, "Chromosomes and Communication: The Discourse of Genetic Counseling," *Medical Anthropology Quarterly* 2 (1988): 143-57; R. Rapp, "Accounting for Amniocentesis," in *Knowledge, Power and Practice: The Anthropology of Medicine and Everyday Life*, ed. S. Lindenbaum and M. Lock (Berkeley: University of California Press, 1993); R. Rapp, "The Powers of 'Positive' Diagnosis: Medical and Maternal Discourses on Amniocentesis," in *Childbirth in America: Anthropological Perspectives*, ed. K. Michaelson (South Hadley: Bergin and Garvey, 1988); R. Rapp, "Moral Pioneers: Women, Men and Fetuses on a Frontier of Reproductive Technology," in *Embryos, Ethics and Women's Rights: Exploring the New Reproductive Technologies*, ed. E.H. Baruch, A.F. D'Adamo, Jr., and J. Seager (New York: Harrington Park Press, 1988). Research looking at prenatal testing from the viewpoint of women with particular disabilities and deaf women is hard to find. There is important work that frames the issues on screening and disability. See, for example, A. Asch and M. Fine, "Shared Dreams: A Left Perspective on Disability Rights and Reproductive Rights," *Radical America* 18 (4)(1984): 51-58.

14. A useful summary of a participatory, feminist approach to research can be found in P. Maguire, *Doing Participatory Research: A Feminist Approach* (Amherst: University of Massachusetts, 1987). See also M. Eichler, *Nonsexist Research Methods: A Practical Guide* (Boston: Allen and Unwin, 1988); S.B. Gluck and D. Patai, eds., *Women's Words: The Feminist Practice of Oral History* (New York: Routledge, 1991); S. Harding, ed., *Feminism and Methodology: Social Science Issues* (Bloomington: Indiana University Press, 1987).

15. Qualitative research in primary health care is a rapidly developing interest in Canada and the United States. See, for example, M. Seifert, "Qualitative Designs for Assessing Interventions in Primary Care: Examples from Medical Practice," in *Assessing Interventions: Traditional and Innovative Methods*, ed. F. Tudiver et al. (Newbury Park: Sage Publications, 1992). Dr. Seifert organizes patient advisory committees to review, help design, and evaluate research and approaches to

treatment. See also P.G. Norton et al., eds., *Primary Care Research: Traditional and Innovative Approaches* (Newbury Park: Sage Publications, 1991).

16. Some specific countries are not mentioned, and some details have been altered since it might be possible to identify some of the women from details in this report.

17. These concerns were borne out in two of the interviews, both with women who had lost previous pregnancies and were worried about test results or confused about whether to proceed with testing. I felt it was too sensitive to ask them about abortion and disability. This does suggest the need for sensitively designed studies focussing on the concerns women raise while waiting for test results.

18. Agencies taking an active role in recruitment were Planned Parenthood Manitoba; Mount Carmel Clinic; Women's Health Clinic; Klinic Community Health Centre; Villa Rosa; Deaf Centre Manitoba; Independent Living Resource Centre; Fort Garry Women's Resource Centre; and Manitoba Association of Childbirth and Family Life Education. They are all based in Winnipeg.

19. The term "disability" is used here as a social category to describe how medical and other institutions would categorize these women and not necessarily how the women perceive themselves.

20. For example, many qualitative research projects on health-related issues focus on in-depth interviews with 10 to 15 persons. This project generated approximately 1 000 pages of transcript.

21. For ease of reading, the report uses the following conventions in discussing the women's perceptions and experiences: where one or two women indicated something, this is noted; 'several' refers to three women; 'some' to four to 10 women; 'many' to more than 10; 'the majority' to over one-half; 'almost all' to over 30 women.

22. The researcher explored the range of issues identified in the sample in further interviews with a variety of health professionals involved in prenatal care in Manitoba.

23. In 1990, 10 362 women were screened in Manitoba, approximately 60 percent of the pregnant women in the province. Of those, 3.8 percent had high elevations, 1 percent had very low levels, and 3.3 percent were at increased risk for Down syndrome and had previously had other prenatal diagnostic tests. Approximately 50 percent of women who have a high AFP level have normal pregnancies and outcomes; about 50 percent have a maternal or fetal complication. With very low AFP levels, 73 percent of women will have normal pregnancies. For those at increased risk of Down syndrome, 97 percent will not be carrying a fetus with a chromosomal abnormality. Source for Manitoba Maternal Serum AFP Program: Dr. Jane Evans, Department of Human Genetics, University of Manitoba. Other Canadian data corroborate the Manitoba data. See Canadian Coordinating Office for Health Technology Assessment, *An Annotated Bibliography of the Costs and Benefits of Prenatal Screening Programs* (Ottawa: CCOHTA, 1991).

24. The number of deliveries in Manitoba for the fiscal year 1990-91 was 17 297. The provincial average for Caesarian delivery was 14 percent. At the two major teaching hospitals in Winnipeg where many of the women in this study delivered their babies, the average Caesarian rate was 19 percent and 17 percent. Source: Manitoba Health Services Commission, *Annual Report for Fiscal Year 1990-91* (Winnipeg: 1991), Table 28.

25. This woman had been born deaf into a hearing family and had not acquired any language, including signing, until she was about seven. She described herself as having learning disabilities and difficulty understanding someone who isn't deaf, including a trained, non-deaf ASL interpreter. The relay interpreter served an intermediary role of clarifying questions and issues.

26. Thirty-one of the 37 interviews were audio-taped. Of the six women who refused, five were immigrant and refugee women and one was Canadian-born.

27. For a good discussion of qualitative methodology and evaluating qualitative data, see M.Q. Patton, *How to Use Qualitative Methods in Evaluation*, 2d ed. (Newbury Park: Sage Publications, 1987); E. Guba and Y. Lincoln, *Effective Evaluation: Improving the Usefulness of Evaluation Results Through Responsive and Naturalistic Approaches* (San Francisco: Jossey-Bass, 1981); and Y. Lincoln and E. Guba, *Naturalistic Inquiry* (Beverly Hills: Sage Publications, 1985).

28. A superb introduction to deaf culture and language is O. Sacks, *Seeing Voices: A Journey into the World of the Deaf* (Berkeley: University of California Press, 1989).

29. There is a growing literature on women's narratives and their meanings and on the uses of oral history in research. See, for example, Personal Narratives Group, ed., *Interpreting Women's Lives: Feminist Theory and Personal Narratives* (Bloomington: Indiana University Press, 1989); M. Jacobus, E.F. Keller, and S. Shuttleworth, eds., *Body/Politics: Women and the Discourses of Science* (New York: Routledge, 1990).

30. The framework adopted here for understanding women's knowledge is influenced by the work of B.F. Crabtree and W. Miller, eds., *Doing Qualitative Research in Primary Care: Multiple Strategies* (Newbury Park: Sage Publications, 1992). They elaborate on the richness of patient discourse within medical encounters. I have added the dimension of power relationships to the discussion here. The framework adopted is also influenced by M.F. Belenky et al., eds., *Women's Ways of Knowing: The Development of Self, Voice, and Mind* (New York: Basic Books, 1986), who, in their work on women and learning, discuss women coming to knowledge.

31. The immigrant women in this study had attended group classes, or had one-to-one information sessions with the health educators. Four of the teenagers had attended prenatal classes at a residential facility or at a community health centre. Two women, one teenager whose first pregnancy ended in abortion and who was currently pregnant, and one deaf woman who was not able to understand hearing prenatal classes, had no formal prenatal education. They were less familiar than the others with basic terms pertaining to pregnancy, labour, and delivery. The women's knowledge of specific tests depended on their experiences and other sources of information.

32. Clinical practice and research on childhood abuse are revealing the links between abuse and addictions and how the body "stores" knowledge and experience. Women who have been sexually abused as children may have flashbacks when they themselves are pregnant or enter certain settings later in life.

33. The maternal serum AFP patient brochure for Manitoba refers to detecting "problems that may affect your baby." It notes that high AFP values may indicate no problem, twins, or the placenta is larger than expected. It notes, "In some cases, birth defects such as spina bifida cause an elevation in the AFP ... Most twins,

incorrect due dates, and babies with spina bifida are detected by high AFP results ... A high AFP result may also suggest increased risk of other complications ... Low AFP values suggest another variety of pregnancy problems. The usual explanation is that the mother is not as far along in her pregnancy as she thought. In other situations, a low value may suggest problems with the baby's development. If you have a low result, you will receive detailed advice regarding the possibility of further investigations regarding your baby's health and development." While spina bifida is mentioned, Down syndrome is not; nor is the word abortion or termination ever used.

34. The conclusions and supplemental recommendations of this report were formulated in close consultation with the members of the Advisory Committee and are supported by the Women's Health Clinic, the sponsor of the research study.

35. Fewer women are being referred for amniocentesis, as guidelines were adjusted. The future goal of screening is to improve specificity of testing and so reduce the numbers of women being referred for counselling and amniocentesis because of positive results (personal communication, Dr. Jane Evans, Department of Human Genetics, University of Manitoba).

36. For example, the Manitoba maternal serum AFP patient brochure is highly directive in its manner. Women are not portrayed as having a choice in deciding about further testing if results are abnormal. The brochure states: "If you have a high AFP result, you will have an ultrasound examination as soon as possible, to help discover the cause ... If your blood test shows an abnormality, you will be contacted by your doctor and further investigations will be organized for you." Women are to inform their doctors if they do not wish to have the maternal serum AFP screening (*Maternal Serum AFP Screening Brochure* [Winnipeg, undated]). In contrast, one community health centre provides a more detailed description of the test and its implications, refers to the need to consider termination of pregnancy in some cases, and discusses anxiety and risks. They stress the need for the client to make the decision concerning whether to have this test (*Alpha Fetoprotein Blood Test — Information Sheet* [Winnipeg: Klinic Community Health Centre, 1991]).

37. Personal communication, Dr. Jane Evans, Department of Human Genetics, University of Manitoba.

38. Discussions with Yvonne Peters, Canadian Disability Rights Council, helped me identify and clarify these issues.

## Bibliography

*Alpha Fetoprotein Blood Test — Information Sheet.* Winnipeg: Klinic Community Health Centre, 1991.

Arnup, K., A. Lévesque, and R.R. Pierson, eds. *Delivering Motherhood: Maternal Ideologies and Practices in the 19th and 20th Centuries.* New York: Routledge, 1990.

Asch, A., and M. Fine. "Shared Dreams: A Left Perspective on Disability Rights and Reproductive Rights." *Radical America* 18 (4)(1984): 51-58.

Belenky, M.F., et al., eds. *Women's Ways of Knowing: The Development of Self, Voice, and Mind.* New York: Basic Books, 1986.

Bishop, J.E., and M. Waldholz. *Genome — The Story of the Most Astonishing Scientific Adventure of Our Time: The Attempt to Map All the Genes in the Human Body.* New York: Simon and Schuster, 1990.

Canadian Coordinating Office for Health Technology Assessment. *An Annotated Bibliography of the Costs and Benefits of Prenatal Screening Programs.* Ottawa: CCOHTA, 1991.

Council for Responsible Genetics. "Position Paper on Genetic Discrimination," and "Position Paper on Human Genome Initiative." *Issues in Reproductive and Genetic Engineering* 3 (1990): 287-95.

Crabtree, B.F., and W.L. Miller, eds. *Doing Qualitative Research in Primary Care: Multiple Strategies.* Newbury Park: Sage Publications, 1992.

Eichler, M. *Nonsexist Research Methods: A Practical Guide.* Boston: Allen and Unwin, 1988.

Faden, R.R., et al. "What Participants Understand About a Maternal Serum Alpha-Fetoprotein Screening Program." *American Journal of Public Health* 75 (1985): 1381-84.

Gluck, S.B., and D. Patai, eds. *Women's Words: The Feminist Practice of Oral History.* New York: Routledge, 1991.

Guba, E.G., and Y.S. Lincoln. *Effective Evaluation: Improving the Usefulness of Evaluation Results Through Responsive and Naturalistic Approaches.* San Francisco: Jossey-Bass, 1981.

Harding, S.G., ed. *Feminism and Methodology: Social Science Issues.* Bloomington: Indiana University Press, 1987.

Jacobus, M., E.F. Keller, and S. Shuttleworth, eds. *Body/Politics: Women and the Discourses of Science.* New York: Routledge, 1990.

Kunisch, J.R. "Electronic Fetal Monitors: Marketing Forces and the Resulting Controversy." In *Healing Technology: Feminist Perspectives,* ed. K.S. Ratcliff et al. Ann Arbor: University of Michigan Press, 1989.

Lincoln, Y.S., and E.G. Guba. *Naturalistic Inquiry.* Beverly Hills: Sage Publications, 1985.

Lippman, A. "Prenatal Genetic Testing and Screening: Constructing Needs and Reinforcing Inequities." *American Journal of Law & Medicine* 17 (1991): 15-50.

McLaren, A. *Our Own Master Race: Eugenics in Canada, 1885-1945.* Toronto: McClelland and Stewart, 1990.

Maguire, P. *Doing Participatory Research: A Feminist Approach.* Amherst: University of Massachusetts, 1987.

Manitoba. Provincial Ultrasound Advisory Committee. "Diagnostic Ultrasound in Manitoba: A Five Year Plan." Winnipeg: Manitoba Health, 1991.

Martin, E. "Science and Women's Bodies: Forms of Anthropological Knowledge." In *Body/Politics: Women and the Discourses of Science,* ed. M. Jacobus, E.F. Keller, and S. Shuttleworth. New York: Routledge, 1990.

—. *The Woman in the Body: A Cultural Analysis of Reproduction.* Boston: Beacon Press, 1987.

*Maternal Serum AFP Screening Brochure.* Winnipeg, undated.

Myerhoff, B. *Number Our Days.* New York: E.P. Dutton, 1978.

Norton, P.G., et al., eds. *Primary Care Research: Traditional and Innovative Approaches.* Newbury Park: Sage Publications, 1991.

Oakley, A. *The Captured Womb: A History of the Medical Care of Pregnant Women.* Oxford: Basil Blackwell, 1984.

—. *Women Confined: Towards a Sociology of Childbirth.* New York: Schocken Books, 1980.

Ontario. Task Force on the Implementation of Midwifery in Ontario. *Report.* Toronto: The Task Force, 1987.

Patton, M.Q. *How to Use Qualitative Methods in Evaluation.* 2d ed. Newbury Park: Sage Publications, 1987.

Personal Narratives Group, ed. *Interpreting Women's Lives: Feminist Theory and Personal Narratives.* Bloomington: Indiana University Press, 1989.

Rapp, R. "Accounting for Amniocentesis." In *Knowledge, Power and Practice: The Anthropology of Medicine and Everyday Life,* ed. S. Lindenbaum and M. Lock. Berkeley: University of California Press, 1993.

—. "Chromosomes and Communication: The Discourse of Genetic Counselling." *Medical Anthropology Quarterly* 2 (1988): 143-57.

—. "Moral Pioneers: Women, Men and Fetuses on a Frontier of Reproductive Technology." In *Embryos, Ethics and Women's Rights: Exploring the New Reproductive Technologies,* ed. E.H. Baruch, A.F. D'Adamo, Jr., and J. Seager. New York: Harrington Park Press, 1988.

—. "The Power of 'Positive' Diagnosis: Medical and Maternal Discourses on Amniocentesis." In *Childbirth in America: Anthropological Perspectives,* ed. K. Michaelson. South Hadley: Bergin and Garvey, 1988.

Reid, M. "Consumer-Oriented Studies in Relation to Prenatal Screening Tests." *European Journal of Obstetrics, Gynaecology and Reproductive Biology* 28 (Suppl.)(1988): 79-92.

Robinson, J.O., B.M. Hibbard, and K.M. Laurence. "Anxiety During a Crisis: Emotional Effects of Screening for Neural Tube Defects." *Journal of Psychosomatic Research* 28 (1984): 163-69.

Romalis, S., ed. *Childbirth, Alternatives to Medical Control.* Austin: University of Texas Press, 1981.

Rothman, B.K. *The Tentative Pregnancy: Prenatal Diagnosis and the Future of Motherhood.* New York: Viking, 1986.

Rusek, S.B. *The Women's Health Movement: Feminist Alternatives to Medical Control.* New York: Praeger, 1979.

Sacks, O. *Seeing Voices: A Journey into the World of the Deaf.* Berkeley: University of California Press, 1989.

Seifert, M.H. "Qualitative Designs for Assessing Interventions in Primary Care: Examples from Medical Practice." In *Assessing Interventions: Traditional and Innovative Methods*, ed. F. Tudiver et al. Newbury Park: Sage Publications, 1992.

Suzuki, D., and P. Knudtson. *Genethics: The Ethics of Engineering Life*. Toronto: Stoddart, 1988.

Trombley, S. *The Right to Reproduce: A History of Coercive Sterilization*. London: Weidenfeld and Nicolson, 1988.

United States. Congress. Office of Technology Assessment. *Mapping Our Genes: Genome Projects — How Big, How Fast?* Washington, DC: U.S. Government Printing Office, 1988.

Wertz, D.C. "What Birth Has Done for Doctors: A Historical View." *Women and Health* 8 (1)(1983): 7-24.

Wertz, R.W., and D.C. Wertz. *Lying-In: A History of Childbirth in America*. New York: Free Press, 1977.

Yoxen, E., and B. Hyde. *The Social Impact of Biotechnology*. Dublin: European Foundation for the Improvement of Living and Working Conditions, 1987.

Zuskar, D.M. "The Psychological Impact of Prenatal Diagnosis of Fetal Abnormality: Strategies for Investigation and Intervention." *Women & Health* 12 (1)(1987): 91-103.

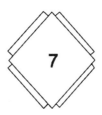

# A Review of Views Critical of Prenatal Diagnosis and Its Impact on Attitudes Toward Persons with Disabilities

## Joanne Milner

**Executive Summary**

This paper reviews and outlines positions critical of the impact that prenatal diagnosis (PND) and selective abortion have on societal attitudes toward persons with disabilities. Many of these positions are that increased use of PND may increase negative attitudes toward persons with disabilities.

It describes the social realities resulting from the availability of PND for women in their childbearing and caregiver roles, and it outlines societal attitudes relating to persons with disabilities. The paper reviews the impact of the medical model of health, disease, and disability on the medicalization of childbirth and disability, including the role of physician education, physician attitudes, and medical terminology.

It also examines the adequacy of PND counselling for informed choice, and delineates the social pressures on women to make the "right" decision. The growing demand for PND services, and concerns about the proliferation of these technologies, are discussed.

The paper concludes by pointing to the need for public discussion about the issues surrounding PND and a role for the organizations that represent people with disabilities in decision making concerning the issues.

---

This paper was completed for the Royal Commission on New Reproductive Technologies in May 1992.

# Introduction

## Submissions to the Royal Commission

Transcripts of the public hearings held across Canada and the briefs submitted to the Royal Commission on New Reproductive Technologies from organizations representing persons with disabilities contribute a range of views concerning new reproductive technologies. They also address the hopes, concerns, and rights of Canadians with disabilities, the rights of women, reproductive choices and how informed those choices are, the significant role of the medical community in providing accurate and unbiased information on congenital disabilities, and the need for social support that fosters more positive attitudes toward persons with disabilities.

Although this paper acknowledges the benefits that prenatal diagnosis (PND) offers to women and society generally, it largely focusses on the views held by advocates of persons with disabilities and the views of women as users of PND services, as it is important to understand these. It discusses a number of key issues frequently raised in the briefs that relate to the topic of PND and attitudes toward persons with disabilities and draws on information provided by the following groups: the Canadian Association for Community Living, DisAbled Women's Network (DAWN) of Canada, the Canadian Disability Rights Council, the Spina Bifida and Hydrocephalus Association of Ontario, the National Tay-Sachs and Allied Diseases Association of Ontario, the Canadian Cystic Fibrosis Foundation, and the Turner's Syndrome Society. The following is a sampling of views that are representative of the critical comments relating to this topic. As such, these views serve as part of the framework for a discussion of PND and attitudes toward persons with disabilities.

### Societal Attitudes

Societal attitudes toward persons with disabilities devalue, discriminate, and oppress. Underlying these attitudes are assumptions about the worth and dignity of these individuals.[1]

### Women's Status in Society

Women, including those with disabilities, remain devalued in today's society. Decision making concerning PND must be freed of sexism and prejudice against women.[2]

### Economic Concerns

The National Tay-Sachs and Allied Diseases Association of Ontario has expressed its support for PND for the prevention of untreatable, fatal genetic diseases and recommends that PND be made more accessible.[3] Other organizations representing people with disabilities — the Prince Edward Island Association for Childbirth and Family Education, and the Spina Bifida and Hydrocephalus Association of Ontario — state that additional health care funding for PND services should go toward more adequate compensation to providers of PND information for the time needed to thoroughly counsel and educate patients (to include, presumably, congenital disability).[4] They also claim that new reproductive technologies are being funded at the expense of basic programs in support of persons with disabilities.[5] The Canadian Disability Rights Council and DAWN, Toronto, have expressed concern that the social, financial, and educative supports for persons with disabilities are currently inadequate; resources and political commitment are needed to redress the social and economic inequities confronting those with disabilities.[6]

As the costs of providing new reproductive technologies are the responsibility of our publicly funded health care system, it is essential that applied knowledge should provide a demonstrable benefit, including that to persons with disabilities. With respect to PND, the Canadian Cystic Fibrosis Foundation states that the desirability and logistics of PND screening programs must be assessed with wisdom and caution.[7]

## Medical Model/Values

The Canadian Disability Rights Council maintains that the medical model or paradigm of health, disease, and disability, which views biology as destiny, contributes to a perception of persons with disabilities as passive, imperfect beings in a society that admires perfection.[8]

## Medical Attitudes

There is an acceptance by society in general and by many physicians that abortion is justified if a serious fetal abnormality is detected using PND. Underlying this is the assumption that the burdens outweigh the benefits of parenting a child with a disability, an assumption that underpins PND and that may contribute to negative attitudes about persons with disabilities. Some believe that medical science has embraced the goal of improving human reproduction and striving for "perfect" babies, and some maintain that this reflects a "eugenic" ideology that is consistent with discriminatory and prejudicial attitudes. As the Prince Edward Island Association for Community Living, the Canadian Disability Rights Council, and the Canadian Association for Community Living point out, the role of physicians as gatekeepers to PND services is extremely important; they have a responsibility to provide families with appropriate information that is unbiased and comprehensive.[9]

## Medical Terminology

DAWN, Canada, asserts that negative terminology (such as the word "defective" to describe a fetus) reflects negative attitudes. Physicians need to examine the language they use and the attitudes that are conveyed through this language.[10]

## Medical Training

The Spina Bifida and Hydrocephalus Association of Ontario is concerned that physicians who provide PND services lack adequate knowledge on how to deal with persons with disabilities, highlighting the

### PND Counselling and Informed Choice

Current counselling services are criticized as emphasizing statistical information on the risk and severity of particular congenital disabilities. Such counselling is viewed as inadequate because, since a "burden" bias is present, personal choice and consent may not be truly informed. The Prince Edward Island Association for Community Living maintains that actual life experiences of those involved with persons with disabilities, including those helping care for them, should also be addressed in counselling sessions.[12] The Spina Bifida and Hydrocephalus Association of Ontario, among others, has also expressed its support for improved counselling and support services, and a standardization of the latter.[13]

### Perceived Pressure to Make the "Right" Decision

DAWN, Canada, contends that there appears to be pressure on some women to agree, before PND, to undergo an abortion should a disorder be discovered. There are fears that there is coercion based on an assumption that abortion is the "right" choice following the detection of a genetic disorder through PND.[14]

### Proliferation of PND Technology

The Manitoba Association for Childbirth and Family Education has expressed its concern about the widespread adoption of PND and the adequacy of the scientific evaluation of the various techniques.[15] The Spina Bifida and Hydrocephalus Association of Ontario has also voiced concern about the impact of a proliferation of PND on those in the community who are disabled,[16] and the Canadian Disability Rights Council cautions that PND technologies can be discriminatory forces contributing to the inequality of people with disabilities. There are fears that the rights they have gained will be eroded as technology proliferates, that "technological fixes" will be preferred over the removal of social and economic obstacles that confront persons with disabilities.[17]

The Canadian Cystic Fibrosis Foundation states that there is a need to temper excitement about advances in new reproductive technologies, because knowledge about their implications remains incomplete. In addition, genetic technology will be driven forward not just by scientific momentum, but by commercial forces. There are potentially large, private financial gains to be made from the proliferation of genetic technologies, and extraordinary care should be exercised in their application.[18]

## The Literature

To examine these views and issues in more detail, a review of the published literature was conducted. The aim was to learn what various critics of PND have written regarding PND and attitudes toward people with disabilities. The attitudes of women, families, and society are discussed in many of the journal articles, research papers, books, and essays reviewed for this paper, which includes material for the years 1969 to 1991. A wide range of disciplines are represented in the literature: genetics, obstetrics, paediatrics, psychiatry, psychology, social work, sociology, anthropology, education, and ethics.

Although many of these sources focus on a particular aspect of genetic counselling, PND, or disability only, they contribute substantially to the development of the themes raised in the briefs to the Commission. Many researchers discuss the increasing range of disorders detectable by PND,[19] and the need to inform individuals and couples about the possibilities of having a child with a disability.[20] Others examine the attitudes of professionals, women, couples, and families toward disability and persons with disabilities; PND and the possibility of aborting fetuses at risk for a serious genetic disorder; the experiences of families who have children with disabilities; the attitudes of families regarding the role of caregiver for a family member with a disability; the responses of women to counselling in terms of reproductive decisions and the factors that might affect the decision making; and the need to educate the public on available PND techniques.[21]

The benefits of PND to pregnant women, families, and society generally are not a focus of this paper, but they are widely acknowledged and well represented in the published literature. For couples known to be at risk of having a child with a serious disorder that can be diagnosed prenatally, PND can remove the uncertainty of having or not having an affected child. This information provides the woman or couple concerned with the option of having an abortion if the fetus is affected, or of continuing the pregnancy with the advantage of being better prepared for the birth of an affected child. Perhaps the most important result is that it enables couples at risk, who would otherwise refrain from having a child at all, to have children without fear of their being affected, because PND can reduce women's or couples' anxiety about having a child with a serious disorder when the fetus is found not to be affected.[22] PND can also serve as a means of preventing the suffering of children who would otherwise be born with serious congenital disorders and that of their families.[23]

With respect to the focus of this paper, several authors maintain that the medical emphasis on the benefits of PND leaves many unanswered questions about some of the costs and the adequacy of scientific evaluations of new PND technologies.[24] These include the medical risk of the procedures (particularly invasive techniques such as amniocentesis and chorionic villus sampling); the financial costs of these technologies to society;[25] the psychological stress that women experience when undergoing testing, or when undergoing an abortion;[26] the family conflict and marital discord that can surface concerning testing and abortion;[27] and the impact that PND may have on attitudes toward disability and persons with disabilities.

There is a call by many for a weighing of these benefits and costs of PND; this paper attempts to contribute in part to that discussion by airing views on the influence that PND may have on attitudes toward persons with disabilities.

## Social Context of Congenital Disability and Prenatal Diagnostic Technologies

### Social Realities for Persons with Disabilities

#### *Societal Attitudes*

Groups representing women and persons with disabilities have expressed concerns that PND technologies are developing in a climate of poor attitudes toward both these sectors of society. The Canadian Disability Rights Council, in its brief to the Commission, suggests that there are negative attitudes underpinning PND, and that the PND technologies reflect discriminatory forces contributing to the inequality of persons with congenital disabilities.[28]

Critics in the relevant literature frequently point out that there has been inadequate attention by both society and medical practitioners to the social context within which PND technologies are developed. They echo statements made in the briefs that decisions concerning PND are being made in a society that is not yet free of prejudice against people with disabilities. Though much progress has been made in the past 15 years or so, persons with disabilities continue to confront negative societal attitudes and to find themselves discouraged from certain places of work, education, housing, and other community facilities.[29]

Various researchers point to the relatively recent attempts to improve attitudes, for example, by working on children's attitudes through integration programs in elementary schools,[30] by studying how contact contributes to positive attitudes,[31] and through de-institutionalization.[32] Such initiatives suggest that society is changing and attitudes are improving;[33] yet stereotypes of persons with disabilities linger, reflecting and contributing to negative societal attitudes.[34] Thus, there is public approval for integration, yet private resistance to it. In this climate, persons with disabilities are struggling to be fully accepted as worthwhile and dignified citizens. This is a difficult struggle, and many authors state that these people are far from attaining equal status.[35]

In discussing the social status of persons with disabilities, several authors point out that these individuals must struggle against society's accumulated fears about disabilities in pursuing and maintaining equal rights.[36] They point out that the climate of fear of disabilities contributes to segregation, isolation, and alienation of persons with disabilities.[37] Some maintain that the stigma experienced by persons with disabilities and by family members caring for them[38] is a social construct that society must challenge by having persons with disabilities participate fully in it.[39]

Regarding the stigma concerning congenital disability and persons with disabilities, Evans and others comment that society is increasingly accepting of an ethic of human accounting and of prescriptive social standards on how people ought to look and behave.[40] Wertz and Sorenson state that long-term societal trends toward an increasing dependence on science and medicine, and an emphasis on the individual, help to foster "this desire for and standard of perfection," which "are likely to increase as ... technological society rewards mental activity"[41] and small families make greater expenditures per child. They assert that the societal value of and large monetary expenditure on efforts to have the "perfect" child are inappropriate.

Kaufmann argues that the striving toward human mental and physical perfection appears to disregard the many other qualities that human beings possess to varying degrees.[42] The social value of persons with disabilities must be better appreciated, and the view of persons with disabilities as burdens must be questioned. As the Canadian Disability Rights Council states, society must "challenge and transform itself" from one that denigrates the worth of those with disabilities to one that supports and values all lives. By so doing, it would change the perception of many that PND technologies can serve as a substitute for the removal of social and economic obstacles still confronting those with disabilities.[43]

## Economic Factors

Economic factors can also have an influence on attitudes toward persons with disabilities. Motulsky and Murray suggest that in more stringent economic times there could be limits on expenditures for those with disabilities.[44] As everyday life becomes more "calibrated," people may become less tolerant of those who deviate from the norm, reflecting an attitude that these individuals are an unnecessary financial burden to the community.[45] The rights gained by persons with disabilities will be eroded.[46]

The current context for PND is that of rapid technological and sociodemographic changes against a backdrop of increasingly scarce resources,[47] pointing to the need to set economic priorities.[48] The Spina Bifida and Hydrocephalus Association has expressed fear that stringent economic conditions will dictate how persons with disabilities are treated, with a potential medical outcome being the tendency to abort a fetus identified with a genetic disorder.[49] Other groups state that funding decisions appear to be made without sufficient consideration of the circumstances of persons with disabilities, and that there is a need to reassess current provincial funding priorities for health and social services.[50]

Conversely, disabilities raise economically based fears about rearing a child with a disability, which can negatively affect attitudes toward persons with disabilities — fears of being financially burdened because there is little financial support available to those with disabilities or to their families who are attempting to care for them, and inadequate support in the way of care facilities and community services; and fear of having to lose the income of one of the parents so that someone may remain at home to care for a child with a disability.[51]

## Social Realities for Women: Childbearing and Caregiver Roles

Society's acceptance of PND technologies can result in the sanctioning and reinforcing of the social role of women as gestators, who feel an obligation to bear healthy babies. Kaufmann asserts that this is an indirect result of women being overly influenced by PND medical technology and its assessments of their pregnancies, whereby she feels they are viewed increasingly in terms of their role to produce healthy newborns — babies who fit socially prescribed physical and mental expectations.[52]

Due to these social norms, which place a lesser value on babies born with certain congenital conditions, the birth of an impaired child is typically viewed as tragic.[53] The prospect of a child with a congenital disability raises fears of social discrimination if one carries a fetus with a congenital disorder to term. Thus, many women find themselves confronted with competing pressures; on the one hand, the expectation to fulfil a biological and social role to produce children and, on the other hand, societal fear or disapproval of disability.

Wertz and Sorenson cite a variety of societal trends that have an impact on women and reproductive decisions:[54] the shift to voluntary parenthood through the use of contraception, smaller families, changes in gender roles, and a higher proportion of women in the workforce. They state that limitations in family size and the decline in infant mortality may contribute to the desire for the "perfect" child, thereby adding to the pressure to have PND.

As well, Rodin and Ickovics suggest that imbalances in social roles, and therefore in equality and control, contribute to added pressures on women. In addition to their increased presence in the workforce, women have greater family responsibilities and experience greater role overload than men. Many women still perform a disproportionate amount of child care and household tasks.[55] Wertz and Sorenson point out that the trend for married women to work outside the home, as well as being a factor in the postponement of childbearing, leaves them with less time and energy to devote to family roles.[56] Yet, because of assumptions about motherhood, it is an expected norm in society that the mother is close to the child and will function in the caregiving role.[57]

Furthermore, the trend toward de-institutionalization of persons with disabilities has resulted in more families assuming the caretaking responsibilities for them.[58] However, the shift away from extended large families means there are fewer helping hands — for example, grandmothers or aunts — should a child with a congenital disability be brought into the family and require greater attention and care.[59]

Women's caregiving role in the context of society's current perception of disability can result in significant stress in raising a child with a disability. However, Baxter claims that it is not the child's deviant appearance or behaviour itself, but society's reaction to the deviant behaviour, that causes much of the stress.[60]

All these realities for women and families — particularly the strain on finances and on the physical and mental health of the caregiver — can make the decision to raise a child with a disability difficult in the absence of adequate social support.

## Medical Attitudes and Influences

### Medical Attitudes Toward Congenital Disability

There is relatively little examination of medical attitudes toward congenital disability and persons with disabilities, or of the factors that may contribute to them, in the medical literature. However, some authors raise the significance of the perception of a disability's severity,[61] the degree of burden it entails, and how this may influence the acceptability of abortion as an option in certain cases. PND is a technology considered by many to be in the best interests of individuals and society alike, partly because of the suffering that can be avoided.[62] Medical professionals reflect societal attitudes, and many physicians appear to consider abortion after PND — the only means, at the moment, to avoid inheritable disorders detectable by PND — the lesser of two evils.[63]

If a serious fetal abnormality is detected, there appears to be a general acceptance of abortion on the part of physicians. For example, a late 1980s survey of physicians in France looked at opinions on and reasons for termination of pregnancy and revealed that termination of pregnancies for Down syndrome appears to be accepted by a majority of French physicians.[64] Similarly, surveys of paediatricians in the United States indicate a widespread acceptance of the practice of withholding treatment if a child has a certain disability.[65] The acceptance of both these approaches to disability appears to be based on the perception that the burdens and sorrows outweigh the benefits of parenting a child with a disability.[66]

Regarding pregnancy as a social role, and all disability as burdensome and tragic, has serious implications for the medical aspects of women's reproductive health, and for attitudes toward disability and persons with disabilities. The availability of PND and possible abortion to avoid congenital disability and the attendant suffering can also reinforce the burden image of those with disabilities.[67]

Underlying this may be expectations on the part of physicians, as on the part of society, that a good citizen will not knowingly give birth to a child with a disability.[68] Several critics, as well as briefs to the Commission, state that the medical focus on PND technologies in reproductive care is an indication that medical professionals and society generally would prefer to eliminate disability rather than learn to live with it and work toward changing societal attitudes.[69] Benham adds that negative attitudes held by health care professionals can actually have the effect of generating fewer options for those with disabilities.[70]

McDonough, writing on the diffusion of genetic amniocentesis in Ontario, states that medical research that has contributed to the development and use of PND reflects medical judgments about socially "undesirable" human attributes, and about technical solutions to the burden of congenital disability.[71] The Science Council of Canada points out that others have even argued that medical science embraces the goal of improving human reproduction and creating "perfect babies," and that this perspective is a eugenic one consistent with discriminatory and prejudicial attitudes.[72]

The claims of some women and families that the PND experience demonstrates this bias about the nature of disabilities find some support in Evans' comments that medical practitioners' first referents to disabilities are often negative stereotypes, and that these are reinforced by a tendency to view the birth of a child with a disability in negative terms.[73]

Conine et al. comment that the medical community may rely on stereotypes due to inadequate education about disabilities. They claim, for example, that medical textbooks offer little or no discussion of the ante-partum, intra-partum, and post-partum needs and problems of women with disabilities.[74] Medical education must address the impact of these stereotyped conceptions on students' attitudes.[75]

Kaufmann states that society's values regarding able-bodied children and women's role in producing normal children are reinforced by the use of PND and subsequent abortion as a means to avoid having children with untreatable disorders.[76] An underlying assumption is that abortion should be the natural outcome of learning that one's fetus has a serious disorder.[77]

## Impact of the Medical Model

Much has been written in recent years about the medicalization of childbirth, that is, medical intervention in a natural process that in many respects has come to be regarded and treated as a disease. Although there is a general acceptance of the medical model of health, disease, and disability, and an acknowledgment of its effectiveness in preventing and treating many diseases, and of the benefits in health status thereby gained, the appropriateness of its application to non-disease states has been called into question. With regard to the reproductive process and the topic of this paper, critics claim that the medical model may reinforce negative attitudes toward reproduction generally and disabled persons specifically, which, in turn, reinforces the legitimacy of the model.

A number of authors from a variety of disciplines have contributed to the discussion of the medical paradigm[78] or model[79] of health, disease, and disability within which scientists, geneticists, and physicians are researching and providing PND services. This model or paradigm implies the following corollaries:

- certain signs and symptoms are indicators of a disorder or disease state that can be classified according to defined criteria;
- disease has a biological source;[80]
- responsibility for certain diseases rests with the individual;[81]
- disease can be prevented, controlled, cured;[82]
- technological developments contribute to human health,[83] and the benefits of these developments should outweigh the costs;[84]
- if technology provides information, this information should be applied;[85]
- there is reliance on technical terms and statistical probabilities regarding the concept of risk;[86]
- training of physicians should emphasize intervention, treatment, and cure, and minimize their uncertainties.[87]

## *The Medicalization of Childbirth and Disability*

Many critics have referred to how the medicalization of various human conditions, implicit in the medical model,[88] has resulted in pregnancy becoming a medical condition to be assessed,[89] so that a couple's reproductive life is dealt with in terms of individual health risk and benefit.[90] There is also, they say, a tendency for society to accept an increasingly medically defined view of "normal"[91] and an expanding classification of genetic "flaws."[92]

A closer study of certain aspects of the medical model is useful in tracing how medicalization of reproduction is postulated by some critics to enhance negative attitudes toward disability.

Bradish asserts that an expanding definition of what constitutes pathologies expands the area in need of medical intervention.[93] Pregnancy, though not termed a pathology, has been increasingly subject to medical intervention and handled in much the same way as a *bona fide* pathology. Motulsky and Murray, in discussing the concept of "normalcy," point out that medical practitioners use a "utilitarian calculus" and majority opinion in deciding which congenital conditions warrant testing and treatment.[94] That is, the standards used to determine what is "normal" are medical standards, and medical professionals are in a position to define normative criteria for fetal function and child development[95] and in so doing to indicate which conditions and disabilities will be remedied and which will come to be stigmatized.[96] Emerging policy in favour of a medical definition of "normalcy" coincides with social norms allowing society to invest selectively in the birth of individuals with characteristics deemed preferable or desirable.[97] Kaufmann refers to the perfectionist ethic in modern medicine that regards physical and mental health as the ultimate good and is reflected in increasing medical intervention in the natural process of conception, gestation, and birth.[98]

It is McDonough's position that a medical focus on "defective genes" obscures the social dimensions of congenital disability — the emphasis on the individual that stems from the view of "biology as destiny" distracts attention from the external influences on a person's health[99] and may limit the ability of medical professionals to understand fully the broader social context of disability and the concerns of persons with disabilities.[100] Similarly, Kaufmann refers to a "neonatology perspective" implying that the woman's action is the primary determiner of the child's health status, and the outcome of a pregnancy her personal responsibility. She maintains that "other social forces beyond the control of the individual pregnant woman are underplayed as primary causes of poor health of the fetus"[101] — for example, poverty, poor nutrition, and physical abuse by a spouse.

These aspects of medicalization may not purposefully neglect the views of women and disabled persons, but the literature suggests that both these sectors of society are concerned about the impact of medicalization on childbirth, disability, and their lives.

### *The Impact of Medical Terminology*

There are claims that the use of certain medical terms, such as "defective" fetus, is an indication of negative attitudes, and that medical practitioners, to better understand the messages this language conveys, should consider more closely the language they use. Since language can label, it can also reinforce stereotyped perceptions or images of persons with disabilities as "wheelchair confined," or being a "burden." Thus, language can reveal not only the parameters of a condition, but the biases of the medical perspective as well.[102]

Critics state that biased attitudes are revealed in terms such as "early assessment and management of pregnancy being required," "abnormal fetus," "pre-termination counselling,"[103] and "fetal malformation"[104] — terms that are common in the medical literature. Similarly, abortion may be referred to as "preventive strategy," or "termination of pregnancy."[105]

When discussing PND, medical professionals speak of fetuses "at risk for genetic defect."[106] The language used in discussing genetic screening and counselling, as it pertains to the diagnosis of late-onset genetic disease, includes terms such as "risk-carriers."[107] There may be good reasons for the continued reliance on these terms, but their use shows that explaining concepts such as "the heterogeneous distribution of deleterious genes among different population groups"[108] means that some individuals may feel fear or guilt, and that any benefits are also inevitably accompanied by the stress of dealing with such knowledge.

Sociological literature also draws attention to the use of this terminology. For example, medical professionals sometimes refer to the "need" to terminate a pregnancy, and Wertz and Sorenson suggest this may be taken to indicate a hierarchy of fetuses[109] that are judged according to their potential to contribute or become a future cost to society.[110]

Leuzinger and Rambert claim that the language of PND also reduces reproductive consequences to individual risks and benefits.[111] Rapp adds that the language of PND may hinder discourse that is meaningful to users of PND services and result in misunderstandings: for example, a diagnosis is labelled "positive" by medical personnel if it indicates the disorder in question is present, while the client may perceive and experience a PND test result indicating a fetus with a genetic disorder as a "negative diagnosis."[112]

Overall, medical terminology places women and pregnancy firmly within a medical discourse.[113] Though there may be valid reasons for this, there is a growing need to discuss and present to women information relating to childbirth and disability in terms that are understandable and as free of bias as possible,[114] with an awareness of the potential impact on attitudes toward disability and persons with disabilities.

## *The Impact of Medical Training*

Evans and others comment on the influence of medical training in encouraging physicians to minimize uncertainty and downplay diagnostic ambiguities.[115] Yet women and physicians are confronted with specific ambiguities when making their decisions about many situations with regard to PND.[116] Fragile-X syndrome, for example, given the current state of knowledge on this syndrome, may leave questions that are unanswerable at this time about the potential mode of inheritance and diversity of expression. This, combined with more accepting attitudes toward abortion, leads Meryash and Abuelo to speculate that too many women might undergo testing and subsequent abortion to avoid congenital disability of uncertain expression.[117] Some critics feel that medical training may leave some practitioners unprepared for the responsibility they must assume when caring for persons with disabilities with chronic conditions,[118] and this may influence physicians to minimize contact with them.

Medical students are trained to regard themselves as objective and learn to repress emotions. In light of the literature that stresses the significance of social and psychological factors in PND counselling, critics think that schools of medicine should reassess this aspect of medical training.[119]

Commenting on the contact that physicians have with persons with disabilities, Conine et al. posit that the concept of normalization and mainstreaming of women with special needs is poorly accepted, and that this is reflected in medical training.[120] The marginalization of persons with disabilities may itself contribute to physicians having insufficient exposure to these people and insufficient knowledge of how to deal with them as patients. The Spina Bifida and Hydrocephalus Association of Ontario and other organizations representing persons with disabilities propose that PND centres could benefit from mutual cooperation, as these groups could serve as resources providing information on lifestyles available to families of children with disabilities. Some also suggest that more comprehensive training of medical personnel would contribute to an improved quality of service.[121]

## Counselling and Informed Choice

In examining PND counselling approaches, genetic counsellors themselves suggest that counselling should focus both on imparting genetic information to the counsellee and on addressing the impact of cultural, religious, and other factors on a counsellee's receptivity to counselling and understanding of the information provided.[122]

However, with respect to congenital disability, some research studies indicate that interviews with women who accept, or who do not accept, PND focussed on the women's knowledge of the genetics of a condition, thus exploring only a narrow area of knowledge concerning the disability.[123] Insufficient discussion may be held about a child's possible disability during interviews with women undergoing PND,[124] yet a person's perception and understanding of the nature and severity of a disability is an important factor in reproductive decision making.[125] There is a need to ensure that the topics counsellors discuss with counsellees go beyond only genetic topics and chances of recurrence, to always include the long-term medical and social implications of disabilities.[126]

Although some medical professionals suggest that an informed choice can exist when primarily statistical information on genetic risk is provided,[127] others counter that informed choice cannot exist without the provision of information on the realities of the life experiences of those involved with persons with disabilities.[128] Families of children with disabilities that can be detected prenatally speak a different discourse than the medical practitioners, one that reflects the meaning of maternity, paternity, and the value of children.[129]

### Range of Information Provided

As the "gatekeeper" to PND services, the geneticist, genetic counsellor, or referring physician is in a position to control the quantity, accuracy, and quality of information on which reproductive decisions are based and has a responsibility to provide unbiased and comprehensive information to counsellees.

Kessler cautions that, because the medical professional is viewed as an authority figure who is assumed to be more knowing, an overemphasis on estimates of risk may shape the counsellee's decision-making processes in the direction of what is perceived to be the counsellor's own beliefs.[130] Frets and Ekwo also point out that there is a distinction to be made between subjective and objective estimates of risk; a woman's estimate of risk is always subjective, and can be influenced by her psychosocial state; and her perception of the degree of severity and "burden" of a congenital disability can vary accordingly.[131]

Psychosocial factors can influence receptivity to information. Ekwo et al. note that the "burden" of a disability may be what women perceive as the degree of severity and psychosocial prognosis of a congenital disorder. They say that counsellees are more likely to act on the information given during counselling if they perceive the burden the family will experience.[132] Meryash, Abuelo, and others say that a poor understanding of statistics on risk, subjective interpretation of risk, and varying perceptions of the severity of a particular disability may result in women perceiving a risk as high that generally would not be perceived as high.[133]

There is growing recognition that the PND counsellor must place emphasis on all the types of information discussed above as well as other aspects of congenital disabilities, such as explaining the variable expressivity and uncertain prognosis of certain congenital disorders,[134] and exploring a counsellee's emotional reactions — for example, feelings about carrying a fetus at genetic risk,[135] feelings of guilt or depression[136] — and the social stigma of raising a child with a disability.[137]

## Pressure on Women to Make the "Right" Decision

Women have to deal with the availability of PND testing, the possibility of having PND, and, if a genetic disorder is detected, the possibility of having an abortion. For many, the reproductive choices available can contribute to perceived pressure on them to make the "right" decision. A number of authors comment on the pressure women experience in terms of two types of "right" decisions.[138] The "right" decision, as it pertains to PND testing and possible abortion, has been described by some as the morally correct decision, wherein all life is valued, whether disability is present or not. On the other hand, the "right" decision has also been described as the practical or socially responsible decision to undergo testing, and possibly an abortion, because of the potential suffering of a child who would otherwise be born, and the burden brought on family members and society by bringing a child with a disability into the world.[139]

The perceived social pressure on women to make the "right" decision to use PND technology is heightened when they have to deal with the option of acting on the information gained. McDonough maintains that there is an "action imperative" built into PND that reduces the right not to have the test, thus adding to the initial pressure. Women may fear being judged adversely by physicians, and society generally, for not acting in a mature, socially responsible way,[140] that is, to make use of PND and not bring into society a child who will require extra care and financial support.[141] Leuzinger and Rambert add that to refuse the information that is available and accessible through PND takes on a negative value.[142] Many groups have commented on the expectation that women over the age of 35 will have PND[143] due to the greater risk of a congenital anomaly, even though some of these women may be willing to assume the risk of having a child with a disability if the pregnancy being assessed is the first and, perhaps, last chance of having a child.[144] Motulsky and Murray speculate that, if there were large declines in the incidence of certain medical conditions or disabilities, it is possible that women might feel further social pressure to conform to trends.[145]

Some have claimed that there is added pressure placed on some women and families by physicians to agree, before PND, to undergo an abortion should a disorder be detected.[146] Groups representing persons with disabilities fear that coercion could result from assumptions or expectations of abortion as the rightful outcome of a "positive" PND finding.[147] The Spina Bifida and Hydrocephalus Association of Ontario says some women may wish to carry to term a fetus with a serious disability, intending to donate the child's organs should it not survive, but they fear there may be pressure to undergo abortion instead.[148]

If congenital conditions are not correctable, physicians may encourage abortion, knowingly or not, as a physician's own set of values may affect the decision-making process during counselling, and there may be pressure perceived by the counsellee to align her attitude with the counsellor's opinions.[149] Kessler, however, says that medical geneticists are generally aware of their status relative to the counsellee, and of their potential to modify the psychological and behavioural states of counsellees regarding decision making.[150]

Rice and Doherty discuss the conflict that can arise within parents from reactions to having to make a decision when a fetus has been identified as having a disorder: there may be conflict between desire to terminate a pregnancy on pragmatic grounds, and desire to continue the pregnancy if they feel that it is morally right. This conflict can become a source of guilt for some parents following abortion.[151]

In the broader context, Niermeijer comments that freedom of choice is a valued principle, but there is also a risk of social pressure to make decisions that are beneficial to society.[152] In a society that offers few resources and supports for those with disabilities, McDonough feels it is not surprising that women would choose to have the diagnostic tests and then possibly undergo an abortion if the test result indicated the presence of a genetic disorder.[153]

Today, women who are having their first child later in life perceive especially strong pressure to have PND because of the greater risk of chromosome disorders in that age group (e.g., Down syndrome). But if the pregnancy being assessed by PND is a woman's first, and perhaps last, chance to have a child, her perception of this event may be quite different from that of the physician counselling her,[154] and she may be willing to assume the risk of having a child with a disability. This range of differing personal situations and values is part of what underlies the statistic that 12 percent of women in Canada over 35 years of age who are referred to have counselling about PND testing opt not to be tested.[155]

## Proliferation of PND Technologies

Technological developments influence medical research and treatment efforts. Medical researchers and practitioners generally regard the new PND techniques as advancements in the assessment of pregnancies.[156] Daya et al. comment that PND technology does a superior job of assessing pregnancies compared to maternal estimates,[157] and its use has increased dramatically due to a growing demand for PND services.[158]

Wertz and Sorenson predict that routine use of PND technology for all pregnancies will eventually result, due to rise in consumer demand,[159] and others warn that its use will continue to escalate. There are already concerns, particularly in some countries without publicly supported health care systems, that PND technology, originally intended for high-risk patients only, will be used by ever-increasing numbers of low-risk women.[160]

These concerns apply in particular to the routine use of ultrasonography. Predictably, in examining attitudes to ultrasound scanning, Hyde reports findings suggesting that women not examined by ultrasound are less likely to approve of its routine use or to regard it as an additional source of reassurance.[161] She holds that the routine use of ultrasound encourages women to believe that physicians consider the scans necessary and, as suggested earlier, may defer to this perceived view. Women feel it is best for them; it is what the physician judges to be the best course of action, and they generally respect their physician's opinion and advice. More generally, McDonough comments that, as a technology becomes routine, the routinization itself becomes a social force;[162] increasingly accessible PND technology is itself seen as a factor in inducing a greater demand for PND services.

Researchers cite several other factors contributing to the proliferation of PND technology and its widespread use. In the view of some,[163] forces shaping diagnostic research are often based on technical feasibility and professional interests without sufficient attention to the social and economic implications, the views and needs of people with disabilities, and societal priorities for the provision of support services. Julian et al. maintain that the dynamics of PND are linked more to technological progress in molecular biology than to a rationalization of health policy and that acceptance of PND by the general public has not been investigated.[164] However, there are numerous surveys in the literature that assess the public's opinion on the use of PND for different situations. Julian et al. point out a need for real social debate on the consequences of the development of PND, including influence on attitudes toward persons with disabilities.

Finkelstein says that the proliferation of PND services reinforces the increasing medicalization of various conditions, which then adds to a climate of encouragement to choose PND.[165] McDonough suggests that, in turn, persistent negative social attitudes and practices toward persons with disabilities may themselves contribute to women responding favourably to PND technology.[166]

Others caution that future increases in the demand for and use of PND services — particularly the advent of newer PND techniques, such as maternal serum alpha-fetoprotein screening,[167] that are simpler, less invasive, more easily accessible, and less costly than amniocentesis and chorionic villus sampling — could lead to adverse social consequences for persons with congenital disabilities and for women and families who may be at higher risk for having children with disabilities. For example, fears have been expressed about the possibility of proliferating PND testing leading to insurance companies and employers obtaining information about their clients or workers,[168] with a potential for misuse and discrimination. As well, some question how it is that some disorders are selected for PND and others are not.[169] Leuzinger and Rambert argue that the act of accepting PND and subsequent abortion to avoid the birth of children with certain disabilities itself becomes institutionalized via the proliferation and routine use of PND technologies.[170] Bradish thinks that the proliferation of PND testing may make it more likely that some women will choose to abort a fetus that is not at risk for a disorder or is at some risk for a disability that results in minor impairment only.[171] Others caution that PND technology is not matched by precise scientific knowledge or optimal detection of disorders, which can lead to uncertainty and error when technology limited in this way is readily available.[172] The Spina Bifida and Hydrocephalus Association of Ontario and other groups representing disabled persons have expressed fear that the proliferation of PND could have a negative impact on people in the community who already have the disability.[173]

The Manitoba Association for Childbirth and Family Education also questions routine use of these technologies in reproduction and the adequacy of PND technology and service evaluation.[174] As one example, Rodin and Ickovics argue that rates of PND use have increased substantially despite their unproven value in reducing the morbidity and mortality of newborns,[175] leaving critics to state that, on the basis of clinical outcome, the major reason to use PND is for the selective abortion of fetuses identified as either having, or being at very high risk of having, serious congenital disability. Various authors believe that, before PND technology is allowed to proliferate further, there should be more thorough evaluation of both short- and long-term risks, the psychological effects on women of the procedures themselves, the anxiety created by PND, and decision making regarding the possibility of abortion.[176]

Some contend that there exists a system of informal social norms and conventions determining when and how new technologies are used — normative standards that are inadequate to address the social and ethical choices generated by new PND technology.[177] They stress that medical scientists need to address the social and ethical implications of their new knowledge,[178] the role of health policy in technology proliferation, and, conversely, the impact of the growing use of PND technology on health care policies and priorities.

## Conclusion

This review of positions critical of the use and impact of PND is helpful in contributing to a well-rounded discussion of PND and its influence on attitudes toward disability and persons with disabilities. Positions supportive of PND have not been dealt with in this paper. It is evident that there is a substantial literature supporting views and claims raised in the briefs to the Royal Commission on New Reproductive Technologies that negative societal attitudes could become more prevalent with increasing use of PND and selective abortion. These expressed views of various groups need to be respected and should become part of a social debate.

Some authors perceive that PND and selective abortion represent a systematic discriminatory selection of human life taking place in society today. The very existence and continuing development of PND technology are seen by them as evidence of assumptions about those with congenital disabilities. Medical technologies are developed on the grounds of avoiding suffering; persons with disabilities are saying that there is more suffering as a result of others' attitudes than by the actual disabilities, and that it is these attitudes that need rectifying.[179]

The social status and realities of those with congenital disabilities, and societal attitudes toward them, warrant serious consideration in the face of advancing PND technologies. There is a need for public discussion about the selection aspect in particular, with a focus on society's fear of disability and the reasons why some disabilities are viewed as socially tolerable, while others are not.[180] As well, society's past and current treatment of those with disabilities, the fears that persist around disability and persons with disabilities, and the question of public policies regarding social and economic support for those with special needs, including women in the caregiving role, deserve closer study. This broader view will allow medicine and society to more adequately address the choices generated by PND.[181]

The medicalization of reproductive aspects of women's lives and the ways in which social trends may be influencing PND research and physician practice also deserve serious attention in the social debate. Society must guard against the determination of rigid or biased criteria for what constitutes serious disability or suffering, and not have perceptions about disability distorted by stereotypes and prejudicial thinking.[182] As practitioners and decision makers, medical professionals should be aware of the part they play in contributing to public policy, which in turn affects many aspects of people's lives.[183]

Many sources stress the importance of informed choice and the need to broaden the range of topics discussed and information provided in PND counselling sessions to include the social aspects of congenital disability and of raising a child with a disability, to explore the emotional and psychosocial factors and how these may affect counsellees' receptivity (e.g., possible anxiety, guilt), and to consider the pressure women may feel to make the "right" decision. Groups such as the Spina Bifida and Hydrocephalus Association of Ontario add that more time should be given in the counselling session to educating users of PND on disabilities.[184] On a wider scale, others suggest that informed choice could be further enhanced by additional genetics education at elementary, secondary, and college levels, and that this would help to promote both personal autonomy and informed public participation.[185]

Many of the briefs from organizations representing persons with disabilities present the view that before true dialogue about their concerns and fears can take place, there must be better representation by them. For example, decision making concerning PND could be improved by representation on hospital ethics committees[186] and at post-clinic conferences.[187] These groups stress the need to reaffirm the principles of equality and self-determination espoused by Canadian society and call on the expressed support of the Commission in articulating these principles on behalf of all individuals who live with congenital disabilities.

## Notes

1. PEI Association for Community Living, brief to the Royal Commission on New Reproductive Technologies (RCNRT).

2. Canadian Abortion Rights Action League, brief to the RCNRT.

3. National Tay-Sachs and Allied Diseases Association of Ontario, brief to the RCNRT.

4. PEI Association for Community Living, Manitoba Association for Childbirth and Family Education, and Spina Bifida and Hydrocephalus Association of Ontario, briefs to the RCNRT.

5. Ibid.

6. Canadian Disability Rights Council and DisAbled Women's Network, Toronto, briefs to the RCNRT.

7. Canadian Cystic Fibrosis Foundation, brief to the RCNRT.

8. Canadian Disability Rights Council, brief to the RCNRT.

9. PEI Association for Community Living, Canadian Disability Rights Council, and Canadian Association for Community Living, briefs to the RCNRT.

10. DisAbled Women's Network, Canada, brief to the RCNRT.

11. Spina Bifida and Hydrocephalus Association of Ontario, brief to the RCNRT.

12. PEI Association for Community Living, brief to the RCNRT.

13. Spina Bifida and Hydrocephalus Association of Ontario, brief to the RCNRT.

14. DisAbled Women's Network, Canada, and Ontario Coalition for Abortion Clinics, briefs to the RCNRT.

15. Manitoba Association for Childbirth and Family Education, brief to the RCNRT.

16. Spina Bifida and Hydrocephalus Association of Ontario, brief to the RCNRT.

17. Canadian Disability Rights Council, brief to the RCNRT.

18. Canadian Cystic Fibrosis Foundation, brief to the RCNRT.

19. M.F. Niermeijer, "Genetic Screening and Counselling — Implications of the DNA Technologies," in *Health Policy, Ethics and Human Values: European and North American Perspectives*, ed. Z. Bankowski and J.H. Bryant (Geneva: Council for International Organizations of Medical Sciences, 1988); World Health Organization, *Genetic Counseling: Third Report of the WHO Expert Committee on Human Genetics*, WHO Technical Report Series No. 416 (Geneva: WHO, 1969), 5-23; F.C. Fraser, "Genetic Counseling," *American Journal of Human Genetics* 26 (1974): 636-61; C. Julian et al., "Physicians' Acceptability of Termination of Pregnancy After Prenatal Diagnosis in Southern France," *Prenatal Diagnosis* 9 (1989): 77-89; C.O. Leonard, G.A. Chase, and B. Childs, "Genetic Counseling: A Consumer's View," *New England Journal of Medicine* 287 (1972): 433-39.

20. P.G. Frets et al., "Model Identifying the Reproductive Decision After Genetic Counseling," *American Journal of Medical Genetics* 35 (1990): 503-509; P. Donnai, N. Charles, and R. Harris, "Attitudes of Patients After 'Genetic' Termination of Pregnancy," *British Medical Journal* (Clinical Research Edition) (21 February 1981): 621-22; Fraser, "Genetic Counseling."

21. World Health Organization, *Genetic Counseling*, 5-23.

22. F.C. Fraser, personal communication, 31 October 1991.

23. Ibid.; Niermeijer, "Genetic Screening"; World Health Organization, *Genetic Counseling*, 5-23; Frets et al., "Model."

24. J. Rodin and J.R. Ickovics, "Women's Health: Review and Research Agenda as We Approach the 21st Century," *American Psychologist* 45 (1990): 1018-34; D.L. Meryash and D. Abuelo, "Counseling Needs and Attitudes Toward Prenatal Diagnosis and Abortion in Fragile-X Families," *Clinical Genetics* 33 (1988): 349-55; United States, President's Commission for the Study of Ethical Problems in Medicine and Biomedical and Behavioral Research, *Screening and Counseling for Genetic Conditions: A Report on the Ethical, Social and Legal Implications of Genetic*

*Screening, Counseling and Education Programs* (Washington, DC: U.S. Government Printing Office, 1983), 5-8, 68-70.

25. Science Council of Canada, "The Need to Know? Genetic Disorders and the Unborn," *Agenda Science Council of Canada* 2 (Autumn 1979): 1-7; D.C. Wertz and J.R. Sorenson, "Sociologic Implications," in *Fetal Diagnosis and Therapy: Science, Ethics and the Law*, ed. M.I. Evans et al. (Philadelphia: J.B. Lippincott, 1989); D. Evans, "The Psychological Impact of Disability and Illness on Medical Treatment Decisionmaking," *Issues in Law and Medicine* 5 (1989): 277-99; A. Kolker and B.M. Burke, "Amniocentesis and the Social Construction of Pregnancy," in *Alternative Health Maintenance and Healing Systems for Families*, ed. D.Y. Wilkinson and M.B. Sussman (New York: Haworth Press, 1987).

26. Meryash and Abuelo, "Counseling Needs"; R. Rapp, "Moral Pioneers: Women, Men and Fetuses on a Frontier of Reproductive Technology," in *Embryos, Ethics and Women's Rights: Exploring the New Reproductive Technologies*, ed. E.H. Baruch, A.F. D'Adamo, Jr., and J. Seager (New York: Harrington Park Press, 1988); Rodin and Ickovics, "Women's Health"; N. Rice and R. Doherty, "Reflections on Prenatal Diagnosis: The Consumers' Views," *Social Work in Health Care* 8 (Fall 1982): 47-57; S. Shiloh, O. Avdor, and R.M. Goodman, "Satisfaction with Genetic Counseling: Dimensions and Measurement," *American Journal of Medical Genetics* 37 (1990): 522-29; P. McDonough, "The Diffusion of Genetic Amniocentesis in Ontario: 1969-1987," *Canadian Journal of Public Health* 81 (1990): 431-35.

27. B. Hyde, "An Interview Study of Pregnant Women's Attitudes to Ultrasound Scanning," *Social Science and Medicine* 22 (1986): 587-92; M. Leuzinger and B. Rambert, "'I Can Feel It — My Baby Is Healthy': Women's Experiences with Prenatal Diagnosis in Switzerland," *Reproductive and Genetic Engineering* 1 (1988): 239-49; Kolker and Burke, "Social Construction of Pregnancy," 95-115.

28. Canadian Disability Rights Council, brief to the RCNRT.

29. Rapp, "Moral Pioneers"; R.E. Verville, "The Americans with Disabilities Act: An Analysis," *Archives of Physical Medicine and Rehabilitation* 71 (1990): 1010-13.

30. V.W. Archie and C. Sherrill, "Attitudes Toward Handicapped Peers of Mainstreamed and Nonmainstreamed Children in Physical Education," *Perceptual and Motor Skills* 69 (1989): 319-22; S.M. King et al., "An Epidemiological Study of Children's Attitudes Toward Disability," *Developmental Medicine and Child Neurology* 31 (1989): 237-45.

31. King, "Children's Attitudes."

32. S.K. Grimes and S.J. Vitello, "Follow-Up Study of Family Attitudes Toward Deinstitutionalization: Three to Seven Years Later," *Mental Retardation* 28 (1990): 219-25.

33. A.G. Motulsky and J. Murray, "Will Prenatal Diagnosis with Selective Abortion Affect Society's Attitude Toward the Handicapped?" *Progress in Clinical and Biological Research* 128 (1983): 277-91.

34. J.J. Tait, "Reproductive Technologies and the Rights of Disabled Persons," *Canadian Journal of Women and the Law* 1 (1986): 446-55.

35. Tait, "Reproductive Technologies"; C. Baxter, "Investigating Stigma as Stress in Social Interactions of Parents," *Journal of Mental Deficiency Research* 33 (1989): 455-66; P.K. Benham, "Attitudes of Occupational Therapy Personnel Toward

Persons with Disabilities," *American Journal of Occupational Therapy* 42 (1988): 305-11; Leuzinger and Rambert, "Women's Experiences"; F.F. Thomas and D. Lee, "Effects of Ethnicity and Physical Disability on Academic and Social Ratings of Photographs," *Psychological Reports* 67 (1990): 240-42.

36. P. McDonough, "Congenital Disability and Medical Research: The Development of Amniocentesis," *Women and Health* 16 (3-4)(1990): 137-53; National Legal Center for the Medically Dependent and Disabled, "Medical Treatment for Older People and People with Disabilities: 1987 Developments," *Issues in Law and Medicine* 3 (1988): 333-60; National Legal Center for the Medically Dependent and Disabled, "Recent Developments in the Law Governing Medical Treatment for Older People and People with Disabilities," *Clearinghouse Review* (May 1988): 31-42; Verville, "Americans with Disabilities Act."

37. Leuzinger and Rambert, "Women's Experiences"; McDonough, "Congenital Disability"; Tait, "Reproductive Technologies."

38. Baxter, "Stigma as Stress"; J.E. Whittick, "Dementia and Mental Handicap: Attitudes, Emotional Distress and Caregiving," *British Journal of Medical Psychology* 62 (1989): 181-89.

39. Baxter, "Stigma as Stress"; McDonough, "Congenital Disability."

40. P. Bradish, "From Genetic Counseling and Genetic Analysis to Genetic Ideal and Genetic Fate?" in *Made to Order: The Myth of Reproductive and Genetic Progress*, ed. P. Spallone and D.L. Steinberg (Oxford: Pergamon Press, 1987); Evans, "Medical Treatment Decisionmaking"; J.L. Finkelstein, "Biomedicine and Technocratic Power," *Hastings Center Report* 20 (July-August 1990): 13-16.

41. Wertz and Sorenson, "Sociologic Implications," 556.

42. C.L. Kaufmann, "Perfect Mothers, Perfect Babies: An Examination of the Ethics of Fetal Treatments," *Reproductive and Genetic Engineering* 1 (1988): 133-39.

43. Canadian Disability Rights Council, brief to the RCNRT.

44. Motulsky and Murray, "Society's Attitude."

45. Finkelstein, "Biomedicine"; Tait, "Reproductive Technologies."

46. Tait, "Reproductive Technologies."

47. Evans, "Medical Treatment Decisionmaking."

48. Science Council of Canada, "Genetic Disorders."

49. Spina Bifida and Hydrocephalus Association of Ontario, brief to the RCNRT.

50. Canadian Disability Rights Council and Manitoba Association for Childbirth and Family Education, briefs to the RCNRT.

51. Leuzinger and Rambert, "Women's Experiences"; McDonough, "Congenital Disability."

52. Kaufmann, "Perfect Mothers."

53. Ibid.

54. Wertz and Sorenson, "Sociologic Implications."

55. Rodin and Ickovics, "Women's Health."

56. Wertz and Sorenson, "Sociologic Implications."

57. Whittick, "Dementia."

58. Ibid.

59. Wertz and Sorenson, "Sociologic Implications."

60. Baxter, "Stigma as Stress."

61. B.F. Seals et al., "Moral and Religious Influences on the Amniocentesis Decision," *Social Biology* 32 (Spring-Summer 1985): 13-30; Shiloh et al., "Satisfaction with Genetic Counseling."

62. McDonough, "Congenital Disability."

63. Science Council of Canada, "Genetic Disorders."

64. Julian et al., "Physicians' Acceptability."

65. Evans, "Medical Treatment Decisionmaking."

66. McDonough, "Congenital Disability."

67. Kaufmann, "Perfect Mothers."

68. Spina Bifida and Hydrocephalus Association of Ontario, brief to the RCNRT.

69. Leuzinger and Rambert, "Women's Experiences"; McDonough, "Congenital Disability."

70. Benham, "Attitudes of Occupational Therapy Personnel."

71. McDonough, "Congenital Disability."

72. Finkelstein, "Biomedicine"; Kaufmann, "Perfect Mothers"; B. Rose, "Diagnosing Defects in the Unborn," *Science Forum* 12 (January-February 1979): 35-38; Science Council of Canada, *Social Issues in Human Genetics: Genetic Screening and Counselling* (Ottawa: Science Council of Canada, 1980).

73. Evans, "Medical Treatment Decisionmaking."

74. T.A. Conine, E.A. Carty, and F. Wood-Johnson, "Provision of Preventive Maternal Health Care and Childbirth Education for Disabled Women," *Canadian Journal of Public Health* 77 (1986): 123-27.

75. B.M. Stafford, J. La Puma, and D.L. Schiedermayer, "One Face of Beauty, One Picture of Health: The Hidden Aesthetic of Medical Practice," *Journal of Medicine and Philosophy* 14 (1989): 213-30.

76. Kaufmann, "Perfect Mothers."

77. Tait, "Reproductive Technologies."

78. Canadian Disability Rights Council, brief to the RCNRT.

79. Evans, "Medical Treatment Decisionmaking."

80. McDonough, "Congenital Disability"; Julian et al., "Physicians' Acceptability"; United States, President's Commission, *Screening and Counseling*, 5-8, 68-70; Science Council of Canada, "Genetic Disorders"; World Health Organization, *Genetic Counseling*, 5-23.

81. Finkelstein, "Biomedicine"; McDonough, "Congenital Disability"; Rapp, "Moral Pioneers." There is discussion of societal trends toward individualism, by Wertz and Sorenson, "Sociologic Implications."

82. Niermeijer, "Genetic Screening"; Kaufmann, "Perfect Mothers"; Tait, "Reproductive Technology."

83. Rodin and Ickovics, "Women's Health"; Finkelstein, "Biomedicine." There is discussion of societal trends toward reliance on high technology, by Wertz and Sorenson, "Sociologic Implications."

84. Rose, "Diagnosing Defects"; Niermeijer, "Genetic Screening"; Kolker and Burke, "Social Construction of Pregnancy."

85. Leuzinger and Rambert, "Women's Experiences."

86. Stafford et al., "One Face of Beauty"; Wertz and Sorenson, "Sociologic Implications"; Rapp, "Moral Pioneers." There is discussion of societal trends toward reliance on medicine and science, by Wertz and Sorenson, "Sociologic Implications."

87. D. Silvestre and N. Fresco, "Reactions to Prenatal Diagnosis: An Analysis of 87 Interviews," *American Journal of Orthopsychiatry* 50 (1980): 610-17; Evans, "Medical Treatment Decisionmaking."

88. Bradish, "Genetic Counselling"; Finkelstein, "Biomedicine"; Hyde, "Pregnant Women's Attitudes"; Kolker and Burke, "Social Construction of Pregnancy"; Silvestre and Fresco, "Reactions."

89. Leuzinger and Rambert, "Women's Experiences"; Kaufmann, "Perfect Mothers."

90. Kolker and Burke, "Social Construction of Pregnancy"; McDonough, "Congenital Disability"; Rapp, "Moral Pioneers"; Rodin and Ickovics, "Women's Health"; Silvestre and Fresco, "Reactions"; Tait, "Reproductive Technologies"; Wertz and Sorenson, "Sociologic Implications."

91. McDonough, "Congenital Disability"; Silvestre and Fresco, "Reactions"; Kaufmann, "Perfect Mothers"; Leuzinger and Rambert, "Women's Experiences"; Rapp, "Moral Pioneers"; Stafford et al., "One Face of Beauty."

92. Finkelstein, "Biomedicine."

93. Bradish, "Genetic Counseling"; Evans, "Medical Treatment Decisionmaking"; Finkelstein, "Biomedicine."

94. Motulsky and Murray, "Society's Attitude."

95. Finkelstein, "Biomedicine"; Kaufmann, "Perfect Mothers."

96. Finkelstein, "Biomedicine."

97. Ibid.; Kaufmann, "Perfect Mothers."

98. Kaufmann, "Perfect Mothers."

99. McDonough, "Congenital Disability"; Evans, "Medical Treatment Decisionmaking."

100. McDonough, "Congenital Disability"; Rapp, "Moral Pioneers."

101. Kaufmann, "Perfect Mothers," 134.

102. Tait, "Reproductive Technologies"; Canadian Disability Rights Council and DisAbled Women's Network, Canada, briefs to the RCNRT.

103. Donnai et al., "Attitudes."

104. Ibid.; J. Lloyd and K.M. Laurence, "Sequelae and Support After Termination of Pregnancy for Fetal Malformation," *British Medical Journal* (Clinical Research Edition) (23 March 1985): 907-909.

105. Donnai et al., "Attitudes"; Kaufmann, "Perfect Mothers."

106. Niermeijer, "Genetic Screening"; Kaufmann, "Perfect Mothers."

107. Niermeijer, "Genetic Screening."

108. World Health Organization, *Genetic Counseling*, 5-23.

109. Wertz and Sorenson, "Sociologic Implications."

110. Finkelstein, "Biomedicine"; Leuzinger and Rambert, "Women's Experiences."

111. Leuzinger and Rambert, "Women's Experiences."

112. Rapp, "Moral Pioneers."

113. Ibid.

114. F.C. Fraser, personal communication, 31 October 1991; Donnai et al., "Attitudes."

115. Evans, "Medical Treatment Decisionmaking"; Conine et al., "Maternal Health Care"; Stafford et al., "One Face of Beauty."

116. Motulsky and Murray, "Society's Attitude."

117. Meryash and Abuelo, "Counseling Needs."

118. Evans, "Medical Treatment Decisionmaking"; Conine et al., "Maternal Health Care"; Stafford et al., "One Face of Beauty."

119. Evans, "Medical Treatment Decisionmaking."

120. Conine et al., "Maternal Health Care."

121. Spina Bifida and Hydrocephalus Association of Ontario, brief to the RCNRT.

122. Fraser, "Genetic Counseling."

123. E.E. Ekwo et al., "Factors Influencing Maternal Estimates of Genetic Risk," *American Journal of Medical Genetics* 20 (1985): 491-504.

124. Silvestre and Fresco, "Reactions."

125. Ekwo et al., "Maternal Estimates"; Frets et al., "Model"; P.G. Frets et al., "Factors Influencing the Reproductive Decision After Genetic Counseling," *American Journal of Medical Genetics* 35 (1990): 496-502.

126. Meryash and Abuelo, "Counseling Needs."

127. Niermeijer, "Genetic Screening"; World Health Organization, *Genetic Counseling*, 5-23.

128. PEI Association for Community Living, Canadian Disability Rights Council, and Ontario Coalition for Abortion Clinics, briefs to the RCNRT.

129. Rapp, "Moral Pioneers."

130. S. Kessler, "The Psychological Paradigm Shift in Genetic Counseling," *Social Biology* 27 (1980): 167-85.

131. Frets et al., "Reproductive Decision"; Ekwo et al., "Maternal Estimates."

132. Ekwo et al., "Maternal Estimates"; Fraser, "Genetic Counseling."

133. Meryash and Abuelo, "Counseling Needs."

134. Fraser, "Genetic Counseling."

135. Shiloh et al., "Genetic Counseling."

136. Ekwo et al., "Maternal Estimates."

137. Meryash and Abuelo, "Counseling Needs"; Kolker and Burke, "Social Construction of Pregnancy."

138. Bradish, "Genetic Counselling"; Hyde, "Pregnant Women's Attitudes"; Science Council of Canada, "Genetic Disorders"; Kaufmann, "Perfect Mothers"; Kessler, "Psychological Paradigm"; Kolker and Burke, "Social Construction of Pregnancy"; Leuzinger and Rambert, "Women's Experiences"; Tait, "Reproductive Technologies"; McDonough, "Congenital Disability"; Rice and Doherty, "The Consumers' Views."

139. Science Council of Canada, *Genetic Screening and Counselling*; Rose, "Diagnosing Defects."

140. Rose, "Diagnosing Defects."

141. Ibid.

142. Leuzinger and Rambert, "Women's Experiences."

143. McDonough, "Congenital Disability."

144. Silvestre and Fresco, "Reactions."

145. Motulsky and Murray, "Society's Attitude."

146. DisAbled Women's Network, Toronto, brief to the RCNRT.

147. Spina Bifida and Hydrocephalus Association of Ontario, brief to the RCNRT.

148. Ibid.

149. Science Council of Canada, "Genetic Disorders"; Kaufmann, "Perfect Mothers"; Donnai et al., "Attitudes."

150. Kessler, "Psychological Paradigm."

151. Rice and Doherty, "The Consumers' Views."

152. Niermeijer, "Genetic Screening."

153. McDonough, "Congenital Disability"; McDonough, "Amniocentesis."

154. Silvestre and Fresco, "Reactions."

155. J.L. Hamerton, J.A. Evans, and L. Stranc, "Prenatal Diagnosis in Canada — 1990: A Review of Genetics Centres," in *Current Practice of Prenatal Diagnosis in Canada*, vol. 13 of the research studies of the Royal Commission on New Reproductive Technologies (Ottawa: Minister of Supply and Services Canada, 1993).

156. Finkelstein, "Biomedicine."

157. S. Daya et al., "Early Pregnancy Assessment with Transvaginal Ultrasound Scanning," *Canadian Medical Association Journal* 144 (1991): 441-46.

158. Fraser, "Genetic Counseling."

159. Wertz and Sorenson, "Sociologic Implications."

160. Ibid.; McDonough, "Congenital Disability."

161. Hyde, "Pregnant Women's Attitudes."

162. McDonough, "Congenital Disability."

163. Ibid.; Kolker and Burke, "Social Construction of Pregnancy."

164. Julian, "Physicians' Acceptability."

165. Finkelstein, "Biomedicine."

166. McDonough, "Amniocentesis."

167. D. Orentlicher, "Genetic Screening by Employers," JAMA 263 (1990): 1005, 1008; Niermeijer, "Genetic Screening"; Science Council of Canada, "Genetic Disorders."

168. Orentlicher, "Screening by Employers"; Niermeijer, "Genetic Screening"; United States, President's Commission, *Screening and Counseling*, 5-8, 68-70.

169. Finkelstein, "Biomedicine."

170. Leuzinger and Rambert, "Women's Experiences."

171. Bradish, "Genetic Counselling."

172. Evans, "Medical Treatment Decisionmaking"; Kaufmann, "Perfect Mothers."

173. PEI Association for Community Living, Manitoba Association for Childbirth and Family Education, and Spina Bifida and Hydrocephalus Association of Ontario, briefs to the RCNRT.

174. Manitoba Association for Childbirth and Family Education, brief to the RCNRT.

175. Rodin and Ickovics, "Women's Health."

176. Kolker and Burke, "Social Construction of Pregnancy"; Leuzinger and Rambert, "Women's Experiences"; McDonough, "Congenital Disability"; Science Council of Canada, "Genetic Disorders."

177. Kaufmann, "Perfect Mothers."

178. Finkelstein, "Biomedicine"; Kaufmann, "Perfect Mothers."

179. McDonough, "Congenital Disability."

180. Ibid.; Leuzinger and Rambert, "Women's Experiences."

181. DisAbled Women's Network, Toronto, and Ontario Coalition for Abortion Clinics, briefs to the RCNRT; Conine et al., "Maternal Health Care."

182. Tait, "Reproductive Technologies."

183. Finkelstein, "Biomedicine."

184. Spina Bifida and Hydrocephalus Association of Ontario, brief to the RCNRT.

185. United States, President's Commission, *Screening and Counseling*, 5-8, 68-70; World Health Organization, *Genetic Counseling*, 5-23; Leonard et al., "Genetic Counselling"; Seals et al., "Amniocentesis Decision"; M.J. Seidenfeld and R.M. Antley, "Genetic Counseling: A Comparison of Counselee's Genetic Knowledge Before and After (Part III)," *American Journal of Medical Genetics* 10 (1981): 107-12.

186. Canadian Association for Community Living, brief to the RCNRT.

187. F.C. Fraser, personal communication, 31 October 1991.

# Bibliography

Archie, V.W., and C. Sherrill. "Attitudes Toward Handicapped Peers of Mainstreamed and Nonmainstreamed Children in Physical Education." *Perceptual and Motor Skills* 69 (1989): 319-22.

Arditti, R., R.D. Klein, and S. Minden, eds. *Test-Tube Women: What Future for Motherhood?* London: Pandora Press, 1989.

Baxter, C. "Investigating Stigma as Stress in Social Interactions of Parents." *Journal of Mental Deficiency Research* 33 (1989): 455-66.

Benham, P.K. "Attitudes of Occupational Therapy Personnel Toward Persons with Disabilities." *American Journal of Occupational Therapy* 42 (1988): 305-11.

Black, R.B., and R. Furlong. "Impact of Prenatal Diagnosis in Families." *Social Work in Health Care* 9 (Spring 1984): 37-50.

Bradish, P. "From Genetic Counselling and Genetic Analysis, to Genetic Ideal and Genetic Fate?" In *Made to Order: The Myth of Reproductive and Genetic Progress*, ed. P. Spallone and D.L. Steinberg. Oxford: Pergamon Press, 1987.

Canadian Abortion Rights Action League. Brief to the Royal Commission on New Reproductive Technologies, 17 October 1990.

Canadian Association for Community Living. Brief to the Royal Commission on New Reproductive Technologies, 19 November 1990.

Canadian Cystic Fibrosis Foundation. Brief to the Royal Commission on New Reproductive Technologies, 19 November 1990.

Canadian Disability Rights Council. Brief to the Royal Commission on New Reproductive Technologies, 28 November 1990.

Citizens' Committee on Biomedical Ethics. *Your Health, Your Choices, Whose Decision, 1985-87*. Summit: New Jersey Citizens' Committee on Biomedical Ethics, 1988.

Conine, T.A., E.A. Carty, and F. Wood-Johnson. "Provision of Preventive Maternal Health Care and Childbirth Education for Disabled Women." *Canadian Journal of Public Health* 77 (1986): 123-27.

Connor, C., ed. *Women with Disabilities Documentation Review and Annotated Bibliography*. Ottawa: Department of the Secretary of State, Status of Disabled Persons Secretariat, Disabled Persons Participation Program, 1989.

Corea, G., et al. *Man-Made Women: How New Reproductive Technologies Affect Women*. Bloomington: Indiana University Press, 1987.

Curtis, D., M. Johnson, and C.E. Blank. "An Evaluation of Reinforcement of Genetic Counselling on the Consultand." *Clinical Genetics* 33 (1988): 270-76.

Day, S., et al. *Four Discussion Papers on New Reproductive Technologies*. Winnipeg and Toronto: Canadian Disability Rights Council (CDRC) and DisAbled Women's Network Canada (DAWN), 1990.

Daya, S., et al. "Early Pregnancy Assessment with Transvaginal Ultrasound Scanning." *Canadian Medical Association Journal* 144 (1991): 441-46.

DisAbled Women's Network, Canada. Brief to the Royal Commission on New Reproductive Technologies, 31 October 1990.

DisAbled Women's Network, Toronto. Brief to the Royal Commission on New Reproductive Technologies, 19 November 1990.

Doerr, A. "Women's Rights in Canada: Social and Economic Realities." *Atlantis* 9 (Spring 1984): 35-47.

Donnai, P., N. Charles, and R. Harris. "Attitudes of Patients After 'Genetic' Termination of Pregnancy." *British Medical Journal* (Clinical Research Edition) (21 February 1981): 621-22.

Ekwo, E.E., et al. "Factors Influencing Maternal Estimates of Genetic Risk." *American Journal of Medical Genetics* 20 (1985): 491-504.

Evans, D. "The Psychological Impact of Disability and Illness on Medical Treatment Decisionmaking." *Issues in Law and Medicine* 5 (1989): 277-99.

Fine, M., and A. Asch, eds. *Women with Disabilities: Essays in Psychology, Culture, and Politics.* Philadelphia: Temple University Press, 1988.

Finkelstein, J.L. "Biomedicine and Technocratic Power." *Hastings Center Report* 20 (July-August 1990): 13-16.

Fraser, F.C. "Genetic Counseling." *American Journal of Human Genetics* 26 (1974): 636-61.

Frets, P.G., et al. "Factors Influencing the Reproductive Decision After Genetic Counseling." *American Journal of Medical Genetics* 35 (1990): 496-502.

—. "Model Identifying the Reproductive Decision After Genetic Counseling." *American Journal of Medical Genetics* 35 (1990): 503-509.

Glover, J., et al. *Ethics of New Reproductive Technologies: The Glover Report to the European Commission.* De Kalb: Northern Illinois University Press, 1989.

Grimes, S.K., and S.J. Vitello. "Follow-Up Study of Family Attitudes Toward Deinstitutionalization: Three to Seven Years Later." *Mental Retardation* 28 (1990): 219-25.

Hamerton, J.L., J.A. Evans, and L. Stranc. "Prenatal Diagnosis in Canada — 1990: A Review of Genetics Centres." In *Current Practice of Prenatal Diagnosis in Canada*, vol. 13 of the research studies of the Royal Commission on New Reproductive Technologies. Ottawa: Minister of Supply and Services Canada, 1993.

Hyde, B. "An Interview Study of Pregnant Women's Attitudes to Ultrasound Scanning." *Social Science and Medicine* 22 (1986): 587-92.

Julian, C., et al. "Factors Influencing Genetic Counseling Attendance Rate: A Geographically Based Study." *Social Biology* 36 (1989): 240-47.

—. "Physicians' Acceptability of Termination of Pregnancy After Prenatal Diagnosis in Southern France." *Prenatal Diagnosis* 9 (1989): 77-89.

Kaufmann, C.L. "Perfect Mothers, Perfect Babies: An Examination of the Ethics of Fetal Treatments." *Reproductive and Genetic Engineering* 1 (1988): 133-39.

Kenyon, S.L., G.A. Hackett, and S. Campbell. "Termination of Pregnancy Following Diagnosis of Fetal Malformation: The Need for Improved Follow-Up Services." *Clinical Obstetrics and Gynecology* 31 (1988): 97-100.

Kessler, S. "The Psychological Paradigm Shift in Genetic Counseling." *Social Biology* 27 (1980): 167-85.

King, S.M., et al. "An Epidemiological Study of Children's Attitudes Toward Disability." *Developmental Medicine and Child Neurology* 31 (1989): 237-45.

Kolker, A., and B.M. Burke. "Amniocentesis and the Social Construction of Pregnancy." In *Alternative Health Maintenance and Healing Systems for Families*, ed. D.Y. Wilkinson and M.B. Sussman. New York: Haworth Press, 1987.

Leonard, C.O. "Counselling Parents of a Child with Meningomyelocele." *Pediatrics in Review* 4 (1983): 317-21.

Leonard, C.O., G.A. Chase, and B. Childs. "Genetic Counseling: A Consumers' View." *New England Journal of Medicine* 287 (1972): 433-39.

Leuzinger, M., and B. Rambert. "'I Can Feel It — My Baby Is Healthy': Women's Experiences with Prenatal Diagnosis in Switzerland." *Reproductive and Genetic Engineering* 1 (1988): 239-49.

Lippman-Hand, A., and F.C. Fraser. "Genetic Counseling: Parents' Responses to Uncertainty." *Birth Defects: Original Article Series* 15 (1979): 325-39.

Lloyd, J., and K.M. Laurence. "Sequelae and Support After Termination of Pregnancy for Fetal Malformation." *British Medical Journal* (Clinical Research Edition) (23 March 1985): 907-909.

McDonough, P. "Congenital Disability and Medical Research: The Development of Amniocentesis." *Women and Health* 16 (3-4)(1990): 137-53.

—. "The Diffusion of Genetic Amniocentesis in Ontario: 1969-1987." *Canadian Journal of Public Health* 81 (1990): 431-35.

Manitoba Association for Childbirth and Family Education. Brief to the Royal Commission on New Reproductive Technologies, 23 October 1990.

Mason, J.K. *Medico-Legal Aspects of Reproduction and Parenthood.* Aldershot (U.K.): Dartmouth Publishing, 1990.

Meryash, D.L., and D. Abuelo. "Counseling Needs and Attitudes Toward Prenatal Diagnosis and Abortion in Fragile-X Families." *Clinical Genetics* 33 (1988): 349-55.

Michaelson, K.L., et al. *Childbirth in America: Anthropological Perspectives.* South Hadley: Bergin & Garvey, 1988.

Miller, C.T., et al. "What Mentally Retarded and Nonretarded Children Expect of One Another." *American Journal on Mental Retardation* 93 (1989): 396-405.

Motulsky, A.G., and J. Murray. "Will Prenatal Diagnosis with Selective Abortion Affect Society's Attitude Toward the Handicapped?" *Progress in Clinical and Biological Research* 128 (1983): 277-91.

National Legal Center for the Medically Dependent and Disabled. "Medical Treatment for Older People and People with Disabilities: 1987 Developments." *Issues in Law and Medicine* 3 (1988): 333-60.

—. "Recent Developments in the Law Governing Medical Treatment for Older People and People with Disabilities." *Clearinghouse Review* 22 (May 1988): 31-42.

National Tay-Sachs and Allied Diseases Association of Ontario. Brief to the Royal Commission on New Reproductive Technologies, 31 October 1990.

Niermeijer, M.F. "Genetic Screening and Counselling — Implications of the DNA Technologies." In *Health Policy, Ethics and Human Values: European and North American Perspectives*, ed. Z. Bankowski and J.H. Bryant. Geneva: Council for International Organizations of Medical Sciences, 1988.

Nova Scotia Advisory Council on the Status of Women. Brief to the Royal Commission on New Reproductive Technologies, 17 October 1990.

Ontario Coalition for Abortion Clinics. "Expanding Women's Choices." Brief to the Royal Commission on New Reproductive Technologies, May 1991.

Orentlicher, D. "Genetic Screening by Employers." *JAMA* 263 (1990): 1005, 1008.

Overall, C. *Ethics and Human Reproduction: A Feminist Analysis*. Boston: Unwin Hyman, 1987.

Paez-Victor, M.E. "Risks and Values: A Study of the Social Context of Prenatal Diagnosis and Counselling." Ph.D. dissertation, York University, 1987.

PEI Association for Community Living. Brief to the Royal Commission on New Reproductive Technologies, 16 October 1990.

PEI Council of the Disabled. Brief to the Royal Commission on New Reproductive Technologies, 16 October 1990.

Rapp, R. "Moral Pioneers: Women, Men and Fetuses on a Frontier of Reproductive Technology." In *Embryos, Ethics and Women's Rights: Exploring the New Reproductive Technologies*, ed. E.H. Baruch, A.F. D'Adamo, Jr., and J. Seager. New York: Harrington Park Press, 1988.

Rice, N., and R. Doherty. "Reflections on Prenatal Diagnosis: The Consumers' Views." *Social Work in Health Care* 8 (1982): 47-57.

Robinson, A., B.G. Bender, and M.G. Linden. "Decisions Following the Intrauterine Diagnosis of Sex Chromosome Aneuploidy." *American Journal of Medical Genetics* 34 (1989): 552-54.

Rodin, J., and J.R. Ickovics. "Women's Health: Review and Research Agenda as We Approach the 21st Century." *American Psychologist* 45 (1990): 1018-34.

Rose, B. "Diagnosing Defects in the Unborn." *Science Forum* 12 (January-February 1979): 35-38.

Sandercock, K. Brief to the Royal Commission on New Reproductive Technologies, 1 November 1990.

Science Council of Canada. "The Need to Know? Genetic Disorders and the Unborn." *Agenda Science Council of Canada* 2 (Autumn 1979): 1-7.

—. *Social Issues in Human Genetics: Genetic Screening and Counselling*. Ottawa: Science Council of Canada, 1980.

Seals, B.F., et al. "Moral and Religious Influences on the Amniocentesis Decision." *Social Biology* 32 (1985): 13-30.

Seidenfeld, M.J., and R.M. Antley. "Genetic Counseling: A Comparison of Counselee's Genetic Knowledge Before and After (Part III)." *American Journal of Medical Genetics* 10 (1981): 107-12.

Shiloh, S., O. Avdor, and R.M. Goodman. "Satisfaction with Genetic Counseling: Dimensions and Measurement." *American Journal of Medical Genetics* 37 (1990): 522-29.

Silvestre, D., and N. Fresco. "Reactions to Prenatal Diagnosis: An Analysis of 87 Interviews." *American Journal of Orthopsychiatry* 50 (1980): 610-17.

Spina Bifida and Hydrocephalus Association of Ontario. Brief to the Royal Commission on New Reproductive Technologies, 20 November 1990.

Stafford, B.M., J. La Puma, and D.L. Schiedermayer. "One Face of Beauty, One Picture of Health: The Hidden Aesthetic of Medical Practice." *Journal of Medicine and Philosophy* 14 (1989): 213-30.

Sultz, H.A., E.R. Schlesinger, and J. Feldman. "An Epidemiologic Justification for Genetic Counseling in Family Planning." *American Journal of Public Health* 62 (1972): 1489-92.

Tait, J.J. "Reproductive Technologies and the Rights of Disabled Persons." *Canadian Journal of Women and the Law* 1 (1986): 446-55.

Thomas, F.F., and D. Lee. "Effects of Ethnicity and Physical Disability on Academic and Social Ratings of Photographs." *Psychological Reports* 67 (1990): 240-42.

Turner's Syndrome Society. Presentation to the Royal Commission on New Reproductive Technologies, Public Hearings, 19 November 1990, Toronto.

United States Commission on Civil Rights. *Medical Discrimination Against Children with Disabilities: A Report of the U.S. Commission on Civil Rights.* Washington, DC: U.S. Commission on Civil Rights, 1989.

United States. President's Commission for the Study of Ethical Problems in Medicine and Biomedical and Behavioral Research. *Screening and Counseling for Genetic Conditions: A Report on the Ethical, Social, and Legal Implications of Genetic Screening, Counseling and Education Programs.* Washington, DC: U.S. Government Printing Office, 1983.

Verville, R.E. "The Americans with Disabilities Act: An Analysis." *Archives of Physical Medicine and Rehabilitation* 71 (1990): 1010-13.

Volodkevich, H., and C.A. Huether. "Causes of Low Utilization of Amniocentesis by Women of Advanced Age." *Social Biology* 28 (1981): 176-86.

Weil, J. "Mothers' Postcounseling Beliefs About the Causes of Their Children's Genetic Disorders." *American Journal of Human Genetics* 48 (1991): 145-53.

Wertz, D.C., and J.R. Sorenson. "Sociologic Implications." In *Fetal Diagnosis and Therapy: Science, Ethics and the Law*, ed. M.I. Evans et al. Philadelphia: J.B. Lippincott, 1989.

Whittick, J.E. "Dementia and Mental Handicap: Attitudes, Emotional Distress and Caregiving." *British Journal of Medical Psychology* 62 (1989): 181-89.

World Health Organization. *Genetic Counseling: Technical Report Series No. 416.* Geneva: World Health Organization, 1969.

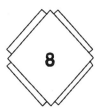

# Parental Reaction and Adaptability to the Prenatal Diagnosis of Genetic Disease Leading to Pregnancy Termination

## Louis Dallaire and Gilles Lortie

**Executive Summary**

The objective of this study was to evaluate the psychological reaction of two groups of parents to a pregnancy termination after they had undergone a prenatal diagnostic procedure. The analysis involved interviews with a study group of 76 patients, who had had an amniocentesis followed by a pregnancy termination because they were at risk of giving birth to a child with a genetic defect or disease; and a comparison group of 124, who had had a pregnancy termination after a major anomaly had been detected by routine ultrasound and who were not at known risk for genetic disease. Patients in the study group had received counselling before the prenatal diagnosis but the patients in the comparison group were unaware that the fetus could have a congenital disease or defect. Patients in the two groups were interviewed by a psychologist to obtain information on the decision to terminate the pregnancy and the experience of the pregnancy termination.

Patients in the study group were aware that the fetus could be affected; such patients experience a period of great anxiety until the results of prenatal investigations are known. They require strong support if there is a termination of the pregnancy, and ongoing support and contact with the medical staff may be needed. The overall reaction

---

This paper was completed for the Royal Commission on New Reproductive Technologies in June 1992.

of the comparison group was one of shock, denial of the fetal abnormality, and guilt over "abandoning the fetus."

The study concludes with several recommendations regarding the approach medical personnel should take during the prenatal diagnostic procedure and presentation of the results, and regarding counselling and support services.

## Introduction

Many papers have dealt with counselling in relation to reproduction in families at risk for a genetic disease (see, for example, American Society of Human Genetics 1975; Boss 1990; Lippman-Hand and Fraser 1979; Pearn 1979; Powledge and Fletcher 1979; Sorenson et al. 1981, 1987; Sorenson and Wertz 1986; Wertz et al. 1986), and some have measured the impact of therapeutic abortion on a couple's mental health and subsequent attitude toward family planning (Galjaard 1989; Iles 1989; Kenyon et al. 1988; Kessler et al. 1984, 1987; Laiho 1988; Rothman 1990; Seidman et al. 1988; Urquhart and Templeton 1991; Wells 1989). Prenatal diagnosis was introduced in 1968 and was offered in most university medical centres by 1976 (Dallaire et al. 1982; Simpson et al. 1976). This study was conducted to evaluate the reactions and adaptability of women who had had a pregnancy termination after a fetal anomaly had been discovered by a prenatal diagnostic technique — either by amniocentesis for a known risk, or by chance from an ultrasound examination.

The main objective of this study was to evaluate the reaction of parents to a pregnancy termination following a prenatal diagnostic procedure. This comprehensive evaluation would allow an analysis of the attitudes and reactions toward the prenatal diagnostic procedure, the impact of pregnancy termination, and the efficacy of genetic counselling or support before and after the diagnostic procedure.

## Materials and Methods

More than 2 000 referrals per year are made to the prenatal diagnosis section of the Service of Medical Genetics at Sainte-Justine Hospital in Montreal. Of these, more than 100 patients request a pregnancy termination for a fetal anomaly. About half (53 percent) of the abnormal pregnancies are first identified by routine ultrasound examination (Dallaire et al. 1991).

For this study, 299 charts were selected at random by the archivist from among the completed charts (which included autopsy reports and completed laboratory results) of patients residing within a 150-kilometre radius of the hospital. Of these 299 patients, 30 had moved without leaving a forwarding address, and 10 never returned a phone message. Therefore, 259 patients were contacted by phone or sent a letter by the nurse coordinator and asked if they would like to participate in the study: 46 declined the invitation for various reasons, including their availability at the time of contact, another pregnancy, or because they did not wish to see a psychologist; 13 refused because they wanted to forget the experience. All respondents were French-speaking, and lived on average 40 kilometres from the hospital. The remaining 200 patients, who agreed to participate, were divided into two groups: the study group, in which there were 76 patients referred for prenatal diagnosis because of an increased risk, and the comparison group, which had 124 patients in whom the abnormal fetus had been discovered by routine ultrasound. It has already been indicated that 53 percent of referred abnormal pregnancies are first identified by routine ultrasound examination. The relative excess in the comparison group (62% compared to 53%) is likely due to the greater availability and willingness of couples in this group to participate in the study.

## Routine Local Procedure

Patients referred for prenatal diagnosis are usually seen first by a staff member of the genetics service. If a patient is clear that she would not terminate a pregnancy if the fetus were abnormal, only ultrasound and routine laboratory tests are done. If a couple wants to make a decision only after the results are available, their wish is always respected; the amniocentesis is then done. No patient is advised to have a pregnancy termination if the fetus is abnormal, and the decision to terminate the pregnancy remains entirely in the hands of the patient. The sole responsibility of medical staff is to offer all medically indicated investigative measures. After permission is received from the patient, a level II or III ultrasound is performed. If an anomaly is detected by ultrasound, or later by molecular, biochemical, or cytogenetic studies after amniocentesis, the referring physician is informed, and the patient is contacted. More information is given if necessary to the couple by one of the medical staff involved (e.g., attending physician, geneticist, obstetrician). When a diagnosis of fetal anomaly is made and pregnancy termination is requested by the couple, the procedure is completed within days of confirmation of the diagnosis. A combination of Laminaria cervical insertion and intra-amniotic injection of prostaglandin is the most commonly used method to induce abortion late in the second trimester of pregnancy. This technique also facilitates confirmation of the fetal pathology. A psychiatrist sees most patients at the time of admission and later if necessary (if possible, those facing pregnancy termination for genetic reasons are offered psychiatric counselling during the pre-abortion period). After abortion, all fetuses are first examined by the geneticist, then shown to the couple if they wish.

Every fetus over 500 g is considered viable and reported as a birth; autopsy consent must be obtained from the parents. Unless otherwise specified, arrangements are made for the burial of the fetus in a common tomb in the city cemetery. The pathology department conducts the autopsy, and the autopsy report and laboratory results (including fetal x-rays) are used by the geneticist for counselling purposes four to six months later. The protocol described here has been the same for the last decade.

## Research Procedure

### Family Contact

A nurse coordinator who knew most of the patients made the initial contact with the families. She explained the aim of the research project to each couple and, if they wished to participate, they were told that a psychologist would contact them to make an appointment. Most interviews were conducted at the patients' homes.

### Psychologists' Training

Two psychologists experienced in interviewing couples were hired and spent time in the prenatal diagnosis clinic to familiarize themselves with ultrasonographic evaluation, amniocentesis/chorionic villus sampling procedures, laboratory techniques (cell culture, cytogenetic, biochemical, and deoxyribonucleic acid analysis), pregnancy termination, psychiatric counselling, and genetic counselling.

### Interviews

A psychologist conducted the two-hour interview at each patient's residence, when possible with the husband present. Further contact by phone with the patient was often made to complete the interview. The interviews were semi-structured, with both closed and open-ended questions. To allow appropriate and sensitive handling of participants, the psychologists were briefed about particular circumstances, such as post-abortion psychological or medical complications or marital difficulties, and they took notes and completed the questionnaire later (Appendix 1). The patients signed an informed consent form (Appendix 2), were given the brochure *A Guide to the Research and Evaluation Program of the Royal Commission on New Reproductive Technologies*, and were told they would receive a summary of the research project's recommendations when they were completed.

### Study Group and Comparison Group

The study group consisted of 76 patients who had had a pregnancy termination after being referred to the prenatal clinic because they were at risk of giving birth to a child with a genetic defect or disease. The comparison group comprised 124 patients who were not known to be at risk of passing on a genetic disease but who had had an unforeseen major anomaly detected by a routine ultrasound examination. The two groups were interviewed and studied in the same manner, but patients from the comparison group had not been counselled before the prenatal diagnostic procedure. The comparison group had an unexpected diagnosis, and had been seen only by ultrasonographers and the technical staff, whereas the study group members were aware of the risk and had been counselled by the genetic counsellors. Any differences between the two groups in intensity of reactions, in the contact between patients and health care professionals after the ultrasound findings, and in communications and reactions during the interviews are likely to be due to their different experiences. It was planned to compare our observations with those of previous studies.

## *Evaluation*

Following is a list of the information and responses we evaluated and the relevant questions asked by the psychologists, which served as a basis for discussion in the interviews:

- individual attitudes of patients and, when possible, their husbands (Q22-24,40-43)
- patients' evaluation of how well they were informed about the reasons for doing the test (Q29,57-59)
- interpretation of genetic risk (Q47,57)
- knowledge of any risk related to the procedure (Q48-50)
- how the test results were preserved (Q27,28)
- who interpreted the results or gave personal advice (Q27,51)
- personal and professional support provided (Q30,37)
- psychiatric support provided before and after the abortion (Q38)
- reaction of the mother to the abortion procedure (Q31-34, 39,52,62,63)
- the follow-up, if any (Q64)
- couples' attitudes about their personal relationship, contraception, future pregnancies, and their living child(ren) (Q36,40, 41,44)
- attitude of patients or couples about the initial psychiatric evaluation, any adverse reaction during the post-pregnancy termination period, and their psychological attitude at the time of the interviewer's visit (Q35,36,38,42,43)

## Results

### General

#### Age of Patients Interviewed
The mean maternal age was 35.2 years for the study group and 27.9 years for the comparison group (Table 1).

#### Reproductive History
The average number of pregnancies was 2.5 in the study group and 2.0 in the comparison group. There was an average of 1.9 live births in the study group and 1.3 in the comparison group (Tables 2 and 3).

Table 1. Distribution of Patients by Maternal Age

| Study group (n = 76) | | Comparison group (n = 124) | |
|---|---|---|---|
| Age (years) | No. of patients | Age (years) | No. of patients |
| 23 | 1 | 17 | 1 |
| 25 | 2 | 19 | 1 |
| 26 | 5 | 20 | 6 |
| 27 | 3 | 21 | 3 |
| 28 | 2 | 22 | 9 |
| 29 | 2 | 23 | 5 |
| 30 | 4 | 24 | 6 |
| 31 | 2 | 25 | 11 |
| 32 | 2 | 26 | 11 |
| 33 | 1 | 27 | 11 |
| 34 | 4 | 28 | 11 |
| 35 | 8 | 29 | 15 |
| 36 | 9 | 30 | 9 |
| 37 | 8 | 31 | 12 |
| 38 | 7 | 32 | 1 |
| 39 | 3 | 33 | 6 |
| 40 | 2 | 34 | 3 |
| 41 | 4 | 35 | 1 |
| 42 | 2 | 37 | 1 |
| 43 | 4 | 38 | 1 |
| 44 | 1 | | |
| | 76 | | 124 |

### Table 2. Parity, Marital Status, and Sterilization in the Study and Comparison Groups

|  | Study group | Comparison group |
| --- | --- | --- |
| Average number of pregnancies | 2.5 | 2.0 |
| Average number of live births | 1.9 | 1.3 |
| Percentage remarried | 10.9 | 7.0 |
| Tubal ligation (%) | 13.1 | 13.0 |
| Vasectomy (%) | 22.4 | 8.9 |

### Table 3. Distribution of Patients According to the Number of Pregnancies

| Gravidity | Study group (n = 76) | Comparison group (n = 124) |
| --- | --- | --- |
| 1 | 16 | 52 |
| 2 | 26 | 40 |
| 3 | 17 | 22 |
| 4 | 8 | 7 |
| 5 | 4 | 3 |
| 6 | 3 | 0 |
| 8 | 2 | 0 |
| Mean | 2.5 | 2.0 |

### Marital Status

In the study group, 10.9 percent had remarried or lived with a second husband at the time of the visit compared to 7 percent in the comparison group.

### Sterilization

In the study group, 22.4 percent of men (mean age 40.8 years) had a vasectomy and 13.1 percent of women (mean age 37.2 years) had a tubal ligation, for a total of 36 percent, after pregnancy termination. In the comparison group, 8.9 percent of men (mean age 29.5 years) and 13 percent of women (mean age 28.0 years) had a sterilization, for a total of 22 percent. The mean number of pregnancies (2.5 in the study group and 2.0 in the comparison group) was similar. In both groups, 80 percent of anomalies that led to pregnancy termination were of unknown cause (renal agenesis, trisomies) or of multi-factorial origin (spina bifida, etc.); 20 percent had a high risk of recurrence (familial chromosomal translocations, skeletal dysplasias, etc.).

## *Diagnoses Leading to Pregnancy Termination*

The diagnoses that led to pregnancy termination in the study and comparison groups are listed in Table 4. The most common anomalies were chromosomal (75 percent) in the study group, and neural tube defects (37 percent) in the comparison group. The numbers are given in Table 5.

**Table 4. Diagnoses in the Study and Comparison Groups (Leading to Pregnancy Termination)**

| Study group | Comparison group |
|---|---|
| *Chromosomal abnormalities* | *Neural tube defects* |
| Trisomy 21 | Anencephaly |
| Trisomy 18 | Dysraphism |
| Trisomy 13 | Hydrocephaly |
| Turner syndrome 45, X | Holoprosencephaly |
| Structural aberrations | |
| Triploidy | *Chromosomal abnormalities* |
| XXXX syndrome | |
| 18p(-) syndrome | Trisomy 21 |
| Fragile X syndrome | Trisomy 18 |
| | Trisomy 13 |
| *Neural tube defects* | Triploidy |
| | Structural abnormalities |
| Anencephaly | Turner syndrome |
| Spina bifida | |
| Hydrocephaly | *Renal anomalies* |
| | Renal agenesis |
| *Skeletal dysplasia* | Hydronephrosis and |
| | associated anomalies |
| Achondroplasia | Polycystic kidneys |
| Osteogenesis imperfecta | |
| | *Other anomalies* |
| *Others* | |
| | Hydrops foetalis |
| Renal dysplasias | Omphalocele |
| Cardiovascular abnormalities | Gastrochisis |
| Myotonic dystrophy | Diaphragmatic hernia |
| Haemophilia | |
| Duchenne-type muscular dystrophy | |

## Table 5. Fetal Anomalies

### Study group (n = 76)

Chromosomal
- Trisomy 21 — 34
- Trisomy 13 — 6
- Trisomy 18 — 9
- Turner syndrome — 2
- Others — 6

Subtotal — 57

- Skeletal dysplasia — 4
- Neural tube defect — 3
- Renal dysplasia — 2
- Others — 10

Total — 76

### Comparison group (n = 124)

- Neural tube defect — 46
- Chromosomal aberrations — 20
- Renal dysplasia — 19
- Skeletal dysplasia — 10
- Gastrointestinal — 6
- Others — 23

Total — 124

## Interviews

### *Interval Since Pregnancy Termination*

Most patients were interviewed at least six months after the pregnancy termination. The mean interval was similar in both groups: more than half of the patients in the two groups were interviewed 24 months or more after the termination (Table 6).

### Were Patients Coerced into Having the Diagnostic Procedure for a Genetic Defect?

This question applied to the study group only. Seventeen percent answered that they had been urged to undergo the prenatal diagnostic procedure because they were at risk of giving birth to a child with a genetic defect or disease. In the study group, most patients had been informed about the prenatal diagnosis by the geneticist, and one in four "felt obligated" to have an amniocentesis (Table 7), while the majority felt it would be better to have the test.

### Table 6. Number of Months Elapsed at the Time of Interview Since Pregnancy Termination

| Months | Study group | Comparison group |
|---|---|---|
| 0-6   | 11 | 1   |
| 6-12  | 5  | 12  |
| 12-18 | 7  | 18  |
| 18-24 | 7  | 17  |
| 24+   | 46 | 76  |
| Total | 76 | 124 |

### Table 7. Origin of Information Received Prior to the Prenatal Diagnostic Procedure

|  | Study group (%) |
|---|---|
| Attending physician | 14 |
| Geneticist | 38 |
| Ultrasonographer | 21 |
| Nurses in genetics | 12 |
| Others | 15 |
| Total | 100 |

## Who Was the Person Who Conveyed the Abnormal Results?

The information about the abnormal result was given to patients in the study group by their own physician (52 percent) or the geneticist (16 percent). In the comparison group, 43 percent were informed by their own physician and 37 percent by the ultrasonographer.

## Were Patients Influenced to Have a Therapeutic Abortion After the Diagnosis of Fetal Anomaly?

Of the women interviewed in both groups, 33 percent said that, although they were free to make their own decision, the urgency to reach a decision and the severity of the defect more or less forced them to decide to have the procedure. Patients in the study group found it hard to accept the diagnosis.

## Length of Gestation at the Time of Diagnosis and Pregnancy Termination

Most diagnoses were made before 20 weeks for the study group; the pregnancy termination took place shortly thereafter at 21.1 weeks. In the comparison group, the termination took place somewhat earlier: the first ultrasound examination was done at 17.9 weeks and the pregnancy termination at 19.0 weeks. Five pregnancies were interrupted after the 23rd week in the comparison group because of a non-viable fetal anomaly (e.g., hydrops foetalis, anencephaly, multiple anomalies, extreme dysraphism) diagnosed during a late first ultrasound examination.

## How Were the Patients Informed of the Diagnosis?

In the study group, the patient herself was informed before her partner in 49 percent of the cases. In the comparison group, the diagnosis was usually made during a routine ultrasound procedure when both spouses were present (69 percent), after which they were informed together of the presence of a fetal anomaly.

## Was the Information About the Anomaly Well Understood?

In general, the information provided by the centre was understood and considered clear. However, 25 percent of the patients in the study group said they thought that the information was insufficient, and 32 percent of the comparison group thought they would have benefited from additional counselling.

# Pregnancy Termination

## Complications

Of patients in the study group, 68 percent said that, during and after the pregnancy termination, they had experienced considerable discomfort and some had had severe complications such as haemorrhage and psychological distress. This was less evident among patients in the comparison group (54 percent).

## Support from Family and Friends

Moral support, sympathy, nursing help, and family relief were offered by family members and friends. This was slightly more evident in the study group (89 percent) than in the other group (81 percent). The knowledge of the fetal anomaly caused a shock, but there was the relief of knowing that the pregnancy could be terminated.

## Did Mourning Occur?

Grief for the dead fetus was prolonged in both groups, especially if it was the result of the only conception of an older mother or if family planning was important to the marital relationship; 82 percent of patients in both groups stated that they were still mourning the loss. However, while 63 percent of patients in the study group wanted to have another child to replace this pregnancy, only 19 percent in the comparison group expressed the same feeling.

### *Usefulness of the Interview with the Psychiatrist*

For several years, a psychiatrist has been a permanent staff member of the prenatal diagnostic program and has acted as a consultant for patients admitted for pregnancy termination for a genetic defect or disease. Most of the patients (73 percent) recalled seeing the psychiatrist at the time of admission and 50 percent of these were satisfied with the interview. For several patients this period had been so traumatic that they did not recall who saw them or why during their 48- to 72-hour stay in hospital. A few of them (8 percent) expressed the need to be seen by a psychiatrist again.

## Overview of the "Obstetrical Experience"

### *In Retrospect, Was the Abortion a Good Decision?*

Most patients felt that the decision to terminate the pregnancy had been the correct choice. A few had had familial problems before the pregnancy and several had experienced unhappiness in the months after the procedure. Some had experienced serious problems, such as legal separation, divorce, and mental health problems. Guilt feelings were also present (10 percent) and were more evident if the counselling offered had indicated a genetic risk associated with that parent's side of the family. In some these feelings of guilt were still present as long as four years after the termination. In 80 percent of the cases in both groups, the decision to terminate the pregnancy had been made for the sake of the unborn child rather than for the parents' own well-being, for the family, or for socioeconomic reasons.

### *Were There Any Feelings of Guilt About the Fetal Anomaly?*

Seventy-one percent of couples in the study group answered "no" without hesitation to this question. Some patients were sad because they were carriers of a mutation (X-linked or recessive gene), others because of their age, but the majority had been informed about a risk and had accepted the fact of this disorder. The picture was entirely different in the comparison group, where 73 percent expressed feelings of guilt in the period immediately following the pregnancy termination. Drug usage by one or both members of the couple, nature of work, medication, family problems, and unknown family history were blamed for this abnormal event. However, the guilt feelings rapidly subsided once the couples understood that they were not to blame or that environmental factors, if any, could not have been avoided.

## Retrospective Views

A few patients in both groups (5 percent) said they had premonitory feelings of fetal demise before the visit to the genetics clinic or the routine ultrasound examination. In reply to the question of how high a risk would be considered "severe," the median response was 10 percent in both groups, but there was great variability, with replies ranging from greater than 1 percent to greater than 50 percent (Table 8). Counselling offered to couples of both groups was found reassuring by 25 percent in the study group and 50 percent in the other group. As many in both groups (50 percent) had received advice from friends. Those with children did not really know how to tell them about the termination, except to say that the "baby" had been sick and was now in heaven.

Table 8. Perception of an "Elevated Risk of Recurrence"

| | % of risk | | | | | | |
|---|---|---|---|---|---|---|---|
| | 1+ | 5+ | 10+ | 15+ | 25+ | 33+ | 50+ |
| Study group (n = 71) | | | | | | | |
| n | 11 | 12 | 13 | 4 | 10 | 8 | 13 |
| % | 16 | 17 | 18 | 6 | 14 | 11 | 18 |
| "No opinion" = 5 | | | | | | | |
| Comparison group (n = 124) | | | | | | | |
| n | 27 | 17 | 21 | 12 | 22 | 6 | 19 |
| % | 22 | 14 | 17 | 9 | 18 | 5 | 15 |

## Suggestions Received from Couples

When couples were asked if they would change the maternal age threshold for amniocentesis, 61 percent in the study group and 53 percent in the comparison group said that the maternal age threshold should be lowered if amniocentesis was not made available to all women. The others favoured the status quo. Most respondents were unaware of the technical difficulty involved in maintaining a universal program and were not influenced by the low incidence of chromosomal aberrations in younger maternal age groups.

## What Was the Most Critical Period for the Patients?

It appears that patients in both groups endured similar psychological pain before and after the abortion; for some, this persisted months and years later. The waiting period before the termination was mentioned by several patients in the study group as the most critical time: the Laminaria cervical insertion is done the day before the prostaglandin injection. During the period between these, the patient is visited by the psychiatrist. For others, the signing of the abortion consent form was the most difficult and felt like an act against nature. If the sex of the fetus corresponded to the sex a couple had wanted, it was more difficult for some; however, most were emotionally attached to the fetus irrespective of its sex. Unlike the comparison group where abnormal findings from the ultrasound were usually divulged to the couple during the initial visit, women in the study group often had to inform their spouse of the "bad news" given to them first by telephone and subsequently at the physician's office.

For many patients the prostaglandin intra-amniotic injection was the most critical event and was described as the "point of no return." The interruption of fetal movements and the expulsion of the fetus were also regarded as traumatic.

Patients in the comparison group had had no reason to think that their fetus would have a congenital disease or defect, whereas most patients in the study group had been resigned to waiting for the results of the prenatal investigation before they could feel completely happy about the pregnancy. We found that couples in the comparison group had often already chosen a name for their child, made plans for the future, and announced the news to family, friends, and children. To them the news was a terrible shock, but although the immediate reaction was intense, it was easier for most of them to overcome the pain because the risk of recurrence was often relatively low, and also mothers were much younger, with an average age of 27.9 years compared to 35.2 years in the study group. Since the mothers had had no reason to suspect that the pregnancy was abnormal, they had already developed a close contact with the "baby," often spoke to it, and had great difficulty in finding words to explain the decision to terminate the pregnancy. They expressed guilt over the "abandonment of the fetus" and found it hard to endure the waiting period from the initiation of the abortion procedure until the termination was completed.

## What Changes Do Couples See as Essential?

There were numerous and varied suggestions originating from the experiences of the study group. They felt that as complete information as possible should be provided at the time of the diagnosis, such as: Would the child live for a long time or be severely mentally retarded? Could the parents get public educational and social services to help them raise the child? The parents did not always fully understand the extent of the anomalies or what exactly they were (e.g., anencephaly, polycystic kidneys). Their questions were relevant and well founded. The confirmation of the fetal anomaly was done in several ways by the attending physician and the geneticist, but the actual diagnosis — the fact that their fetus was identified as having the anomaly — almost always shocked the couple. This was not particularly criticized by the couples. They suggested that the interval between the news and the pregnancy termination should be reduced, more should be explained about the anomaly, and there should be more opportunity for the mothers to confide in a person on the ward who would care for them during hospitalization, because the spouse is often too affected to be able to help.

Patients appreciated being in a private room away from other women having abortions for "social reasons" or from those bearing a normal fetus. Patients in the study group had known they were at risk, because of their age or for other reasons, but they had always hoped that their pregnancy would be a normal one. Local anaesthesia at the time of expulsion should not be overlooked or not given because of a lack of personnel. Any way of making the experience less painful should not be neglected. Patients wanted to know more about the termination and possible complications. A follow-up, preferably at home, would be welcomed by many. Patients suggested that, within a month, a visit from a nurse, psychologist, or expert counsellor would have been appreciated to help them review and accept the past events. Such visits should be followed by an appointment with the geneticist to explain the results of the autopsy, laboratory tests, and the risks for a future pregnancy.

Patients in the study group knew they were at risk but the actual diagnosis and pregnancy termination had a compounding effect on their life: they feared another pregnancy and were in great need of support during the following period. They also wanted to hear that there had been no real alternative and that their decision had been the right one.

For the parents in the comparison group, because the finding of anomaly was unexpected, there had been no need to discuss the termination before the day when the diagnosis was made. They felt that they would have liked more time spent with them to explore the various options, such as proceeding with the termination, or carrying the fetus to term or carrying it until it died *in utero*. More severe structural anomalies were found in this group (e.g., anencephaly, rachischisis, gastrochisis). Like the study group, they wanted to shorten the interval between the diagnosis and the abortion, but they also wanted more time to digest the "catastrophic" event and to make their decision in their own time, instead of feeling time pressure regarding the need to decide about pregnancy termination as soon as the ultrasound diagnosis was confirmed. Patients in this group were often informed of the fetal anomaly minutes after the initiation of a routine ultrasound by a technologist or physician ultrasonographer; this meant the etiology or the implications of the diagnosis may not have been discussed until they met, after the termination, with the geneticist. The women in this group generally wanted to be told as soon as possible that they could become pregnant again.

## Discussion

The literature on reactions of women to termination of their pregnancies for genetic reasons is scanty. More than a decade ago, Donnai et al. (1981) studied the attitudes of 12 patients after a termination of pregnancy for genetic reasons and found persistent psychological and social reactions. Jones et al. (1984) analyzed the reactions of 14 women and 12 men and found that in 70 percent of the cases the marital relationship improved. Most of the couples relied on relatives, friends, and counsellors to help them cope with the adverse situation. In a group of women who had experienced a pregnancy termination for a fetal neural tube defect, 82 percent were satisfied with the prenatal procedure and the availability of the service when they left the hospital; however, their post-partum reaction was not so positive (White-Van Mourik et al. 1990). More than 50 percent of the patients were dissatisfied with the follow-up and the lack of professional information concerning their later reproductive status.

An acute grief reaction in 80 percent of patients has been mentioned by several authors (Dagg 1991; Elder and Laurence 1991; Jonsen 1988; Lloyd and Laurence 1985; White-Van Mourik et al. 1990). In Lloyd and Laurence's (1985) retrospective study of reactions after termination of pregnancy for a fetal malformation, 77 percent of women interviewed had an immediate acute grief reaction and 46 percent of them remained symptomatic six months after the event. The authors also remarked that the genetic counselling given at amniocentesis was not very helpful as compared to counselling given up to 16 weeks after the termination. They suggested that patients be seen three months after the pregnancy termination by a skilled genetic counsellor. Support from genetic field workers was perceived as essential by 83 percent of those patients who were visited after pregnancy termination. The authors stated that "improved follow-up support and counselling have lessened the adverse emotional consequences, and support should therefore be offered to all women undergoing termination for fetal malformation."

Provision of this support may be easier said than done, given the resource implications. They and others also found that there is a need for informing the couples on the etiology of the fetal anomaly, the risk for future pregnancies, and the availability of prenatal diagnostic services (Black 1990; Couch-Hockedy 1989; Drugan et al. 1990; Frets et al. 1990; Furlong and Black 1984; Jones et al. 1984; Jonsen 1988). However, there is an irreducible minimum period of time needed to analyze the pathological, laboratory, and radiological data in order to reach a final diagnosis. In our experience couples can interpret this apparent delay as a means of escape or a refusal to divulge information about the post-mortem findings. The prenatal diagnostic service must ensure that every case is followed up and that the geneticist or the attending physician has interpreted the results to the couple as soon as they are available. General recommendations were made by other authors (Kenyon et al. 1988), who stressed the need for organized follow-up in prenatal diagnostic clinics.

More recently, chorionic villus sampling has been introduced into current prenatal diagnostic practice. This is done earlier than amniocentesis. Black (1990) mentioned that, as expected, losses at the later stage of gestation in those who had amniocentesis were associated with greater mood disturbance than in the group who had chorionic villus sampling, but this difference, based on a small sample, was not statistically significant. In the post-counselling sessions, several points merit consideration and should be addressed. These include anticipation of a high risk level, the presence or not of living child(ren), handicapped or in good health, and the accuracy of the diagnosis and any risk for future pregnancies. Guilt feelings are more likely to surface if a precise final diagnosis has not been reached. The influence of relatives may alter the perception of the problem as it really exists; this may interfere with the couple's decision to contemplate another pregnancy. It is interesting to note (Frets et al. 1990) that few couples come back to a centre for supportive counselling; most of those who contact the centre again want more technical and clinical information. From this Dutch study, it appears that the availability of prenatal diagnostic services may influence a couple's decision if the risk is over 15 percent. The desire to have children, if they have none, usually predominates, irrespective of the genetic risk, especially if a prenatal diagnostic service is available.

The two groups studied had their own particular characteristics. Patients at risk for a genetic disease or defect were aware that the fetus might be affected. Such couples will usually wait until after the results are available before letting themselves feel committed and close to their fetus and enjoying the pregnancy with family members and friends. This makes the period before test results are available very difficult. They require strong support if there is a termination; close contact with the medical staff is essential until the level of risk involved in another pregnancy is identified. If they have decided against another pregnancy, they still need a final evaluation of the genetic findings and familial consequences.

In both groups studied, few expressed guilt or thought that they had made the wrong decision. Several couples in the study group decided to refrain from another pregnancy and 36 percent requested a tubal ligation or vasectomy compared to 22 percent in the comparison group. It could be that the higher frequency of sterilizations in the study group was related to their older age; nevertheless, among couples who opted for a sterilization, parental age, gravidity, or a high risk of recurrence seemed to have little effect on their decision. The overall reaction of the comparison group was sudden and acute, and they expressed denial about the abnormal finding. In the study group, couples were already anxious, somewhat prepared for the news, but they still experienced a long-lasting grief reaction.

Up to the point when the diagnosis was made, the medical management was acceptable; then both groups had to deal with several unexpected and avoidable situations. In general, patients thought the personnel, the support, information, and follow-up after the abortion were all satisfactory, but there were some distinct exceptions. Presented here is a summary of remarks and suggestions made by patients from both groups. This information should be used to learn the lessons necessary to structure better care, which will also be influenced by availability of local personnel, technical availability, and feasibility related to the type of anomaly.

We found the pregnancy had often been planned and was usually welcomed. There was little time for couples to decide whether they wanted to continue the pregnancy; the decision had to be made because the pregnancy was usually already in or near the 20th week at diagnosis. Patients in the comparison group often had to endure the uncertainty and uneasiness of the personnel in the ultrasound department when the anomaly was identified. They felt they were treated as numbers and as curious specimens. Repeated scans and films were taken without explanation and technical personnel came to look at the screen, ignoring the patient undergoing the examination.

When they were admitted to hospital for the abortion, they had to sign a medical and surgical consent form, and the Laminaria were inserted into the cervix. Within hours, they saw the psychiatrist, received an injection of prostaglandin, and aborted in the next 6 to 24 hours. The spouse could be present, but few other people were specifically assigned to take care of the patient's needs other than medical ones. The abortion was attended by nursing staff, and often no analgesia or epidural anaesthesia was given. The fetus was shown to the parents in a "plastic" box, rather than wrapped in a blanket, which was found to be cold and uncaring. The patient left the hospital within 24 to 28 hours, often still in doubt about the confirmation of the exact diagnosis and the implications of it.

When patients left the hospital, they had little information about time allowed off from work, how to handle complications such as bleeding, how to control mastitis, and who would see them in a few weeks to check the uterus. The burial had to be arranged and papers signed if the fetus was over 500 g. All this occurred while the mourning process was beginning. The psychiatrist visited once and, unless asked, did not return. There is a parents' association for those who have lost living children, but some patients found it provides little support for people who have lost a fetus. For some individuals, the worst feeling was not knowing exactly where the fetus was buried: was it cremated or buried in a common grave in an unknown site, and when did this take place? Most couples would have liked to pray at the grave. Many said that they expected the same kind of support from medical personnel and to be treated in the same manner as parents who had lost a child.

The parental reaction to a pregnancy termination is even more complex than already described in the literature. Some authors (White-Van Mourik et al. 1992) describe a "state of emotional turmoil" after a second-trimester termination of pregnancy. Parents do not adapt without pain to the loss of a desired pregnancy. Their defence mechanisms are not yet in place, and this is even more evident in those, like the patients in the comparison group, whose pregnancy has seemed to be uneventful and where no problem is anticipated. Almost all couples sometimes forget the seriousness of the malformation or disease and convince themselves that the infant could, with care and treatment, recover after birth. Those lapses and parental ambivalence about the choice made, and their overall compliance to the situation strongly suggest a modified approach to the "prise en charge" of couples who have a fetal anomaly identified. The problems linked to the availability of medical services for the handicapped child have already been raised elsewhere (Dallaire 1984). Even if an acceptable solution to the care of these handicapped children is found, many parents will likely continue to choose pregnancy termination instead of an anticipated difficult parenthood. In our study, psychological interviews of 200 patients have shed some light on the deficiencies in care surrounding the procedure of pregnancy termination for a genetic disease or congenital anomaly. These are the recommendations that follow from what we have learned.

## Recommendations

1. When applicable, university and hospital teaching programs should include information sessions addressed to students and newly arrived medical and paramedical staff on the emotional impact that a pregnancy termination for a fetal genetic disease or congenital anomaly has. Couples should receive support in the same way as parents who have lost a child.

2. During the ultrasound sessions or at the time of communication of the laboratory results, the patient's right to privacy should be respected. A respectful and personal approach should be used, and unexplained discussion of the findings among the staff in the presence of the patient (or couple) who are usually unaware of the presence of a fetal anomaly should be avoided. Recorded image displays are better used later for teaching purposes.

3. Audio, video, or written information on the specific anomaly or disease identified in the fetus should be offered to couples. This information could help them before or even after they have made their decision concerning the outcome of pregnancy.

4. Relevant research should be encouraged to help develop the means to offer ultrasonographic or biological diagnoses earlier in gestation. Early amniocentesis and the use of biological or ultrasound signs of disease may eventually improve methods of prenatal diagnosis. In the

meantime, any unnecessary delays in confirming a diagnosis or informing the couples should be avoided.

5. Couples should be supported if they wish to carry the pregnancy to spontaneous delivery, even if the fetus is affected by a lethal disease or defect.

6. If the patient is offered a medical termination late during the second trimester of pregnancy, local anaesthesia (when indicated) should be offered; during the expulsion period, a competent and compassionate nursing and medical staff should actively support and assist the patient.

7. The mourning reaction should be anticipated and respected. A psychiatric consultation in the pre-termination period should be followed by a contact with the couple sometime later at home. Patients suggested that this contact be initiated by the medical team because people often do not feel comfortable contacting the psychiatric team themselves.

8. A social worker (or trained volunteer) should be present and available to the patients during their stay in hospital and should ensure liaison between the patients and nursing or medical staff.

9. A counsellor or clinical nurse should, within a few weeks, contact the couple to arrange for a genetic consultation when the final laboratory results and pathology reports are available. This appointment or telephone conversation will allow confirmation of laboratory results and reassessment of the possible need of psychological support.

10. All procedures surrounding the care of the fetus after expulsion, its preparation for viewing by the parents, and the paperwork for burial should be completed with compassion and respect.

11. Involvement with a parents' group or association could prevent the feeling of isolation expressed by many couples. Family members and friends often do not understand the sorrow as well as people who have had a similar experience.

# Appendix 1. Questionnaire

## Questionnaire*

**INFORMATION SHEET**

1. Identification (laboratory #)

2. Date of birth:
   Day _____ Month _____ Year _____

3. Obstetrical history:
   G _____ P _____ A _____ EA _____

   |   | YES | NO |
   |---|-----|-----|

4. Was this a first relationship?  ___ ___

5. A second?  ___ ___

6. A third or later?  ___ ___

7. Pregnancy after tubal ligation  ___ ___

8. Pregnancy after vasectomy  ___ ___

9. Occupation (hers): _____

10. Occupation (his): _____

11. Abnormal pregnancy:
    **LMP:** Day _____ Month _____ Year _____

12. Date of termination:
    Day _____ Month _____ Year _____

13. Reason for consultation for the group under study:
    1. AMA  _____
    2. Previous NTM  _____
    3. Previous aneuploidy  _____
    4. Familial translocation  _____

---

* All information already included in the file will be entered directly on the questionnaire.

5. Metabolic disease          _____
6. Other                      _____

14. Abnormality revealed during routine ultrasonography in the control group:
    1. Malformation syndrome     _____
    2. Other (for example, fetal death)    _____

15. Final diagnosis for both groups:
    1. Chromosomal abnormality    _____
    2. Malformation of the neural tube    _____
    3. Hereditary malformation syndrome    _____
    4. Malformation syndrome of indeterminate etiology    _____
    5. Metabolic disease    _____
    6. Other    _____

Specify _____
_____
_____
_____

**INTERVIEW**

16. Interval since termination of pregnancy:
    1. 0 - 6 months    _____
    2. 6 - 12 months   _____
    3. 12 - 18 months  _____
    4. 18 - 24 months  _____
    5. over 24 months  _____

|  |  | YES | NO |
|---|---|---|---|
| 17. Ligation | since termination | \_\_\_ | \_\_\_ |
| 18. Vasectomy | "         " | \_\_\_ | \_\_\_ |

19. Wanted pregnancy:   Patient          ___  ___
                         Spouse           ___  ___
                         Couple           ___  ___

20. If currently pregnant:
        a) Unplanned pregnancy
        b) Planned pregnancy

21. Complications following termination          ___  ___

    Specify (infections, haemorrhaging, psychological complications and so on):

    a) physical _____

    _____

    b) psychological _____

    _____

22. In the couple's view, was the prenatal assessment
    imposed or strongly recommended by the medical
    staff (perception of each of the parents)?          ___  ___

    _____

    _____

    _____

23. Did you agree with the prenatal diagnosis procedure?
                         1. patient              ___  ___
                         2. spouse               ___  ___

24. Did any of the following people influence your decision?
                         1. attending physician  _____
                         2. geneticist           _____
                         3. nurse                _____
                         4. counsellor           _____
                         5. spouse               _____
                         6. others               _____

    _____

    _____

    _____

    _____

25. Advancement of the pregnancy as of the date of the diagnosis
                    ___ weeks

26. Advancement of the pregnancy as of the date of the termination

    _____ weeks

27. Announcement made by:
    1. attending physician      _____
    2. geneticist               _____
    3. medical sonographer      _____
    4. resident                 _____
    5. obstetrician on call     _____
    6. other                    _____

28. News announced to:
    1. patient                  _____
    2. patient and spouse       _____
    3. spouse                   _____

29. Diagnosis clearly understood at the time of the announcement:
    1. clear                    _____
    2. unclear                  _____
    3. insufficient information _____

**IMPACT OF DIAGNOSIS**

30. Did you receive support from those around you?

    |            | YES | NO |
    |------------|-----|----|
    | 1. friends | ___ | ___ |
    | 2. family  | ___ | ___ |
    | 3. others  | ___ | ___ |

    _____
    _____

31. What was the most critical period following the announcement of the news (provide psychological details for both)?

    _____
    _____
    _____
    _____

32. Termination psychologically accepted by the patient at the time of the announcement:

    a) patient _____

    _____

    b) spouse _____

    _____

33. Influence of the sex of the fetus on the reaction (detail for both)

    _____
    _____
    _____
    _____

34. Influence of the number of children on the couple's reaction

    _____
    _____
    _____
    _____

|  | YES | NO |
|---|---|---|

35. Was there a period of "mourning" for the child?     ___   ___

    Describe the process (6 months, 12 months, 24 months)

    _____
    _____
    _____
    _____

36. Is this baby a replacement?     ___   ___

    (if subsequent pregnancy) _____

    _____
    _____
    _____
    _____

|   | YES | NO |
|---|---|---|

37. Did you see a psychiatrist at the time of the termination?  ___ ___

   Did this visit help you?  1. patient  ___ ___
   2. couple  ___ ___
   3. spouse  ___ ___

38. The following would like to be seen by a psychiatrist or a therapist now (or later) for follow-up.
   1. patient  ___ ___
   2. couple  ___ ___
   3. spouse  ___ ___

   _____
   _____
   _____

39. Do you feel you made a good decision at the time?  ___ ___

   _____
   _____
   _____

40. Did you have marital problems before this abnormal pregnancy?  ___ ___

   _____
   _____
   _____

41. Unfortunate personal events related to the termination (such as separation):

   Specify _____
   _____
   _____
   _____

42. Did one of you feel guilty? If so, in what way?

   _____
   _____
   _____

43. If yes, is this feeling still there?

   _____
   _____
   _____
   _____

44. Unfortunate events in the immediate family (bereavement, family guilt):

   Specify _____
   _____
   _____
   _____

## RETROSPECT AND ATTITUDES

|  | YES | NO |
|---|---|---|
| 45. Did you sense an abnormality? | ___ | ___ |
| 46. Was this your first pregnancy by this spouse? | ___ | ___ |
| 47. Do you know the risk for a future pregnancy? | ___ | ___ |
| 48. If you become pregnant, will you undergo prenatal diagnosis? | ___ | ___ |

   _____
   _____
   _____
   _____

49. For you, which of the following constitutes a high risk (%)?

   | 1+ | 5+ | 10+ | 15+ | 25+ | 33+ | 50+ | ___ |
   | (1) | (2) | (3) | (4) | (5) | (6) | (7) | |

50. Were you reassured by the information on the risks related to the procedure?   ___  ___

   _____
   _____
   _____
   _____

|  | YES | NO |
|---|---|---|
| 51. Did you receive advice from friends? | ___ | ___ |

_____
_____
_____
_____

52. How do you feel about your children?

_____
_____
_____
_____

**SUGGESTIONS FROM THE COUPLE REGARDING PRENATAL DIAGNOSIS INDICATIONS**

53. Regarding advanced maternal age:
    1. status quo          _____
    2. < 35                _____
    3. > 35                _____
    4. other               _____

54. Regarding ultrasounds (manner of reception and so on):

    Specify _____
    _____
    _____

55. Regarding amniocentesis:

    Specify _____
    _____
    _____

56. Regarding the method of termination (anaesthesia):

    Specify _____
    _____
    _____

## OVERALL IMPRESSION

|  | YES | NO |
|---|---|---|
| 57. Did you receive enough information before undergoing your examination? | ___ | ___ |

Specify _____

_____

_____

_____

58. Did you receive enough information before having your pregnancy terminated?   ___   ___

Specify _____

_____

_____

_____

59. Who provided you with the most information on prenatal diagnosis?
    1. attending physician  _____
    2. geneticist  _____
    3. medical sonographer  _____
    4. genetic counsellors or nurses  _____
    5. others  _____

_____

_____

60. What did you perceive the medical staff's attitude to be toward amniocentesis?
    1. in favour of the test  _____
    2. not in favour of the test  _____

|  | YES | NO |
|---|---|---|
| 61. Did you feel obliged to decide in favour of amniocentesis? | ___ | ___ |

_____

_____

_____

_____

|  | YES | NO |
|---|---|---|

62. Did you feel obliged to decide to have an abortion?
    1. before the amniocentesis ___ ___
    2. after the amniocentesis ___ ___

63. What motivated you most to decide to terminate the pregnancy? The quality of life of:
    1. yourself        _____
    2. you as a couple _____
    3. your family     _____
    4. other children  _____
    5. society         _____

64. Post-termination follow-up (genetic counselling, interpretation of the abnormality and so on)

_____
_____
_____

**SUMMARY AND INTERPRETATION OF THE INTERVIEW**

_____
_____
_____
_____
_____

**PSYCHOLOGIST'S PERCEPTION**

a) regarding the bereavement
b) regarding the environment
c) overall assessment of the intervention


Date: _____

Signature: _____
         (Psychologist responsible for the interview)

## Appendix 2. Consent Form

**Consent**

**Prenatal diagnosis program — Hôpital Sainte-Justine**

*Study on accessibility to prenatal diagnosis and
the services offered at the time
of pregnancy termination due to fetal abnormality*

We agree to meet with a psychologist and to respond to the best of our knowledge to the questions asked concerning follow-up of the prenatal diagnosis of genetic disease. All answers provided will remain entirely anonymous.

We would like to be informed of the *conclusions* of this study:

        YES \_\_\_   NO \_\_\_

Patient _____Witness _____

Date: _____

## Appendix 3. Letter of Endorsement

### ETHICS SUBCOMMITTEE

A committee at the Hôpital Sainte-Justine composed of the following members:

| | |
|---|---|
| Philippe CHESSEX, MD | Neonatology |
| Hubert LABELLE, MD | Orthopaedics |
| Georges Etienne RIVARD, MD | Haematology |
| Michel VANASSE, MD | Neurology |
| Sylvie VANDAL | Outpatient Services |

At their meeting of August 1, 1991, the members of the Ethics Subcommittee reviewed the clinical research project entitled *Parental reaction and adaptability to the prenatal diagnosis of genetic disease leading to pregnancy interruption*, submitted by <u>Louis Dallaire, MD and Gilles Lortie, MD</u> and found it to conform to the standards established by the Ethics Committee of the Sainte-Justine Hospital. The project is therefore accepted by the committee.

_____  <u>August 29, 1991</u>
Hubert Labelle, MD  Date
Chair of the Ethics Subcommittee


cc: Claude C. Roy, MD
    Chair of the Ethics Committee

## Appendix 4. Project Personnel

| | |
|---|---|
| Micheline Des Rochers | Nurse Coordinator |
| Rachel Clermont | Psychologist |
| Christina Vachon | Psychologist |
| Jocelyne Roussin | Secretary |
| Françoise Dagenais | Archivist |
| Bernard Grignon | Administrator (Department of Medical Genetics) |
| Richard Maheu | Administrator (Research Centre) |

## Bibliography

American Society of Human Genetics. 1975. "Genetic Counseling." *American Journal of Human Genetics* 27: 240-42.

Black, R.B. 1990. "Prenatal Diagnosis and Fetal Loss: Psychosocial Consequences and Professional Responsibilities." *American Journal of Medical Genetics* 35: 586-87.

Boss, J.A. 1990. "How Voluntary Prenatal Diagnosis and Selective Abortion Increase the Abnormal Human Gene Pool." *Birth* 17 (June): 75-79.

Couch-Hockedy, S. 1989. "Women's Experiences of Gynaecology." *Professional Nurse* 4 (January): 173-76.

Dagg, P.K.B. 1991. "The Psychological Sequelae of Therapeutic Abortion — Denied and Completed." *American Journal of Psychiatry* 148: 578-85.

Dallaire, L. 1984. *Étude et évaluation des services médicaux disponibles aux jeunes enfants (0 à 5 ans) souffrant de déficience et rapport sur l'utilisation et l'accessibilité de ces services: Enquête sur l'accueil à l'enfant handicapé.* Sillery: Conseil des affaires sociales et de la famille.

Dallaire, L., et al. 1982. "Le diagnostic prénatal des maladies génétiques au second trimestre de la grossesse. Partie I: Les indications." *Union Médicale du Canada* 111: 189-205.

—. 1991. "Prenatal Diagnosis of Fetal Anomalies During the Second Trimester of Pregnancy: Their Characterization and Delineation of Defects in Pregnancies at Risk." *Prenatal Diagnosis* 11: 629-35.

Donnai, P., N. Charles, and R. Harris. 1981. "Attitudes of Patients After 'Genetic' Termination of Pregnancy." *British Medical Journal* (21 February): 621-22.

Drugan, A., et al. 1990. "Determinants of Parental Decisions to Abort for Chromosome Abnormalities." *Prenatal Diagnosis* 10: 483-90.

Elder, S.H., and K.M. Laurence. 1991. "The Impact of Supportive Intervention After Second Trimester Termination of Pregnancy for Fetal Abnormality." *Prenatal Diagnosis* 11: 47-54.

Frets, P.G., et al. 1990. "Factors Influencing the Reproductive Decision After Genetic Counseling." *American Journal of Medical Genetics* 35: 496-502.

Furlong, R.M., and R.B. Black. 1984. "Pregnancy Termination for Genetic Indications: The Impact on Families." *Social Work in Health Care* 10 (Fall): 17-34.

Galjaard, H. 1989. "Early Diagnosis and Prevention of Genetic Diseases." In *Reviews in Perinatal Medicine*. Vol. 6, ed. E.M. Scarpellis and E.V. Cosmi. New York: Alan R. Liss.

Iles, S. 1989. "The Loss of Early Pregnancy." *Baillières Clinical Obstetrics and Gynaecology* 3: 769-90.

Jones, O.W., et al. 1984. "Parental Response to Mid-Trimester Therapeutic Abortion Following Amniocentesis." *Prenatal Diagnosis* 4: 249-56.

Jonsen, A.R. 1988. "Women's Choices — The Ethics of Maternity." *Western Journal of Medicine* 149: 726-28.

Kenyon, S.L., G.A. Hackett, and S. Campbell. 1988. "Termination of Pregnancy Following Diagnosis of Fetal Malformation: The Need for Improved Follow-Up Services." *Clinical Obstetrics and Gynecology* 31: 97-100.

Kessler, S., H. Kessler, and P. Ward. 1984. "Psychological Aspects of Genetic Counseling. III. Management of Guilt and Shame." *American Journal of Medical Genetics* 17: 673-97.

Kessler, S., et al. 1987. "Attitudes of Persons At Risk for Huntington Disease Toward Predictive Testing." *American Journal of Medical Genetics* 26: 259-70.

Laiho, A. 1988. ["My Unborn Child."] *Katilolehti: Tidskrift for Barnmorskor* 93 (October): 28-33.

Lippman-Hand, A., and F.C. Fraser. 1979. "Genetic Counseling — The Post-Counseling Period: II. Making Reproductive Choices." *American Journal of Medical Genetics* 4: 73-87.

Lloyd, J., and K.M. Laurence. 1985. "Sequelae and Support After Termination of Pregnancy for Fetal Malformation." *British Medical Journal* (23 March): 907-909.

Pearn, J. 1979. "Decision-Making and Reproductive Choice." In *Counseling in Genetics*, ed. Y.E. Hsia et al. New York: Alan R. Liss.

Powledge, T.M., and J. Fletcher. 1979. "Guidelines for the Ethical, Social and Legal Issues in Prenatal Diagnosis." *New England Journal of Medicine* 300: 168-72.

Rothman, B.K. 1990. "Commentary: Women Feel Social and Economic Pressures to Abort Abnormal Fetuses." *Birth* 17 (June): 81.

Seidman, D.S., et al. 1988. "Child-Bearing After Induced Abortion: Reassessment of Risk." *Journal of Epidemiology and Community Health* 42: 294-98.

Simpson, N.E., et al. 1976. "Prenatal Diagnosis of Genetic Disease in Canada: Report of a Collaborative Study." *Canadian Medical Association Journal* 115: 739-46.

Sorenson, J.R., and D.C. Wertz. 1986. "Couple Agreement Before and After Genetic Counseling." *American Journal of Medical Genetics* 25: 549-55.

Sorenson, J.R., et al. 1981. "Reproductive Pasts, Reproductive Futures. Genetic Counseling and Its Effectiveness." *Birth Defects: Original Article Series* 17 (4): 1-192.

—. 1987. "Reproductive Plans of Genetic Counseling Clients not Eligible for Prenatal Diagnosis." *American Journal of Medical Genetics* 28: 345-52.

Urquhart, D.R., and A.A. Templeton. 1991. "Psychiatric Morbidity and Acceptability Following Medical and Surgical Methods of Induced Abortion." *British Journal of Obstetrics and Gynaecology* 98: 396-99.

Wells, N. 1989. "Management of Pain During Abortion." *Journal of Advanced Nursing* 14: 56-62.

Wertz, D.C., J.R. Sorenson, and T.C. Heeren. 1986. "Clients' Interpretation of Risks Provided in Genetic Counseling." *American Journal of Human Genetics* 39: 253-64.

White-Van Mourik, M.C., J.M. Connor, and M.A. Ferguson-Smith. 1990. "Patient Care Before and After Termination of Pregnancy for Neural Tube Defects." *Prenatal Diagnosis* 10: 497-505.

—. 1992. "The Psychosocial Sequelae of a Second-Trimester Termination of Pregnancy for Fetal Abnormality." *Prenatal Diagnosis* 12: 189-204.

# Contributors

**Julie Beck**, B.Sc., B.Ed.

**Michael H. Butler**, M.A., Department of Geography, Queen's University.

**Louis Dallaire**, M.D., Ph.D., FRCPC, FCCMG.

**F. Clarke Fraser**, O.C., Ph.D., M.D., FRCPC, FCCMG.

**Karen R. Grant**, Ph.D., Associate Professor, Department of Sociology, University of Manitoba.

**Susan J. Koval**, M.A., Division of Medical Genetics, Department of Paediatrics, Queen's University.

**Gilles Lortie**, M.D., CSPQ.

**Ian Ferguson MacKay**, M.Sc.

**Patrick M. MacLeod**, M.D., FRCPC, FCCMG, DABMG, Division of Medical Genetics, Department of Paediatrics, Queen's University.

**Joanne Milner**, B.A.

**Mark W. Rosenberg**, Ph.D., Department of Geography, Queen's University.

**Sari Tudiver**, Ph.D., Resource Coordinator and researcher, Women's Health Clinic, Winnipeg.

# Mandate

(approved by Her Excellency the Governor General
on the 25th day of October, 1989)

The Committee of the Privy Council, on the recommendation of the Prime Minister, advise that a Commission do issue under Part I of the Inquiries Act and under the Great Seal of Canada appointing The Royal Commission on New Reproductive Technologies to inquire into and report on current and potential medical and scientific developments related to new reproductive technologies, considering in particular their social, ethical, health, research, legal and economic implications and the public interest, recommending what policies and safeguards should be applied, and examining in particular,

(a) implications of new reproductive technologies for women's reproductive health and well-being;

(b) the causes, treatment and prevention of male and female infertility;

(c) reversals of sterilization procedures, artificial insemination, *in vitro* fertilization, embryo transfers, prenatal screening and diagnostic techniques, genetic manipulation and therapeutic interventions to correct genetic anomalies, sex selection techniques, embryo experimentation and fetal tissue transplants;

(d) social and legal arrangements, such as surrogate childbearing, judicial interventions during gestation and birth, and "ownership" of ova, sperm, embryos and fetal tissue;

(e) the status and rights of people using or contributing to reproductive services, such as access to procedures, "rights" to parenthood, informed consent, status of gamete donors and confidentiality, and the impact of these services on all concerned parties, particularly the children; and

(f) the economic ramifications of these technologies, such as the commercial marketing of ova, sperm and embryos, the application of patent law, and the funding of research and procedures including infertility treatment.

# The Research Volumes

## Volume 1: New Reproductive Technologies: Ethical Aspects

| | |
|---|---|
| Approaches to the Ethical Issues Raised by the Royal Commission's Mandate | W. Kymlicka |
| Assisted Reproductive Technologies: Informed Choice | F. Baylis |
| Medicalization and the New Reproductive Technologies | M. Burgess/A. Frank/ S. Sherwin |
| Prenatal Diagnosis and Society | D.C. Wertz |
| Roles for Ethics Committees in Relation to Guidelines for New Reproductive Technologies: A Research Position Paper | J.B. Dossetor/J.L. Storch |
| Economic, Ethical, and Population Aspects of New Reproductive Technologies in Developing Countries: Implications for Canada | P. Manga |

## Volume 2: Social Values and Attitudes Surrounding New Reproductive Technologies

| | |
|---|---|
| An Overview of Findings in This Volume | RCNRT Staff |
| Social Values and Attitudes of Canadians Toward New Reproductive Technologies | Decima Research |
| Social Values and Attitudes of Canadians Toward New Reproductive Technologies: Focus Group Findings | Decima Research |
| Key Findings from a National Survey Conducted by the Angus Reid Group: Infertility, Surrogacy, Fetal Tissue Research, and Reproductive Technologies | M. de Groh |

Reproductive Technologies, Adoption, and
  Issues on the Cost of Health Care:
  Summary of Canada Health Monitor Results         M. de Groh

Survey of Ethnocultural Communities on New
  Reproductive Technologies                         S. Dutt

World Religions and New Reproductive
  Technologies                                      H. Coward

Personal Experiences with New Reproductive
  Technologies: Report from Private Sessions        RCNRT Staff

## Volume 3: Overview of Legal Issues in New Reproductive Technologies

The Constitution and the Regulation of New
  Reproductive Technologies                         M. Jackman

An Overview of the Legal System in Canada           S.L. Martin

Overview of Canadian Laws Relating to Privacy
  and Confidentiality in the Medical Context        E.L. Oscapella

Reproductive Technology: Is a Property Law          M.M. Litman/
  Regime Appropriate?                               G.B. Robertson

New Reproductive Technologies:                      K.M. Cherniawsky/
  Commercial Protection                             P.J.M. Lown

The Limits of Freedom of Contract:
  The Commercialization of Reproductive             M. Martin/A. Lawson/
  Materials and Services                            P. Lewis/M. Trebilcock

Appropriating the Human Being: An Essay on
  the Appropriation of the Human Body and of
  Its Parts                                         J. Goulet

The Civil Code of Quebec and New
  Reproductive Technologies                         M. Ouellette

New Reproductive Technologies: International
  Legal Issues and Instruments                      R.J. Cook

## Volume 4: Legal and Ethical Issues in New Reproductive Technologies: Pregnancy and Parenthood

| | |
|---|---|
| Juridical Interference with Gestation and Birth | S. Rodgers |
| Reproductive Hazards in the Workplace: Legal Issues of Regulation, Enforcement, and Redress | J. Fudge/E. Tucker |
| The Challenge of the New Reproductive Technologies to Family Law | E. Sloss/R. Mykitiuk |
| "Surrogate Motherhood": Legal and Ethical Analysis | J.R. Guichon |
| Surrogate Parenting: Bibliography | J. Kitts |

## Volume 5: New Reproductive Technologies and the Science, Industry, Education, and Social Welfare Systems in Canada

| | |
|---|---|
| Discovery, Community, and Profit: An Overview of the Science and Technology System | L. Edwards, with the assistance of R. Voyer |
| An Overview of Select Social and Economic Forces Influencing the Development of *In Vitro* Fertilization and Related Assisted Reproductive Techniques | A. Rochon Ford |
| Commercial Involvement in New Reproductive Technologies: An Overview | J. Rowlands/ N. Saby/J. Smith |
| The Role of the Biotechnology Industry in the Development of Clinical Diagnostic Materials for Prenatal Diagnosis | G. Chaloner-Larsson/ F. Haynes/C. Merritt |
| Report on a Survey of Members of the Pharmaceutical Manufacturers Association of Canada and Biotechnology Companies | SPR Associates Inc. |
| Canada's School Systems: An Overview of Their Potential Role in Promoting Reproductive Health and Understanding of New Reproductive Technologies | Shannon and McCall Consulting Ltd. |
| Social Welfare and New Reproductive Technologies: An Overview | S. Torjman |

## Volume 6: The Prevalence of Infertility in Canada

| | |
|---|---|
| Historical Overview of Medical Perceptions of Infertility in Canada, 1850-1950 | W.L. Mitchinson |
| The Prevalence of Infertility in Canada, 1991-1992: Analysis of Three National Surveys | C.S. Dulberg/T. Stephens |
| Infertility Among Canadians: An Analysis of Data from the Canadian Fertility Survey (1984) and General Social Survey (1990) | T.R. Balakrishnan/ R. Fernando |
| Infertility, Sterilization, and Contraceptive Use in Ontario | T.R. Balakrishnan/ P. Maxim |
| Adoption as an Alternative for Infertile Couples: Prospects and Trends | K.J. Daly/M.P. Sobol |
| Annotated Bibliography on the Prevalence of Infertility | M.R.P. de la Roche |

## Volume 7: Understanding Infertility: Risk Factors Affecting Fertility

| | |
|---|---|
| Sexually Transmitted Infections: Their Manifestations and Links to Infertility and Reproductive Illness | A.R. Ronald/R.W. Peeling |
| The Physiological Effects of Aging on Fertility Decline: A Literature Review | J. Jantz-Lee |
| Effects of Licit and Illicit Drugs, Alcohol, Caffeine, and Nicotine on Infertility | H. Boyer |
| A Literature Review of the Physiological Manifestations Related to Infertility Linked to Weight, Eating Behaviours, and Exercise | S.E. Maddocks |
| Contraception: An Evaluation of Its Role in Relation to Infertility — Can It Protect? | B.N. Barwin/W. Fisher |
| The Physiological Links Between Endometriosis and Infertility: Review of the Medical Literature and Annotated Bibliography (1985-1990) | A. Ponchuk |
| The Impact of Medical Procedures on Fertility | S. Dumas/ É. Guilbert/J-É. Rioux |

| | |
|---|---|
| Occupational and Environmental Exposure Data: Information Sources and Linkage Potential to Adverse Reproductive Outcomes Data in Canada | P.K. Abeytunga/ M. Tennassee |
| Evaluation of an Environmental Contaminant: Development of a Method for Chemical Review and a Case Study of Hexachlorobenzene (HCB) as a Reproductive Toxicant | J.F. Jarrell/ J. Seidel/P. Bigelow |
| Pilot Study on Determining the Relative Importance of Risk Factors for Infertility in Canada | P. Millson/K. Maznyk |

## Volume 8: Prevention of Infertility

| | |
|---|---|
| Prevention of Infertility: Overcoming the Obstacles | A. Thomson |
| The Effectiveness of Sexually Transmitted Disease Infertility-Related Prevention Programs | L. McIntyre |
| The Burden of Chlamydial and Gonococcal Infection in Canada | R. Goeree/P. Gully |
| Social Factors Relevant to Sexually Transmitted Diseases and to Strategies for Their Prevention: A Literature Review | L. Hanvey/D. Kinnon |
| Feasibility of Economic Evaluations of Sexually Transmitted Disease Prevention Programs in Canada | R. Goeree |
| Issues in Evaluating Programs to Prevent Infertility Related to Occupational Hazards | A. Yassi |
| The Integration of Theoretical Approaches to Prevention: A Proposed Framework for Reducing the Incidence of Infertility | B. Hyndman/A. Libstug/ I. Rootman/N. Giesbrecht/ R. Osborn |

## Volume 9: Treatment of Infertility: Assisted Reproductive Technologies

**Part 1: Overview of Assisted Reproductive Technologies**

| | |
|---|---|
| Medically Assisted Reproductive Technologies: A Review | M.A. Mullen |
| A Socio-Historical Examination of the Development of *In Vitro* Fertilization and Related Assisted Reproductive Techniques | A. Rochon Ford |
| The Professions Involved in New Reproductive Technologies: Their Present and Future Numbers, Training, and Improvement in Competence | L. Curry |
| Legislation, Inquiries, and Guidelines on Infertility Treatment and Surrogacy/Preconception Contracts: A Review of Policies in Seven Countries | L.S. Williams |

**Part 2: Assisted Insemination**

| | |
|---|---|
| Donor Insemination: An Overview | R. Achilles |
| Issues and Responses: Artificial Insemination | D. Wikler/N. Wikler |
| The Social Meanings of Donor Insemination | R. Achilles |
| Lesbian Women and Donor Insemination: An Alberta Case Study | F.A.L. Nelson |
| Self-Insemination in Canada | R. Achilles |
| The Conceptual Framework of Donor Insemination | D. Wikler |
| Artificial Insemination: Bibliography | M. Musgrove |

## Volume 10: Treatment of Infertility: Current Practices and Psychosocial Implications

| | |
|---|---|
| Survey of Canadian Fertility Programs | T. Stephens/J. McLean, with R. Achilles/L. Brunet/ J. Wood Catano |
| An Evaluation of Canadian Fertility Clinics: The Patient's Perspective | SPR Associates Inc. |

| | |
|---|---|
| Infertile Couples and Their Treatment in Canadian Academic Infertility Clinics | J. Collins/E. Burrows/ A. Willan |
| Implementing Shared Patient Decision Making: A Review of the Literature | R.B. Deber, with H. Bouchard/A. Pendleton |
| The Psychosocial Impact of New Reproductive Technology | J. Wright |
| Life Quality, Psychosocial Factors, and Infertility: Selected Results from a Five-Year Study of 275 Couples | A. Abbey/L.J. Halman/ F.M. Andrews |
| Review of the Literature on the Psychosocial Implications of Infertility Treatment on Women and Men | E. Savard Muir |

## Volume 11: New Reproductive Technologies and the Health Care System: The Case for Evidence-Based Medicine

| | |
|---|---|
| The Canadian Health Care System | M.M. Rachlis |
| Framework for Technology Decisions: Literature Review | A. Kazanjian/K. Cardiff |
| Infertility Treatment: From Cookery to Science — The Epidemiology of Randomized Controlled Trials | P. Vandekerckhove/ P.A. O'Donovan/ R.J. Lilford/T.W. Harada |
| Meta-Analysis of Controlled Trials in Infertility | E.G. Hughes/ D.M. Fedorkow/J.A. Collins |
| Treatment of Male Infertility: Is It Effective? A Review and Meta-Analyses of Published Randomized Controlled Trials | P. Vandekerckhove/ P.A. O'Donovan/ R.J. Lilford/E. Hughes |
| Adverse Health Effects of Drugs Used for Ovulation Induction | J.F. Jarrell/J. Seidel/ P. Bigelow |
| Methodological Challenges in Evaluating a New and Evolving Technology: The Case of *In Vitro* Fertilization | R. Goeree/J. Jarrell/ R. Labelle |
| Cost-Effectiveness of an *In Vitro* Fertilization Program and the Costs of Associated Hospitalizations and Other Infertility Treatments | R. Goeree/R. Labelle/ J. Jarrell |

Public Preferences Toward an *In Vitro*
Fertilization Program and the Effect of the
Program on Patients' Quality of Life
    R. Goeree/R. Labelle/
    J. Jarrell

The Child Health Study: Record Linkage
Feasibility of Selected Data Bases:
A Catalogue
    L. Hayward/D.E. Flett/
    C. Davis

Infertility Treatment — Epidemiology, Efficacy,
Outcomes, and Direct Costs: A Feasibility
Study, Saskatchewan 1978-1990
    C. D'Arcy/N.S.B. Rawson/
    L. Edouard

## Volume 12: Prenatal Diagnosis: Background and Impact on Individuals

The History and Evolution of Prenatal Diagnosis
    I.F. MacKay/F.C. Fraser

Risk Assessment of Prenatal Diagnostic Techniques
    RCNRT Staff

A Survey of Research on Post-Natal Medical
and Psychological Effects of Prenatal
Diagnosis on Offspring
    J. Beck

A Demographic and Geographic Analysis of the
Users of Prenatal Diagnostic Services in
Canada
    P.M. MacLeod/
    M.W. Rosenberg/
    M.H. Butler/S.J. Koval

Perceptions, Attitudes, and Experiences of
Prenatal Diagnosis: A Winnipeg Study of
Women Over 35
    K.R. Grant

Manitoba Voices: A Qualitative Study of
Women's Experiences with Technology in
Pregnancy
    S. Tudiver

A Review of Views Critical of Prenatal Diagnosis
and Its Impact on Attitudes Toward Persons
with Disabilities
    J. Milner

Parental Reaction and Adaptability to the
Prenatal Diagnosis of Genetic Disease
Leading to Pregnancy Termination
    L. Dallaire/G. Lortie

## Volume 13: Current Practice of Prenatal Diagnosis in Canada

| | |
|---|---|
| Prenatal Diagnosis in Canada — 1990: A Review of Genetics Centres | J.L. Hamerton/ J.A. Evans/L. Stranc |
| An Assessment of the Readability of Patient Education Materials Used by Genetic Screening Clinics | J. Wood Catano |
| Canadian Physicians and Prenatal Diagnosis: Prudence and Ambivalence | M. Renaud/L. Bouchard/ J. Bisson/J-F. Labadie/ L. Dallaire/N. Kishchuk |
| An Analysis of Temporal and Regional Trends in the Use of Prenatal Ultrasonography | G.M. Anderson |
| Maternal Serum AFP Screening Programs: The Manitoba Experience | B.N. Chodirker/J.A. Evans |

## Volume 14: Technologies of Sex Selection and Prenatal Diagnosis

| | |
|---|---|
| Ethical Issues of Prenatal Diagnosis for Predictive Testing for Genetic Disorders of Late Onset | M. Cooke |
| Prenatal Testing for Huntington Disease: Psychosocial Aspects | S. Adam/M.R. Hayden |
| Screening for Genetic Susceptibilities to Common Diseases | L. Prior |
| Preference for the Sex of One's Children and the Prospective Use of Sex Selection | M. Thomas |
| Bibliography on Preferences for the Sex of One's Children, and Attitudes Concerning Sex Preselection | M. Thomas |
| Attitudes of Genetic Counsellors with Respect to Prenatal Diagnosis of Sex for Non-Medical Reasons | Z.G. Miller/F.C. Fraser |
| Preimplantation Diagnosis | F.C. Fraser |
| Somatic and Germ Line Gene Therapy: Current Status and Prospects | L. Prior |

## Volume 15: Background and Current Practice of Fetal Tissue and Embryo Research in Canada

| | |
|---|---|
| The Use of Human Embryos and Fetal Tissues: A Research Architecture | M.A. Mullen |
| Legal Issues in Embryo and Fetal Tissue Research and Therapy | B.M. Dickens |
| Human Fetal Tissue Research: Origins, State of the Art, Future Applications, and Implications | A. Fine |
| Report on a Survey of Use and Handling of Human Reproductive Tissues in Canadian Health Care Facilities | SPR Associates Inc. |
| Report on a Follow-Up Survey of Use and Handling of Human Reproductive Tissues (Survey of Medical Laboratories and Medical Waste Disposal Firms) | SPR Associates Inc. |
| Embryo Transfer and Related Technologies in Domestic Animals: Their History, Current Status, and Future Direction, with Special Reference to Implications for Human Medicine | K.J. Betteridge/D. Rieger |
| Human Embryo Research: Past, Present, and Future | A. McLaren |

# Commission Organization

## Commissioners

Patricia Baird
Chairperson
Vancouver, British Columbia

Grace Jantzen
London, United Kingdom

Bartha Maria Knoppers
Montreal, Quebec

Susan E.M. McCutcheon
Toronto, Ontario

Suzanne Rozell Scorsone
Toronto, Ontario

## Staff

John Sinclair
Executive Director

Mimsie Rodrigue
Executive Director (from July 1993)

### Research & Evaluation

Sylvia Gold
Director

Nancy Miller Chénier
Deputy Director
Causes and Prevention of Infertility

Janet Hatcher Roberts
Deputy Director
Assisted Human Reproduction

F. Clarke Fraser
Deputy Director
Prenatal Diagnosis and Genetics

Burleigh Trevor Deutsch
Deputy Director
Embryo and Fetal Tissue Research

### Consultations & Coordination

Dann M. Michols
Director

Mimsie Rodrigue
Deputy Director
Coordination

Anne Marie Smart
Deputy Director
Communications

Judith Nolté
Deputy Director
Analysis

Denise Cole
Deputy Director
Consultations

Mary Ann Allen
Director
Administration and Security

Gary Paradis
Deputy Director
Finance